NURSING CARE
IN RADIATION ONCOLOGY

NURSING CARE
IN RADIATION ONCOLOGY
SECOND EDITION

Karen Hassey Dow, RN, PhD, FAAN
Associate Professor, School of Nursing
College of Health and Public Affairs
University of Central Florida
Orlando, Florida

Jennifer Dunn Bucholtz, RN, MS, OCN
Clinical Specialist/Nurse Manager
Division of Radiation Oncology
The Johns Hopkins Oncology Center
Baltimore, Maryland

Ryan R. Iwamoto, ARNP, MN, AOCN
Clinical Nurse Specialist
Department of Radiation Oncology
Virginia Mason Medical Center
Seattle, Washington

Vickie K. Fieler, RN, MS, AOCN
Advanced Practice Nurse/Senior Associate
University of Rochester Cancer Center and School of Nursing
Rochester, New York

Laura J. Hilderley, RN, MS
Clinical Nurse Specialist
Radiation Oncology Services of Rhode Island
Warwick, Rhode Island

W. B. Saunders Company
A Division of Harcourt Brace & Company
PHILADELPHIA   LONDON   TORONTO   MONTREAL   SYDNEY   TOKYO

W. B. SAUNDERS COMPANY

A Division of Harcourt Brace & Company
The Curtis Center
Independence Square West
Philadelphia, Pennsylvania 19106

Library of Congress Cataloging-in-Publication Data

Nursing care in radiation oncology / [edited by] Karen Hassey Dow . . .
[et al.]. — 2nd ed.
     p.   cm.
   Includes bibliographical references and index.
   ISBN 0-7216-2347-6
   1. Cancer—Radiotherapy.   2. Cancer—Nursing.   I. Dow, Karen
Hassey.
   [DNLM: 1. Oncologic Nursing.   2. Radiation Oncology—nurses'
instruction.   WY 156 N9724 1997]
RC271.R3N87   1997
616.99′40642—dc21
DNLM/DLC   96-37239

NURSING CARE IN RADIATION ONCOLOGY   ISBN 0–7216–2347–6

Printed in the United States of America

Last digit is the print number: 9   8   7   6   5   4   3   2   1

To my husband, Norman, for his support, perseverance, and love. To my daughter, Lauren, who was a child during the editing of the first edition and is now a teenager. Thanks for the developmental patience, humor, and joy.

KHD

To my husband, Frank, for his unending support, encouragement, and love; and to my twin sister, Jeanette, who shares my commitment to caring for others.

JB

To my family, friends, colleagues, and patients who continue to teach me lessons on living life with richness and depth.

RI

In loving memory of Clint Wise, 1942–1997.

VF

As in the first edition of this text, my thanks go to my husband, Dave, and to my employer and colleague, Philip Maddock, for their patience and support of my writing and editing efforts. In addition, my deep appreciation to Karen and our three new editors, Jennifer, Ryan, and Vickie, for so ably bearing the greater responsibility for the second edition.

LH

Contributors

Allison Blackmar, RN, BSN, MSHP, OCN
Inpatient Nursing Coordinator
Cancer Institute of New Jersey
New Brunswick, New Jersey
Radiation Oncology Nursing Documentation

Patricia Bieck, RN, BSN, OCN
Staff Nurse, Radiation Oncology
University of Rochester Cancer Center
Rochester, New York
Care Maps in Radiation Oncology

Barbara E. Bodansky, RN, MSN, AOCN
Associate Professor
Columbia University School of Nursing
Clinical Nurse Specialist
Department of Radiation Oncology
Memorial Sloan-Kettering Cancer Center
New York, New York
The Advance Practice Nurse in Radiation Oncology

Jennifer Dunn Bucholtz, RN, MS, OCN
Adjunct Faculty
Department of Advanced Nursing Science
University of Delaware
Newark, Delaware
Clinical Specialist/Nurse Manager
Division of Radiation Oncology
The Johns Hopkins Oncology Center
Baltimore, Maryland
Radiation Carcinogenesis

Karen Hassey Dow, RN, PhD, FAAN
Associate Professor
School of Nursing, College of Health and Public Affairs
University of Central Florida
Orlando, Florida
Nursing Research in Radiation Oncology

Carrie F. Dunne-Daly, RN, MS
Oncology Clinical Nurse Specialist
Radiation Oncology Department
Saint Joseph Hospital
Chicago, Illinois
Principles of Brachytherapy

Vickie K. Fieler, RN, MS, AOCN
Doctoral Candidate
University of Rochester School of Nursing
Advanced Practice Nurse
University of Rochester Cancer Center
Rochester, New York
Radiation Oncology Research in Clinical Trials

Joseph D. Giuliano, RN, BA, BSN
Senior Research Nurse/Program Coordinator
The Johns Hopkins University School of Medicine
Baltimore, Maryland
Skin Cancer

Michele Haller, RN, BSN
Nurse Leader
University of Rochester Cancer Center
Rochester, New York
Care Maps in Radiation Oncology

Laura J. Hilderley, RN, MS
Clinical Nurse Specialist
Radiation Oncology Services of Rhode Island
Warwick, Rhode Island
Radiation Oncology: Historical Background
Principles of Teletherapy

Ryan R. Iwamoto, ARNP, MN, AOCN
Clinical Instructor, School of Nursing
University of Washington
Clinical Nurse Specialist, Radiation Oncology
Department of Radiation Oncology
Virginia Mason Medical Center
Seattle, Washington
Cancers of the Head and Neck

Joanne Frankel Kelvin, RN, BSN, MSN
Instructor in Clinical Nursing
Columbia University
Manager/Clinical Nurse Specialist
Department of Radiation Oncology
Memorial Sloan-Kettering Cancer Center
New York, New York
Gastrointestinal Cancer

Joy Miller Knopp, BS, MN, ARNP
Clinical Faculty, Department of Radiation
  Oncology
University of Washington School of Medicine and
  School of Nursing
Seattle, Washington
Oncology Adult Nurse Practitioner
Eastside Radiation Oncology
Bellevue, Washington
Lung Cancer

Karen Kugel, RN, BSN
Staff Nurse, Medical Oncology
University of Rochester Cancer Center
Rochester, New York
Care Maps in Radiation Oncology

Anne E. Lara, RN, MS, CS, OCN
Adjunct Faculty
University of Delaware College of Nursing
Nurse Manager
Department of Radiation Oncology
Medical Center of Delaware
Newark, Delaware
*Continuous Process Improvement—One Department of
Radiation Oncology's Experience*

Catherine Comeau Lew, RN, BSN
Staff Nurse, Pediatric Oncology Nurse
Department of Radiation Oncology
Brigham and Women's Hospital
Boston, Massachusetts
Pediatric Cancer

Karen E. Maher, RN, MS, ANP, OCN
Instructor, School of Medicine
Radiation Therapy Technologist Program
Oregon Health Sciences University
Adult Nurse Practitioner
Department of Radiation Oncology
Legacy Portland Hospitals
Portland, Oregon
Male Genitourinary Cancers

Susan R. Mazanec, RN, MSN
Clinical Instructor, Frances Payne Bolton School of
  Nursing
Case Western Reserve University
Clinical Nurse Specialist
Division of Radiation Oncology
University Hospitals of Cleveland
Cleveland, Ohio
Breast Cancer

Stephanie Mitchell, RN, BSN
Senior Clinical Nurse
The Johns Hopkins Oncology Center
Baltimore, Maryland
Gynecologic Cancer

Lisa Noll, RN, MS, OCN
Former Associate, Radiation Therapy
Former Research Nurse
Joint Center for Radiation Therapy
Harvard Medical School
Boston, Massachusetts
Chemical Modifiers of Radiation Therapy

Linda Price, RN, BSN
Staff Nurse, Radiation Oncology
University of Rochester Cancer Center
Rochester, New York
Care Maps in Radiation Oncology

Nancy E. Riese, RN, BS, MS, MPH
Instructor in Radiation Oncology
Harvard Medical School
Director, Chemical Modifier Clinical Trials Program
Joint Center for Radiation Therapy
Boston, Massachusetts
Chemical Modifiers of Radiation Therapy

Ellen Sitton, RN, MSN, OCN, RT(T)
Clinical Nurse Specialist Radiation Oncology
USC/Kenneth Norris Jr. Cancer Hospital
Los Angeles, California
*Managing Side Effects of Skin and Fatigue
Hodgkin's Disease and Non-Hodgkin's Lymphoma*

Rosalie Smith, RN
Nurse Manager, Surgical Oncology/Immunotherapy
  Unit and Radiation Oncology Clinic
National Institutes of Health
Warren G. Magnuson Clinical Center
Nursing Department, Critical and Acute Care Patient
  Service
Bethesda, Maryland
Hyperthermia and Intraoperative Radiation Therapy

Elyse Sporkin, RN, MPH, OCN
Administrative Director
Melanoma and Skin Center
M. D. Anderson Cancer Center
Houston, Texas
*Administrative Issues in Today's Managed Care
Environments*

Jayne S. Waring, RN, BSN, OCN
Nurse Oncologist
Florida Radiation and Oncology Group
Florida Cancer Center
Palatka, Florida
Rural Care Issues in Radiation Oncology

Fred Wojtas, RN, BS, RTT
Assistant Professor
Erie Community College
Supervising Radiotherapy Nurse
Radiation Medicine Department
Roswell Park Memorial Institute
Buffalo, New York
Hyperthermia and Intraoperative Radiation Therapy

Foreword

It is with great pleasure and pride that I write this foreword to the second edition of *Nursing Care in Radiation Oncology* edited by Karen Hassey Dow, Jennifer Bucholtz, Ryan Iwamoto, Vickie Fieler, and Laura Hilderley. Over the course of my own career, I have seen nursing in radiation oncology evolve from a rare presence with an undefined role to a full partnership with physicians and other health-care providers in the management of radiation oncology patients. This evolution occurred despite some resistance, but succeeded because of the persistence and vision of the nurses involved in this effort. The editors and contributors to this book are among the leaders who have facilitated this evolution.

Nurses in radiation oncology have assumed major responsibilities in patient education, symptom management, and psychosocial support. Increasingly, nurses function as the patient's primary link in coordinationg care across multiple specialties and settings. More broadly, nurses contribute to quality of life by helping patients improve their physical, psychological, social, and spiritual well-being. At the Harvard Joint Center for Radiation Therapy where I practice, nurses also play important roles in administration, resident training, and research. This text provides the definitive source for information in these various areas and is a clear and comprehensive statement of the breadth and depth of nursing care in radiation oncology.

The major beneficiaries of this expertise and effort in radiation oncology are, of course, the patients. Perhaps less apparent to some is the benefit to physicians. Sharing patient care with committed and talented nurses has been among my most gratifying professional relationships. Physicians increasingly have come to realize that collaborative patient care enhances their effectiveness, professionalism, and even quality of life. I am personally indebted to the nurses with whom I have collaborated, many of whom have contributed to this text.

Jay R. Harris, MD
Clinical and Education Director
Joint Center for Radiation Therapy
Professor of Radiation Oncology
Harvard Medical School
Boston, Massachusetts

Preface

The title of our book, *Nursing Care in Radiation Oncology*, is the same. However, the content of the second edition has been changed significantly to reflect changes in oncology care and radiation oncology practice over the past five years. While the debate continues over the radical shifts occurring in the delivery of cancer care to our patients and their families, the editors recognized the need to make a radical departure in the conceptualization of the sections and chapters of the second edition. These changes were needed to provide nurses in many different practice settings with the knowledge necessary to provide safe and compassionate care for patients receiving radiation therapy. We further acknowledge that many more nurses who are not working specifically in radiation oncology centers or departments will be providing care in the future.

Given these assumptions, we embarked on our new project. The reader will note new faces among our editors and contributors. First, we are very pleased to be joined by three additional editors, Jennifer Bucholtz, Ryan Iwamoto, and Vickie Fieler, who are expert clinicians, excellent writers, and skilled editors. They are widely known and well respected both individually and collectively for their work in radiation oncology. Their clinical experience, thoughtful critiques, and scholarly endeavors contributed substantially to the second edition.

We are also delighted to have 15 new contributors to the second edition. These expert clinicians represent diverse geographic locations and practice domains supporting the comprehensive, substantive nature of this textbook.

The book is divided into three major sections. Section I, *History and Application of Radiation Oncology*, combined Sections 1 and 5 of the first edition with a new twist. The content of the chapters

was reviewed, condensed, and updated. Information on the historical background of radiation therapy became a separate chapter. Specialized treatments of intraoperative radiation therapy and hyperthermia were combined into one chapter to reflect the decreased use of these treatment modalities since the first edition. A new chapter on radiation oncology research in clinical trials was also added to reflect the expansion in the basic science of radiation therapy.

Section 2 constitutes the major portion of our content and is now titled *Treatment of Cancer with Radiation Therapy*. We modified the chapter titles from nursing diagnoses (as noted in the first edition) to the different types of cancer treated with radiation therapy. The change reflects the move toward a more interdisciplinary and multidisciplinary focus. The section begins with a chapter on general effects of treatment on skin and fatigue. These are common nursing problems seen in the majority of cancers treated with radiation. Each chapter includes how radiation is used for the specific cancer (from early stage disease through palliative care), types of radiation delivery, major side effects and nursing interventions, relevant research, and future directions. Information on nursing diagnoses, radiation treatment for oncological emergencies, and late effects that was included in separate sections in the first edition is now incorporated under the different chapters on cancer sites.

Section 3, *Dimensions of Oncology Nursing Practice in Radiation Oncology* is also expanded and updated from the first edition. This section reflects the increasing breadth and depth of nursing practice in radiation oncology. We have included new information on advanced practice issues, innovative practice models in radiation oncology, and administrative issues in today's managed care environment. We have added a unique chapter on the radiation oncology nurse's role in the rural setting, documentation concerns in radiation oncology, and quality improvement issues using care maps as examples. The book concludes with a chapter on research conducted by nurses in radiation oncology.

The second edition retains much of the distinct flavor of our first edition. The chapters are written by practicing nurses in radiation oncology who have upfront knowledge of the dilemmas and rewards of cancer care today. The second edition is also a comprehensive textbook that continues to fulfill the need for the science, art, and rationale of nursing practice in the care of patients receiving radiation therapy. We believe the major reorganization of content in the second edition reflects cancer treatment and care that will be delivered in the future.

Additionally, the second edition is the result of the collective talents of the editors and contributors who gave up valuable personal time toward the project. Most often, after long hours spent in the clinical setting, they sat at their computers to write their chapters and edit their manuscripts just one more time. We would also like to thank our families, friends, and significant others who encouraged us and sacrificed their time so that we could meet our publishing deadlines. We are indebted to our editor, Barbara Nelson Cullen, and the staff at W. B. Saunders for their publishing expertise and patience.

Finally, we dedicate this book to our patients and their families who teach us what really counts, who give us countless rewards, and who keep us focused on why we continue to care in nursing.

KHD
JB
RI
VF
LH

Contents

III
Dimensions of Oncology Nursing Practice
in Radiation Oncology

Color Plates follow

Notice

Radiation oncology is an ever-changing field. Standard safety precautions must be followed, but as new research and clinical experience broaden our knowledge, changes in treatment and drug therapy become necessary or appropriate. The editors of this work have carefully checked the generic and trade drug names and verified drug dosages to ensure that the dosage information in this work is accurate and in accord with the standards accepted at the time of publication. Readers are advised, however, to check the product information currently provided by the manufacturer of each drug to be administered to be certain that changes have not been made in the recommended dose or in the contraindications for administration. This is of particular importance in regard to new or infrequently used drugs. It is the responsibility of the treating physician, relying on experience and knowledge of the patient, to determine dosages and the best treatment for the patient. The editors cannot be responsible for misuse or misapplication of the material in this work.

The Publisher

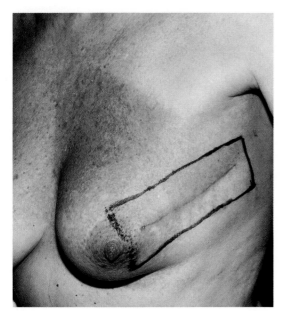

Color Plate 1 • Erythema secondary to breast irradiation.

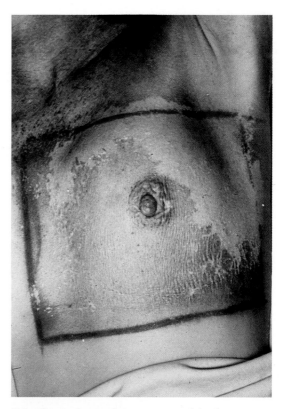

Color Plate 2 • Increased pigmentation and dry desquamation secondary to breast irradiation.

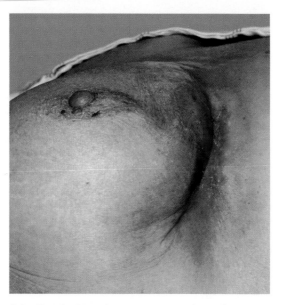

Color Plate 3 • Moist desquamation secondary to breast irradiation. Note increased skin reaction in skin fold in inframammary region.

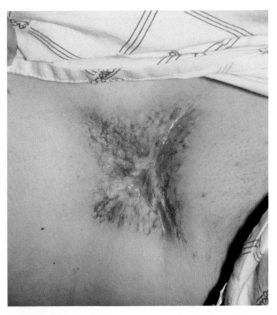

Color Plate 4 • Late skin changes including fibrosis, pigmentation changes, telangiectasia, and retraction in the axilla approximately 2 years after 45Gy (5Gy × 9 in 4½ weeks) plus hyperthermia for recurrent melanoma.

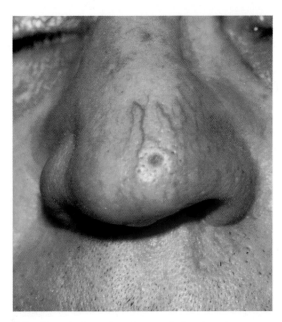

Color Plate 5 • Late skin changes of telangiectasia approximately 2 years after interstitial implant for squamous cell carcinoma of the nasal vestibule.

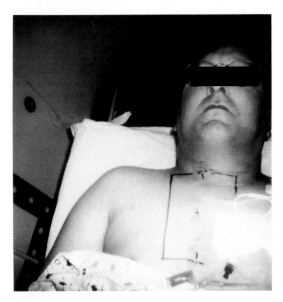

Color Plate 6 • A patient with classic superior vena cava syndrome signs.

I

History and Application
of Radiation Therapy

Radiation Oncology: Historical Background

LAURA J. HILDERLEY

Development of Radiation Therapy

Although radiation therapy had its beginnings in the late nineteenth century with the discoveries by such eminent scientists as Roentgen, Becquerel, and the Curies, the groundwork for their discoveries had already been laid. In 460 B.C. Democritus proposed the idea that tiny particles called atoms were the building blocks of all materials. Medieval alchemists were intrigued by fluorescence, a chemical property of certain elements that played a significant role in Roentgen's discovery of x rays. Similarly, early work by Sir Isaac Newton (1642–1727) and Benjamin Franklin (1706–1790) on the nature and production of electricity provided vital information leading to the development of generators, motors, and transformers to produce the current for Roentgen's experiments almost a century later. One additional development, the vacuum tube and subsequent cathode ray, attributed to Sir William Crookes (1832–1919), was to play a major part in the discovery of x rays by Roentgen.

Wilhelm Konrad Roentgen (1845–1923), a German physicist at the University of Wurzburg, was particularly interested in working with cathode ray tubes. Late in the afternoon of November 8, 1895, Roentgen was at work in his laboratory experimenting with a fluorescent barium compound, when he made his renowned discovery. An electrical charge was passed through a cathode ray tube that had been shielded with black cardboard; it produced a fluorescent glow extending a few feet from the tube. Because cathode rays were known to have limited distance, Roentgen concluded that a new type of ray was being produced and continued to investigate its penetrating power. This powerful ray was given the designation X, the scientific symbol for the unknown. Roentgen was subsequently honored with the first Nobel Prize for physics and by the naming of this new science as *roentgenology*.

Paralleling the events in Germany that led to Roentgen's discovery of the x ray were the activities of Antoine Henri Becquerel (1852–1908) in France. Becquerel was particularly interested in the chemical properties of the elements; he is credited with the discovery in 1896 that uranium is naturally radioactive. Becquerel's publication on this phenomenon caught the attention of Marie Curie (1867–1934), who was looking for a subject to research in her pursuit of a doctoral degree. With her husband and fellow scientist, Pierre Curie (1859–1906), Marie determined to explain the origin of this newly recognized energy produced by uranium. Although the answer to that question eluded the scientific community for many years, the investigations of the Curies led very quickly to the discovery of polonium and radium in 1898. For the next 35 years Madame Curie concentrated her efforts on the investigation of radium and radioactivity, until her death from aplastic anemia in 1934.

During the early 1900s the therapeutic use of x rays became widely popular. In Chicago, Emil Grubbe developed a dermatitis on his hands while working with x ray tubes. He then decided to apply this tissue-damaging effect to a patient with an ulcerating breast cancer and claimed, years later, that the treatment improved the lesion noticeably.

Although the discovery of radium and its ionizing radiation paralleled the discovery of x rays, application of radium in medical practice evolved more slowly, largely because of the great

3

difficulty in extracting even small amounts of radium from pitchblende. However, by 1900 sufficient amounts of radium were being prepared, and its widespread therapeutic application was underway. Interstitial radium needles were implanted, and the first reports of tumor sterilization were issued.

In the first decade of the twentieth century radiation was employed in the treatment of benign as well as malignant disease. Thyrotoxicosis, rheumatism, herpes, and gout were treated with the same vigor as was applied to the treatment of cancer. Radium's apparent curative powers soon had the public and the scientific world hailing it as a restorative, rejuvenating panacea. Over the next decade, growing concern was expressed about the adverse effects of radiation and the documented cases of radiation-induced cancer. Cures were also documented, but results could not be duplicated because there was no way of measuring a given dose of radiation. Technical development continued, and more penetrating x ray machines were produced.

Between 1920 and 1940 the development of deep-therapy x ray machines with a range of 180,000 to 250,000 volts allowed treatment of more deeply seated tumors with maximum tumor destruction. Such doses, however, frequently caused destruction of normal tissue, sometimes resulting in tissue necrosis and death. Lung damage following the treatment of breast cancer was recognized, and attempts were made to devise methods of avoiding lung tissue by rearranging the direction of treatment beams. Treatment reproducibility and dosage measurement were still a problem. The use of skin erythema as a biological indicator of dose was a common but unsatisfactory method, particularly to the radiologists.

During this period, radium was available in many forms, such as creams, powders, and suppositories; mail-order business in radium products was booming. Radon toothpaste was advertised as a plaque preventive by a German manufacturer (Grigg, 1965). It was not until the mid-1930s that the American Radium Society declared that mail-order distribution of radium treatments was unethical. Despite such seemingly unscientific applications of this new technology, radiotherapy was beginning to be recognized as an established science. An international dose unit for x ray was defined and called the *roentgen* or *R unit*. With this definition, the search for a method of measuring dose in air and in tissues was launched. Radiobiology also emerged as a science concerned with the effects of radiation on all tissues.

The development of the atomic bomb during World War II was among the most significant events of the 1940s for its effect on all of society as well as on the science of radiation. Following the war, medicine and engineering combined to produce high-powered treatment machines, including the betatron and linear accelerator. Radioactive isotopes resulting from neutron bombardment of stable elements, such as cobalt and cesium, helped to refine nuclear medicine for both diagnostic and therapeutic purposes. The cobalt teletherapy machine became standard equipment in most radiation treatment facilities, generating high-energy gamma radiation from the radioactive cobalt-60 source.

Use of megavoltage equipment became a practical reality between 1950 and 1970. Computers were employed to calculate isodose distributions and later for analysis of data when controlled clinical trials were introduced in the late 1950s. In 1953 the Seventh International Congress of Radiology met in Copenhagen and adopted the rad as the unit of absorbed dose of any ionizing radiation. Combined therapy and efforts to increase the radiosensitivity of tumors led to remarkable improvement of results in the treatment of some tumors.

By 1970 radiation therapy was an accepted, highly scientific, and still growing discipline within the practice of oncology. Advances and improvements in machine design, refinement of techniques, and ever-increasing application of computer science brought about remarkable progress in cancer treatment, while sparing normal tissue and minimizing side effects. The trend toward the use of the term *radiation oncology* to describe the practice of radiotherapy reflected the greater emphasis on all aspects of the study of malignant tumors and not just the delivery of ionizing radiation.

During the 1980s and early 1990s oncology care was enhanced by attention to the team approach to cancer management. Quality radiation treatment became increasingly available outside of hospitals and medical centers as private, freestanding practices were established. Radiation oncology nurses increased in numbers and, in many settings, moved into an advanced practice role.

Intraoperative radiation, hyperthermia, and the use of radiolabeled antibodies underwent careful scrutiny in clinical trials, many of which continue today (Cox, 1994; Goff & Griffin, 1995; Gunderson et al., 1995; Johnstone et al., 1994; Macklis, 1994; Oleson, 1994; Waldman, 1991). Brachytherapy techniques, particularly high-dose rate brachytherapy, have been optimized allowing treatment on an outpatient basis (Arterbery, 1993; Hilaris, 1994; Orton, 1991). Further refinement of stereotactic radioneurosurgery using either the gamma knife or specially adapted linear accelerators has provided an option for treatment of some intracranial lesions that were previously not accessible by standard radiation techniques (Flickinger et al., 1994; Thapar & Laws, 1995). Conformal radiotherapy, which allows increased intensity of radiation by reducing the volume of normal tissues within the overall treatment volume, has been given continued and renewed attention—especially with the development of three-dimensional treatment planning computer equipment.

Terminology also underwent changes when the term *Gray* replaced *rad* (1 Gray = 100 rad) in 1985. Other changes in terminology adapted in 1985 by the International Commission on Radiation Units and Measurements included *Becquerel* in place of *Curie* and *Sievert* instead of *Rem*.

Radiation oncology today is characterized by continual refinement of treatment techniques and expanded application of combined modality therapy. Numerous cooperative group studies employ radiation as primary or adjuvant therapy. Other sections of this book detail some of the contemporary applications of radiation in cancer treatment, such as in the use of radiolabeled antibodies, altered fractionation schemes, and intraoperative radiotherapy.

References

Arterbery VE. (1993). High dose rate brachytherapy for carcinoma of the cervix (Review). *Current Opinion in Oncology*, 5(6), 1005–1009.

Cox JD. (1994). Clinical applications of new modalities. In JD Cox (Ed.), *Moss' radiation oncology: Rationale, technique, results.* (7th ed., pp. 971–986). St. Louis, MO: Mosby—YearBook.

Flickinger JC, Lunsford LD, & Kondziolka D. (1994). Radiosurgery. In PM Mauch & JS Loeffler (Eds.), *Radiation oncology: Technology and biology.* (pp. 198–215). Philadelphia: WB Saunders.

Goff BA, & Griffin DW. (1995). The use of intraoperative radiation therapy in radical salvage for recurrent cervical cancer: Outcome and toxicity. *American Journal of Obstetrics & Gynecology, 172,* 1881–1886; discussion 1886–1888.

Grigg ERN. (1965). *The trail of the invisible light, from x-strahlen to radiobiology.* Springfield, IL: Charles C Thomas.

Gunderson LL, Nagorney DM, Martenson JA, Donohue JH, Garton GR, Nelson H, & Fieck J. (1995). External beam plus intraoperative irradiation for gastrointestinal cancers (Review). *World Journal of Surgery, 19*(2), 191–197.

Hilaris B. (1994). Evolution and general principles of high dose rate brachytherapy. In S. Nag (Ed.), *High dose rate brachytherapy: A textbook.* (pp. 3–10). Armonk, NY: Futura Publishing.

Johnstone PA, Sindelar WF, & Kinsella TJ. (1994). Experimental and clinical studies of intraoperative radiation therapy (Review). *Current Problems in Cancer, 18*(5), 249–290.

Macklis R. (1994). Radioimmunoconjugates and other target-selective therapeutic radiopharmaceuticals. In PM Mauch & JS Loeffler (Eds.), *Radiation oncology: Technology and biology.* (pp. 357–381). Philadelphia: WB Saunders.

Oleson JR. (1994). Hyperthermia. In PM Mauch & JS Loeffler (Eds.), *Radiation oncology: Technology and biology.* (pp. 276–299). Philadelphia: WB Saunders.

Orton CG. (1991). High and low dose rate remote afterloading: A critical comparison. In R Sauer (Ed.), *International radiation therapy techniques—brachytherapy.* (pp. 53–57). Berlin, Germany: Springer-Verlag.

Thapar K, & Laws ER. (1995). Tumors of the central nervous system. In GP Murphy, W Lawrence, & RE Lenhard (Eds.), *Clinical Oncology.* (2nd ed., pp. 378–410). Atlanta, GA: American Cancer Society.

Waldman TA. (1991). Monoclonal antibodies in diagnosis and therapy. *Science, 252,* 1657.

Principles of Teletherapy

LAURA J. HILDERLEY

Radiation Oncology

Radiation oncology is the term used to describe the clinical as well as scientific discipline dedicated to the treatment of a person with cancer using ionizing radiation. As a clinical discipline, radiation oncology focuses on treatment of the individual while providing care and support for the individual patient and family. As a science, radiation oncology encompasses education of personnel, research, and other academic pursuits designed to increase knowledge and further refine the application of ionizing radiation in malignant disease. *Radiation therapy* or *radiotherapy* refers to the treatment modality used in radiation oncology. The goal of treatment is delivery of a therapeutic dose of ionizing radiation to the tumor while minimizing injury to surrounding healthy tissues. Achieving this therapeutic ratio requires application of the many clinical and scientific principles of radiation oncology, including physics, radiobiology, pathology, radiology, medicine, and nursing.

Indications for Radiation Therapy

Radiation therapy may be used as the primary treatment for certain cancers, such as early laryngeal lesions and prostate cancers. The goal of primary treatment is cure of disease. Radiation is also effective in achieving long-term control when cure is not possible. In the adjuvant setting, radiation often precedes or follows definitive surgery to ensure local control. Examples include preoperative radiation for colorectal cancers and radiation following lumpectomy for early breast cancer. Treatment for palliation of symptoms (pain, bleeding, obstruction, neurological compromise) constitutes approximately 50 percent of all treatments given in radiation facilities.

When planning the course of therapy, the radiation oncologist must consider the individual patient's needs, desires, and life expectancy as well as the principles of physics and radiobiology (Lenhard et al., 1995). Generally, the treatment course is shorter when the intent is palliative, giving only enough radiation to accomplish palliation without causing undue side effects. When life expectancy is short, the quality of that life must be maximized, and this would be incompatible with a lengthy course of radiation.

When cure or long-term control of cancer is the goal, total radiation dosage and length of the treatment course are greater. Differential doses are used because the primary tumor may require a higher dose than lymphatic drainage sites that require prophylactic treatment. Planning is more complex than that required for most palliative treatments, and one is usually more willing to risk inducing acute side effects. Of course, with the anticipation of increasing the patient's life span, the risk of late (chronic) side effects must also be weighed (Ritter, 1994). Modern radiation oncology requires a team effort. Treatment decisions and planning of any course of radiotherapy involve a joint approach and thorough patient and family education. Informed consent is essential. Incorporation of the principles of physics, radiobiology, dosimetry, treatment technique, anatomy and physiology, psychosocial factors, and patient-family needs requires input from many disciplines when available.

Workup and Evaluation

The decision to treat with radiation therapy should be preceded by a thorough patient workup. History and physical examination, laboratory and diagnostic radiological studies, and pathological confirmation of tumor type are considered essential. On rare occasions, radiotherapy may be given without biopsy-proven disease when the tumor is either inaccessible or when there is risk of serious injury in attempting to obtain a biopsy specimen.

Selecting Treatment Modalities and Intent

A multidisciplinary tumor conference may be employed to help in the decision to treat and in determining the best plan of therapy, particularly in the present era of multimodal therapy. The intent of therapy (curative, palliative, adjuvant) must be determined before physical planning is begun.

When radiotherapy is to be preceded by several cycles of chemotherapy (e.g., for small-cell carcinoma of the lung) or is to be given following resection of an operable lesion, the radiation oncologist and other team members should have the opportunity to meet and examine the patient before chemotherapy or surgery. From the patient's perspective, meeting the various specialists and visiting the radiation facility before any treatments

are given allows an opportunity to ask questions and explore the risks versus the benefits of the proposed treatment.

Teletherapy

The most common method of delivering radiation therapy is by external beam (Mansfield, 1990; Schray et al., 1990). *Teletherapy*, or external beam radiotherapy, refers to radiation treatment delivered by a radioactive source or electromagnetic energy from a machine placed at some distance from the target site. Teletherapy (from the Greek *tele*, meaning "from a distance") is distinguished from brachytherapy, or the use of implanted or injected radioactive sources. (*Brachytherapy* is discussed in Chapter 3.)

Teletherapy equipment can be categorized according to energy produced and depth of penetration within the target area. Table 2-1 lists types of

Table 2-1 • Teletherapy Equipment and Its Use

Equipment	Emission	Beam Characteristics and Radiobiological Effects	Clinical Application, Advantages, Disadvantages
KILOVOLTAGE 40–150 kV	X rays	Superficial, limited range, poor skin tolerance	Skin cancers or other very superficial lesions, if electrons are not available
ORTHOVOLTAGE 150–1000 kV	X rays	Deep penetration, high skin dose, high bone absorption	Limited because of poor skin tolerance and potential for bone necrosis
^{137}Cesium radioisotope teletherapy (600 kV)	Gamma rays	Large source size with wide penumbra	Long half-life Low energy and output Used in head and neck treatment
MEGAVOLTAGE/SUPERVOLTAGE ^{60}Cobalt 1.25–2 MeV	Gamma rays	Deeply penetrating Skin-sparing as a result of maximum dose buildup beneath the skin Produces penumbra area at edge of beam that receives less dose	Deep-seated tumors Ease of mechanical operation Slower dose rate (longer treatment time) as source decays
LINEAR ACCELERATORS 4–20 MeV	Photons	Deeply penetrating Skin-sparing Increased versatility and precision of dose distribution	Deep-seated tumors Large field capability Complex electronics with tendency for "down time"
6–30 MeV	Electrons (optional)	Electrons give maximum dose on skin and a few centimeters beneath, falling off rapidly thereafter	Skin lesions, chest wall recurrence, superficial nodes
BETATRON 10–30 MeV	Electrons	High-velocity electrons with deep penetration	High dose rate with shorter treatment time Limited field size
18–40 MeV	Photons	High-energy photons	Bulky equipment Low dose rate photons

equipment, emissions, beam characteristics, and clinical applications.

Kilovoltage (low voltage) machines with a range of 40 to 150 kV were some of the earliest available sources of ionizing radiation and are still in use today for treating very superficial skin cancers. A kilovoltage unit that operates with only a 2 cm or less source-to-skin distance (SSD) is called a contact unit. Those operating at a 15 to 20 cm SSD are called superficial units.

Orthovoltage (deep therapy) equipment in the range of 150 to 1000 kV was introduced in the 1920s and 1930s. Although capable of reaching deep-seated tumors, orthovoltage x rays produced severe late effects because of high bone absorption, leading to osteonecrosis. Skin tolerance was also very poor with these machines, which operated at an SSD of approximately 50 cm.

Megavoltage (supervoltage) machines evolved during the period immediately after World War II. Nuclear reactors allowed production of sufficient quantities of radionuclides for medical usage. The cobalt teletherapy unit was first introduced in 1951 in Canada and became the mainstay of most radiotherapy treatment facilities until the 1960s.

Cobalt machines are mechanically simple and have the ability to penetrate deep within the target site. A typical cobalt source emits gamma radiation with an energy range of 1.17 to 1.38 MeV (million electron volts) and operates at an SSD of 80 to 100 cm. Cobalt is a radioactive element that emits energy through a process of constant decay or disintegration (half-life of 5.26 years). Therefore efficiency of output decreases over time, and the radioactive source must be replaced every few years.

Cesium teletherapy machines, like the cobalt machine, utilize a radioactive source (137 Cs) to produce gamma radiation. The radioactive nuclide of cesium is reactor produced and readily available. However, cesium has low energy output (0.662 MeV), and a cesium teletherapy machine is technically categorized as orthovoltage rather than megavoltage equipment. Because of the characteristic low energy of cesium, the source size must be considerably larger than a cobalt source, and with a low output, the SSD must be shortened to 20 to 40 cm. Combining these three physical characteristics (low energy, large source size, and short SSD) results in a large penumbra for the cesium teletherapy machine. *Penumbra* refers to that area at the edges of a radiation beam that receives a somewhat lower dose of radiation than the area within the primary beam as outlined at the target site.

The linear accelerator is the predominant teletherapy equipment in use in most treatment centers throughout the world. The linac or clinac generates electrons using high-frequency electromagnetic waves to accelerate the electrons to high energy before striking a tungsten target and producing photons. Photon radiation is then directed at the target volume in a defined, shaped beam as it emerges at a very high speed from the linac. Photon energy is equivalent to gamma radiation (produced by a cobalt source) in its energy range and penetrating power.

Many linear accelerators are equipped with an electron mode that allows use of the electron energy itself for treatment of surface lesions or those within a few centimeters of the surface. The electron beam is characterized by rapid dose buildup followed by rapid dose falloff beyond the target volume. Electrons are equivalent to beta radiation in depth of penetration and have useful energies ranging from 6 to 35 MeV. Because of the rapid dose buildup at the surface of the target, electron therapy characteristically produces more intense skin reactions than does photon therapy. An example of a linear accelerator with photon and electron capacity is shown in Figure 2-1.

Figure 2-1 • A Varian Clinac 2300 C/D linear accelerator (© Varian Associates, Inc.) with dual photon energies between 6 and 25 MV and six electron energies between 4 and 22 MeV available. Photo courtesy of Varian Associates, Inc., Palo Alto, CA.

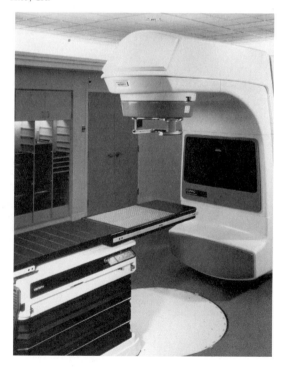

High LET and Heavy Charged Particle Beams

Linear energy transfer (LET) refers to the quality of different types of ionizing photons and particles. LET describes the rate and amount of energy transfer of a given radiation as it passes through a target substance. High LET beams expend most of their energy (and thus have their greatest impact) on tissues within a few centimeters of the skin surface. Low LET sources may be of equal energy to high LET sources but deposit or transfer that energy much more slowly as the beam passes through tissue, thus continuing to have significant effect on tissues deep within the body.

Megavoltage teletherapy equipment, as previously described (see Table 2-1), is the most common means of delivering radiation therapy. There are situations, however, in which a distinct therapeutic advantage can be gained through the use of heavy charged particle beams or high LET radiations (Cox, 1994; Griffin, 1992; Munzenrider & Crowell, 1994).

Relative Biological Effectiveness (RBE)

Equal doses of ionizing radiation from different energy sources do not produce equal biological effects (Hall & Cox, 1994). The ratio of dose required of any given source to produce an effect equal to that of a standard dose of 250 kilovoltage x ray is known as the relative biological effectiveness (RBE). RBE increases with LET up to a certain point. However, with very high LET, there is a decrease or loss of RBE as each succeeding lethal hit on a given cell becomes redundant (Hall & Cox, 1994).

Clinical trials using protons, helium ions, fast neutrons, heavy ions (carbon, neon, argon), and negative pi-mesons (pions) have been under way at a number of sites around the world since the 1950s (Griffin, 1992; Hall, 1994; Munzenrider & Crowell, 1994). Characteristics of high LET and heavy charged particle beams are described in Table 2-2. The two major advantages to these sources of ionizing radiations are (1) deposition of large doses of radiation in small volumes of tissue, with sparing of surrounding normal tissue (proton beams, heavy ions, and negative pi-mesons), and (2) biological advantages, including more effective killing of hypoxic cells and decreased fluctuation in radiosensitivity throughout the cell cycle (fast neutrons, heavy ions, and pi-mesons).

Fast neutron therapy was first introduced in the 1930s. Although tumor response in these early studies was encouraging, late sequelae in long-term survivors were severe enough to discourage further usage for a number of years. When in vitro cell culture techniques became available in the 1950s, neutron studies were resumed and important information regarding RBE of high LET radiation was made clear. Essentially, a given dose of high LET neutron therapy was capable of much greater cellular damage than conventional therapy in spite of tumor hypoxia.

Table 2-2 • High Linear Energy Transfer (LET) and Heavy Charged Particle Beams

Energy Source	Beam Characteristics and Radiobiological Effects	Use in Clinical Trials
FAST NEUTRONS 16–50 MeV deuterons	Fixed field size and beam position Wide penumbra Absorbed dose decreases exponentially with depth Low OER RBE higher with small dose increments	Advanced cancers of the head, neck, and pelvis, gliomas, and melanoma Esophageal cancer and osteosarcomas
PROTONS AND HELIUM IONS 600 MeV	Precise dose distribution with ability to deliver very high tumor dose with sparing of adjacent normal tissues RBE and OER similar to that obtained with gamma and photon sources	Pituitary tumors, chondrosarcoma, cordoma, abdominal and pelvic tumors Soft tissue sarcomas Head and neck tumors
NEGATIVE PI-MESONS 40–70 MeV	Absorbed dose increases slowly with depth, then rises sharply Lowered OER Enhanced RBE	Tumors of the head and neck, brain, prostate, pancreas Skin metastases

Clinical research using physics laboratory-based cyclotrons flourished during the 1970s to mid-1980s. Griffin (1992) summarized the many clinical trials from that era as follows: fast neutrons are significantly more effective in treating inoperable and recurrent salivary gland tumors than conventional therapy; locoregional control and three-year survival in lung cancer patients exhibiting complete or partial response at six months was significant; improved disease-free survival with no difference in acute or late normal tissue sequelae was achieved using neutron therapy for prostate cancer; 53 percent overall control rate was achieved with neutron treatment of soft tissue sarcomas versus 38 percent using photon/electron therapy; osteogenic and chondrosarcomas treated with neutrons showed 55 and 49 percent local control rates versus 21 and 33 percent, respectively, using photon irradiation.

Neutron therapy continues to hold promise, particularly with the introduction of hospital-based neutron therapy systems with improved dose-distribution. Boron neutron capture therapy (BNCT) is also being utilized to increase delivery of thermal neutrons to deep-seated tumors (Wazer et al., 1994). An isotope of boron, ^{10}B, is known to have an affinity for slow or thermal neutrons. Pharmacologic delivery systems have been developed to aid in the concentration of ^{10}B in tumor tissue, thus increasing the neutron dose at the target site.

Heavy charged particle clinical studies began in the United States during the mid-1970s at the University of California—Lawrence Berkeley Laboratory (helium ions) and at Massachusetts General Hospital with the Harvard cyclotron (protons). The precise nature of the heavy charged particle beam (its ability to deliver a high dose to the tumor while sparing surrounding tissues) makes this method of irradiation particularly suitable for treating central nervous system tumors. Local control rates for tumors of the uveal tract, those near the base of the brain, or those lying near the spinal cord have been quite encouraging (Hug et al., 1995; Munzenrider & Crowell, 1994).

The physical and biological advantages of high LET and heavy charged particle beams are offset somewhat by the complexity and costs of the equipment and facilities required. Munzenrider and Crowell (1994) summarize results of the various studies conducted throughout the United States and worldwide. Results vary with different tumor sites and energy sources; however, it is generally agreed that despite slow accumulation of data, sparse population groups in any given tumor category, and complexity and cost of equipment, research into the clinical application of high LET and charged particle beam therapy should continue and expand (Griffin, 1992; Hall & Cox, 1994; Munzenrider & Crowell, 1994).

Principles of Radiation Physics

Understanding ionizing radiation requires a basic understanding of atomic and molecular structure. All matter is composed of atoms, and atoms combine to form molecules. An atom consists of a central core or nucleus containing positively charged protons and neutrons that have no charge. Orbiting about the nucleus are negatively charged electrons equal in number to the number of protons. The atom maintains a stable state through the balance between the number of protons $(+)$ and electrons $(-)$.

Electromagnetic energy is characterized by vibrations of electric and magnetic intensity in space called electromagnetic waves. The distance from the peak of one wave to the peak of the next is called the wavelength. *Frequency* refers to the number of vibrations of the wave in one second. Electromagnetic waves are a form of energy, and as the length of a wave increases, the intensity of its energy decreases. This is explained by the fact that the farther an electromagnetic wave (beam) travels from its source, the wider the area over which its energy is spread. The electromagnetic spectrum is made up of energies of decreasing wavelength as follows: Radio waves, infrared light, visible light, ultraviolet light, ionizing radiations. Ionizing radiation, then, is electromagnetic energy with very short wavelength and very high energy intensity.

Therapeutic radiation is either electromagnetic or particulate in nature and is capable of the ionization of matter. Electromagnetic radiations are characterized by high energy and absence of mass. They can be thought of as bundles of available energy. X rays and gamma rays are two forms of electromagnetic radiation that are roughly equivalent and differ only in their means of production. X rays are generated electrically by machine (linac, betatron, orthovoltage, kilovoltage) and are also referred to as *photons*, particularly as generated by megavoltage machines (see Table 2-1). Gamma radiation is produced through spontaneous emission by radioactive materials undergoing nuclear transition. Radioactive cobalt and cesium are the primary sources of gamma emissions used for teletherapy.

Electromagnetic radiation interacts with matter at the molecular level, causing a disruption of the atom's stability through three potential processes known as the photoelectric effect, the Compton effect, and pair production.

Photoelectric effect occurs when a photon collides with an orbiting electron, transferring the photon's energy to that electron and causing it to be ejected from the atom. Part of the photon energy is used up in overcoming the attractive force between the atomic nucleus and its electron, and the remainder is carried by the electron. The photoelectric effect, therefore, results in true absorption of the radiation.

The Compton effect describes the partial loss of energy from the photon in ejecting an electron, resulting in a secondary photon of less energy than the original but nonetheless capable of proceeding to cause further ionizations.

Pair production, the third potential action of ionizing radiation with atoms, involves interaction of the photon with the nucleus of the atom (as opposed to its orbiting electrons), producing two electron particles, one with a positive charge and one with a negative charge. Electromagnetic energy (the photon) has now been converted to particulate (electron) energy. Because the electron pair have opposite and equal electrical charges, they do not affect the net electrical charge of the atom, and therefore ionization does not take place at this point. As the electron pair continue to seek a stable state, they may subsequently produce ionization through interaction with other atoms.

Particulate radiations that are used in therapy include electrons, neutrons, protons, helium ions, heavy ions (carbon, neon, argon), and negative pions (see Table 2-2). As noted earlier, electrons are the most commonly used form of particulate radiation. The interaction of electrons with atoms is one of direct collision. The electron (characterized by its properties of mass and low energy) loses energy constantly through many collisions with matter, thus expending its energy after penetrating only a short distance within the target substance.

Biological Effects of Ionizing Radiation

Radiobiology is that aspect of radiation oncology that examines and integrates the principles of mammalian biology with the physical and chemical effects of ionizing radiation. Principles of radiobiology are an essential part of radiotherapy planning and constitute a major part of the specialty training for radiation oncologists.

Whereas the goal of radiation treatment is to destroy or inactivate cancer cells, a parallel goal is to preserve and maintain the integrity of the normal tissues being treated. Any local tissue change caused by ionizing radiation can have systemic effects with alterations in various physiological processes. For example, mediastinal radiation is likely to cause esophagitis—a local tissue reaction. The resulting dysphagia, however, can affect the patient's intake and compromise nutrition. Similarly, high-dose radiation for a squamous cell carcinoma in the head and neck region can produce an intense skin reaction. In addition to the local discomfort of this reaction, moist desquamation alters the protective mechanism of the integumentary system.

Understanding and integration of radiobiological principles into nursing care helps to assure the desired patient outcome. As nurses assume greater responsibility for managing treatment and disease-related symptoms and side effects, the science of radiation oncology becomes integral to planning appropriate care.

Cell Survival/Cell Kill

Ionizing radiation has both a direct and an indirect effect on the target cells. Direct damage refers to actual ionizing events affecting the DNA. Ionization may cause breakage in one or both chains of the DNA molecule, faulty cross-linking of the chains after breakage, damage or loss of a nitrogenous base (thymine, adenine, guanine, cytosine), or actual breakage of the hydrogen bond between the two chains of the DNA molecule. In addition to the direct effect on chromosomal structures, a complex chain of chemical reactions takes place in the medium (mostly water) surrounding the cells. The ionization of water (Figure 2-2) results in significant toxic changes that ultimately affect the cell's function and survival. Loss of the cell's reproductive capacity is considered to be the most biologically significant end point of radiation damage.

Cellular Response to Radiation Injury

The relative radiosensitivity of a given tumor is closely related to its proliferative activity. Radiosensitivity is an expression of the response of a tumor to radiation in terms of degree and speed of response (Hall & Cox, 1994). Some tumors may therefore be classified as very radiosensitive, but this does not necessarily correlate with

---

The final products of the ionization of water molecules (HOH) by radiation are an ion pair (H$^+$, OH$^-$) and free radicals (H$^•$, OH$^•$), which are capable of damaging the cell. The ionization of water is shown in the following steps:

$$HOH \xrightarrow{\text{Radiation}} HOH^+ + e^-$$

The free electron (e$^-$) is then captured by another available water molecule and, as shown in the next step, forms the second ion:

$$HOH + e^- \rightarrow HOH^-$$

Because the two ions (HOH$^+$, HOH$^-$) produced by these reactions are unstable, rapid breakdown occurs (in the presence of other normal water molecules), forming yet another ion and a free radical as follows:

$$HOH^+ \rightarrow H^+ + OH^•$$

$$HOH^- \rightarrow OH^- + H^•$$

Although the resulting ion pair (H$^+$, OH$^-$) have some potential for cellular damage through chemical reactions, they are more likely to recombine and form water (HOH). The free radicals (H$^•$, OH$^•$) are extremely reactive, and they too may simply recombine to form water. However, free radicals appear to be more likely to undergo chemical interactions with other free radicals, forming cytotoxic agents, as shown in this reaction:

$$OH^• + OH^• \rightarrow H_2O_2 \text{(hydrogen peroxide)}$$

Free radicals that result from the interaction of radiation with water are capable of triggering a variety of chemical reactions within the cell and are therefore believed to be a major factor in the production of damage in the cell.

Figure 2-2 • The ionization of water by radiation. Water, which constitutes 80 percent of the mammalian cell content, undergoes a series of chemical reactions when exposed to ionizing radiation. In this illustration, water (HOH) is converted to hydrogen peroxide (H$_2$O$_2$). From Hilderley LJ. (1993). Radiotherapy. In S. Groenwald et. al. (Eds.), *Cancer nursing: Principles and practice* (3rd ed., p. 245). Boston: Jones & Bartlett Publishers. Reprinted with permission.

radiocurability, which is the local or regional eradication of tumor. For example, although non-Hodgkin's lymphoma is very radiosensitive, it is not necessarily radiocurable. Adenocarcinoma of the prostate requires high-dose radiation and may not regress for months following a course of treatment, yet it is considered radiocurable.

Following radiation, a given population of cells in any tumor will sustain lethal injury, and some cells will maintain indefinite reproductive capacity. For the fatally damaged cell, several pos-

sibilities are present. There may be immediate lysis or interphase death without an attempt at mitosis. The number of cells undergoing immediate lysis increases with the dose of radiation. Other cells, which have not undergone postradiation lysis but have sustained lethal damage, will exhibit the lethal effects after one or two attempts at mitosis.

The radiosensitivity of normal tissue encompassed by the radiation beam is vitally important. All tissues within the body have a known degree of radiosensitivity, and it is this characteristic of the healthy tissues surrounding the tumor site that largely determines the maximum dose as well as the expected side effects.

The Oxygen Effect

Although the exact mechanism of the oxygen effect is not fully understood, it is generally agreed that oxygen acts at the level of the free radicals, as seen in Figure 2-2. As radiation passes through biological material, ion pairs are formed that very quickly progress to the production of free radicals. These free radicals are characterized by an unpaired electron and are therefore highly reactive. Free radicals then break chemical bonds, trigger chemical changes, and ultimately stimulate the chain of events leading to biological damage. Oxygen (if available) reacts with free radicals, binding them into organic compounds that essentially make them unavailable for reparative function.

Oxygen Enhancement Ratio

The oxygen enhancement ratio (OER) describes the magnitude of the dose required to produce a given level of biological damage under oxygenated versus hypoxic conditions. Low LET radiations, which are sparsely ionizing (x rays and gamma rays), require three times the dose under hypoxic conditions as under oxygenated conditions (OER of 2.5 to 3). Neutron therapy (intermediate ionizing density) has a very low OER of 1.6, thus making this a more effective treatment under anoxic conditions than x ray or gamma radiation (see Table 2-2).

Sublethal injury may be repaired after an initial cycle delay, allowing mitosis and regrowth to occur. Sublethal damage repair may also be faulty, with chromosomal aberrations resulting. If the surviving cell is capable of undergoing mitosis, the chromosomal damage is likely to result in genetic mutation.

As the science of radiobiology developed, certain phenomena were observed that led to the increased ability to achieve eradication of the tumor while sparing healthy tissue. The four Rs of radiobiology have served to define the biochemical and physiological parameters of radiosensitivity:

1. *Repair* refers to the ability of cells to recover from sublethal radiation injury.
2. *Reproduction* occurs when irradiated cells are able to complete the cell cycle and undergo successful mitosis between radiation doses.
3. *Redistribution* of cells in the cell cycle theoretically brings surviving cells into synchrony, with more of them in the most sensitive (M) phase of the cell cycle with each successive radiation dose.
4. *Reoxygenation* is the process in which radio-resistant hypoxic tumor cells become radiosensitive aerated cells between doses of a fractionated course of radiotherapy.

Fractionation

A single dose of ionizing radiation produces a greater effect on tissue than that same dose divided into several fractions. This can be viewed as both a positive and a negative effect when considering the concept of therapeutic ratio in planning a course of radiation therapy. If the goal of treatment is to eradicate tumors while sparing normal tissues, then fractionation becomes crucial to achieving this goal.

Fractionation of total dose is planned to take advantage of the four *Rs* of radiobiology. *Repair* of sublethal injury generally occurs within 24 hours and possibly in as few as 4 hours. Normal cells therefore can repair between daily doses of radiation. Tumor cells may do so initially but become less capable of repair as treatment is protracted. *Repopulation* or regeneration of healthy cells continues after repair of sublethal injury allows mitosis to take place. Tumor cells are more likely to die during mitosis as the result of lethal radiation damage.

Successive daily doses of radiation given at regular intervals help to disrupt the tumor cell cycle, causing division delay. *Redistribution* of tumor cells in their cycle theoretically enhances the effectiveness of each succeeding radiation dose because more cells are likely to be in mitosis at the same time. Healthy cells are less likely to be subject to redistribution.

The single most important advantage of fractionation is the opportunity it provides for *reoxygenation* of the tumor cells. The presence of oxygen in the cell at the time of irradiation greatly

increases the lethal effect of ionization; according to Coleman et al. (1994), adding oxygen even 1/100 of a second after exposure produces no sensitization to radiation, because the lifetime of a free radical is measured in microseconds.

In addition to allowing time for reoxygenation, fractionation has an advantage when treating large tumors with necrotic (anoxic) central components. As daily radiation gradually destroys the outer (oxygenated) layers of the tumor mass, the central core is thus exposed to capillary oxygenation and becomes more radiosensitive to the latter portion of the protracted course of treatment. This assumes, of course, that good microcirculation exists in the target site. Preexisting factors such as compromised circulation (due to radical surgical procedures or radiation fibrosis) as well as anemia can effectively reduce radiosensitivity.

Recent studies have introduced new insights into biological factors affecting radiation response in both normal and tumor tissues (Peters et al., 1990). As a result, various fractionation schedules have been introduced that deviate from the standard single daily fraction.

Alternative Fractionation

Daily single fractions given five times a week is the standard fractionation schedule for radiation therapy with a dose range from 1.8 to 2.0 gray (Gy). Alternative fractionation schemes continue to receive attention as the search continues to achieve greater cell kill and tumor control. Prolonging treatment in order to administer higher doses of radiation and spare acute reactions may, however, lead to excessive late injury. In addition, there is some evidence that prolonged treatment time allows for proliferation of surviving tumor cells (Fowler & Tepper, 1992; Hall & Cox, 1994).

Two strategies have been developed involving multiple fractions per day: hyperfractionation and accelerated fractionation. In both approaches, four to six hours between doses must be allowed for repair of sublethal damage from the first dose before the second is given (Fowler, 1992; Hall & Cox, 1994; Peters & Ang, 1994).

Hyperfractionation refers to the use of several smaller than standard doses given more than once daily in the standard overall treatment time. Daily dose and total dose are usually greater than that used in conventional treatment (see Table 2-3). The goal is to reduce (or at least not increase) late effects and gain better tumor control. Two and sometimes three fractions per day are administered with the appropriate time interval between

Table 2-3 • Comparison of Conventional Fractionation with Hyperfractionation and Accelerated Fractionation

	Conventional	Hyperfractionation	Accelerated Fractionation
Overall treatment time	5–8 weeks	5–8 weeks	2.5–7 weeks
Fractions per day	1	2–3	1–3
Total number of fractions	25–38	60–80	25–38
Dose per fraction	1.2–2.0 Gy	1.0–1.2 Gy	1.2–2.0 Gy
Total dose	45–65 Gy	60–81 Gy	25–76 Gy

each dose. Total daily dose approximates that given for the same tumor treated with a standard single fraction per day.

Accelerated fractionation refers to a shortened overall treatment time in which standard total doses are given in a shorter time period by increasing the number of standard fractions per day (see Table 2-3). The rationale for accelerated fractionation is based upon the fact that reducing overall treatment time reduces the opportunity and probability of tumor cell regeneration during the treatment course and therefore increases the likelihood of tumor control. As long as the overall time is not markedly reduced, acute reactions are usually tolerable. However, if overall time is significantly shortened, then total dose must also be reduced to prevent severe acute reactions. Four approaches to accelerated fractionation are under current study and usage (Peters & Ang, 1994). Type A accelerated fractionation calls for a short course of treatment with a correspondingly reduced total dose. Type B accelerated fractionation uses a less reduced time frame than Type A to deliver multiple fractions per day and a split course to decrease severity of reactions. Type C fractionation uses the technique of administering the boost as the second daily fraction during two or more weeks of the standard single daily dose. Finally, Type D accelerated fractionation calls for a

steady increase in the dose each week throughout the course of treatment. Theoretically, this regime is thought to prepare the mucosa to tolerate intensive treatment by stimulating a regenerative response in the target tissue with lower than usual daily dose in the first weeks of treatment. This dose-intensification technique allows reduction in overall time without significantly decreasing the total dose. Table 2-4 compares the four types of accelerated fractionation.

Although alternative fractionation schemes show some promise and potential for further study, there has been evidence of unexpected late sequelae in normal tissue, usually seen after protracted recovery from acute reactions. Nursing support is an essential component for all patients undergoing hyperfractionated or accelerated treatment. Because of the relatively high risk of complications and the complexity of treatment scheduling, such regimens are usually reserved for major centers and are employed on a study basis.

Systemic Radiotherapy

Systemic radiation has been used in the treatment of malignancies since the beginning of this century. Early therapy involved the whole body or a major part of it and was administered in low,

Table 2-4 • Comparison of Four Types of Accelerated Fractionation

	Type A	Type B	Type C	Type D
Overall treatment time	2–4 weeks	4–7 weeks	5–6 weeks	5–6 weeks
Fractions per day	2–3	1–3	1–2	1–3
Dose per fraction	1–3.75 Gy	1.6–2 Gy	1.8–2 Gy	1–2 Gy (*progressively escalated*)
Total dose	25–55 Gy	60–72 Gy	68.4–74 Gy	66–76 Gy

fractionated doses, often with excellent palliative results. Today this technique, known as total body irradiation (TBI), has several applications, including the treatment of occult metastases, palliation of disseminated disease, and in conjunction with multimodality therapy. TBI is currently employed as part of the preparatory regimen for bone marrow transplantation, as well as therapy for generalized superficial malignant disease. Systemic radiotherapy is also used in reference to the treatment of large volumes of the body in a single dose, called hemibody irradiation (HBI).

Total Body Irradiation

Total body irradiation (TBI) was first used in the early 1900s as a systemic treatment approach for a variety of malignancies. The use of TBI was, however, greatly limited by the resulting severe bone marrow toxicity. The median lethal dose of TBI in humans is approximately 300 centigray (cGy) in a single dose (Lin & Drzymala, 1992). Therefore, until bone marrow transplant became technically feasible in the 1970s, TBI was used primarily for obtaining short-term remission or palliation of symptoms (Lawton, 1994).

Clinical Applications

TBI is currently being used for the treatment of lymphopoietic malignancies and in preparation for marrow transplantation. The goals of the procedure are twofold: eradication of malignant cells throughout the body and the suppression of the immune response to permit survival of the engrafted stem cell.

Before 1979, TBI in humans was predominantly administered as a single treatment, totaling approximately 1000 cGy at various dose rates. Later, a fractionated regimen was adopted in an effort to exploit the more rapid repair rates of normal tissues as well as decrease the associated toxicity. Although the fractionation schedule and the entire preparatory regimen for bone marrow transplantation are not universally established, the total body radiation is likely to be fractionated into at least three treatments; many centers employ a twice-daily schedule for three days, administering 200 cGy fractions to a total of 1200 cGy (Tarbell et al., 1994; Thomas, 1990). The use of large-body fields creates a unique set of problems requiring sophisticated physics support for dose calculation and a high degree of accuracy in the clinical setup. In most situations the patient is placed in a side-lying position. Mid-

way through each fractionated treatment, the patient changes position (e.g., side to side or abdomen to back). Total treatment time per fraction is approximately 20 minutes, depending on machine energy, dose rate, fraction size, and clinical setup. A decreased radiation dosage to the lungs may be accomplished by anatomic positioning (arms across the chest) or by the use of lead blocks.

TBI caused both acute and delayed toxicities. In patients who are to receive marrow transplantation (because marrow suppression is a goal and not a problem in this case), acute gastrointestinal (GI) and delayed pulmonary toxicity are the limiting factors (Emami et al., 1991). In nontransplantation patients (e.g., those treated for non-Hodgkin's lymphoma), marrow suppression is the dose-limiting toxicity (Hoppe, 1994). Acute toxicities tend to be immediate and rather short lived. Nausea is experienced by almost all patients but tends to subside after the first 48 hours. Three to five days after radiation therapy, more pronounced GI side effects develop, including severe vomiting and diarrhea, but these may also be related to other factors, including the administration of chemotherapeutic drugs such as methotrexate and cyclophosphamide. Most patients experience a fever but are afebrile after 24 hours. Transient episodes of parotitis and pancreatitis may result in mild otalgia and abdominal pain, respectively, and tend to resolve spontaneously in two to three days. Skin erythema occurs in most patients initially. More severe skin changes, along with complete alopecia and severe oral mucositis, occur within four to ten days postradiation, related to the concomitant use of certain chemotherapeutic agents as well as the TBI itself.

As the success of treatment improves and the number of long-term survivors increases, the incidence of late effects and chronic toxicity associated with TBI become matters of concern. The development of pulmonary toxicity appears to be related to dose rate as well as to total dose. The interstitial pneumonitis seen in these patients is thought to be the result of the combined toxicity of the radiation and chemotherapy. While recent studies indicate that these changes may be reversible over time, delayed pulmonary toxicity remains the primary dose-limiting factor in the administration of TBI. Other long-term side effects that remain under investigation are impaired growth and development, gonadal dysfunction and infertility, cataract formation, and the development of second malignancies (Tarbell et al., 1994).

TBI has been used in the treatment of myelo-proliferative (lymphoproliferative) disease, specifically chronic lymphocytic leukemia, with a goal of depleting circulating cells. TBI, administered in fractionated doses of 5 to 10 cGy per day, three to five times per week, for a dose of 100 to 400 cGy, has been successful in producing clinical and hematological remissions and in achieving prolonged survival for a substantial number of patients.

TBI is also used in the treatment of mycosis fungoids (MF), a neoplasm of T-lymphocytes. Because of the extreme radiosensitivity of these lesions, radiation has long been established as an effective therapy in their treatment. The development of treatment techniques using electrons represented a major breakthrough in the treatment of this disease. Electrons, which penetrate to a depth of 1 to 2 cm, enabled treatment to be administered to the epidermis and dermis over the entire body surface while sparing deeper normal tissues. This limited penetration also spares the mucous membrane, bone marrow, GI tract, and other vital organs. Most patients are treated in a standing position by multiple field techniques. Generally, two treatment cycles per week are administered for a total dose of 3000 to 3600 cGy in 8 to 9 weeks. Additional treatment with separate electron fields or with orthovoltage radiation may be required for areas not directly exposed to the electrons, or those shielded by overlapping skin folds (soles of the feet, perineum, and top of the head). Organs that are intentionally shielded from the electron beam include the eyes and the nail beds. Nearly all patients experience some skin dryness and development of erythema and desquamation in doses greater than 3000 cGy. Short-term application of topical steroids or systemic diuretics may be helpful in reducing lower extremity or generalized skin edema. Total hair loss occurs by the end of treatment, with complete regrowth occurring within 4 to 6 months following completion of treatment. Temporary impairment of sweat-gland function resulting from direct radiation injury is also common. In patients who have received courses of topical chemotherapy in addition to skin irradiation, telangiectasia and other changes of chronic radiodermatitis may be noted. The potential of total-skin, low-energy electron irradiation to deliver an adequate and uniform therapeutic dose to a depth of 0.25 to 1.0 cm while sparing underlying tissue has also made it an effective mode of treatment for other generalized skin lesions such as lymphoma cutis and Kaposi's sarcoma.

Hemibody Irradiation

Hemibody irradiation (HBI) is a technique in which a large single dose of radiation is administered to a large volume of the body in a single treatment. HBI has been used in major treatment centers since the late 1970s and is most often used to achieve pain relief in areas of disseminated disease or to reduce bulky, locally advanced disease in the abdomen or pelvis. It also offers the potential to treat both halves of the body sequentially in larger doses than could be accomplished with total body irradiation. Because both halves of the body are included in this technique, it is often called sequential hemibody radiation therapy (SHRT). This approach has also been used in the palliation of advanced multiple myeloma with moderate treatment-related toxicity (Singer et al., 1989). HBI is sometimes selected to treat solid tumors that are without clinical evidence of metastases but are at high risk for early dissemination, particularly when effective systemic therapy is not established. Such examples include non-small-cell lung carcinomas, esophageal tumors, prostatic cancer, and GI tumors (Rubin & Scarantino, 1994). This treatment approach has also been used effectively as a consolidation technique in patients with tumors that have responded to chemotherapy and have a high tendency to progress or recur. Large single fractions of irradiation are also thought to have value as combined modality treatment with radiosensitizers and demonstrate an improved therapeutic ratio by increasing the oxygen enhancement ratio of these drugs (Rubin & Scarantino, 1994).

The efficacy of systemic HBI for the palliation of cancer-related pain has been firmly established in the literature. Because disseminated disease most often occurs as metastases to many areas of the body, frequent courses of radiation therapy are required. Often, previously treated areas must be reirradiated to adequately encompass symptomatic areas. HBI as a single dose to a large volume (one half) of the body offers a suitable alternative and is an advantage to patients who are debilitated and for whom daily treatments may involve additional discomfort and inconvenience. HBI as palliative treatment for advanced disease has been used by several investigators over the past decade, with positive results in more than 75 percent of cases. Relief is usually obtained within 24 to 48 hours following the administration of 600 to 800 cGy to a single treatment field. Treatment fields are generally classified as one of three areas. The upper hemibody field extends from the head to the level of the fourth lumbar vertebrae at the umbilicus; the head may or may not be included. Midbody radiation is administered to a field that includes the abdomen and pelvis from the top of the diaphragm to the obturator formina. Lower hemibody radiation includes the torso below the iliac crest and the lower extremities to the ankle. Frequently, premedication with an analgesic is advisable, particularly for patients who are experiencing severe pain.

Side effects are both acute and chronic, with pulmonary dysfunction constituting the major dose-limiting toxicity. Toxicities associated with upper hemibody irradiation are generally more severe than those experienced with mid- or lower-body treatment fields. Various pretreatment regimens have been used to minimize radiation-induced nausea and vomiting (Lawton, 1994).

Recent studies have shown that abdominal radiation stimulates the release of serotonin by the enterochromaffin cells in the GI tract. Serotonin in turn stimulates hydroxytryptamine receptors (HT3), with emesis resulting (Rubin & Scarantino, 1994). Specific HT3 antagonists (ondansetron) effectively prevent or reduce radiation-induced vomiting resulting from abdominal treatment. Pretreatment with effective antiemetics has allowed most HBI to be given on an outpatient basis.

Because bone marrow toxicity occurs in all three types of HBI, monitoring of blood counts is essential. Toxicity primarily involves the platelets and white blood cells, with greatest depression noted 10 to 14 days after treatment. Blood cell counts generally return to normal 6 to 8 weeks following completion of HBI. Subacute toxicity, occurring 3 weeks to 3 months after treatment, includes such side effects as dry mouth, alopecia, radiation pneumonitis, and prolonged bone marrow depression. Chronic side effects may occur for up to two years after upper hemibody irradiation (Awwad et al., 1990).

Treatment Planning and Simulation

Treatment with ionizing radiation is based on a body of knowledge accumulated over many years of research. Achieving the desired therapeutic outcome involves application of careful planning techniques, integration of radiobiological knowledge, understanding of the physics of radiation, selection of the appropriate treatment machine, prescription of the exact treatment specifications, and ultimate supervision of the process. Evalua-

tion of results and patient follow-up are no less important than planning and carrying out the treatment.

The radiation oncologist is responsible for treatment planning, and in most facilities other professionals are involved as well. Radiation physicists, radiobiologists, computer scientists, radiation therapists, dosimetrists, and possibly others may have a role in the planning process.

The nurse's role in treatment planning is primarily as an educator for the patient and family (Greenburg et al., 1990). Explaining the treatment and potential side effects, exploring patient concerns and communicating them to the appropriate team member, and assuring the patient of continued support throughout treatment and follow-up are some of the primary nursing priorities.

Glasgow and Purdy (1992) and Kijewski (1994) address the many aspects of treatment planning, emphasizing the care and complexity of this process. Although tumor control or eradication of disease is the desired goal of treatment, consideration must be given to quality and quantity of life as well. Combined-modality treatment is quite common. Multidisciplinary conferences may precede actual radiation therapy treatment planning, and decisions regarding other modalities (chemotherapy and surgery) will be factored into the radiation plan.

Factors considered in treatment planning include the following: Histology, tumor size and location, route(s) of spread, anticipated side effects, age and general health of the patient, stage of disease and prognosis, and available equipment (teletherapy and brachytherapy). With this information on hand, the process of planning proceeds and usually includes the following steps.

Standard Practice

Defining target volume and normal structures involves study of x rays, computerized tomography (CT) scans, other radiographic studies, and, in many instances, palpation of the tumor. Normal anatomical landmarks are used to further define the treatment field, particularly when gross tumor is not visible or palpable. Fluoroscopy and ordinary radiographs taken on the simulator machine help to define the field and reproduce the portal to be targeted by the treatment beam.

Drawing of the patient's contour can be used to generate computer cross-sections through the treatment volume and determination of dose distribution within that volume. Several alternative plans may be generated from which the radiation oncologist selects the one that provides the desired dose distribution.

Verification films are taken, and skin markings are placed on the patient to define the field(s). These inked lines are usually replaced by tiny permanent marks (tattoos) that can be used to reconstruct the field at any time. Patient objection to skin markings is common and certainly understandable, particularly when such lines are on a visible area. Careful and thorough explanation regarding the importance of the marks should be a part of skin care instructions given to the patient at the time of simulation. It is also important to convert the lines to permanent marks (which are barely visible) as soon as position is confirmed and reproducible on a daily basis.

The most common means of ensuring treatment reproducibility is through placement of three coordinate points on the patient's skin. Light beams (often laser lights) are mounted from three positions in the simulator room, all of which intersect at a given point on the target (patient). Skin marks identify these three points of entry on the patient. These same three coordinates are mounted in the treatment room, and the patient's position is set up daily to align the three laser light points with the skin markings. If the treatment position is relatively simple, no further positioning device is needed. However, when it is difficult for the patient to lie perfectly still and rigid, additional techniques must be employed.

Immobilization and positioning devices may be necessary to ensure reproducibility of the exact treatment portal. Various techniques have been developed to facilitate positioning; these include the use of casts, plastic masks, bite-blocks, tape, arm boards, and other devices. Safety belts help in positioning and also provide security for the patient while lying on the narrow treatment and simulator table (couch). Immobilization or restraining devices are used most commonly for head and neck treatment sites, for pediatric patients, and for the confused patient who is unable to remain in position.

Organ shielding and beam modification are also important parts of the treatment planning and simulation process. All structures encompassed by a radiation beam do not need to be treated; indeed, many should not be treated. A radiation beam can be pictured as a rectangle on the surface of the material at which it is aimed. The rectangle can be made larger or smaller, and the length of its sides can be adjusted by a shaping device, called the collimator, contained in the head of the treatment machine. However, many fields are irregular and are carefully shaped to block normal tissues. Lead blocks are cut and poured, then mounted on a template placed between the energy source and the patient, thus protecting normal tissues from the radiation.

Other beam modifiers include wedges and tissue compensators, such as a wax bolus. These devices are sometimes necessary when treating a surface with an uneven contour to achieve the desired dose distribution within the target volume.

Dose distribution in the target site and surrounding tissues is determined next. This process, once done by hand calculation, is now accomplished with sophisticated computer programs. Determining dose distribution is critical to finalizing the field arrangement, assuring maximum dose to the tumor volume, and minimizing radiation dose to surrounding healthy tissues. Standard treatment planning produces, in effect, a two-dimensional treatment plan (Kijewski, 1994).

Meticulous technique in setting the patient up for treatment each day is the responsibility of the radiation therapist. The therapist must carefully document all aspects of the treatment technique, including position, use of support or immobilization devices, and, of course, daily and cumulative dose. One means of verifying that the position is accurate is by taking a portal film, an actual x ray film taken with the patient in the treatment position. Although these are not diagnostic-quality films, the portal film does provide a means of comparison with the simulator film to ensure proper treatment positioning.

Conformal Therapy

Advances in computer simulation and three-dimensional (3-D) treatment planning have led to a renewed interest in conformal therapy for specific tumors and body sites. Conformal irradiation is defined as integration of CT with the planning computer to determine a beam configuration that conforms precisely to the target organ or site (Hanks et al., 1993; Lichter & TenHaken, 1995). The concept that radiation planning should be based on multiple sections through the anatomic volume of interest rather than a single section through the center is not new (Kijewski, 1994). Three-dimensional treatment planning has been explored since the 1950s, at which time planning and calculations were done mechanically. With the continued development of computer software and improved algorithms, conformal 3-D treatment planning may soon become standard practice.

Conformal therapy limits the high dose volume to the 3-D shape of the target site thus restricting dose to surrounding tissues even more so than with standard treatment planning. This ability to limit the target volume allows delivery of an even higher dose than that used in standard treatment. A major benefit from 3-D conformal therapy is the increased probability of delivering a tumorcidal dose and decreasing local failure. A second major benefit is more effective sparing of normal tissues with reduced short-term and late complication rates. Conformal radiation therapy may not be suitable for all clinical situations. The potential benefit must be such that the additional time, effort, and cost of 3-D conformal therapy is warranted.

Examples of treatment that would not be suitable for conformal therapy include situations in which an accurate tumor volume cannot be determined, or in which anatomic landmarks can readily be used to define volume. However, ongoing trials with conformal radiation and dose escalation are currently under way for treatment of brain, lung, liver, and prostate cancers (Armstrong et al., 1993; Hanks, 1994; Leibel et al., 1994; Lichter & TenHaken, 1995). Nasopharynx, parotid, and other head and neck tumors are also being treated with conformal treatment techniques (Essers et al., 1994; LoSasso et al., 1993).

Conformal treatment can be accomplished through use of multiple (5 to 6) fields and conventional lead alloy blocks. A second set of blocks must be prepared to treat the smaller target volume included in the cone-down boost. Kijewski (1994) notes, however, that when more than four fields are used, the treatment process itself becomes quite unwieldy and time consuming.

Because of the complexity and time-consuming nature of multifield conformal therapy, the multileaf collimator was developed. The multileaf collimator consists of 20 to 40 matched pairs of thin lead leaves mounted on either side of the jaw in the head of the machine. Each leaf is operated by its own motor and responds to computer commands controlling the precise shape of the treatment field by movement of individual leaves in and out of the beam. Changing the field shape takes only a few seconds.

The multileaf collimator supports dose intensification trials currently under way to determine new levels of maximally tolerated dose (MTD) to various organ sites (Leibel et al., 1994; Lichter & TenHaken, 1995; Ling et al., 1993). Increases of 10 to 20 percent MTD have already been accomplished. It is hoped that ongoing clinical trials will ultimately prove that three-dimensional treatment planning and conformal therapy enhance the effectiveness of radiation treatment.

Dose Prescription

Radiation dose is prescribed in units called grays (Gy) or in centigrays (cGy). Until the mid-1980s, the unit of dose was called a rad; thus the literature reflects mixed usage of the two terms. The radiation oncologist prescribes the treatment including the treatment site, number of fields, daily dose fraction, total radiation dose, total elapsed time, number of fractions, use of beam modifiers, and energy source. The radiation treatment record includes field size, description of fields, SSD, simulation information, machine output, treatment time, drawings, diagrams, photos of the patient in treatment position, and clear documentation of any changes in the prescribed plan, including any missed treatments.

Summary

In today's sophisticated cancer treatment environment, radiation oncology plays a major role in cure, control, and palliation of cancer symptoms. More than 60 percent of all persons diagnosed with cancer receive radiation treatment at some time during the course of the disease. The person with cancer who is referred for radiation therapy can best be supported by a nurse who understands the history, physical and chemical principles, and biological effects of radiation therapy and is prepared to provide the education and information needed.

References

Armstrong JG, Burman C, Leibel S, Fontenla D, Kutcher G, Zelefsky M, Fuks Z. (1993). Three-dimensional conformal radiation therapy may improve the therapeutic ratio of high-dose radiation therapy for lung cancer. *International Journal of Radiation Oncology, Biology, Physics*, 26(4), 685–689.

Awwad HK, El Badawy S, Ghamrawy K. (1990). Late tissue reactions after single fraction sequential half-body irradiation (HBI) in patients with non-Hodgkin's lymphoma. *International Journal of Radiation Oncology, Biology, Physics*, 19(5), 1229–1232.

Coleman CN, Beard CJ, Hlatky L, Kwok TT, Bump E. (1994). Biochemical modifiers; Hypoxic cell sensitizers. In PM Mauch and JS Loeffler (eds.). *Radiation oncology: Technology and biology*, 55–89. Philadelphia: W. B. Saunders.

Cox JD. (1994). Clinical applications of new modalities. In JD Cox (ed.). *Moss' radiation oncology: Rationale, technique, results* (7th ed.), 971–986. St. Louis: Mosby YearBook.

Emami B, Lyman J, Brown L, Coia L, Goitein M, Munzenrider JE, Shank B, Solin LJ, Wesson M. (1991). Tolerance of normal tissue to therapeutic irradiation. *International Journal of Radiation Oncology, Biology, Physics, 21*(1), 109–122.

Essers M, Keus R, Lanson JH, Mijnheer BJ. (1994). Dosimetric control of conformal treatment of parotid gland tumors. *Radiotherapy and Oncology, 32*(2), 154–162.

Fowler JF. (1992). Brief summary of radiological principles in fractionated radiotherapy. *Seminars in Radiation Oncology, 2,* 16–21.

Fowler JF & Tepper JE. (1992). Fractionation in radiation therapy. *International Journal of Radiation Oncology, Biology, Physics, 2,* 1–72.

Glasgow GP and Purdy JA. (1992). External beam dosimetry and treatment planning. In CA Perez and LW Brady (eds.), *Principles and Practice of Radiation Oncology* (2nd ed), 208–243. Philadelphia: J. B. Lippincott.

Greenburg S, Petersen J, Hanson-Peters I, Baylinson W. (1990). Interstitially implanted ^{125}I for prostate cancer using transrectal ultrasound. *Oncology Nursing Forum, 17*(6), 849–854.

Griffin TW. (1992). Particle beam radiation therapy. In CA Perez and LW Brady (eds.). *Principles and Practice of Radiation Oncology* (2nd ed.), 368–395. Philadelphia: J. B. Lippincott.

Hall E. (1994). Time, dose and fractionation in radiotherapy. In *Radiobiology for the Radiologist* (4th ed.), 211–229. Philadelphia: J. B. Lippincott.

Hall EJ & Cox JD. (1994). Physical and biologic basis of radiation therapy. In JD Cox (ed.), *Moss' Radiation oncology: Rationale, technique, results* (7th ed.), 3–66. St. Louis: Mosby YearBook.

Hanks GE. (1994). The prostate. In JD Cox (ed.). *Moss' radiation oncology: Rationale, technique, results* (7th ed.), 587–614. St. Louis: Mosby YearBook.

Hanks GE, Myers CE, Scardino PT. (1993). Cancer of the prostate. In VT DeVita, S Hellman, SA Rosenberg (eds.). *Cancer principles and practice of oncology,* 1073–1113. Philadelphia: J. B. Lippincott.

Hilderley LJ. (1993). Radiotherapy. In S Groenwald et al. (Eds.), Cancer nursing: Principles and practice (3rd ed., p. 245). Boston: Jones & Bartlett Publishers.

Hoppe RT. (1994). Total lymphoid irradiation. In PM Mauch and JS Loeffler (eds.). *Radiation oncology: Technology and biology,* 419–436. Philadelphia: W. B. Saunders.

Hug EB, Fitzek MM, Liebsch NJ, et al. (1995). Locally challenging osteo and chondrogenic tumors of the axial skeleton: Results of combined proton and photon radiation therapy using three dimensional treatment planning. *International Journal of Radiation Oncology, Biology, Physics, 31*(3), 467–476.

Kijewski P. (1994). Three-dimensional treatment planning. In PM Mauch & JS Loeffler (eds.). *Radiation oncology: Technology and biology,* 10–33. Philadelphia: W. B. Saunders.

Lawton C. (1994). Radiation therapy for bone marrow transplant. In JD Cox (ed.). *Moss' radiation oncology: Rationale, technique, results* (7th ed.), 937–950. St. Louis: Mosby YearBook.

Leibel SA, Heimann R, Kutcher GJ, Zelefsky MJ, Burman CM, Melian E, Orazem JP, Mohan R, LoSasso TJ, Lo YC, Wiseberg BA, Chapman DS, Ling CC, Fuks Z. (1994). Three-dimensional conformal radiation therapy in locally advanced carcinoma of the prostate: Preliminary results of a Phase I dose-escalation study. *International Journal of Radiation Oncology, Biology, Physics, 28*(1), 55–65.

Lenhard RE, Lawrence W, McKenna RJ. (1995). General approach to the patient. In GP Murphy, W Lawrence, RE Lenhard (eds.). *Clinical oncology* (2nd ed.), 64–74. Atlanta: American Cancer Society.

Lichter AS & TenHaken R. (1995). Three-dimensional treatment planning and conformal radiation dose delivery. In VT Devita, S Hellman, SA Rosenberg (eds.). *Important advances in oncology,* 95–109. Philadelphia: J. B. Lippincott.

Lin H & Drzymala RE. (1992). Total-body and hemi-body irradiation. In CA Perez and LW Brady (eds.). *Principles and practice of radiation oncology* (2nd ed.), 256–264. Philadelphia: J. B. Lippincott.

Ling CC, Burman C, Chui CS, Jackson A, Kutcher GJ, Leibel S, LoSasso T, Mageras G, Mohan R, York E, Fuks Z. (1993). Prospectives of multidimensional conformal radiation treatment. *Radiotherapy Oncology, 29*(2), 129–139.

LoSasso T, Chui CS, Kutcher GJ, Leibel SA, Fuks Z, Ling C. (1993). The use of a multileaf collimator for conformal radiotherapy of carcinomas of the prostate and nasopharynx. *International Journal of Radiation Oncology, Biology, Physics, 25*(2), 373–375.

Mansfield CM. (1990). Intraoperative Ir-192 implantation for early breast cancer: Techniques and results. *Cancer, 66*(1), 1–5.

Munzenrider JE & Crowell C. (1994). Charged particles. In PM Mauch & JS Loeffler (eds.). *Radiation oncology: Technology and biology,* 34–55. Philadelphia: W. B. Saunders.

Peters LJ & Ang KK. (1994). Altered fractionation schemes. In PM Mauch & JS Loeffler (eds.). *Radiation Oncology: Technology and biology,* 545–565. Philadelphia: W. B. Saunders.

Peters LJ, Brock WA, Travis EL. (1990). Radiation biology at clinically relevant fractions. In VT DeVita, S Hellman, SA Rosenberg (eds.). *Important advances in oncology 1990,* 65–83. Philadelphia: J. B. Lippincott.

Ritter MA. (1994). Cell proliferation. In PM Mauch & JS Loeffler (eds.). *Radiation oncology: Technology and biology,* 525–544. Philadelphia: W. B. Saunders.

Rubin P and Scarantino CW. (1994). Hemibody irradiation. In PM Mauch & JS Loeffler (eds.). *Radiation oncology: Technology and biology,* 405–418. Philadelphia: W. B. Saunders.

Schray MF, Gunderson LL, Sim FH, Pritchard DJ, Shives TC, Yeakel PD. (1990). Soft tissue sarcoma: Integration of brachytherapy, resection and external irradiation. *Cancer, 66*(3), 451–456.

Singer CRJ, Tobias, JS, Giles F, Rudd GM, Blackman GM, Richards JDM. (1989). Hemibody irradiation: An effective second line therapy in drug resistant multiple myeloma. *Cancer, 63,* 2446–2451.

Tarbell, NJ, Chin LM, Mauch PM. (1994). Total body irradiation for bone marrow transplantation. In PM Mauch & JS Loeffler (eds.). *Radiation oncology: Technology and biology,* 387–418. Philadelphia: W. B. Saunders.

Thomas ED. (1990). TBI regimens for marrow grafting. *International Journal of Radiation Oncology, Biology, Physics, 19*(5), 1285–1288.

Wazer DE, Zamenhos RG, Harling OK, Madoc-Jones H. (1994). Boron neutron capture therapy. In PM Mauch & JS Loeffler (eds.). *Radiation oncology: Technology and biology,* 167–191. Philadelphia: W. B. Saunders.

Principles of Brachytherapy

CARRIE DUNNE-DALY

Brachytherapy is the temporary or permanent placement of a radioactive source either on or within a tumor. Also called internal radiation therapy or implant therapy, brachytherapy offers the advantage of delivering a high dose of radiation to a specific tumor volume, with a rapid falloff in dose to adjacent normal tissues. The most common methods used to provide a therapeutic dose of internal radiation therapy include interstitial implant, intracavitary treatment, and systemic therapy. In an interstitial implant, the radioactive source is contained in the form of a needle, seed, wire, or catheter that is implanted directly into the tumor. In an intracavitary treatment, the radioactive source is placed directly into the body cavity and held in place by an applicator. In systemic therapy (radiopharmaceutical therapy), an unsealed radioactive source is given orally or intravenously.

Brachytherapy has been used since the early 1900s, following the discovery of radium by Marie and Pierre Curie. Treatment with brachytherapy began with the use of surface applicators of radium to treat skin lesions. Since then, many developments, both beneficial and destructive, have occurred in the therapeutic use of radioactive sources.

In the early days of brachytherapy, physicians had limited knowledge of the destructive effects from improper handling of radioactive sources. In the 1950s, afterloading methods were developed in which source holders are placed during the operative procedure but the radioactive sources are not added until later when the patient has been returned to his or her room. This technique protects nurses and other health care workers from undue radioactive exposure. In the 1960s and 1970s, the development of the linear accelerator led to a decline in the popularity of brachytherapy. The 1980s witnessed a renewed interest in the use of brachytherapy, either alone or in combination with other modalities, such as hyperthermia (Glasgow & Perez, 1992).

Today, knowledge about the long-term effects of radiation exposure has led to highly regulated guidelines on the safe use and handling of radioactive isotopes. In a comprehensive study done by Nag et al. (1995), it was found that 819 facilities in the United States practice brachytherapy. The most common radioactive sources used are cesium-137, iridium-192, iodine-125, and iodine-131. The most common techniques used are intracavitary, interstitial, intraluminal, and plaques. The most common sites treated are cervix, endometrium, head and neck, and lung. High-dose rate (HDR) remote afterloading brachytherapy or low-dose rate (LDR) remote afterloading brachytherapy was used in approximately 25 percent of the facilities that responded to the survey (Nag et al., 1995). With the advent of improved safety and protection techniques and increased knowledge about the care of implant patients, occupational exposure to radiation has declined significantly.

This chapter discusses the basic principles of the radiobiology of brachytherapy, reviews the use of brachytherapy in the treatment of selected cancers and the related nursing interventions, and discusses the properties of radioactive isotopes and specific radiation safety guidelines needed in the care of brachytherapy patients.

Radiobiology of Brachytherapy

The basic radiobiological principles of repair, repopulation, redistribution, and reoxygenation (the four Rs) have a different tissue response when radiation is administered on a continuous basis either in high- or low-dose rate (brachytherapy), as opposed to being fractionated on a daily basis (external beam radiation).

Repair is an intracellular process that is thought to be equally efficient in both normal and cancer cells. Normally, repair is complete within a few hours after external beam radiation. Theoretically, with brachytherapy techniques, there should be a decreased ability of malignant cells to repair damage. Thus, when external beam radiation is combined with brachytherapy, tumor cells in the irradiated volume that may survive with external beam radiation are less likely to undergo repair.

Repopulation involves the replacement of dead or dying cells through cell multiplication. Both normal and malignant cells are able to recover from radiation injury; however, repopulation rates vary with different tissues. Theoretically, continuous-dose rate radiation, when targeted to a specific tumor volume, would decrease the ability of malignant cells to repopulate. The rapid falloff in radiation dose to normal surrounding tissues would have less interference with the ability of normal tissues to repopulate after radiation damage.

Redistribution of cells throughout the cell cycle occurs after a dose of fractionated radiation. Irradiated cells may be blocked in the late G2 phase of the cell cycle and are more susceptible to radiation damage. With brachytherapy, a greater percentage of cancer cells accumulate in the G2 phase. Although cellular proliferation can occur during brachytherapy, these new cells are still blocked in the G2 phase and continue to be susceptible to radiation damage. Redistribution of a significant proportion of the cell population into G2 phase can result in an increased sensitization effect.

Reoxygenation is the process in which hypoxic tumor cells become sensitized as a result of the redistribution of oxygen after radiation exposure. Reoxygenation occurs as a result of decreased tumor burden and changes in the blood flow patterns of tumors. Less oxygen is needed to sensitize cells to damage with continuous radiation. Hence brachytherapy techniques may be more effective with anoxic tumors than conventional fractionated external beam radiation (Perez et al., 1992).

Brachytherapy in Specific Cancers

Brachytherapy can be used alone or in combination with external beam radiation, surgery, chemotherapy, or hyperthermia. It is used to im-

prove control of local disease, treat areas at high risk for tumor recurrence, enhance comfort with recurrent disease, preserve vital organ function, and spare normal surrounding tissues from damage. Implantation techniques have been used in a wide variety of cancers of the endometrium, cervix, breast, head and neck, lung, liver, colon, bladder, prostate, and brain. Table 3-1 lists the types of cancers in which brachytherapy techniques have been used.

Gynecological Cancer

Brachytherapy has been used for temporary intracavitary insertion of a sealed radioactive source into the cervix and uterus for gynecological cancers. Although brachytherapy may be used alone, it is most often combined with external beam radiation therapy to treat bulky disease and improve local control.

Cervical Cancer

In the treatment of cervical cancer, it is very important for the radiation oncologist to select the appropriate cylinder or colpostat and the appropriate length for the intrauterine tandem. A colpostat or vaginal cylinder with the largest possible diameter provides the greatest tumor dose at the depth for a given mucosal dose. Three systems have been used for brachytherapy of cervical cancer: the Paris, the Swedish, and the Manchester systems. These systems differed in the type of applicator used, the strength of the radioactive source, and the time in which the radioactive source is administered.

TYPES OF APPLICATORS

Applicators used to insert intracavitary sources in the uterus and vagina include rubber catheters and ovoids (Paris system), metallic tandems and plaques (Swedish system), and plastic tandems and ovoids (Manchester system). In the 1940s

Table 3-1 • Cancers Treated with Brachytherapy

Cancer	Technique	Radioactive Source
Endometrial	Intracavitary	Radium, cesium
Cervical	Intracavitary	Radium, cesium
Prostate	Interstitial	Iodine, gold
Breast	Interstitial	Iridium
Ocular melanoma	Plaque therapy	Cobalt, iodine, palladium
Head and neck	Interstitial thermal	Iridium, cesium
Rectal	Interstitial	Cesium
Esophageal	Intraluminal	Cesium
Bronchogenic	Endobronchial	Iridium, iodine

Fletcher designed a preloaded, cylindrical colpostat that was longer than the Manchester ovoids. It had partial shielding at both ends, with handles that facilitated the insertion of the colpostat and helped to maintain its position. Suit further modified the design so that the colpostat could be afterloaded. Tungsten shields were placed in the colpostats to decrease the radiation dose to the bladder and to the anterior rectal wall without compromising the radiation dose to the uterine, sacral, and broad ligaments (Glasgow & Perez, 1992). Today the Fletcher-Suit applicator is the standard applicator used in brachytherapy of cervical cancer.

The Fletcher-Suit applicator may not be suitable in every patient situation. Thus other applicators such as the Henschke and minicolpostats have been developed. The Henschke applicator's configuration conforms better to a patient with a narrow vagina. However, the radioactive sources are placed parallel to the long axis of the bladder and rectum and do not provide for any shielding, such that potentially higher doses of radiation could be delivered to these organs.

If the vagina is narrow or if an anatomical distortion occurs as a result of tumor growth, minicolpostats may also be used. Minicolpostats have a smaller diameter and a flat surface to allow for easier insertion. Similar to the Henschke applicator, many minicolpostats have no shielding. This can result in a higher dose to the bladder and rectum, which requires an adjustment in the activity or strength of the radioactive source or the specified time in which the radiation is delivered.

Interstitial implants with needles are also used to increase the radiation dose to the parametrium after external beam or intracavitary radiation. Metallic needles containing radium-226, cobalt-60, or cesium-137, and plastic needles containing iridium-192 seeds or wires, have been implanted into the parametrium. The interstitial implant procedure is similar to that of the intracavitary insertion. The radiation oncologist must exercise special care to avoid inserting the needles into the bladder. Packing the vagina with iodoform gauze helps to anchor the needles once they are in place. A cystoscopy and rectal examination may be done after the placement to identify whether any needles have been misplaced; if so, they should be withdrawn and replaced immediately.

Endometrial Cancer

Endometrial cancers may grow irregularly into the uterine cavity and produce a deformity of the lumen of the uterus as a result of exophytic tumor spread, thickening of the uterine wall caused by myometrial infiltration, or uterine enlargement (Glasgow & Perez, 1992). The radiation oncologist first determines the size and shape of the patient's uterus by rotating a uterine sound and measuring the width and depth of the uterine cavity.

The different types of applicators used for cervical cancer are also employed in brachytherapy for endometrial cancer. The radiation oncologist may pack the uterus with capsules. Therapeutic advantages of packing the uterus are that a bulky tumor can be flattened out, which allows the base of the lesion to be radiated more effectively; the stretching of the uterine wall makes it thinner and permits higher radiation doses to be delivered to the serosa, and a more uniform distribution can be delivered to the entire myometrium.

Heyman capsules may also be afterloaded to decrease radiation exposure to the radiation oncologist and to allow for improved verification of the radioactive sources in the uterus before loading with the radioactive source.

Vaginal Cancer

In patients with vaginal cancer, specific vaginal cylinders or applicators may be used. Vaginal cylinders have a central, hollow metallic cylinder in which the radioactive sources are placed. Some vaginal cylinders have lead shielding to protect parts of the vagina from radiation.

Type and Strength of Radioactive Sources in Gynecological Cancers

The most common radioactive sources used in the treatment of gynecological cancers are cesium-137, iridium-192. The selection of the strength of the radioactive source is important, because an excessive radiation dose to the vaginal mucosa (over 14,000 cGy total dose) may lead to severe mucosal atrophy, fibrosis, vaginal stenosis, or necrosis.

Intracavitary Implant Procedure

The insertion of the applicators (tandem into the uterus and ovoids into the vagina) is performed by the radiation oncologist while the patient is under general anesthesia. Once the applicators are in place, the vagina may be packed with iodoform gauze to stabilize the tandem and ovoids. Sutures may also be secured loosely to assist in holding the applicator in place. Verification films are taken to ensure proper placement of the applicators using a "dummy" source of radiation so the radiation dose to the tumor bed is maximized and the radiation dose to the bladder and colon is minimized.

The radioactive source is inserted or afterloaded when the patient returns to her hospital room which minimizes radiation exposure to health care workers.

NURSING CARE OF PATIENTS WITH INTRACAVITARY IMPLANTS

Nurses must plan direct patient care keeping their own safety in mind. Nurses need to minimize the time spent close to the patient and maximize their distance from the patient. Preimplant teaching should include detailed information regarding the implant procedure, afterloading, self-care activities, nursing care, visitors' time limitations, and possible adverse effects if any. A description of sensations that the patient may experience is helpful in relieving anxieties. Patients also benefit from seeing what the applicator and a "dummy" radioactive source look like before the implant procedure. Numerous pamphlets and patient education materials available from the American Cancer Society, National Cancer Institute, and the Oncology Nursing Society help to reinforce teaching by the nurse.

Several precautionary measures must be taken to prevent displacement of the radioactive source and to ensure patient comfort. During the implant period, patients are on bed rest, and the head of the bed should be elevated no more than 15 degrees. For comfort and to reduce pressure on the lower back while on bed rest, patients may log roll from side to side but should avoid twisting and turning. It may also be helpful to place a small pillow behind the lower back to relieve pressure. Patients may also prefer to bring a favorite pillow from home to use while in the hospital. Bed linens are not changed unless they become soiled.

During the implant period, patients' usual self-care activities will be altered. They may sponge bathe from the waist up. They will not be able to void in the usual manner or move their bowels. A Foley catheter will keep the bladder constantly drained to prevent unusual displacement of the radioactive source. Patients should be encouraged to maintain a high fluid intake to prevent bladder irritation. They will also be on a low-residue diet and will be given an antidiarrheal medication (such as Lomotil or Imodium) to prevent bowel movements from occurring during the implant period. It is important for patients to wear thigh-high antiembolic stockings and to flex their toes and feet while in bed to minimize venous stasis.

Patients may feel abdominal fullness, a dull abdominal cramping, low backache, and the urge to void. These are common discomforts experienced during intracavitary implant and are usually related to the placement of the applicator or the Foley catheter. Mild analgesics can help to relieve the discomfort. Sharp, or extreme pain is unlikely, and an uncommon reaction that should be reported.

Patients may often feel that time progresses very slowly during the implant period. Quiet, diversional activities such as reading, listening to tapes, watching television, or talking to family and friends on the telephone may help. Visitors are encouraged, but they must be at least 18 years old, not be pregnant, and may visit for a 30-minute period or less each day. The family can call the patient by phone occasionally so she does not feel isolated.

Once the implant time is completed, the radiation oncologist and radiation safety officer will remove the radioactive source and the applicators in the patient's room. Patients should be offered a pain reliever before implant removal to lessen any discomfort. Once the radioactive source is removed and the radiation safety officer surveys the room to ensure that there is no residual radiation, linen and dressings can be disposed of in the usual manner (Dunne-Daly, 1994a). The Foley catheter is then removed, and the patient may slowly get out of bed and resume her normal self-care activities. The nurse should assist the patient to ambulate before patient is discharged. Some patients may experience weak legs or feel dizzy after being on bed rest.

Patients are given instructions on postimplant care as well as a follow-up appointment in the radiation therapy department. Discharge instructions include information about normal changes in elimination, vaginal discharge, and voiding. Normal bowel activities may not return for a few days. If patients have a feeling of abdominal fullness and constipation, natural laxatives such as prune juice or bran may be recommended. Patients can expect a small to moderate amount of light vaginal spotting and light cramping. The patient should contact the radiation oncologist or primary nurse if heavy bleeding or sharp abdominal cramping occurs. Patients may also experience frequent voiding in small amounts for the first day, but this should improve quickly. Malodorous, foul-smelling urine and pain during urination are symptoms of infection and need to be reported to the radiation oncologist. Tiredness may persist for a few weeks. Resuming normal work, family, and household routines depend on the individual, as there is no contraindication from the implant itself. Nurses need to assess the level of patient and family understanding about the radiation treatment. It should be stressed that patients have no residual radiation and are not radioactive. Sexual activity may be resumed when the patient feels comfortable. Patients may require a vaginal dilator with instructions on how to use it and how often, to prevent vaginal stenosis. Use of a dilator or having sexual intercourse on a regular basis will allow the patient to be sexually active in the future and will prevent painful, poorly visualized pelvic exams.

Remote Afterloading Brachytherapy

Remote afterloading brachytherapy for interstitial and intracavitary applications is becoming a widely used technology for both low-dose-rate (LDR) and high-dose-rate (HDR) implants (Brady, Micarly, et al., 1993; Jones et al., 1994). LDR systems use cesium-137 or iridium-192 with dose rates in the range of 0.4 to 2.0 Gy per hour. HDR systems are built for cobalt-60 or iridium-192 sources with rates greater than 12 Gy per hour. Medium-dose rates range from 2 to 12 Gy per hour (Brady, Micarly, et al., 1993; Brady, Rotman, & Calvo, 1993).

There are distinct advantages to using such systems:

1. Brachytherapy treatment may be given on an outpatient basis, which reduces cost.
2. The applicator is inserted in a treatment room, which eliminates the need for an operating room procedure.
3. There isn't a need for special radioactive source preparation, so radiation exposure to the staff is minimal.
4. A remote afterloading system allows for loading and unloading of the radioactive sources and recording of the times when the source is in the patient.
5. A wide range of dose distributions is available.
6. Treatment times are shorter, which allows for a greater degree of patient comfort and reduces complications from prolonged bedrest, such as pulmonary embolism or deep vein thrombosis (Bauer & Schultz-Wendtland, 1993, Brady, Micarly, et al., 1993; Brady, Rotman, & Calvo, 1993).

HDR brachytherapy units are used in a shielded room. The applicators are first inserted into the patient, and the radioactive sources are then loaded using a remotely activated system. Built-in safety mechanisms check the placement of the applicator and the position of the radioactive source. Both fractionation and total radiation dose are important factors in decreasing complications without compromising the results of HDR brachytherapy. Early in the development of HDR, there were reports of increased pelvic complications, bladder, rectosigmoid, and small intestine complications in comparison with patients treated with conventional brachytherapy. This was likely related to the greater biological effectiveness of the higher radiation dose rate. Technical factors such as perforation, asymmetrical positioning of the tandem, and suboptimal placement of the ovoids may have been contributing factors in the development of complications. In today's use, the dose per fraction of HDR intracavitary radiation and the number of fractions are important factors in the development of complications, local tumor control, and residual disease. When a 10 to 15 percent adjustment is made in total dose (TD), the rate of complications decreased without compromising the results of therapy.

Breast Cancer

Brachytherapy for breast cancer involves the use of temporary interstitial implants of iridium-192 to the original tumor site to decrease the likelihood of tumor recurrence. LDR wires have been exchanged to an HDR iridium source in some institutions (Hammer et al., 1994). It is administered as a radiation boost in conjunction with primary external-beam breast radiation. The use of radioactive breast implants has declined with the widespread use of electron boosts and patients' desire not to undergo surgery. However, breast implants may still be used to treat larger fields or deep areas in the breast that are not as easily accessible with electrons.

The Breast Implant Procedure

The breast implant procedure is performed with the patient under local or general anesthesia. A one- to two-day hospital stay is typically required. The breast implant procedure is performed by the radiation oncologist. The implant site is marked on the skin after the volume of tissue to be implanted is determined. Rigid, metallic needles are inserted to serve as conduits for the placement of narrow, hollow plastic catheters. The hollow plastic catheters are secured with buttons at each end, and then the hollow metal needles are removed. Unlike intracavitary implants, verification films are not required. The afterloading technique is used to insert strands of iridium-192 seeds into the catheters after the patient returns to the hospital room.

NURSING CARE OF PATIENTS WITH BREAST IMPLANTS

Implant time is variable and usually lasts for approximately 48 hours. The usual radiation dose rate is 50 to 60 cGy per hour. Generally, breast implants are well tolerated and often look more painful than they reportedly feel by patients. The patient may experience heaviness or slight throbbing pain or discomfort in the implanted breast for the first day. The pain and discomfort gradually subside. Patients may be out of bed as tolerated, but they are restricted from leaving their hospital room for radiation safety reasons. There are no dietary restrictions. Patients are not allowed to shower or get the implant site wet. As with patients undergoing gynecological implants, the use of diversionary activities helps patients to pass the time more easily.

Once the radiation dose rate per hour is completed, the iridium and catheters are removed in the patient's room, and the patient is discharged. Linens and dressings may be disposed of in the usual manner once the room is surveyed. Post-implant teaching includes information on skin care, fatigue, and return to daily activities. Patients may note slight skin dryness and crusting at the implant site that gradually subside within a few weeks. They should be encouraged to wear a firm-fitting bra, since the implanted breast may continue to feel full and heavy for a few weeks. Patients are given a schedule for follow-up in the radiation therapy department. Patients may resume other work and family and household responsibilities based on their preferences and needs.

Head and Neck Cancers

Brachytherapy for head and neck cancers is often combined with external beam radiation and other treatment modalities to achieve local tumor control. Temporary interstitial or intracavitary implants are usually used, but permanent interstitial implants have also been used for treatment of tumors extending into the base of the skull. Radioisotopes that have been used in brachytherapy for head and neck cancers are cesium-137, iridium-192, radium-226, and cobalt-60.

Head and Neck Implant Procedure

Head and neck implants are performed in the operating room with the patient under general anesthesia. General anesthesia via nasotracheal intubation is preferred for implants of the oral cavity and lips. Although rare, a tracheostomy may be performed for extensive lesions requiring

large radioactive implants and for tumors arising from the base of tongue or vallecula, because the resulting edema may cause breathing difficulties. During the procedure the oral cavity is kept dry with preanesthetic medication and suctioning.

Lesions beneath the tongue are usually implanted through the dorsum of the tongue. The anterolateral needles emerge from the undersurface of the tongue and are reinserted into the floor of the mouth. For lesions of the posterolateral tongue border, the tongue is pulled forward so that the implant may be started at the base of the tongue. Implantation of the base of the tongue is usually done by inserting long metallic guides into the submaxillary/subdigastric region. The radiation oncologist must exercise great care in implanting the anterolateral needles away from the thin mucous membrane that covers the bone in the upper and lower gum, as well as the periosteum, teeth, and bone, to prevent osteoradionecrosis. Afterloading may be done with iridium-192 wires once patients return to their rooms. Verification films are taken to check the position of the radioactive source.

NURSING CARE OF PATIENTS WITH HEAD AND NECK IMPLANTS

Head and neck implants are generally uncomfortable. Offering pain medication is very important. Steroids can be administered to decrease or prevent local swelling. The head of the bed is elevated to a 45-degree angle, and patients are encouraged to be out of bed. Physical activities are restricted to within the patient's room. Diet restrictions depend on the type of implant. Some patients tolerate a liquid or soft diet; others may require intravenous fluids, nasogastric tube feeding, or gastrostomy tube feedings.

Patients with intraoral implants may be unable to speak clearly. In addition, the limitation on time that the nurse can spend with a brachytherapy patient may add to the patient's sense of isolation. A plan for communication should be carefully set up during the preimplant teaching. Using a pad of paper and pencil, picture cards, a magic slate, or picture board are different ways in which patients may communicate (Dunne-Daly, 1994a).

Implants of the anterior oral cavity may be removed in the radiation therapy department instead of the patient's room. Precautions are taken, because bleeding at the implant site may occur.

Brachytherapy head and neck implants may be done in the radiation oncology department with the patient under local anesthesia if preloaded or "hot" cesium implants are used. Some patients receive a split-course of radiation, which consists of external beam radiation followed by one or two outpatient implants, and then the final course of external beam treatment. Patients may be treated as outpatients with "hot" implant needles (generally cesium-137 needles). Patients stay in the radiation oncology department for several hours. Once the specified radiation dose has been delivered, the needles are removed and the patient may go home.

Side effects depend on the specific area of the head and neck treated. Generally, localized pain and nutritional, swallowing, and eating problems are ongoing from the external beam radiation and may increase slightly from the implant procedure. As with other patients, brachytherapy patients need to have access to the staff in the radiation oncology department so that their many concerns and questions can be addressed promptly.

Prostate Cancer

Prostate cancer is the most common cancer in men today (Stahlinski et al., 1994). Interstitial implants for prostate cancer have been used since 1914. The use of brachytherapy for prostate cancer is controversial because of mixed results reported with older implant techniques and because of the large number of competing treatment methods available (Porter & Foreman, 1993). Advances in prostate brachytherapy include introduction of new radioisotopes, innovative afterloading techniques, computer-based dosimetry analysis, and modern imaging modalities (Porter et al., 1995). Currently, low-energy permanent implants with iodine-125 seeds with a half-life of 59.6 days or palladium-103 with a half-life of 17 days are the two most common radioactive sources used (Grimm et al., 1994; Porter et al., 1995; Porter & Foreman, 1993). The most common treatment of prostate cancer with brachytherapy is the use of iodine-125 as a permanent implant. In prostate cancer, brachytherapy is generally not used as primary radiation therapy but as a supplemental boost to areas in the prostate that are at high risk for recurrence. Interstitial implantation into the prostate may be done at the time of staging laparotomy, but it most often follows a course of external beam radiation therapy.

In certain patient conditions, iodine-125 seeds or palladium-103 seeds have been used instead of external beam radiation. The rationale is that a higher dose of radiation can be delivered to the prostate with a correspondingly smaller radiation dose delivered to the adjacent bladder and rectum; treatment can be delivered in a shorter time period compared with conventional external beam radiation; continuous LDR radiation may be more effective than conventional external beam radiation for a slow-growing tumor such as prostate cancer; and low-dose-rate radiation with iodine-125 or palladium-103 has limited penetration in tissues and thus presents less of a radiation protection problem than use of other radioisotopes (Glasgow & Perez, 1992; Stahlinski et al., 1994). These sources deliver a more confined dose to the prostate but must be placed with great precision to avoid underdosage (cold spots). Also, adverse effects associated with brachytherapy—particularly impotence, incontinence, and bowel injury—are considerably fewer and milder with an implant as compared to external beam radiation and radical prostatectomy.

The Prostate Implant Procedure

Regardless of whether iodine-125 seeds or palladium-103 seeds are used adjuvantly with external beam or as the sole radiation treatment of choice, they are implanted permanently into the prostate either through the perineum or with an open retropubic laparotomy technique. These seeds may also be implanted via transrectal ultrasound in selected patients with localized disease or transperitoneally using ultrasound and C-arm guidance (Greenburg et al., 1990; Stahlinski et al., 1994). The radiation oncologist and the radiation dosimetrist review transrectal ultrasound volume studies and determine the radiation source best suited for the tumor type, how many seeds are required for the tumor size, and the placement of the seeds.

The radioactive seeds are placed within an implant needle. With the patient under general anesthesia and in lithotomy position, a Lucite template is placed against the perineum, which serves as a guide for the arrangement and spacing of the implant needles. With the use of transrectal ultrasound, the implant needles are viewed on the ultrasound screen and are positioned according to the preimplant plan. After the desired area in the prostate is located, the needle is withdrawn, leaving the radioactive seeds in the tissue; as many as 100 or more seeds can be implanted. A cystoscopy may be performed after the procedure by the urologist to determine if any seeds were accidently left in the urethra or bladder. Verification films are taken to determine where the radioactive seeds settled after implantation and to calculate the radiation dose to the site.

NURSING CARE OF PATIENTS WITH PROSTATE IMPLANTS

Patients usually remain in the hospital for a few days or until the radioactive iodine seeds decay to less than 30 millicuries of radioactivity. During hospitalization, patients are capable of full self-care but are restricted to their room (National Council on Radiation Protection and Measurements, 1990). The patient may have a Foley catheter in place initially. Patients may experience minor perineal discomfort that can be relieved with a mild pain medication. Generally, they have little difficulty in urination but may experience a slight amount of hematuria within the first day after implant (Greenburg et al., 1990). The patient may experience mild urinary frequency or urgency as well as obstruction caused by the needle insertion and presence of the radioactive seeds. Approximately 3 percent of patients need recatheterization and are discharged with catheters in place.

Infrequently, the radioactive seeds may become dislodged, so for additional safety reasons, all urine must be strained to retrieve any lost radioactive seeds. Patients and their families need radiation safety information. They must be reassured that the patient is not radioactive. They need to understand that the radioactive seeds will decay over a period of a few months and that there is no long-term danger from radiation exposure with this type of implant. However, young children and pregnant women should maintain a safe distance (three feet) from the patient for the first month. Patients may resume sexual intercourse when they are comfortable but should use a condom for about three months (Greenburg et al., 1990).

Interstitial Brain Implants

Brachytherapy has been used in the adjuvant radiation treatment of malignant brain tumors. It is often delivered as a "boost" to brain tumors after external beam radiation, for recurrent primary brain tumors, and metastatic brain disease that has progressed (Shetiata et al., 1994). Additional radiation for brain tumors by implants, although not curative, can improve survival and performance in selected patients (Kreth et al., 1995; Shetiata et al., 1994). A stereotactic technique is used to implant radioactive sources into brain tissue. With the patient under anesthesia, a Lucite template is attached to a stereotactic frame and to the patient's head. The template is a thick acrylic block that contains holes spaced at 1-cm intervals. Through the template, multiple burr holes are made through the cranium. The tumor is outlined on a CT scan with the aid of contrast material. After the grid pattern has been created, catheters are placed in each hole under CT visualization to encircle the entire tumor volume. Teflon catheters are inserted through the burr holes and into the brain tissue. Once the tumor volume is implanted, the length of the radioactive sources is determined and x ray films are obtained for dosimetry, dummy seeds and ribbons are inserted into the catheters.

When the catheters are secured, the patient is transferred to the intensive care unit, where the dummy sources are replaced by ribbons of iridium-192 seeds. Metal buttons are attached to the catheters to fasten them to the scalp. In general, the duration of the implant lasts from 70 to 100 hours to deliver 6000 to 7000 cGy total dose to the tumor. Implants using iodine-125 seeds or gold-198 seeds have been used as permanent implants after debulking surgery.

Choroidal Melanoma

Radiation therapy has been widely employed in the treatment of choroidal melanoma. Custom-designed plaques using radioactive iodine-125, iridium-192, cobalt-60, radioactive gold-192, and ruthenium-106 have been used for treatment of choroidal melanomas. In these instances, brachytherapy is used as an alternative to enucleation. During surgery, a dummy plaque, which serves as a guide, is placed within a specific area over the sclera. The dummy plaque is then removed, a radioactive plaque is anchored to the sclera, and the conjunctiva is closed over the plaque. Tumors may be treated with 8000 to 10,000 cGy to the apex of the lesion. Once the defined radiation dose is delivered, the plaque is removed under local anesthesia (Markoe et al., 1992). It has been cited that as little as a 200-cGy single dose or 800 cGy in fractionated doses can result in radiation-induced cataracts (Merriam & Focht, 1957). Improved radioactive plaque therapy techniques with three-dimensional dosimetry are needed to reduce the overall incidence of treatment complications. Transpupillary thermotherapy (TTT) is a new treatment for choroidal melanoma used as an adjunct to brachytherapy, which needs further evaluation (Oosterhuis et al., 1995).

Bronchogenic Malignancies

Traditionally, brachytherapy has involved the use of LDR sources that are implanted in the patient temporarily, for two to seven days. HDR brachytherapy is frequently used in the management of that primary and recurrent bronchogenic malignancies (Speiser & Spratling, 1993). It provides direct treatment to the primary site of the lung cancer and improves palliative management of recurrent disease when conventional treatments have failed (Jordan & Mantravadi, 1991; Rector et al., 1992). HDR brachytherapy allows patients to be treated with a high dose of radiation in a short period of time as outpatients, with minimal radiation exposure to health care providers.

Researchers have strived to standardize endobronchial brachytherapy and continue to evaluate the effectiveness of this treatment in decreasing obstructive disease in patients with intraluminal endobronchial carcinomas.

The patient is not to drink or eat for 8 to 12 hours before the procedure. Vital signs are monitored and an intravenous (IV) started. The nurse prepares the patient for the insertion of a bronchoscope, which will be used to guide the catheter to the tumor area. A local anesthetic is used to numb the area, and the patient may be lightly sedated. Additional medications may be given through the IV to help the patient relax or to decrease the gag reflex.

Usually a pulmonologist assists the radiation oncologist during the procedure. A flexible bronchoscope is passed transnasally and a small catheter with a guide wire is passed through the working channel of the bronchoscope; then the bronchoscope is removed. The guide wire is replaced with ribbon dummy seeds. Additional catheters can be added for entire tumor coverage. The catheters are taped to the nose and x rays obtained to check placement.

The radiation is delivered through the catheter, which is connected by a cable to the computerized HDR brachytherapy afterloading machine. The computer sends the radiation source through the catheter to the tumor area (Jordan & Buck, 1991). A high-activity iridium-192 source is most commonly used. A dose of 700 cGy is usually given in the first fraction (Gustafson et al., 1995). After treatment is completed, the catheters are removed. One to four fractions are given generally one week apart. The actual treatment time is about 5 to 10 minutes, but the patient is usually in the radiation therapy department for several hours pre- and postprocedure.

Radioisotope for Metastatic Bone Pain

The control of bone pain in patients with multiple skeletal metastasis is a significant clinical problem in patients with advanced cancer of the breast, lung, and prostate. Strontium-89 (Metastron) is a radiopharmaceutical agent recently available for palliative therapy for pain associated with metastatic cancer of the bone. Strontium-89 has a half-life of 50.5 days (McEwan et al., 1994). In the body, strontium-89 acts like calcium, clearing rapidly from the blood and healthy bone, but localizes preferentially at sites of osteoblastic metastases. Strontium-89 delivers useful doses of beta radiation to the lesions while selectively sparing healthy bone and bone marrow (Crawford et al., 1994).

Strontium-89 is administered on an outpatient basis by a radiation oncologist who has been licensed to administer radiopharmaceutical agents, or by a nuclear medicine physician. It is given intravenously; the usual dose is 4 mCi. The dose can be repeated if necessary after 90 days or longer. In order to receive strontium-89: the patient must have osteoblastic skeletal metastases as seen on a bone scan, WBC of greater than 2.4×10^3, platelet count greater than 6.0×10^4, and normal BUN and creatinine levels.

Patients receiving strontium-89 are instructed to flush the toilet twice after use, wash hands after using the toilet, and wash linens or clothes that become exposed to body excretions for the first 24 hours. Patients need to be reassured they are not radioactive.

The most common adverse reaction is mild bone marrow toxicity, which has a nadir at 4 to 8 weeks following the injection, with a partial return to baseline in 12 weeks. A complete blood count should be monitored periodically. Approximately 10 percent of patients will experience "flare" pain, which occurs up to 72 hours after the injection, requiring additional analgesics until pain subsides. This "flare" pain can last up to one week (Robinson et al., 1995).

A decrease in the original bone pain is not generally observed until the second or third week following the injection, possibly due to the relatively long half-life of strontium-89. Pain relief has been reported to last from 3 to 6 months.

Brachytherapy in Benign Conditions

Brachytherapy techniques have also been used to treat benign conditions such as pterygium, a nonmalignant ocular condition. A pterygium is an elastotic degeneration of collagen that produces a fleshy mass in the bulbar conjunctiva that grows across the cornea and replaces the epithelium and Bowman's membrane (Markoe et al., 1992). Although the primary treatment for this condition is surgical excision, there are high recurrence rates associated with surgery. Brachytherapy can be used to decrease the recurrence rate. Treatment consists of a weekly surface application of strontium-90 for 3 to 4 weeks (Hilderley, 1993; Markoe et al., 1992).

Unsealed Radioactive Sources

Iodine-131, an unsealed radioisotope, is employed in the treatment of diseases of the thyroid, such as hyperthyroidism, thyroid ablation, and thyroid cancer. Special radiation precautions are required, because iodine-131 presents a potential contamination hazard. Iodine-131 is administered systemically and can be excreted in feces, urine, vomitus, saliva, sweat, and other body fluids. Half of the radioactive iodine-131 is excreted within the first two days after administration. During this time, nurses need to wear gloves while providing direct care. Such articles as the telephone, call light, and the floor must be covered with plastic. Patients can be up and about but are restricted to their room. Patients are taught to flush the toilet several times after each bowel movement or urination (Dunne-Daly, 1994a; Dunne-Daly, 1994b). Linen and patient gowns may be contaminated, and are kept in separate isolation bags in the patient's room. Disposable plastic or paper products are used for dietary trays and utensils (National Council on Radiation Protection and Measurements, 1990).

Patient Teaching and Support

Nurses play a critical role during the preimplant, implant, and postimplant periods. Patient and family education is essential. Nurses caring for patients anticipating stressful treatments such as brachytherapy assist patients to become knowledgeable and to participate in their care (Brandt, 1991). Information on sensations that patients are likely to experience reduces the patients' and families' fears, anxieties, and concerns. Many patients find it helpful to read pamphlets or booklets about the implant. Other patients find it useful to see what the brachytherapy equipment will look like. It can be useful to have a "dummy" kit of the gynecological implant or "dummy" iridium wires available in the radiation therapy department for patient teaching.

During the implant period, radiation oncology nurses are vital in teaching the inpatient nursing staff. Maintaining contact with the staff and being available to answer questions ensures a smooth inpatient transition for the patient and provides reassurance for the nursing staff. Inpatient nursing staff find it invaluable to have the radiation oncology nurses' assessment and patient plan of care during external beam radiation available in the patient record. In addition, daily documentation of the remaining length of implant time helps to keep the inpatient nursing staff informed. Inservices are valuable in providing information about implants that are frequent on a particular unit.

Teaching about the postimplant period is also very critical for the patient and family. Although the physical side effects may subside, this time can be emotionally draining for patients, because another aspect of their treatment is completed. Nurses can be available by telephone and can make sure that the patient has an appointment for follow-up in the radiation therapy department.

Properties of Radioactive Isotopes

A review of basic properties of radioactive isotopes will assist the reader in understanding why additional precautionary techniques are needed with brachytherapy. After the initial discovery of x rays by Roentgen, radioactive isotopes were found to emit three distinct types of radiation: alpha particles, beta particles, and gamma rays. Since the discovery of these radioactive elements, several other particles—such as neutrons, positrons, neutrinos, pi-mesons, mu-mesons, and K-mesons—have been detected. Several of these particles are of research interest rather than clinical interest. Of the 103 known radioactive elements, the first 92 occur naturally; the remaining have been produced artificially. All elements with an atomic number greater than 82 (lead) are radioactive.

The decay constant of a radioactive nucleus is defined as the fraction of the total number of atoms that decay per unit time. Radioactivity is defined as the total number of disintegrations per unit time interval. The curie (Ci) is a unit of activity that is equal to 3.7×10^{10} disintegrations per second. The becquerel (Bq) is a special name for the SI unit for activity and is equal to one disintegration per second. The half-life of a radioactive isotope is the time required for the number of atoms in a particular sample to decrease by one-half.

Gamma decay occurs when a nucleus undergoes a transition from a higher to a lower energy level. During this process, high-energy photons called x rays are emitted. Related to gamma decay is a process called internal conversion. Rather than emitting gamma rays, excess energy from the excited nucleus is transferred to an electron in one of the inner atomic shells, which causes the ejection of the electron from the atom and the resulting emission of characteristic x rays.

In beta decay, a neutron within the nucleus is converted into a proton, which results in an electron and an antineutrino being emitted. With beta decay, the emitted particles vary in their kinetic energy. Half-lives for beta decay are longer than gamma decay half-lives.

Alpha decay occurs when the ratio of neutrons to protons is low and in nuclides with atomic numbers greater than 82 (Purdy et al., 1992). Alpha particles have high linear energy transfer (LET), which means that they lose their energy quickly when they collide with electrons in their path. With a high LET, alpha particles are unable to penetrate more than 0.04 mm into tissue.

Mechanism of Radiation Injury in Cells

Alpha and beta particles and gamma rays exert damage in tissue by transferring energy to living matter. They ionize molecules in cells to cause physical and chemical changes that ultimately alter the biological processes responsible for cellular reproduction. Irradiated cells are either destroyed or are left unable to reproduce. The extent of radiation injury is partly a function of the ionizing capabilities of the isotope. Alpha and beta particles are directly ionizing radiations. They are electrically charged and produce ionization at small intervals along their paths through collision with other particles. Gamma rays are indirectly ionizing and have no electrical charge. Gamma rays transfer energy to directly ionizing particles, ionize and liberate electrons in the atom with low energy loss, and proceed to ionize other particles in their path. The net result is that indirectly ionizing gamma rays transfer energy to directly ionizing particles deeper within tissue. Because gamma emitters possess the greatest capacity to produce damage deep in tissue, they also present the greatest hazard to care providers. Table 3-2 lists commonly used radioisotopes in brachytherapy and their radioactive emission.

Federal Regulations Regarding Radiation Exposure

Federal regulations on radiation exposure stipulate that the maximum permissible dose for whole-body occupational exposure is 50 mSv per year (National Council on Radiation Protection

Table 3-2 • Radioisotopes and Their Properties

Radioisotope	Symbols	Half-Life	Type
Cesium-137	^{137}Cs	30 years	Beta, gamma
Gold-198	^{198}Au	2.7 days	Beta, gamma
Iodine-125	^{125}I	60 days	Beta, gamma
Iodine-131	^{131}I	8 days	Beta, gamma
Iridium-192	^{192}Ir	74.4 days	Beta, gamma
Phosphorus-32	^{32}p	14.3 days	Beta
Radium-226	^{226}Ra	1620 years	Alpha, gamma
Strontium-90	^{90}Sr	28.1 years	Beta

From National Council on Radiation Protection and Measurements: Report #40, Protection against radiation from brachytherapy sources, 1972, Bethesda, Md.

and Measurements, 1990). These standards are based on risk versus benefit criteria and take into account factors such as age, occupational versus nonoccupational exposure limits, and critical organ exposure. The permissible dose equivalents listed in Table 3-3 represent maximum limits.

Table 3-3 • Recommendations on Limits for Exposure to Ionizing Radiation

A. Occupational exposures*	
1. Effective dose limits	
a) Annual	50 mSv
b) Cumulative	10 mSv × age
2. Equivalent dose annual limits for tissues and organs	
a) Lens of eye	150 mSv
b) Skin, hands, and feet	500 mSv
B. Guidance for emergency occupational exposure*	
C. Public exposures (annual)	
1. Effective dose limit, continuous or frequent exposure*	1 mSv
2. Effective dose limit, infrequent exposure*	5 mSv
3. Equivalent dose limits for tissues and organs*	
a) Lens of eye	15 mSv
b) Skin, hands, and feet	50 mSv
4. Remedial action for natural sources:	
a) Effective dose (excluding radon)	>5 mSv
b) Exposure to radon decay products	$>7 \times 10^{-3}$ Jh m^{-3}
D. Education and training exposures (annual)*	
1. Effective dose limit	1 mSv
2. Equivalent dose limit for tissues and organs	
a) Lens of eye	15 mSv
b) Skin, hands, and feet	50 mSv
E. Embryo-fetus exposures* (monthly)	
1. Equivalent dose limit	0.5 mSv
F. Negligible individual dose (annual)*	0.01 mSv

*Sum of external and internal exposures but excluding doses from natural sources. From National Council on Radiation Protection and Measurements: Report #116. Limitation of exposure to ionizing radiation, 1993, Bethesda, Md.

Despite federal standards regarding maximum limits, occupational exposure is recommended to be "as low as reasonably achievable," designated by the acronym ALARA. In practice, nurses working with brachytherapy patients receive less than 1 mSv or 2 percent of the maximum permissible dose limit per year. This low level of exposure is achieved by close collaboration and monitoring by the radiation safety officer and careful observation of safety measures by nurses (Dunne-Daly, 1994b).

General Radiation Safety Guidelines for Nursing

Implants have been a source of fear and misunderstanding for nurses and other health care workers. This fear and misunderstanding is highly communicable and can negatively affect patient care (Sticklin, 1994). The most common fears are related to fertility and pregnancy, as well as skepticism regarding the accuracy of information supplied by the radiation safety officer or department.

Staff education is necessary to alleviate unfounded concerns and fears, providing the staff with basic knowledge needed to care safely for implant patients. Topics include principles of radiation biology and brachytherapy, radiation safety, and emergency measures (Sticklin, 1994).

Nurses caring for patients with radiation implants must adhere to safety precautions (Table 3-4). It is important to know the specific radioisotope, whether sealed or unsealed, and whether temporary or permanent (Dunne-Daly, 1994b).

Designated radiation implant rooms with lead lining in the walls are provided at many institutions that have a high volume of implant patients. Other institutions may use an automatic remote control device located next to the patient's room, where radioactive sources can be inserted by remote afterloading for short periods. Institutions that are not equipped with lead-lined rooms have designated appropriate rooms by the radiation safety officer. These are generally located at the ends of halls or corridors, not next to a stairwell or open area, therefore reducing potential radiation exposure to others.

The maximum radiation dose limit to the public is 500 millirem a year. When families or friends visit patients, certain restrictions are imposed so that radiation exposure is minimized. Visitors must be over the age of 18 and must not be pregnant. Visit time is limited to no more than 30 minutes and a distance of at least 6 feet needs to be maintained between the visitor and the radioactive source.

Nurses assigned to care for these patients should be rotated to prevent any one person from constant exposure. Nurses rarely have been reported to receive more than 100 mrem per year, which is less than the average annual background dose (Sticklin, 1994). Nurses wear a dosimeter film badge that measures exposure when caring for the patient and limit their patient care to 30 minutes per 8-hour shift. Pregnant nurses are not assigned to care for these patients. A sign specifying isolation and "Caution: Radioactive Material" is placed on the patient's door and chart, alerting all to radiation safety precautions.

Although implants are placed securely and are unlikely to become dislodged, a pair of long-handled forceps and a lead container is kept in the patient's room if this should occur. Nurses need to know that the forceps, and not bare hands, are used to retrieve the radioactive source that may have become dislodged. The source is then placed in the lead container (Dunne-Daly, 1994a). All dressings and bed linens must be saved until the radioactive source is removed. They can be removed in the usual manner after being checked by the radiation safety officer.

Specific Nursing Guidelines for Radiation Safety

By following three simple and key principles, nurses can keep their own occupational exposure to radiation "as low as reasonably achievable."

Time

The shorter the time interval that one is exposed to the radioactive source, the less the amount of radiation that will be absorbed. It is important to stress minimum exposure time, because nurses cannot feel or sense the radiation or any physical discomfort that reminds them to limit their working times. A general rule of thumb is to limit direct nursing care to 30 minutes per 8-hour shift (Dunne-Daly, 1994b).

Table 3-4 • Commonly Used Radioactive Sources That Are Hazardous to Health Care Workers

Radium-226
Iridium-192
Iodine-131
Cesium-137
Gold-198

Distance

Radiation exposure and distance are inversely related. In other words, the intensity of radiation decreases as the square of the distance from the source increases. The following rule can be used to calculate exposure: Amount of radiation exposure at 1 meter from the radioactive source × distance squared = the amount of radiation exposure at any distance from the source × distance squared.

Shielding

The type of shielding device recommended depends on the specific radioactive source. The maximum distance that radioactive sources can penetrate is called the range. Alpha particles cannot penetrate the outermost layers of skin, and a thin sheet of paper can sufficiently shield from alpha particles. Alpha particles, therefore, are not an external hazard. Most beta particles, like alpha particles, are not external hazards, because they cannot penetrate the outermost layer of skin. For example, the range in tissue of phosphorus-32, a beta emitter, is 0.8 cm.

The penetrability of brachytherapy sources is commonly expressed in their half-value layer (HVL) or their tenth-value layer (TVL) in lead or tissue. The percentage of radiation that can penetrate decreases as the thickness of the shield increases. Thus the HVL is the thickness required for a shield to reduce the exposure rate by a factor of 2, and the TVL is the thickness required for a shield to reduce the exposure rate by 10 (Glasgow & Perez, 1992).

In practice, the use of lead shielding has both advantages and disadvantages. When used properly, lead shielding provides additional safety from radiation exposure. When used improperly, lead shielding provides a false sense of security. In practice, nurses have found that lead shielding is very cumbersome to work around. Often nursing staff may spend more time in a patient's room maneuvering around lead shields. On the other hand, the presence of a lead shield may serve as a constant reminder to limit one's radiation exposure. If nurses maintain maximum distance from the radioactive source and maximize efficient use of time, they can protect themselves with or without shielding.

Personnel Monitoring Devices

Personnel monitoring devices are required by law. Monitoring devices do not protect the individual from radiation; they simply record the amount of radiation exposure. Monitoring devices should be worn only within the hospital or work area. Occupational exposure rates are closely monitored by the institution's radiation safety officer. To reduce fear of radiation exposure, the radiation safety officer can share film badge reports that indicate amount of exposure by nurses working with implant patients (Sticklin, 1994).

When caring for implant patients, nurses must always wear some type of monitoring device. Different types of monitoring devices or detectors are used for personnel and environmental monitoring. These include the nuclear emulsion monitor or film badge, the thermoluminescent dosimeter detector (TLD) or ring badge, and the pocket ion-chamber dosimeter (Glasgow & Perez, 1992; Dunne-Daly, 1994b).

The film badge, the most widely used personnel monitoring device, is accurate, reliable, and inexpensive to use. The film badge is made of a photographic emulsion mounted in a plastic holder and provides a measure of whole-body exposure. The film darkens in proportion to exposure to radiation and is changed every month by the radiation safety officer.

The TLD is used for personnel monitoring, similar to the film badge. Because of its small size, the TLD is very useful for monitoring radiation doses to the hand; thus the term *ring badge* is used interchangeably with TLD. A TLD contains a thermoluminescent powder such as lithium fluoride. Electrons in the lithium are raised to an excited state when exposed to the radioactive source. The excited energy appears in the form of visible light, and the amount of light is proportional to the energy absorbed by the radiation. The major disadvantage of the TLD is that it does not document an individual's cumulative exposure.

A pocket ion-chamber dosimeter is shaped like a pen and can be attached to clothing. This ionization chamber must be charged before use. Exposure of the chamber to radiation results in loss of the charge in proportion to the amount of radiation exposure. It is a self-reading monitor that provides immediate information on one's radiation exposure. The nurse records the reading on the pocket ion-chamber before entering the patient's room, wears the chamber while in the room, and then records a reading when leaving the patient's room. Similar to TLDs, once readings are taken and values recorded, it is not possible to double-check the radiation exposure.

A Geiger-Mueller counter (G-M counter) is used for environmental monitoring, not for personnel monitoring because it does not measure exposur or dose rate. The G-M counter reacts to the presence of ionizing particles by producing electrical pulses that are triggered by the transfer of energy of the radioisotope to electrons in the G-M counter. The G-M counter is the most popular survey meter because it is easy to operate, sensitive, and reliable. The radiation safety officer will survey the room, linen, and garbage with a G-M counter after the source is removed and before the room is cleaned.

Future Directions for Brachytherapy

Brachytherapy techniques continue to be used in innovative capacities alone or with external beam radiation therapy, chemotherapy, or surgery. There is a move toward outpatient brachytherapy with the use of remote afterloading devices for interstitial and intracavitary applications, using both LDR and HDR applications. The majority of new brachytherapy technologies are based on the use of cesium-137 or iridium-192 and high-intensity iodine-125 seeds. New isotopes are currently being evaluated for their use for specific cancers (Brady, Rotman, & Calvo, 1993).

Summary

There are numerous brachytherapy techniques that employ a wide variety of both sealed and unsealed radioactive sources for cancer treatment. These techniques may be used singly or in combination with external beam radiation therapy, surgery, and chemotherapy to improve control of local disease and preserve normal surrounding tissues from damage. Although nursing care of patients may differ, depending on the particular cancer site implanted and the radioactive isotope used, general guidelines can be followed. The most important consideration in caring for patients with implants is the effective teaching of patients, families, and nursing staff and close collaboration with the radiation safety officer, the radiation oncology nurses, and the radiation oncologist. Radiation protection is based on three key principles of time, distance, and shielding.

References

Bauer M, Schulz-Wendtland R. (1993). Technical note: A new afterloading applicator for primary brachytherapy of endometrial cancer. *British Journal of Radiology, 66*(783), 256–259.

Brady L, Micarly B, Miyamoto C, et al. (1993). Therapeutic advances in radiologic treatment of cancer. *Cancer Supplement, 72*(11), 3463–3469.

Brady L, Rotman M, Calvo F. (1993). New advances in radiation oncology for gynecologic cancer. *Cancer* Supplement, *71*(4), 1652–1659.

Brandt B. (1991). Informational needs and selected variables in patients receiving brachytherapy. *Oncology Nursing Forum, 18*(7), 1221–1229.

Crawford E, Kozlowski J, Debruyne F, et al. (1994). The use of strontium-89 for palliation of pain from bone metastases associated with hormone-refractory prostate cancer. *Urology, 44*(4), 481–485.

Dunne-Daly C. (1994a). Brachytherapy. *Cancer Nursing, 17*(4), 355–364.

Dunne-Daly C. (1994b). Education and nursing care of brachytherapy patients. *Cancer Nursing, 17*(5), 434–445.

Glasgow P, Perez C. (1992). Physics of brachytherapy. In C. Perez & L. Brady. *Principles and practice of radiation oncology.* (2nd ed.); 265–299 Philadelphia: J. B. Lippincott.

Greenburg S, Petersen J, Hansen-Peters I, Baylinson W. (1990). Interstitially implanted I-125 for prostate cancer using transrectal ultrasound. *Oncology Nursing Forum, 17*(6), 849–854.

Grimm P, Glasko J, Ragde H. (1994). Ultrasound-guided transperineal implantation of iodine-125 and palladium-103 for the treatment of early stage prostate cancer. *Atlas of the Urologic Clinics of North America, 2*(2), 113–125.

Gustafson G, Vicini F, Freedman L, et al. (1995). High-dose-rate endobronchial brachytherapy in the management of primary and recurrent bronchogenic malignancies. *Cancer, 75*(9), 2345–2350.

Hammer T, Seewald D, Track C. (1994). Breast cancer: Primary treatment with external beam radiation therapy and high-dose-rate iridium implantation. *Radiology, 193*, 573–577.

Hilderley L. (1993). Radiotherapy. In SL Groenwald, MH Frogge, M Goodman, CH Yarbro (Eds). *Cancer nursing: Principles and practice.* (3rd ed.); 235–267. Boston: Jones & Bartlett.

Jones G, Lukka H, O'Brien B. (1994). High-dose-rate versus low-dose-rate brachytherapy for squamous cell carcinoma of the cervix: An economic analysis. *British Journal of Radiology, 67*(803), 1113–1120.

Jordan L, Buck S. (1991). A teaching booklet for patients receiving high-dose-rate brachytherapy. *Oncology Nursing Forum, 18*, 1235–1238.

Jordan L, Mantravadi R. (1991). Nursing care of the patient receiving high-dose-rate brachytherapy. *Oncology Nursing Forum, 18*,(7), 1167–1171.

Kreth F, Faist M, Warnke P, et al. (1995). Interstitial radiosurgery of low grade gliomas. *Journal of Neurosurgery, 82*(2), 418–429.

Markoe A, Brady L, Carlsson U, Shields J, Augsburger J. (1992). Eye. In C. Perez & L. Brady. *Principles and practice of radiation oncology.* (2nd ed.). 595–609. Philadelphia: J. B. Lippincott.

McEwan A, Amyotte G, McGowan D, et al. (1994). A retrospective analysis of the cost effectiveness of treatment with Metastron (89Sr-Chloride) in patients with prostate cancer metastatic to bone. *Nuclear Medicine Communications, 15*, 499–504.

Merriam GR, Focht E. (1957). A clinical study of radiation cataracts and their relationship to dose. *American Journal of Roentgenology and Radiation Therapy, 77*, 759.

Nag S, Owen J, Farnan N, et al. (1995). Survey of brachytherapy practice in the United States: A report of the clinical research committee of the American Endocurietherapy Society. *International Journal of Radiation Oncology, Biology, Physics, 31*(1), 103–107.

National Council on Radiation Protection and Measurements. (1993). NCRP Report #116. Limitation of exposure to ionizing radiation. Washington, DC: U.S. Government Printing Office.

National Council on Radiation Protection and Measurements. (1974). NCRP Report #39. Basic radiation protection criteria. Washington, DC: U.S. Government Printing Office.

Oosterhuis J, Korver H, Kakebeeke-Kemme H, Bleeker J. (1995). Transpupillary thermotherapy in choroidal melanomas. *Archophthalmology, 113,* 315–321.

Perez C, Garcia D, Grigsby P, Williamson J. (1992). Clinical applications of brachytherapy. In C. Perez & L. Brady *Principles and practice of radiation oncology.* (2nd ed.), 300–367. Philadelphia: J. B. Lippincott.

Porter A, Basko T, Grimm P, et al. (1995). Brachytherapy for prostate cancer. *Ca-A Cancer Journal for Clinicians, 45*(3), 165–178.

Porter A, Forman J. (1993). Prostate brachytherapy: An overview. *Cancer, 71*(3), 953–958.

Purdy J, Lightfoot D, Glasgow G. (1992). Principles of radiologic physics, dosimetry, and treatment planning. In C. Perez & L. Brady. *Principles and practice of radiation oncology.* (2nd ed.); 183–207. Philadelphia: J. B. Lippincott.

Rector K, Knapp M, Brant T. (1992). Endobronchial brachytherapy. *Gastroenterology Nursing,* 104–106.

Robinson R, Preston D, Schiefelbein B, et al. (1995). Strontium-89 therapy for the palliation of pain due to osseous metastases. *Journal of the American Medical Association 274,* 420–424.

Shetiata W, Sunantha S, Ploysongsang S, et al. (1994). Interstitial brain brachytherapy. *Applied Radiology, 1,* 11–14.

Speiser B, Spratling L. (1993). Remote afterloading brachytherapy for the control of endobronchial carcinoma. *International Journal of Radiation Oncology, Biology, Physics, 25*(4), 579–587.

Stahlinski C, Friedman F, Finklestein S. (1994). Brachytherapy: A minimally invasive option for treating prostate cancer. *Minimally Invasive Surgical Nursing, 8*(3), 106–109.

Sticklin L. (1994). Strategies for overcoming nurses' fear of radiation exposure. *Cancer Practice, 2*(4), 275–279.

Hyperthermia and Intraoperative Radiation Therapy

FRED WOJTAS AND ROSALIE SMITH

Within the field of radiation oncology, new technologies are constantly being developed; as new specialized forms of treatment become available, older forms gradually fall from use. Some technologies and treatment procedures never live up to their expectations. Hyperthermia and intraoperative radiation therapy (IORT) are examples of treatments that seem to be fading from use. The enthusiasm once seen by a broad spectrum of practitioners is now held by only a few solid believers. However, because these treatment techniques are still being used, it is important for nurses to know how to care for patients receiving them. This chapter will review hyperthermia and IORT and briefly outline their history. Clinical applications and nursing care issues will also be discussed.

Hyperthermia

Interest in and use of hyperthermia have declined in the United States over the past ten years for a number of reasons, ranging from financial to political. However, there are some radiation centers in the United States offering hyperthermia. In Europe there is a stronger interest, and current investigations with randomized studies are under way, under the sponsorship of the European Society of Hyperthermia Oncology (ESHO), the Medical Research Council (MCR) in the United Kingdom, and the Dutch Health Insurance Fund Council (Gonzales-Gonzalea, 1993).

History

Heat has been used to treat cancers for hundreds of years. Records dating back to Homer's era (800 B.C.) describe the healing qualities of hot steam baths in the treatment of many illness (Hornback, 1984).

One of the first written reports on the effects of hyperthermia was by Busch, reporting the disappearance of tumors after episodes of high fever caused by erysipelas (Busch, 1866). Other authors also reported similar occurrences of tumor regression following periods of fever. William Coley began his experiments with fever-producing toxins in the 1890s. Coley reported excellent responses to patients with attenuated cultures of *Streptococcus erysipelatis* (Coley, 1896). Coley describes a case of round-cell sarcoma, previously excised five times, that completely regressed after an erysipelas infection. The patient was alive seven years later. Warren (1935) described the effects of heating patients after irradiation. Warren produced hyperthermia by using a heating cabinet that contained carbon filament bulbs. Immediate improvement in the patient's condition and tumor shrinkage was observed. However, this treatment was not a cure.

Meyer and Mutscheller (1937) observed the synergistic effects of radiation and hyperthermia. They used half the usual dose of radiation plus heat to control skin tumors. Hornback (1984) noted that although there was continued interest in hyperthermia during the first half of the twentieth century, the development of radiation therapy was under way, and many scientists were more enthusiastic about improving x rays than continuing hyperthermia studies.

The 1970s and 1980s brought about new interest in the field of hyperthermia. Significant improvements were made in equipment, techniques, and thermometry (measurement of temperatures). International societies were developed to promote the growth and knowledge of hyperthermia. Grant funding increased. Commercial interests and development were instrumental in the progression of hyperthermia to an accepted treatment modality (see Figures 4-1 and 4-2).

In the late 1980s and early 1990s funding for hyperthermia research decreased. The Food and Drug Administration (FDA) increased regulations on manufacturers of hyperthermia equipment. Insurance reimbursements also decreased. The results of the Radiation Therapy Oncology Group (RTOG) trial 81-04 (a comparison between radiation alone and radiation combined with hyperthermia) did not support adjuvant hyperthermia. The complete response rate (CR) in patients treated with combined hyperthermia and radiation was only 32 percent, not significantly different from the 28 percent CR rate observed in patients treated with radiation alone. The poor quality control and overall outcome of the RTOG trial dealt clinical hyperthermia a possibly lethal blow in this country (Storm, 1993). No hyperthermia trials are currently being conducted by U.S. cooperative groups (Sapozink, 1994). The past enthusiasm for hyperthermia in this country has virtually disappeared.

Biology

Hall and Roizin-Towle (1984) stated that the biological effects of heat are favorable for its use as a cancer treatment modality and discussed seven specific points.

1. *Heat kills cells in a predictable and repeatable way.* It has been shown that temperatures of 42°C produce cell killing. A rapid increase in the rate of killing occurs with a temperature increase to 44°C (Robinson & Wizenberg, 1974), a temperature range tolerated by humans in local and regional anatomical areas.
2. *The relatively radioresistant S phase cells are selectively killed and radiosensitized by heat.* The combination of hyperthermia and radiation has been shown to have a synergistic effect (Dewey et al., 1972). Cells in the S phase of reproduction are radioresistant; however, this is the most sensitive phase for hyperthermia. Therefore, tumor cells that are unaffected by radiation are killed by the addition of hyperthermia.
3. *Cells that are nutrient deficient or have a low pH are more sensitive to heat.* Tumors tend to have hypoxic cores because of poor vascularity. These hypoxic components are radioresistant

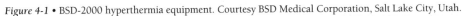

Figure 4-1 • BSD-2000 hyperthermia equipment. Courtesy BSD Medical Corporation, Salt Lake City, Utah.

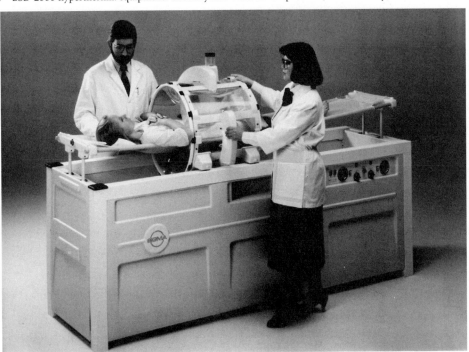

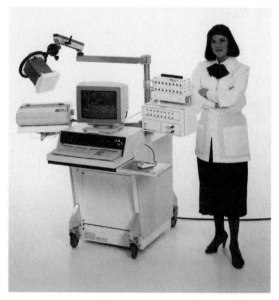

Figure 4-2 • BSD-500 hyperthermia equipment. Courtesy of BSD Medical Corporation, Salt Lake City, Utah.

yet sensitive to hyperthermia. By combining the two modalities, the x rays will destroy the vascular (nutrient and oxygen) enriched peripheral cells, whereas the hyperthermia will be effective on the hypoxic components.

4. *Heated cells develop a thermotolerance (resistance to further heating).* This has been shown to be a significant effect. Cell thermotolerance does decrease. However, it has been shown to last as long as 100 hours and is associated with cell cycling time and lowered pH. Using radiation therapy and hyperthermia in combination also reduces the amount of radiation needed, a phenomenon called thermal enhancement ratio (TER). For example, if 1000 cGy of radiation are required to destroy 50 percent of tumor cells and only 500 cGy are required for 50 percent destruction when heat is added, then the thermal enhancement ratio is 2.

5. *Heat inhibits the repair of radiation damage.*

6. *The effects of some chemotherapy agents are enhanced by hyperthermia.* The use of chemotherapy agents in conjunction with hyperthermia has been investigated. Studies have shown that heat potentiates the action of alkylating agents, nitrosoureas, and cisplatin (Dewhirst, 1994; Hahn, 1978). Under investigation is the use of hyperthermia to treat central nervous system tumors. Hyperthermia can alter the permeability of the blood-brain barrier, allowing drugs to cross in addition to enhancing their actions

(Thuning et al., 1980). Further work is needed to appreciate these effects, to control them, and to employ these effects in clinical practice.

7. *Hyperthermia by itself has never been shown to be carcinogenic and is only slightly mutagenic.* However, the combined effects of hyperthermia and radiation therapy have not been fully evaluated.

Hyperthermia's Effect on Blood Flow

A contributing factor to the effectiveness of hyperthermia is its effect on blood flow. In normal tissue, heat produces a rapid increase in blood flow with the dilation of blood vessels. However, this effect is not as apparent in the neovasculature of growing tumors (Song, 1984). The increased blood flow in normal tissue during heating produces a cooling effect as it carries away the absorbed heat. Tumors, however, do not exhibit as great an increase in blood flow during heating, thus leading to heat retention. This tendency for tumor tissue to hold heat results in more dramatic temperature elevations than in normal tissue. The vessels in tumors exhibit damage at a lower temperature than that of normal tissue, which renders the cellular environment acidic, hypoxic, and nutritionally deprived and may contribute to the cell's destruction (Song, 1984).

Methods of Administering Hyperthermia

There are three distinct classifications for hyperthermia: local, regional, and whole body, using both radiofrequencies and ultrasound applicators. The type of applicator is chosen based on tumor size, depth, and site, and not on the method of heating per se (Ben-Yosef & Kapp, 1995). Each method has its own purpose, technique, effect, and nursing challenges. Local hyperthermia pertains to heating only a tumor-bearing area. In most cases these are superficial skin or subcutaneous masses that can be easily defined and evaluated. The primary target is only the tumor mass, with very little margin of normal tissue included in the heating field. Local hyperthermia may also be used for deep-seated tumors, such as intracranial malignancies that can be defined and treated with invasive interstitial techniques (Edwards et al., 1991).

Regional hyperthermia refers to treating a tumor site and surrounding normal tissue. These are usually situations in which the tumor volume is diffuse and difficult to define, necessitating treatment of a whole region rather than a localized area. Whole-body hyperthermia is a method that elevates the temperature of the whole body (core temperature) and is used for disseminated disease.

Table 4-1 summarizes the various methods of inducing hyperthermia.

Nursing Implications

Workup

A complete workup should be performed and reviewed before hyperthermia begins. Seizure disorders need to be noted and under control. Paralysis or paresthesia, especially when it occurs in the treatment area, presents a concern. Subjective evaluation of the treatment is the best gauge the radiation oncology team has of assessing acute side effects. The heated area should be assessed for metallic objects (surgical clips, prosthesis, shrapnel, foreign bodies), because all will cause excessive heat, resulting in pain and tissue damage. The presence of any of these objects may be a contraindication for treatment (BSD Medical Corporation, 1988). Pacemakers also present a contraindication to any type of radiofrequency hyperthermia.

Preparing for Treatment

Psychological support and preparation for this procedure through patient education is an essential nursing function. Patients should empty their bladder before the procedure to alleviate discomfort. It is important to assure the patient's comfort as the duration of the procedure is 60 to 90 minutes. Baseline vital signs are obtained, thermometry probes are inserted, and applicators are positioned properly before treatment begins. Frequent communication with patients during the procedure is essential to assess any discomfort or emotional distress that may be experienced.

For regional abdominal or pelvic hyperthermia, a bowel prep is given to evacuate the

Table 4-1 • Summary of Methods of Inducing Hyperthermia

	Techniques	Possible Applications
RF APPLICATORS		
Local	Unit positioned directly against tumor at body surface	Small superficial tumors
Multiple external arrays	Units positioned around tumor or surround point for regional heating	Large or multiple tumors; deep tumors
Interstitial	Single or arrays of antenna inserted into tumors externally or surgically implanted	Tumor masses accessible for direct implantation
Intracavitary	Antennae inserted into involved body cavity	Tumors of pharynx, esophagus, vagina, cervix, prostate, rectum
Inductive external	Electromagnetic loops or coils positioned against body surface or surround patient	Large or deep tumors in several body regions
Inductive interstitial	Ferromagnetic seeds implanted directly into tumor and heated by external inductive unit	Any site accessible for implantation, especially during surgical exposure
Capacitive external	Pairs of electrical plates placed across body region	Various sites
Capacitive interstitial	Arrays of needle or wire electrodes inserted across tumor volume	Any site accessible for implantation
ULTRASOUND APPLICATORS		
Single external	Unit positioned directly against tumor at body surface	Small superficial tumors
Multiple external arrays	Units positioned against body with beams focused at tumor volume	Deep tumors of abdomen, pelvis, extremities; large superficial tumors
Intracavitary	Unit inserted into involved body cavity	Tumors of vagina, cervix, prostate, rectum
LOCAL AND REGIONAL PERFUSION METHODS		
Saline perfusion	Warmed saline constantly perfused across mucosa via catheters	Superficial mucosal tumors
Blood perfusion	Warmed blood constantly infused into catheterized vessel	Tumors supplied by regional vessels, especially tumors of extremities
Systemic methods	Whole-body heating induced by various methods (warming blankets, heat boxes, space suits, perfusion of warmed blood)	Metastatic disease

Adapted from J Meyer. (1983). Hyperthermia in cancer therapy: What's new in cancer care. *Practicing Physicians, VI*(1).

intestinal contents. A Foley catheter is inserted to continuously drain the bladder and to create a temperature-monitoring avenue for insertion of a sterile temperature probe. The area of treatment should be exposed and any clothes with metal trim (buckles, snaps, zippers) and jewelry must be removed. Saline bags may be placed around the neck, under the arms, and between the legs to alleviate hot spots caused by resonance (BSD Medical Corporation, 1988).

Treatment Monitoring

The importance of continuous monitoring and documentation during treatment cannot be stressed enough. Blood pressure, pulse, applicator position, patient comfort, and acute symptoms must be observed.

At termination of treatment, the treated area is inspected for any sign of thermal changes (erythema, blisters, extremely warm to touch). Cannula sites are cleaned and an antibiotic ointment and dry sterile dressing applied. Patients are instructed to contact the physician or nurse if they experience an elevation of temperature, pain, sign of infection, or cannula displacement. At the conclusion of the hyperthermia course, cannulas are removed and tips sent for culture to evaluate the possibility of local infection.

Side Effects

Acute toxicity and late effects associated with hyperthermia have been acceptable; however, severe toxicity has been reported with the retreatment of recurrent sites, brain tumors, whole-body hyperthermia, and hyperthermia used adjuvantly with chemotherapy (Sapozink, 1994).

Skin reaction is the most prevalent side effect when local superficial hyperthermia is used. Reactions range from no visible reaction to complete skin breakdown. Pain may be associated with a burn, infection, or irritation at the cannula site.

In regional and whole-body hyperthermia, larger volumes of tissue and deeper planes are heated. The areas, depth of heating, blood flow, power, frequency, and temperature are components that could cause potential side effects. Specific anatomical regions and organs are known to be sensitive to hyperthermia:

1. *Testicles.* A single high dose of microwave radiation or prolonged period may result in temporary or permanent sterility (Murca et al., 1976).
2. *Cataracts.* During hyperthermia of the head and neck area, inadvertent heating of the eye may occur. A single high dose of microwave radia-

tion or repeated exposure over a long period may result in cataract formation that may not be observable for several weeks (BSD Medical Corporation, 1984).

3. *GI.* Nausea, vomiting, and diarrhea were observed in many patients receiving whole-body hyperthermia approximately 12 hours after the procedure (Bull, 1982).
4. *Liver.* Damage to the liver, as demonstrated by Blair and Levin (1978), was related to temperature. The higher the temperature (in excess of 42°C), the greater the damage. Temporary elevation of liver enzymes has also been reported (Short, 1979).
5. *Circulatory system.* Disseminated intravascular coagulation was seen in patients treated with whole-body hyperthermia (Ludgate et al., 1976).
6. *Cardiac side effects.* Cardiac arrhythmias are frequently seen, usually as premature ventricular contractions or bigeminy (Short, 1979).
7. *CNS.* Seizures rarely occur (Barlogie et al., 1979), peripheral neuropathies have been seen (Scott et al., 1985).
8. *Fever.* Temperature elevation of unknown origin has been observed in several patients 18 to 24 hours after whole-body hyperthermia (Smith et al., 1980), which resolved in 3 days.
9. *Drug enhancement.* Hyperthermia is known to enhance the pharmacological activity of some drugs, with unpredictable results. It may exacerbate pre-existing disease (cardiopulmonary) and overexceed the patient's temperature-controlling systems, leading to unpredictable sequelae (BSD Medical Corporation, 1984).

The careful evaluation of candidates, monitoring of equipment and treatment temperatures, and continuing observation of patients is essential to reduce the incidence of adverse reactions.

Quality Assurance

The goal of a comprehensive quality assurance program for hyperthermia is to ensure proper delivery of heat treatment to a specific area at a specific temperature for a specific time. Strict guidelines are necessary to accomplish this repeatedly. Nurses, as well as physicians, physicists, and therapists, must evaluate their roles and responsibilities to establish optimum patient treatment practices. An effective quality assurance plan must incorporate reliable methods of assuring proper function of equipment and personnel. Each procedure should be reviewed in light of its safety and efficacy.

Intraoperative Radiation Therapy

Historical Perspective

Intraoperative radiation therapy (IORT) is the delivery of a large single dose of radiation to surgically exposed tumors or resected tumor beds that are considered to have residual microscopic disease or are at risk for regional spread. The technique of IORT allows for direct visualization of the tumor to maximize the radiation dose delivered and minimize the radiation effects to adjacent normal tissue.

Although IORT is considered an innovative approach to cancer treatment, it is not new. As early as 1915, Finisterer described a laparotomy procedure and intraoperative delivery of orthovoltage radiation in a patient with locally advanced gastric carcinoma and called the procedure eventration treatment (Finisterer, 1915). In 1937, Eloesser at Stanford University treated six patients with locally advanced gastrointestinal cancers using limited surgery and IORT (Eloesser, 1937). Small clinical trials were conducted during the 1940s and 1950s, but widespread use of IORT was limited by x ray energy and equipment. With the beginning of the megavoltage era in the 1960s, interest in the potential advantages of IORT began to diminish (Kinsella & Sindelar, 1985). High-energy equipment and sophisticated treatment planning allowed the radiation oncologist to treat deep-seated tumors with more accuracy.

Abe et al. (1975) pioneered the reintroduction of IORT in Japan. In 1976 Goldson and Henschke at Howard University performed their first IORT procedure and also introduced the concept of a "dedicated intraoperative suite," in which the surgical procedure and radiation therapy were performed in the same room (Goldson, 1982).

In the late 1970s and continuing through the mid 1980s, the National Cancer Institute (NCI) pioneered the design of studies addressing technology development (Fraass et al., 1985), animal models (Barnes, et al. 1990; Kinsella et al., 1985), and two prospective randomized trials (Sindelar, Kinsella, Chen, et al., 1993; Sindelar, Kinsella, Tepper, et al., 1993). To date, most of the clinical experience with IORT has been in phase I toxicity studies and phase II efficacy studies using historical controls as comparison. The Radiation Therapy Oncology Group (RTOG) investigated IORT with the development of six phase II trials in the mid 1980s, five of which have been completed and reported (Avizonis et al., 1995; Kiel et al., 1991; Lanciano et al., 1993; Tepper et al., 1991; Wolkov et al., 1992).

Current Clinical Applications

IORT is commonly used to treat cancers of the stomach, pancreas, and colorectum. Typically, these are sites where local control is difficult to achieve. The size of the primary tumor and extent of spread to lymph nodes or adjacent structures often preclude a curative resection or may result in the need for gross resection with residual disease. The administration of high-dose external beam radiation therapy alone rarely provides long-term local control and has significant toxicity, particularly to the gastrointestinal tract. Surgery in combination with external beam radiation therapy may provide improved local control for some abdominal tumors. However, the effects of combined treatment on normal tissue are still a major concern. Other sites for which IORT can be administered are the bladder, retroperitoneum, breast, extremities, and brain.

Two major indications for the use of IORT are (1) use with surgery to irradiate a tumor bed or areas of unresectable gross tumors and (2) as a "boost" in combination with large-field external beam radiation therapy and surgical resection (Abe et al., 1975). Although several institutions have developed and participated in phase I/II protocols, many more have used IORT without benefit of an established protocol to evaluate efficacy (Leffall, 1992).

Requirements for Clinical IORT

Although treatment protocols vary widely, several general requirements are recommended if IORT is to be done safely and reproducibly (Kinsella & Sindelar, 1985). The first requirement is a team approach that begins with a mutually shared treatment philosophy between the surgical and radiation oncologists. As the protocols are written and implemented, members of other disciplines must be identified and incorporated into the team. Personnel from anesthesiology, radiation oncology, surgery, nursing, and environmental services offer support to an IORT program. The team approach begins with the surgeon's decision on the type of surgical incision to use as the first step in planning for optimal exposure of the surgical bed for IORT delivery (Sindelar et al., 1988).

Technical factors for IORT include a radiation treatment machine with a high-energy electron beam (12 to 20 MeV) with an attenuated orthovoltage beam (250 to 300 kV), specialized applicators with precise dosimetry and capability of field matching, and a field verification system. The advantage of high-energy electrons is the flat dose distribution over several centimeters, followed by a rapid falloff in dose. The homogeneous dose distribution level, as measured in centimeters, is usually about one-third of the maximum energy of the electrons used.

Advantages of an orthovoltage unit (Bane & Shurkus, 1983; Rich et al., 1984) include that it is less expensive, more mobile, and requires less shielding of the room. Its usefulness is limited, however, because of the inhomogeneous dose distribution at depths of over 5 cm. Two other drawbacks are the long treatment times required to deliver the radiation dose and the increased absorption of radiation in bone at standard orthovoltage energies (Tepper & Sindelar, 1981).

A second requirement for a successful IORT program is to define strict criteria for patient selection and assessment of tumor response and normal tissue tolerance.

The third requirement is the physical environment in which the IORT is performed. The two options are a dedicated intraoperative suite and geographically separate surgical and radiation oncology treatment areas. Dedicated suites are specifically designed or modified radiation therapy treatment rooms where both the operative procedure is performed and IORT is delivered. Although there are safety advantages in the use of a dedicated suite, there are also considerable costs of equipment, personnel, and resources. Most institutions have geographically separate areas for surgery and for radiation treatment. This requires a safe, efficient transport system with cooperation from all disciplines (Campbell & Iwamoto, 1992). The housekeeping staff must clean and disinfect the radiation therapy suite, supply staff must provide appropriate sterile supplies, and designated monitoring staff must coordinate the transfer time with clear hallways and elevator access.

Extreme care should be exercised at all times during patient transfer to avoid sudden changes in positioning. The Surgilift sheet or other similar moving devices can be used to move the anesthetized patient and should be in place before surgery begins. The patient can then be lifted from the operating table to a bed for transfer to the radiation oncology department. Another method for transport uses an operating room table equipped with wheels and a hydraulic-electric lift system as devised at Loma Linda University (Archambeau et al., 1988).

A major consideration during transfer is the risk of contamination or evisceration of the surgical wound. The surgical incision is temporarily closed with a continuous running suture. The incision is then liberally covered with a sterile, impervious, self-adhesive barrier and multiple layers of sterile drapes. When the patient arrives in the radiation oncology department, the surgical field is reprepped and redraped. The continuous running suture is removed and the patient is prepared for the IORT treatment.

The IORT Procedure

After the surgical wound is reopened, the surgical and radiation oncologists ascertain the specific number and size of radiation treatment fields required based on the tumor volume and the individual patient's anatomy, using field matching techniques when necessary. Customized sets of Lucite applicators in various shapes, lengths, and circumference sizes are selected and attached to the linear accelerator (McCullough & Gunderson, 1988).

The Lucite applicators are gas rather than steam sterilized, because steam will alter their shape and render them useless. Most applicators have a beveled edge that aids in placing them against sloping surfaces, such as the pelvic side wall. Self-retaining retractors that are versatile in direction, depth, and degree of tension are necessary to provide continued exposure of the tumor or tumor bed. Continuous suction is maintained to prevent fluid accumulation, which can alter the depth of the treated area and interfere with the radiation dose.

Docking is the process of attaching one end of the Lucite applicator to the head of the treatment machine with the other end positioned in the patient's exposed surgical wound. The end of the applicator to be positioned in the patient is placed into a stainless steel shield to further minimize scatter radiation dose to surrounding normal tissue. Extreme care and caution must be exercised until the docking is completed to prevent any sudden changes in the position of retractors and Lucite applicators. Movement could result in tears or other damage to blood vessels and organs.

Once the docking is completed, all personnel leave the radiation treatment room and the treatment is delivered. Members of the surgical team must maintain sterility during the treatment time. The patient is continuously monitored and observed via a television camera. If necessary, the treatment can be interrupted for repositioning of the patient and equipment.

IORT doses have ranged from 1000 to 4000 cGy, with 1500 to 2000 cGy being the most commonly prescribed dose. The time for treatment delivery depends on the electron energy used, number of fields, dose per field, and total dose. The IORT procedure adds a minimum of 2 hours to the patient's operative and anesthetic exposure (Kinsella & Sindelar, 1985). After the IORT treatment is delivered, the surgical procedure is completed, either in the radiation oncology department or in the main surgical suite.

Preoperative Care

In an effort to define the tumor size, location, and extent of disease preoperatively, the patient will require numerous invasive and noninvasive procedures. Included in the preoperative evaluation are a comprehensive history and physical examination, serum chemistries to include appropriate tumor markers, hematology, and coagulation profiles, chest x ray evaluation, and computed tomography and contrast studies of the primary site of disease. Liver scanning or ultrasonography, computed tomography and contrast studies of adjacent structures, thin-needle biopsies, peritoneoscopy, and angiography may be required on a selective basis. The nurse must be aware of the patient's specific preoperative schedule of studies to provide accurate instructions for care before and after the procedure. It is important that the patient know and understand where the tests will be performed, length of time required for the study, and expected sensations and side effects.

Using visual aids and easily understood written information, the nurse must provide individual or group teaching sessions for patients who may receive preoperative radiation therapy prior to the IORT boost. An explanation of the treatment schedule, site-specific side effects, and symptom management should be included in the teaching. Nursing diagnoses related to nutrition, protective mechanisms, and elimination must also be identified as the plan of care is further defined.

Intraoperative Care

During the intraoperative period all members of the IORT team maintain safety of the anesthetized patient. Safe and accurate delivery of the radiation therapy is the primary responsibility of the staff of the radiation oncology department.

It is helpful for the nurse to identify two liaison persons. One liaison should be at the intraoperative treatment site and the second in the recovery room or surgical intensive care unit. These individuals can provide information about progress of the procedure and arrival times. The nurse can convey this information to the waiting family to allay some of their anxieties (Liming, 1993).

Postoperative Care

The postoperative plan of nursing care depends on the specific surgical procedure performed and whether IORT was given. When IORT is used in patients undergoing major surgical procedures, it is difficult to evaluate whether and how the addition of IORT may affect the postoperative course. The nurse armed with an awareness and understanding of the specific surgical procedure performed, what normal structures were partially or totally resected, and what type of reconstruction and anastomoses were performed will be better prepared to observe and evaluate the patient.

Complications that could occur in any patient receiving a major surgical procedure include infection, abscess, fistula, bleeding, or obstruction. The nurse must develop and maintain especially keen observation skills while caring for the postoperative patient who also received IORT. The nurse's accurate documentation of the postoperative progress provides vital information on incidence and onset of complications.

The addition of postoperative external beam radiation therapy demands a complex plan of nursing care. The focus of care becomes broader as more nursing diagnoses are identified. Again, the nurse must provide patient teaching regarding site-specific side effects and symptom management. Some patients will also receive concomitant chemotherapy with 5-FU alone or in combination with other agents such as leucovorin, levamisole, cisplatin, and mitomycin-C. The nurse must be aware of the specific agents administered and how they interact with radiation therapy, because combined modality therapy can provide a greater challenge to symptom management.

Follow-Up Care

After the completion of the postoperative course of radiation therapy, some patients may continue to receive adjuvant therapy. The nurse must evaluate and modify the plan of nursing care because many chemotherapeutic agents can alter the postoperative recovery period. At regularly prescribed intervals during follow-up, the patient must receive a complete medical evaluation.

At the completion of the adjuvant therapy, the acute side effects of external beam radiation therapy or chemotherapy begin to diminish, and the patient often focuses on issues that perhaps were not given high priority during active treatment. Issues of sexuality, confidence in the workplace and society, and survival from the cancer diagnosis can begin to take on new meaning for the patient at this time. Continued modification of the care plan by the nurse is necessary as the patient progresses toward optimal recovery and reintegration at an altered level of functioning.

Summary

Hyperthermia

The use of heat alone (Gabriele et al., 1990) or adjunctively with radiation or chemotherapy has been shown to increase local and regional tumor control (Suit, 1992), but there is much to improve upon:

1. Equipment must be constantly improved, and new methods must be devised to deliver heat.
2. New and improved techniques in thermometry, both invasive and noninvasive (Delannoy et al., 1990), must be established.
3. Cooperative group clinical trials must be promoted and supported. Collaboration among researchers is needed to test and evaluate the efficacy of different procedures. A multi-institutional contract was sponsored by the National Cancer Institute (NCI) at the same time RTOG initiated radomized trials. Its purpose was to evaluate available hyperthermia equipment. The conclusion of this study was that the equipment was inadequate for proper heating of many of the tumors larger than 3.0 cm entered on the RTOG study, and inappropriate quality assurance and thermometry procedures were used (Dewhirst & Corry, 1992).

In controlled clinical studies in Europe, hyperthermia has demonstrated the ability to dramatically increase local and regional control, without an increase in toxicity, for both superficial and deep tumors (Suit, 1992).

It is possible that convincing demonstration of efficacy enhancement by hyperthermia will require clinical trials of multi-institutional or even multinational scale. The recent clinical reports suggest that the greatest chance for success might involve coordination of American, European, and Asian resources for technology and data management, financial support and administration, and larger appropriate patient bases (Sapozink, 1994).

The current state of hyperthermia in the 1990s gives cause for both optimism and pessimism (Sapozink, 1994). Hyperthermia will continue to play a role in the management of cancer patients, so nurses must be knowledgeable about the clinical aspects of this treatment modality to function as an effective member of the radiation therapy team.

IORT

IORT is carried out in more than 250 U.S. and foreign centers. Researchers from 21 countries presented on the results of IORT administration at an international meeting in Kyoto, Japan, in 1990. The 1990 Patterns of Care study conducted by the RTOG (Coia & Hanks, 1992) revealed that of the 1,293 radiation oncology facilities in the United States, 108 reported using IORT. None of the identified facilities is devoted primarily to IORT administration, nor is there any nationally organized society or journal devoted to IORT.

The greatest amount of experience with IORT (with or without external radiation, chemotherapy, or maximal resection) has been in adults with gastrointestinal cancers, with lesser experience in patients with locally advanced retroperitoneal sarcoma and recurrent genitourinary and gynecological cancers. The addition of IORT to aggressive multimodality treatment plans has resulted in improved local control and long-term survival in patients with unresectable and locally recurrent colorectal cancers. Treatment with IORT has provided long-term salvage of approximately 30 percent in patients with genitourinary and gynecological cancers. In contrast, the addition of IORT in patients with locally unresectable pancreatic cancer has made no impact on survival, presumably because of the high incidence of liver and peritoneal involvement (Gunderson, 1994). The NCI experience (Sindelar, Kinsella, Chen, et al., 1993; Sindelar, Kinsella, Tepper, et al., 1993) with two randomized protocols—one for gastric cancer and one for abdominal and pelvic soft tissue sarcomas—demonstrated no improvement in local control and long-term survival in the patients randomized to the arm containing IORT. In both protocols, a higher percentage of patients who received IORT maintained local disease control.

The question of complications and long-term sequelae has been evaluated and answered through these experiences. Cromack et al. (1988) reported on 119 patients undergoing extensive abdominal or pelvic surgical procedures in four randomized studies at the NCI. The majority of complications involved the gastrointestinal system to include enteritis, bowel obstruction, and hemorrhage. No significant differences were noted between groups receiving IORT versus surgery alone. Noyes et al. (1992) reported on the RTOG experience of 220 patients treated on three phase II studies. The leading complications in patients receiving IORT were anastomotic leak (gastric cancer), wound infection (pancreatic cancer), and operative hemorrhage (rectal cancer). These complications appear to be more closely related to the extensive type of surgery as opposed to IORT.

Although the data suggest that IORT has a salutary effect in certain patients with a malignant diagnosis, there is a lack of adequate numbers of patients in prospective randomized clinical trials to document efficacy. Despite a long-term and sincere commitment from a large number of investigators in multiple institutions in the United States, the phase I/II RTOG studies were never able to proceed to phase III prospective trials due to lack of patient accrual. The RTOG has decided not to pursue indications for the use of IORT.

Hanks and Lanciano (1996) advise that single institutions that continue to pursue IORT need to see it as part of a multimodality approach with surgery and chemotherapy if survival is to be improved. In addition, the issue of quality of life for patients treated with IORT must also be evaluated and documented if no survival improvement is expected.

References

Abe M, Takahashi M, Yabumoto E, Onoyama Y, Torizuka K, Tobe T. (1975). Techniques, indications, and results of intraoperative radiotherapy of advanced cancers. *Radiology*, 116, 693–702.

Archambeau JO, Aitken D, Potts TM, Slater JM. (1988). Cost-effective, available-on-demand intraoperative radiation therapy. *International Journal of Radiation Oncology, Biology, Physics*, 15, 775–778.

Avizonis VN, Buzydlowski J, Lanciano R, Owens JC, Noyes RD, Hanks GE. (1995). Treatment of adenocarcinoma of the stomach with resection, intraoperative radiotherapy, and adjuvant external beam radiation: A phase II study from Radiation Therapy Oncology Group 85-04. *Annals of Surgical Oncology*, 2, 295–302.

Bane CL, Shurkus LM. (1983). Caring for intraoperative radiation patients. *Association of Operating Room Nurses Journal*, 37, 840–846.

Barlogie B, Corry PM, Yip E, Lippman L, Johnson DA, Khalil K, Tenczynski TF, Reilly E, Lawson R, Dosik G, Rigor B, Hankenson R, Freireich EJ. (1979). Total-body hyperthermia with and without chemotherapy for advanced human neoplasms. *Cancer Research*, 39, 1481.

Barnes M, Duray P, DeLuca A, Anderson W, Sindelar W, Kinsella T. (1990). Tumor induction following intraoperative radiotherapy: Late results of the National Cancer Institute canine trials. *International Journal of Radiation Oncology, Biology, Physics*, 19, 651–660.

Ben-Yosef R, Kapp DS. (1995). Direct clinical comparison of ultrasound and radioactive electromagnetic hyperthermia applicators in the same tumours. *International Journal of Hyperthermia*, 11(1), 1–10.

Blair RM, Levin W. (1978). Clinical experience of the induction and maintenance of whole-body hyperthermia. In C Steffer (ed). *Cancer therapy by hyperthermia and radiation*. Baltimore: Urban & Schwarzenberg.

BSD Medical Corporation. (1984). *Indication and use of the BSD 400/500 hyperthermia system*. Salt Lake City: BSD Corporation.

BSD Medical Corporation. (1988). *BSD 2000 Operators Manual*. Salt Lake City: BSD Corporation.

Bull JMC. (1982). Whole-body hyperthermia as an anticancer agent. *CA-A Cancer Journal for Clinicians*, 32(2), 123.

Busch W. (1866). Uber den Einfluss Welchen Heftigere Erysipein Zuweillen Auf Organisierte Neubildunge Ausuben. *Verhandlung-gen des Naturhistorischen Vereines der Preussischen Rheinlande und Westphalens*, 23, 28.

Campbell C, Iwamoto R. (1992). Intraoperative radiation therapy *Today's O.R. Nurse*, 14(9), 19–23.

Coia LR, Hanks GE. (1992). The need for subspecialization: Intraoperative radiation therapy. *International Journal of Radiation Oncology, Biology, Physics*, 24(5), 891–893.

Coley WB. (1896). The therapeutic value of the mixed toxins of the streptococcus of erysipelas and bacillus prodigious in the treatment of inoperable malignant tumors. *American Journal of Medical Science*, 112, 221, 255.

Cromack DT, Maher MM, Hoekstra H, Kinsella T, Sindelar WF. (1988). Are complications in intraoperative radiation therapy more frequent than in conventional treatment? *Archives of Surgery*, 124, 229–234.

Delannoy J, LeBihan D, Hoult DI, Levin RL. (1990). Hyperthermia system combined with a magnetic resonance imaging unit. *Medical Physics*, 17, 855–860.

Dewey WC, Hopwood LE, Saparetto SA, Gerweck LE. (1972). Cellular responses to combinations of hyperthermia and radiation. *Radiology*, 123, 472.

Dewhirst MW. (1994). Future direction of hyperthermia biology. *International Journal of Hyperthermia*, 10(3), 339–345.

Dewhirst M, Corry P. (1992). Future directions for multi-institutional clinical trials in hyperthermia. *A National Cancer Institute Workshop*, Washington DC: NCI.

Edwards DK, Stupperich TK, Welsh DM. (1991). Hyperthermia treatment for malignant brain tumors: Nursing management during therapy. *Journal of Neuroscience Nursing*, 23(1), 34–38.

Eloesser L. (1937). The treatment of some abdominal cancers by irradiation through the abdomen combined with cautery excision. *Annals of Surgery*, 106, 645–652.

Finisterer H. (1915). Zur therapie inoperabler Magen-und Darmkarzinome mit freilegund und nachfolgender Rontgenbestrahlung. *Strahlentherapie*, 6, 205–213.

Fraass BA, Miller RW, Kinsella TJ, Sindelar WF, Harrington FS, Yeakel K, et al. (1985). Intraoperative radiation therapy at the National Cancer Institute: Technical innovations and dosimetry. *International Journal Radiation Oncology, Biology, Physics*, 11, 1299–1311.

Gabriele P, Orecchia R, Ragona R, Tseroni V, Sannazzari L. (1990). Hyperthermia alone in the treatment of recurrences of malignant tumors. *Cancer*, 66, 2191–2195.

Goldson AL. (1982). Intraoperative radiation therapy. In VT DeVita et al. (eds.). *Principles and practice of oncology*, 1856–1861. Philadelphia: J. B. Lippincott.

Gonzalez-Gonzalea D. (1993). Current status of clinical trials in Europe. *Abstract of the Hyperthermia in Clinical Oncology Meeting*. Munich, Germany.

Gunderson LL. (1994). Rationale for and results of intraoperative radiation therapy. *Cancer*, 74(2), 537–540.

Hahn GM. (1978). Interaction of drugs and hyperthermia in vitro and in vivo. In C Steffer (ed.). *Cancer therapy by hyperthermia and radiation*. Baltimore: Urban & Schwarzenberg.

Hall E, Roizin-Towle L. (1984). Biological effects of heat. *Cancer Research, 44*(suppl. 10), 4708, 4713.

Hanks GE, Lanciano RM. (1996). Intraoperative radiation therapy: Cut bait or keep on fishing? *International Journal of Radiation Oncology, Biology, Physics, 34*(2), 515–517.

Hornback N. (1984). *Hyperthermia and cancer: Human clinical trial experience, 1*, Boca Raton, FL: CRC Press.

Kiel KD, Won MH, Witt TR, Noyes D, Sause WT, Lanciano R, et al. (1991). Preliminary results of protocol RTOG 85-07: Phase II study of intraoperative radiation for retroperitoneal sarcomas. In M Abe, M Takahashi (eds.). *Proceedings of the Third International Symposium of Intraoperative Radiation Therapy*, 371–372. Tokyo: Pergamon Press.

Kinsella TJ, Sindelar WF. (1985). Newer methods of cancer treatment: Intraoperative radiotherapy. In VT DeVita et al. (eds.). *Principles and Practice of Oncology*, 2293–2304. Philadelphia: J. B. Lippincott.

Kinsella TJ, Sindelar WF, DeLuca AM, Pezeshkpour G, Smith R, Maher M, et al. (1985). Tolerance of peripheral nerve to intraoperative radiotherapy (IORT): Clinical and experimental studies. *International Journal of Radiation Oncology, Biology, Physics, 11*, 1579–1585.

Lanciano RM, Calkins AR, Wolkov HB, Buzydlowski J, Noyes D, Sause W, et al. (1993). A phase I/II study of intraoperative radiotherapy in advanced unresectable or recurrent carcinoma of the rectum: A Radiation Therapy Oncology Group (RTOG) study. *Journal of Surgical Oncology, 53*, 20–29.

Leffall LD. (1992). Is it time yet to invest in an intraoperative radiation therapy facility? *Journal of Surgical Oncology, 49*(3), 139.

Liming PR. (1993). IORT perioperative nursing challenges: One hospital's experience. *Today's O.R. Nurse, 15*(3), 35–38.

Ludgate CM, Webber RG, Pettigrew RT, Smith AW. (1976). Coagulation defects following whole-body hyperthermia in the treatment of disseminated cancer: A limiting factor in treatment. *Clinical Oncology, 2*, 219–225.

McCullough EC, Gunderson LL. (1988). Energy as well as applicator size and shape utilized in over 200 intraoperative electron beam procedures. *International Journal of Radiation Oncology, Biology, Physics, 15*, 1041–1042.

Meyer J. (1983). Hyperthermia in cancer therapy: What's new in cancer care. *Practicing Physician, VI*(1), 5.

Meyer WH, Mutscheller A. (1937). Heat as a sensitizing agent in radiation therapy of neoplastic diseases. *Radiology, 28*, 215.

Murca GJ, Ferris ES, Buchta FI. (1976). A study of microwave radiation of the rat testis. In CC Johnson, MI Shores (eds.). *Biological effects of electromagnetic waves*, 484–494. Washington, DC: Hew Publications (FDA-778010).

Noyes RD, Weiss SM, Krall JM, Sause WT, Owens JR, Wolkov HB, et al. (1992). Surgical complications of intraoperative radiation therapy: The Radiation Therapy Oncology Group experience. *Journal of Surgical Oncology, 50*(4), 209–215.

Rich TA, Cady B, McDermott WV, Kase KR, Chaffey JT, Hellman S. (1984). Orthovoltage intraoperative radiotherapy: A new look at an old idea. *International Journal of Radiation Oncology, Biology, Physics, 10*, 1957–1965.

Robinson JE, Wizenberg MJ. (1974). Thermal sensitivity and the effects of elevated temperatures on the radiation sensitivity of Chinese hamster cells. *ACTA Radiologica (Therapy, Physics, Biology), 13*, 243.

Sapozink MD. (1994). Clinical hyperthermia in the 1990s: Does the buck stop here? *International Journal of Hyperthermia, 10*(3), 395–401.

Scott R, Clay L, Story K, Johnson R. (1985). Transient microwave-induced neurosensory reactions during superficial hyperthermia treatment. *International Journal of Radiation Oncology, Biology, Physics, 11*, 561–566.

Short G. (1979). Hyperthermia and cancer: A brief review of its history, status, and potential. Salt Lake City: BSD Corporation.

Sindelar WF, Hoekstra HJ, Kinsella TJ. (1988). Surgical approaches and techniques in intraoperative radiotherapy for intra-abdominal, retroperitoneal, and pelvic neoplasms. *Surgery, 103*, 247–256.

Sindelar WF, Kinsella TJ, Chen PW, DeLaney TF, Tepper JE, Rosenberg SA, et al. (1993). Intraoperative radiotherapy in sarcomas of the retroperitoneum. Final results of a prospectively randomized clinical trial. *Archives of Surgery, 128*, 402–410.

Sindelar WF, Kinsella TJ, Tepper JE, DeLaney TF, Maher MM, Smith R, et al. (1993). Randomized trial of intraoperative radiotherapy in carcinoma of the stomach. *American Journal of Surgery, 165*, 178–187.

Smith R, Bull J, Lees D, Schuette W. (1980). Whole-body hyperthermia: Nursing management and interventions. *Cancer Nursing, 3*, 185–188.

Song CW. (1984). Effects of local hyperthermia on blood flow and microenvironment; A review. *Cancer Research, 44*(suppl. 10) , 4721S.

Storm FK. (1993). What happened to hyperthermia and what is its current status in cancer treatment? *Journal of Surgical Oncology, 53*, 141–143.

Suit HD. (1992). Potential for improving survival rates for the cancer patient by increasing the efficacy of treatment of the primary lesion. *Cancer, 50*, 1227–1234.

Tepper J, Sindelar W. (1981). Summary of the workshop on intraoperative radiation therapy. *Cancer Treatment Reports, 65*, 911–918.

Tepper JE, Noyes D, Krall JM, Sause WT, Wolkov HB, Dobelbower RR, et al. (1991). Intraoperative radiation therapy of pancreatic carcinoma: A report of RTOG 85-05. *International Journal of Radiation Oncology, Biology, Physics, 21*, 1145.

Thuning CA, Bakir NA, Warren J. (1980). Synergistic effects of combined hyperthermia and a nitrosourea in treatment of a murine ependymoblastoma. *Cancer Research, 40*, 2726.

Warren SL. (1935). Preliminary study of the effect of artificial fever upon hopeless cases. *American Journal of Roentgenology, 33*, 75.

Wolkov HB, Graves GM, Won M, Sause WT, Byhardt RW, Hanks GE. (1992). Intraoperative radiation therapy of extrahepatic biliary carcinoma: A report of RTOG 85-06. *American Journal of Clinical Oncology, 15*, 323–327.

Chemical Modifiers
of Radiation Therapy

LISA NOLL AND NANCY RIESE

Chemical modifiers are drugs that are not necessarily cytotoxic but may be effective in altering the sensitivity of cells to the effects of ionizing radiation. Over the past 15 to 20 years, a number of compounds have been identified that appear to provide either selective enhancement of radiation damage to tumor cells (radiosensitization) or protection of normal tissue (radioprotection).

The goal of chemical modification is to achieve a therapeutic gain, i.e., an increase in tumor cell killing without a proportional increase in normal tissue damage. In general, combined-modality therapy refers to regimens that use more than one cytotoxic therapy—e.g., radiation therapy and antineoplastic drugs—to achieve an effect greater than that of either therapy alone. There may or may not be a direct interaction between the two modalities, and the sequencing of therapies varies. The term *chemical modifier* has generally been reserved for agents that are in themselves nontherapeutic but enhance or mitigate the action of another effective therapy. Modifiers are invariably used concurrently with the primary therapy.

This chapter reviews the historical background of chemical modification of radiation therapy and the radiobiological basis, summarizes clinical research in the field, and outlines implications for nursing care of patients participating in investigations of radiosensitizing and radioprotective drugs.

History of the Use of Chemical Modifiers

The clinical development of chemical modifiers for use in radiation therapy has roots in radiobio-

logical research. Since the late 1950s, progress has been made in understanding the mechanisms of radiation damage. A variety of experimental evidence supports the hypothesis that radiation effects are the result of damage to the cell's genetic material, DNA (Coleman, 1996). It has also been established that the response of cells to ionizing radiation can be influenced by manipulations of the cellular environment, including variations in oxygenation and temperature, and the addition of numerous chemical compounds. There has been steady progress in the laboratory in understanding tumor physiology along with an expanding recognition of the multiplicity of factors that determine treatment response. Earlier research that focused on oxygen deprivation has shifted to the broader concept of "nutritional deficiency" as a contributor to radiation resistance (Coleman et al., 1994).

Radiosensitizers

The term *radiosensitizer* refers to compounds that enhance the damaging effects of ionizing radiation. A radiation sensitizer must be present at the time of irradiation for it to be effective. A large number of chemical compounds have been demonstrated to alter the biochemical and biological events occurring at the time of radiation or in the period immediately following radiation, when the cell attempts to repair damage. It has been known for more than 50 years that oxygen is a potent sensitizer of hypoxic cells. Radiosensitizing agents have been broadly classified, therefore, as either hypoxic cell sensitizers or nonhypoxic cell sensitizers. Further categorization is done on the basis of chemical structure and mechanism of action. Table 5-1 summarizes current approaches to radiosensitization.

Dose Modification

The term *dose modification factor* (DMF) is used to quantify the magnitude of a particular modifying effect. A DMF is the ratio of the dose required to produce a given measure of cell damage in the absence and presence of a given modifying agent. For example, if it takes 2,500 cGy to kill 99 percent of hypoxic cells in the absence of a sensitizer, and 1,000 cGy to kill 99 percent of hypoxic cells in the presence of a sensitizer, the DMF = 2500/1000 = 2.5. This is also called the sensitizer enhancement ratio (SER). In cases where the sensitizer is oxygen, it is called the oxygen enhancement ratio (OER) (Hall, 1994).

Hypoxic Cell Sensitizers

The term *hypoxic cell sensitizer* is used to describe compounds that restore the radiosensitivity of

Table 5-1 • Current Clinical Uses of Chemical Modifiers

Clinical Setting	Agent/Maneuver
RADIATION THERAPY	
Oxygen mimetic sensitizers	Etanidazole
	Nimorazole
Increased oxygen delivery	Perfluorochemical with hyperbaric oxygen
	Transfusion, erythropoietin
Decreasing hemoglobin affinity for O_2	BW12C
Alteration in blood flow	Nicotinamide
	Hydralazine
MODULATION OF INTRACELLULAR THIOLS	
Decrease glutathione (GSH)	BSO
Increase thiol radioprotection	WR-2721
Altered radiosensitivity of DNA	IUdR, BUdR
CHEMOTHERAPY	
Chemosensitization	Etanidazole
Chemoprotection	WR-2721
Thiol depletion	BSO
APPLICABLE TO BOTH	
Agents toxic to hypoxic cells	Di N-oxides, e.g. tirapazamine (SR 4233)
	Mitomycin-C and newer analogues, e.g. EO9
	Bifunctional nitroimidazoles e.g. RB 6145

Reprinted with permission from CN Coleman. (1996). Radiation and chemotherapy sensitizers and protectors. In BA Chabner & DL Longo (eds). *Cancer chemotherapy and biotherapy: Principles and practice* (2nd ed) Philadelphia: Lippincott Raven.

hypoxic cells. They are designed to replace oxygen in the chemical reactions following irradiation and are therefore sometimes called oxymimetic sensitizers. Hypoxic cell sensitizers have been tested in the clinic more extensively than other agents and so will be the main focus of this chapter. It is increasingly recognized that numerous processes besides hypoxia play a role in tumor response. From a historical perspective, attempts to exploit the "oxygen effect" stand as models for subsequent strategies for modifying treatment response.

The Oxygen Effect

The relative radioresistance of hypoxic cells and the sensitizing effect of oxygen were first observed in the early years of radiation therapy. In 1955, Thomlinson and Gray described the appearance in human bronchogenic carcinoma of areas of necrosis at distances of 150 to 200 microns from the nearest capillaries. The measured distance corresponded to the distance oxygen can diffuse across respiring tissue before being metabolized by cells. The observation led to the hypothesis that a subpopulation of chronically hypoxic but viable cells exists at the border between well-oxygenated tumor cells and necrotic regions of tumors. Because well-oxygenated cells are more sensitive to damage by radiation, they are killed preferentially. Figure 5-1 is a schematic representation of tumor hypoxia.

Studies of tumor vasculature have demonstrated abnormalities in tumor blood flow, and a variety of laboratory methods have been developed to demonstrate hypoxia in human tumors (Coleman, 1996). Recent laboratory evidence suggests that tumors probably contain both cells that are chronically hypoxic and cells that are acutely hypoxic as a result of transient disruptions in tumor blood flow (Coleman et al., 1994).

Although the exact mechanism of the oxygen effect is not known, one explanation is that the presence of oxygen during radiation favors the production and persistence of chemically unstable molecules known as free radicals. Free radicals interact with DNA resulting in damage. By increasing the production and stability of free radicals, the presence of oxygen appears to decrease the likelihood that damaged DNA will be repaired (Pizzarello & Witcofski, 1982).

The term *oxygen enhancement ratio* (OER)— the ratio of the doses of radiation required to produce a given biological effect in the absence and presence of oxygen—is used to describe the magnitude of the effect in various cells and tumor

Figure 5-1 • The diffusion of oxygen from a capillary through tumor tissue. The distance to which oxygen can diffuse is limited largely by the rapid rate at which it is metabolized by respiring tumor cells. For some distance from a capillary, cells are well oxygenated (*white*). At greater distances oxygen is depleted, and tumor cells become necrotic (*black*). Hypoxic tumor cells form a layer, perhaps one or two cells thick, in between (*gray*). In this region the oxygen concentration is high enough for the cells to be viable but low enough for them to be relatively protected from the effects of x-rays. These cells may limit the radiocurability of the tumor. The distance to which oxygen can diffuse is about 70 μm at the arterial end of a capillary and less at the venous end. From E Hall (1994). *Radiobiology for the Radiologist* (4th ed) Philadelphia: JB Lippincott.

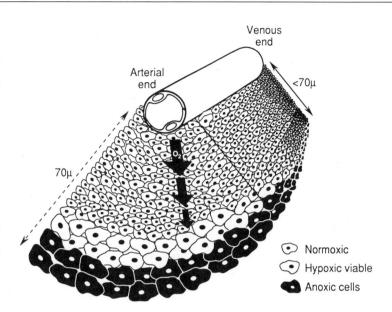

models. For mammalian cells irradiated with gamma or x rays, OERs range from 2.5 to 3.0. Expressed in another way, two-and-a-half to three times more radiation dose is required to cause the same amount of damage in hypoxic cells compared to well-oxygenated cells. Figure 5-2 shows typical survival curves for cells irradiated under hypoxic and oxygenated conditions.

There is a variety of indirect evidence suggesting that tumor cell hypoxia is important in clinical radiation therapy. Early in this century, it was learned that so-called fractionated treatment—multiple small daily doses given over a prolonged period of time—led to better tumor control than large single-dose treatment (Coleman, 1996). This results in part from a process known as reoxygenation. As well-oxygenated tumor cells die, hypoxic cells become better oxygenated and therefore more sensitive to radiation therapy.

Further evidence that tumor cell hypoxia may be important in clinical radiation therapy comes from observations indicating that high preirradiation hemoglobin concentration is a factor in improved response to irradiation. Several clinical studies in the 1980s found statistically significant associations between hemoglobin concentration and local tumor control for patients undergoing radiation therapy (Bush, 1984; Overgaard et al., 1986; Quilty & Duncan, 1986).

A number of clinical and laboratory efforts to overcome hypoxic cell radioresistance either by

increasing oxygen delivery to tissues or by the use of oxymimetic agents have been made. In the 1950s, attempts were made to increase the oxygen concentration of tumor cells by administering radiation to patients in high-pressure oxygen chambers called hyperbaric oxygen. The technique has largely been abandoned because of the technical complexity and its relatively small benefits. However, the results have served to strengthen the idea that tumor cell hypoxia is a clinically significant problem (Henk, 1986).

Increasing Tumor Oxygenation

Alternative methods to increase tumor oxygenation are being developed. One approach uses perfluorocarbon agents that increase the oxygen-carrying ability of the blood. A prototype agent is Fluosol-DA, used as a blood substitute. Early trials were inconclusive because toxicity limited the amount of drug that could be given (Lustig et al., 1989). However, newer, less-toxic compounds are under investigation.

A second approach now in clinical trials in Europe is called ARCON-accelerated radiation therapy using carbogen and nicotinamide. Carbogen is a gas containing 95 percent oxygen and 5 percent carbon dioxide. Nicotinamide is a consolidating agent that improves tumor oxygenation (Zackrisson et al., 1994). A third approach is the use of erythropoiten to increase hemoglobin concentrations. This method requires 4 to 6 weeks of treatment before radiation therapy (Lavey &

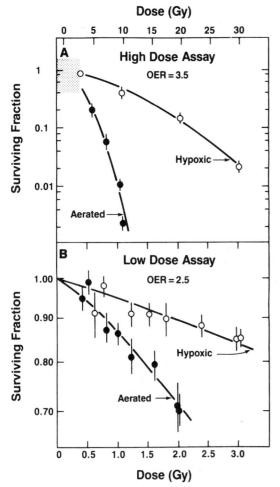

Figure 5-2 • Cells are much more sensitive to x-rays in the presence of molecular oxygen than in its absence (ie, under hypoxia). The ratio of doses under hypoxia to aerated conditions necessary to produce the same level of cell killing is called the oxygen enhancement ratio (OER). It has a value close to 3 at high doses but may have a lower value of about 2 at x-ray doses below about 2 Gy (200 rads). From Palcic B & Skarsgard LD. (1984). *Radiation Research 100*, 328-339. Redrawn in Hall E. (1994). *Radiobiology for the radiologist.* (4th ed). Philadelphia: JB Lippincott.

Dempsey, 1993). Additional approaches that alter hemoglobin affinity for oxygen to increase the release of oxygen in tissues are being developed.

Nitroimidazoles

In the 1960s, several laboratories in England and the United States began a search for chemical agents that would mimic the radiosensitizing effects of oxygen but would diffuse across cells without being metabolized. In theory, such compounds would cause a selective enhancement of damage to hypoxic tumor cells, because normal

tissues are not hypoxic. A group of compounds known as nitroimidazoles have undergone extensive testing. The two-nitroimidazole compound metronidazole underwent clinical evaluation in the 1970s. Although toxicity limited the dosages that could be given, there was sufficient evidence of clinical efficacy to stimulate interest in developing more efficient, less toxic radiosensitizers.

ETANIDAZOLE

Etanidazole has been evaluated in a series of clinical trials (Coleman, Noll, et al., 1992). As with the other nitroimidazoles, toxicity limits the number of radiation treatments that can be sensitized, which in turn limits the potential efficacy of the compound.

The dose-limiting toxicity of this compound is peripheral neuropathy that consists of sensory loss and paresthesias, primarily affecting the extremities. The paresthesias affect the soles of the feet, toes, and occasionally the hands. Symptoms are described variably as numbness, tingling, burning, loss of temperature sensation, or an intermittent ache. When the drug was given as a continuous intravenous infusion over one to two days, a syndrome described as "cramping/arthralgia" was observed (Riese et al., 1994). Although objective neurological changes—such as heightened sensitivity to pinprick and decreased vibratory sense—may occur, the changes are primarily subjective in nature, making it important to be alert for patient complaints. Mild neuropathies resolve rapidly over a period of a few days. More severe paresthesias may be long-lasting or permanent, so it is crucial that early subtle symptoms of neuropathy be detected and drug therapy discontinued. The same is true for the "cramping/arthralgia" syndrome, so that those involved in administering the drug must be very vigilant.

Occurrence of neurotoxicity is related to cumulative drug exposure, as calculated by serum drug pharmacokinetics measured over a 24-hour period. Pharmacokinetic monitoring and dose modification of the individual patient will decrease the risk of neuropathy (Coleman, Buswell, et al., 1992). Figure 5-3 shows a sample pharmacokinetic profile.

Other side effects are unusual, consisting of nausea and vomiting, rash, transient arthralgias, and rare transient granulocytopenia. No central nervous system toxicity or ototoxicity has been observed. In the phase I trial there were no observations of enhanced damage to normal tissue.

A randomized trial conducted by the Radiation Therapy Oncology Group (RTOG) compared radiation therapy with or without etanidazole in

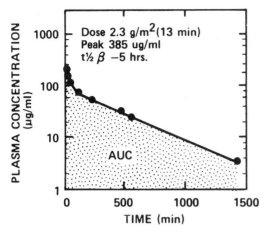

Figure 5-3 • Sample pharmacokinetic profile of a patient treated with etanidazole. The pharmacokinetic parameter area-under-the-curve (AUC) of serum concentration over time is calculated from serum drug levels taken at selected intervals following a single drug administration. Etanidazole drug level measurements may be useful in assessing the likelihood of developing neurotoxicity. Reprinted with permission from the publisher from CN Coleman. (1985). Hypoxic cell radiosensitizers: Expectations and progress in drug development. *International Journal of Radiation Oncology, Biology, Physics, 11*(2): 323–329. Copyright 1985 by Elsevier Science Inc.

patients with locally advanced head and neck cancers. No overall benefit to the use of etanidazole was observed, though there was a suggestion of benefit for a subset of patients with N0–N1 disease (Lee et al., 1995). A similarly designed trial in Europe also failed to demonstrate a significant benefit from etanidazole in head and neck cancers (Chassagne et al., 1992).

A phase II study using etanidazole in locally advanced prostate cancer found that the use of etanidazole was associated with a more rapid onset of complete clinical response. However, the overall treatment outcome was found to be similar to that of patients receiving radiation alone (Beard et al., 1994). A phase I study of etanidazole as a continuous infusion during brachytherapy for malignant glioma demonstrated that etanidazole does penetrate into brain tumors (Hurwitz et al., 1992) and established a maximum tolerated dose for continuous infusions (Riese et al., 1994).

Nimorazole is a five-nitroimidazole compound. Although it is less potent than etanidazole, it has less toxicity so it can be administered every day as opposed to every other day.

A meta-analysis that included 50 randomized trials of nitroimidazoles found some benefit to the use of hypoxic sensitization, while acknowledging that the magnitude of the benefit has not been

great (Overgaard, 1994). A challenge for the future is to identify patients in whose tumors hypoxia is most likely to be present, as well as to develop multiple strategies for overcoming hypoxia (Coleman, 1996). The future use of etanidazole depends on results of ongoing trials involving early stage head and neck cancers, and single dose use with stereotactic radiosurgery.

Thiol Depletion

The competition theory of radiation damage suggests that oxygen molecules compete with reducing compounds (such as those with sulfhydryl groups) at the time of irradiation (Coleman, 1996). An excess of oxygen leads to the propagation of damaging free radicals, while an excess of sulfhydryl-containing compounds leads to chemical restitution of radiation damage, as shown in Figure 5-4. In accordance with the competition theory, there has been interest in depleting levels of intracellular sulfhydryl compounds to improve the efficiency of radiation therapy. There is also interest in thiol augmentation for radioprotection of normal tissue.

A number of intracellular compounds known as thiols contain a sulfhydryl (-SH) group and are believed to have a role in the restitution of radiation-induced injury by means of their ability to scavenge free radicals (Hei et al., 1984). In preclinical experimentation, agents that deplete cellular thiol levels have been demonstrated to have a role in modifying radiosensitivity. Glutathione (GSH) is a sulfhydryl-containing tripeptide that is a major intracellular component and appears to be important in detoxifying cytotoxic agents. Numerous experiments have suggested that GSH depletion can modify the effects of certain antineoplastic agents as well as enhance radiosensitivity of hypoxic cells. There is ongoing interest in how manipulation of sulfhydryl biochemistry might be used in clinical treatment, in combination with both chemotherapy and radiation therapy (Coleman et al., 1994). Because GSH is an important component of numerous intracellular processes, clinical use will require careful observation for drug-induced toxicity.

Nonhypoxic Cytotoxics

McGinn and Kinsella (1994) have recently reviewed the history of the use of nonhypoxic cell sensitizers including the halogenated pyrimidines and fluorinated pyrimidines. Because of their similarity to thymidine, the analogs bromodeoxy-

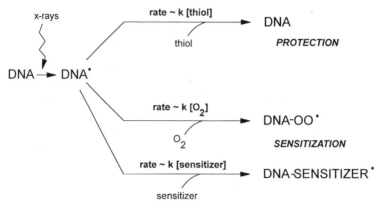

Figure 5-4 • Competition model. This theoretical model has been useful in the development of hypoxic cell radiosensitizers. The oxygenmimetic sensitizer is designed to take the place of oxygen in hypoxic tumors. Although depletion of thiols (-SH, protectors) is not a very effective means of radiosensitization by itself, thiol depletion may enhance the efficacy of the hypoxic cell sensitizers. Reprinted with permission from CN Coleman, EA Bump, RA Kramer. (1988). Chemical modifiers of cancer therapy. *Journal of Clinical Oncology*, 6:709.

uridine (BUdR) and iododeoxyuridine (IUdR) are taken up by actively dividing cells and incorporated into newly synthesized DNA. The exact mechanism of enhanced radiosensitivity is not fully understood.

Drug incorporation into DNA is a determinant of sensitization, with radiosensitivity being proportional to the numbers of tumor cells that incorporate the IUdR or BUdR and the percentage of thymidine replaced. Because incorporation requires DNA synthesis, attainment of a therapeutic gain depends on the cell-cycling activity of various tissues within the radiation fields. Generally speaking, the ideal target for the halogenated pyrimidines would be tumors that contain large numbers of actively dividing cells, surrounded by normal tissues that divide relatively infrequently. These principles have been important in guiding the development of clinical strategies.

Bromodeoxyuridine (BUdR) was first tested in the clinic in the late 1960s in the United States and Japan. Despite some promising results in the treatment of brain tumors in the Japanese studies, there were significant problems with normal tissue toxicity (e.g., mucosal damage with head and neck cancers), poor tumor perfusion due to abnormal vasculature, and hepatic deactivation of the drugs. A series of clinical trials employed differing dose levels, routes of administration (intra-arterial versus intravenous), and schedules of administration in various disease sites (McGinn & Kinsella, 1994). There have been some promising results in sarcomas and anaplastic astrocytomas.

Current work is directed toward optimizing drug uptake by modulating thymidine metabolism to improve drug incorporation into DNA.

Antineoplastic Compounds with Radiosensitizing Properties

In contrast to the sensitizers discussed above, hypoxic cytotoxic agents have antitumor activity independent of radiation. Improved therapeutic results are based on the model of either "spatial cooperation" (each modality targets tumor cells in different parts of the body as in primary breast radiation and adjuvant chemotherapy) or "enhancement" in which a drug adds to disease response within the irradiated tissue volume (Phillips, 1994). Similar to other chemical modification strategies, success depends on achieving an improved "therapeutic ratio" in which the improvement in disease reduction exceeds the increase in normal tissue damage.

Ongoing research efforts are directed toward developing new drugs and to refining doses and scheduling for known agents. Several classes of agents are now undergoing initial evaluation including the so-called hypoxic cytotoxics. Tirapazamine (SR4233) is a bioreductive agent with preferential toxicity to hypoxic cells (Coleman et al., 1994). Analogs of the antineoplastic agent Mitomycin C also appear to have selective toxicity for hypoxic cells (Coleman, 1996). A third group of agents known as "dual function" compounds act both as oxymimetic sensitizers and as direct toxins to hypoxic cells (Coleman, 1996).

Radioprotectors

The term *radioprotector* refers to compounds that protect cells and tissues against the damaging effects of radiation (see Figure 5-4). Near the end of World War II, concerns about the effects of radiation exposure in the event of nuclear war stimulated research to identify agents capable of protecting against radiation injury. Patt et al. (1949) reported that administration of cysteine before irradiation could protect rats against death from bone marrow suppression. During the late 1950s and early 1960s a number of highly effective sulfhydryl-containing radioprotective drugs were developed through the U.S. Army Antiradiation Drug Development Program.

These sulfhydryl compounds demonstrated protection to cells in culture and to mice exposed to potentially lethal doses of radiation. Although the precise mechanism of the radioprotection is not understood, a widely accepted explanation of the effect of the sulfhydryl compounds is that they act as "radical scavengers" (Hall, 1994). To be useful, a protector must have a selective effect on normal tissue, allowing a larger dose of radiation to be delivered to the tumor without a proportionate increase in normal-tissue damage. Factors that may contribute to the preferential effect of radioprotectors on normal tissue include differential uptake by tumors and normal tissues as a result of abnormalities in tumor blood flow and variations among tissues with respect to cellular distribution and metabolism (Yuhas et al., 1984).

Clinical Use of Radioprotectors

In 1986, Turrisi et al. reviewed data on WR-2721 (amifostine), a phosphorylated aminothiol that provides selective protection of normal tissue. Amifostine has now been evaluated in a series of clinical trials as a protector of normal tissue against both radiation and chemotherapy. The drug is given as an intravenous infusion before radiation therapy or chemotherapy. Dose-limiting side effects are emesis and reversible hypotension; minor side effects include somnolence and sneezing. The incidence of hypotension was related to the interval of drug administration, tending to be more common with longer infusion periods. Hypotension is manageable in most patients with postural changes and infusion of saline (Turrisi et al., 1986).

Effectiveness appears to be related to tissue concentration of the drug at the time of radiation. A phase I/II study using WR-2721 given as an enema showed that it could be administered safely in enema form. The drug did not protect the rectosigmoid mucosa from radiation damage at the dose levels administered (Montana et al., 1992). Although success has been limited, ongoing clinical trials are evaluating the efficacy of the drug in a variety of clinical settings involving both radiation therapy and chemotherapy (Coleman, 1996).

Nursing Implications

At present, chemical modification of radiation remains largely within the area of investigational therapeutics. Most patients receiving modifiers do so in the setting of a clinical trial, according to a well-defined treatment plan or protocol. The following discussion will outline some of the issues in the nursing care of patients receiving chemical modifiers.

Direct Care

Direct care responsibilities include patient and family education, administration of investigational agents, observation of response to treatment, and management of side effects.

Nurses who care for patients receiving investigational agents require specialized knowledge about the rationale for the treatment approach as well as a thorough familiarity with the treatment plan. Such knowledge makes it possible to participate effectively in the process of informed consent, helping the patient and family to understand the proposed treatment, the procedures involved, and the potential risks and benefits. In addition to providing information, nurses may counsel patients who have concerns about taking part in a clinical trial of an investigational therapy.

Daugherty et al. (1995) reported that patients participating in phase I trials understand the risks of participating but in general do not understand the real purpose of the study (dose-escalation). The patients believe they will have a therapeutic benefit if they participate. It is important for the nurse and radiation oncologists to explain that the primary goal of a phase I trial is not for therapeutic benefit.

The NCI publishes a booklet designed for patients that describes the clinical research process, called "What are Clinical Trials All About?" (Office of Cancer Communications, 1995). The booklet was developed with assistance from patients and health care professionals. It addresses many of the common questions that arise and includes the term *radiosensitizer* in the glossary.

Familiarity with the rationale for the proposed treatment and the details of the procedure are necessary to ensure that the investigational therapy is administered correctly and that accurate assessments of effects and side effects are made. The activity of many chemical modifiers depends on the concentration of drug present at the time of radiation. Nurses who administer agents such as etanidazole, tirapazamine, and amifostine must be aware of the importance of careful coordination and documentation of the interval between drug administration and time to radiation therapy or chemotherapy. Expertise in intravenous therapy is required because many protocols require repeated venous access thus it may be necessary to coordinate care with home care or visiting nurses.

Depending on the particular clinical investigation, very little or a great deal may be known about possible adverse reactions. It is important that both expected and unexpected responses suspected to be caused by the investigational treatment be carefully observed, accurately documented, and promptly reported. Nurses need to become familiar with the guidelines used for the reporting and grading of toxicity. The Radiation Therapy Oncology Group (RTOG) developed a set of toxicity criteria specifically for radiosensitizers, radioprotectors, and chemotherapy given in conjunction with radiation therapy.

Management of expected side effects of treatment may be dictated by the clinical protocol. Interventions may also need to be developed in response to newly observed responses. For this reason, the importance of both formal and informal sharing of information among nurses in different institutions cannot be overestimated. Observations made during the course of a given study may help guide the development of new treatment plans.

Indirect Patient Care

Nurses who work with modifiers may serve as a resource to other health care professionals and to patients and families. Given the dual modality approach of chemical modifiers, nurses can coordinate the various disciplines required for the provision of treatment.

In many institutions, nurse coordinators have broad-reaching responsibility for study conduct, which includes communicating with investigational review boards and cooperative study groups, reporting to regulatory agencies, and managing data. Many nurses also function as data managers. This role combined with clinical knowledge and an understanding of research methodology can help ensure success of the clinical protocols (Cassidy, 1993).

Participation in the development of new therapeutic modalities provides opportunities for independent nursing research. Several of the national cooperative study groups have formed nursing committees to foster nursing research, specifically in the areas of symptom management and quality of life.

Sources of Information

Depending on the stage of clinical development and testing, various information about an experimental therapy can be accessed in the medical and nursing literature. The introduction to clinical protocols is usually an excellent source of background information and will provide additional references as well. For all drugs sponsored by the NCI, the Cancer Therapy Evaluation Program (CTEP) has a document known as a clinical brochure, which describes preclinical data, pharmaceutical data, and observed clinical toxicity to date. Pharmaceutical companies may also have such information, which is usually incorporated in the body of clinical protocols. Another vitally important resource is the experience of other nurses working in similar areas of investigation. Cooperative oncology groups, for example RTOG in the case of radiosensitizers and protectors, serve as a network for the sharing of information in more or less formal ways. Opportunities for nurses to attend national meetings and to publish their experiences further extend the possibilities for sharing information and expertise.

Future Directions

Results of ongoing clinical trials will be necessary to evaluate the potential contribution of the newest generation of radiosensitizers and radioprotectors. Although there is reason to expect that sensitizers will contribute to improved local control in some disease sites, the mechanisms of radioresistance are almost certainly multiple, and overcoming them will require a variety of strategies. At present there is ongoing development of new agents as well as investigation of the efficacy of existing agents. Given the effort involved in bringing new agents to the clinic, an equally important area of investigation is the development of strategies for optimizing the use of known agents, including combinations of sensitizers, and possibilities for combining sensitizers and protectors with other treatment modalities such as chemotherapy and hyperthermia.

Summary

The use of chemical and biochemical agents designed to modify radiation therapy points to the need for close collaboration between radiation oncology and medical oncology nurses. Oncology nurses who work primarily with chemotherapy have expertise in drug administration, familiarity with pharmacokinetic concepts, and experience in the clinical testing of new agents. Radiation oncology nurses are particularly expert in managing problems of local effects of treatment. As with any combined-modality approach, to deliver high-quality patient care there will need to be a sharing of skills and knowledge. Furthermore, nurses have a central role in the design, conduct, and analysis of experimental clinical trials.

References

Beard C, Buswell L, Rose MA, Noll L, Johnson D, Coleman CN. (1994). Phase II trial of external beam radiation with etanidazole (SR2508) for the treatment of locally advanced prostate cancer. *International Journal of Radiation Oncology, Biology, Physics, 29*, 611–616.

Bush RS. (1984). Current status of treatment of localized disease and future aspects. *International Journal of Radiation Oncology, Biology, Physics, 10*, 1165–1174.

Cassidy J. (1993). The role of the data manager in clinical cancer research: An opportunity for nurses. *Cancer Nursing, 16*(2), 131–138.

Chassagne D, Charreau I, Sancho-Garnier H, Eschwege F, Malaise EP. (1992). First analysis of tumor regression for the European randomized trial of etanidazole combined with radiation therapy in head and neck carcinomas. *International Journal of Radiation Oncology, Biology, Physics, 122*, 581–584.

Coleman CN. (1985). Hypoxic cell radiosensitizers: Expectation and progress in drug development. *International Journal of Radiation Oncology, Biology, Physics, 11*, 323.

Coleman CN. (1996). Radiation and chemotherapy sensitizers and protectors. In BA Chabner & DL Longo (Eds). *Cancer chemotherapy and biotherapy: Principles and practice* (2nd ed.). Philadelphia: Lippincott Raven.

Coleman CN, Beard CJ, Hlatky L, Kwok TT, Bump E. (1994). Biochemical modifiers: Hypoxic cell sensitizers. In P Mauch & J Loeffler (eds.). *Radiation oncology: Technology and biology*, 56–89. Philadelphia: W. B. Saunders.

Coleman CN, Buswell L, Noll L, Riese N, Rose M. (1992). The efficacy of pharmacokinetic monitoring and dose modification of etanidazole on the incidence of neurotoxicity: Results from a phase II trial of etanidazole and radiation therapy in locally advanced prostate cancer. *International Journal of Radiation Oncology, Biology, Physics, 22*, 565–568.

Coleman CN, Noll L, Riese N, Buswell L, Howes AE, Loeffler JS, Alexander E, Wen P, Harris JR, Kramer R, Hurwitz SJ, Neben TY, Grigsby P. (1992). Final report of the phase I trial of continuous infusion etanidazole (SR 2508): A Radiation Therapy Oncology Group Study. *International Journal of Radiation Oncology, Biology, Physics, 22*, 577–580.

Daugherty C, Ratain MJ, Grochowski E, Stocking C, Kodish E, Mick R, Siegler M. (1995). Perceptions of cancer patients and their physicians involved in phase I trials. *Journal of Clinical Oncology, 13*(5), 1062–1072.

Hall EJ. (1994). *Radiobiology for the radiologist.* (4th ed.). Philadelphia: J. B. Lippincott, 134–135.

Hei TK, Geard CR, Hall EJ. (1984). Effects of cellular nonprotein sulfhydryl depletion in radiation induced oncogenic transformation and genotoxicity in mause C3H 10T 1/2 cells. *International Journal of Radiation Oncology, Biology, Physics, 10*, 1255–1259.

Henk JM. (1986). Late results of a trial of hyperbaric oxygen and radiation therapy in head and neck cancer: A rationale for hypoxic cell sensitizers? *International Journal of Radiation Oncology, Biology, Physics, 12*, 1339–1341.

Hurwitz SJ, Coleman CN, Riese N, Loeffler JS, Alexander A III, Buswell L, Neben TY, Shargel L, Kramer RA. (1992). Distribution of etanidazole into human brain tumors: Implications for treating high-grade gliomas. *International Journal of Radiation Oncology, Biology, Physics, 22*, 573–576.

Lavey RS, Dempsey WH. (1993). Erythropoietin increases hemoglobin in cancer patients during radiation therapy. *International Journal of Radiation Oncology, Biology, Physics, 27*, 1147–1152.

Lee DJ, Cosmatos D, Marcial VA, Fu KK, Rotman M, Cooper JS, Ortiz HG, Beitler JJ, Abrams RA, Curran WJ, Coleman CN, Wasserman TH. (1995). Results of an RTOG phase III trial (RTOG 85-27) comparing radiation therapy plus etanidazole with radiation therapy alone for locally advanced head and neck carcinomas. *International Journal of Radiation Oncology, Biology, Physics, 32*, 567–576.

Lustig R, McIntoshLowe LN, Rose C, Haas J, Krasnow S, Spaulding M, Prosnitz L. (1989). Phase I/II study of Fluosol DA and 100% oxygen as an adjuvant to radiation in the treatment of advanced squamous cell tumors of the head and neck. *International Journal of Radiation Oncology, Biology, Physics, 16*, 1587–1593.

McGinn CJ, Kinsella TJ. (1994). Biochemical modifiers: Nonhypoxic cell sensitizers. In P Mauch & J Loeffler (eds.). *Radiation oncology: Technology and biology*, 90–112. Philadelphia: W. B. Saunders.

Montana GS, Anscher MS, Mansbach CM, Daly N, Delannes M, Clark-Pearson D, Gaydica EF. (1992). Topical application of WR-2721 to prevent radiation-induced proctosigmoiditis: A Phase I/II Trial. *Cancer, 69*(11), 2826–2830.

Overgaard J, Hansen HS, Jorgensen K, Hansen MH. (1986). Primary radiation therapy of larynx and pharynx carcinoma: An analysis of some factors influencing local control and survival. *International Journal of Radiation Oncology, Biology, Physics, 12*, 515–521.

Overgaard J. (1994). Clinical evaluation of nitroimidazoles as modifiers of hypoxia in solid tumors. *Oncology Research, 6*, 509–518.

Patt H, Tyree EB, Straube RL. (1949). Cysteine protection against X-irradiation. *Science, 110*, 213–214.

Phillips TL. (1994). Biochemical modifiers: Drug-radiation interactions. In P Mauch & J Loeffler (eds.). *Radiation oncology: Technology and biology*, 113–151. Philadelphia: W. B. Saunders.

Pizzarello DJ, Witcofski RL. (1982). *Medical radiation biology.* (2nd ed), 106. Philadelphia: Lea & Febiger.

Quilty PM, Duncan W. (1986). Primary radical radiation therapy for T3 transitional cell cancer of the bladder: An analysis of survival and control. *International Journal of Radiation Oncology, Biology, Physics, 12*, 853–860.

Riese NE, Loeffler JS, Wen P, Alexander E, Black PM, Coleman CN. (1994). A phase I study of etanidazole and radiation therapy in malignant glioma. *International Journal of Radiation Oncology, Biology, Physics, 29*, 617–620.

Turrisi AT, Glover DJ, Hurwitz S, Glick J, Norfleet AL, Weiler C, Yuhas JM, Kligerman MM. (1986). Final report of the phase I trial of single-dose WR-2721. *Cancer Treatment Reports, 70*, 1389–1393.

Yuhas JM, Afzal SM, Afzal V. (1984). Variation in normal tissue responsiveness for WR-2721. *International Journal of Radiation Oncology, Biology, Physics, 10*, 1537–1539.

Zackrisson B, Franzen L, Henuriksson R, Littbrand B, Stratford M, Dennis M, Rojas AM, Denekamp J. (1994). Acute effects of accelerated radiotherapy in combination with carbogen breathing and nicotinamide (ARCON). *Acta Oncologica 33*, 377–381.

Radiation Carcinogenesis

JENNIFER DUNN BUCHOLTZ

Since the early discoveries of the harmful effects of x rays, ionizing radiation has been one of the most widely studied carcinogens by the scientific community. The emergence of nuclear power for weapons and energy production, as well as the increasing use of radiation in medicine, have perpetuated the studies concerning radiation carcinogenesis. This chapter will present historical studies concerning radiation carcinogenesis, the current thinking about the mechanism of radiation carcinogenesis, factors relating to risk assessment and risk estimates, and a review of the literature concerning radiation-induced tumors. A perspective on the use of this information by nurses will be offered.

Historical Studies

Early Findings

Early observations of skin cancer among handlers of the early, crude forms of radiation first demonstrated the carcinogenic abilities of radiation. Shortly after the first uses of x rays for diagnosis and therapy in the late 1890s, untoward radiation injuries were noticed. Before 1900, most of the documented injuries involved skin reactions on the hands of individuals who operated the new, primitive x ray equipment. Figure 6-1 depicts an early x-ray machine showing a fluoroscope held with an unprotected hand. Acute untoward reactions included reddening and blistering of the skin followed by throbbing, tenderness, and paresthesias of the involved hands. Over time, chronic changes occurred, including atrophy of the epidermis and skin cancers. In 1902, Freiben reported the first case of skin cancer presumed to be caused by x rays (Upton, 1986). Hesse documented 94 cases of skin cancer by 1911. These were found among physicians and other handlers of radium and x ray equipment (Upton, 1975). In *American Martyrs to Science Through the Roentgen Rays*, Percy Brown pays tribute to 27 American physicians who died from cancer triggered by their years of pioneering work with x rays (Brown, 1936).

In 1911, von Jagie reported a high incidence of leukemia in five radiation workers in the same occupational group (Upton, 1975). Other studies of people exposed to various occupational sources of radiation also demonstrated a higher than normal incidence of cancers. One of the most noted is the development of osteosarcomas and other head and neck cancers in radium dial clock painters. In the 1920s, employees of a clock company painted luminous radium crystals on clocks and other timepieces. A common practice among these employees, mostly women, was to hold brushes containing a radioactive source between their teeth (Looney, 1958; Martland, 1931). Thorough follow-up of these employees demonstrated a high incidence of osteosarcomas and head and neck cancers.

These early studies, though important, cannot be used to deduce any quantitative risk associated with occupational radiation exposure and cancer induction, because radiation doses were not measured (Hall, 1994).

Effects of Atomic Weapons

Perhaps the most noted and consciousness-raising examples of radiation carcinogenesis occurred during World War II in the aftermath of the atomic bombings of Hiroshima and Nagasaki, Japan. A high incidence of leukemias in survivors appeared within five years. All types of leukemia, except chronic lymphocytic leukemia, were found (Okada, 1975). In addition, a higher incidence of solid tumors was also noted (National Academy of Sciences, 1972). Through the Radiation Effects Research Foundation (RERF), follow-up studies

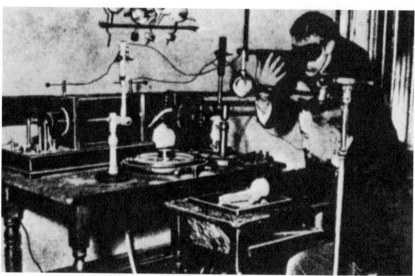

Figure 6-1 • Operation of an early x ray machine showing a hand-held fluoroscope. From Brown P. (1936). *American martyrs to science through the roentgen rays.* Courtesy Charles C. Thomas, Publisher, Springfield, IL.

on these survivors and their offspring continue today, more than fifty years after the explosions (Mabuchi et al., 1994; Preston et al., 1994; Thompson et al., 1994). The most recent report from the Committee on the Biologic Effects of Ionizing Radiation (BEIR V) identifies higher than previously reported estimates of cancer risk in Japanese survivors (National Academy of Sciences, 1990). Schull's long-term follow-up studies of the Japanese atomic bomb survivors point to significant increases in cancer mortality from leukemias (except chronic lymphocytic) and cancers of the breast, colon, liver, lung, ovary, skin, stomach, and thyroid (Schull, 1995). Of interest is that the age of exposure made a difference in the induction of solid tumors: Those exposed at earlier ages showed more susceptibility to radiation-induced cancers.

Additional information was gained on carcinogenic effects of ionizing radiation after World War II. During a 1954 thermonuclear weapons test in the central Pacific conducted by the United States, nuclear fallout accidentally diverged from its expected path and fell on the Marshall Islands, exposing the inhabitants to cesium-137 and strontium-90. Follow-up studies have shown a higher than expected incidence of benign and cancerous thyroid tumors in the island people exposed to this radiation (Conard et al., 1980). A recent report of more than 8,500 Navy veterans who participated in an atmospheric nuclear test in 1958 showed no significantly elevated numbers of cancers in this group compared to a group of more than 14,600 Navy veterans who did not participate in any nuclear weapons test (Watanabe et al., 1995).

Follow-up studies of nuclear power plant disasters, such as the one that occurred on April 26, 1986, in Chernobyl, Russia, are just beginning to unravel those affected by the long-term effects of the radiation. A sharp increase in the number of thyroid cancers in children in Belarus has been reported (Balter, 1995). Uncertainty and debate continue regarding which radioactive isotopes or other contributing factors, such as industrial pollution or a genetic predisposition to thyroid cancers in these children, may be responsible.

Effects of Therapeutic Radiation

Perhaps the most significant studies to document the possible induction of tumors by therapeutic ionizing radiation were those that showed both benign and malignant tumors that developed at higher than expected rates in patients treated for a variety of benign conditions. Court Brown and Doll (1957, 1965) found that a higher than normal incidence of cancer deaths occurred in patients who were treated with radiotherapy for ankylosing spondylitis. Their sample included 14,554 patients treated with x rays in England from 1935 to 1954. Besides a higher incidence of leukemia than normally expected, patients also had a higher than expected increase in the incidence of death from other cancers. The solid tumors were most likely to occur in tissues treated by the radiation (i.e., lung, bone, stomach, pancreas, pharynx). The most recent report of the follow-up continues to show significant increases in leukemias, non-Hodgkin's lymphoma, multiple myeloma, and solid tumors of the esophagus, colon, pancreas, lungs, bone, connective and soft tissue, prostate, bladder, and kidney (Weiss et al., 1994).

Other historically significant studies, showing the occurrence of cancer after therapeutic radiation cited in the National Academy of Sciences' 1972 BEIR report, include (1) women treated for postpartum mastitis showing higher than expected incidences of breast cancer, (2) women treated for menorrhagia showing higher than expected incidences of gastrointestinal tumors, (3) persons treated with iodine-131 for thyroid cancers and persons treated with phosphorus-32 for polycythemia showing higher than expected incidences of leukemias, and (4) infants given radiation therapy to the chest for enlarged thymus glands showing higher than expected incidences of leukemia, thyroid tumors, and other neoplasms.

Even frequently administered low doses of diagnostic radiation have suggested the cancer-induction properties of ionizing radiation. Women in Canada and in the United States who received frequent fluoroscopic examination of the chest for pulmonary tuberculosis were found in follow-up to have a much higher than expected incidence of breast cancer (MacKenzie, 1965; Boice et al., 1991). Stewart proposed that children whose mothers received diagnostic pelvic x rays during pregnancy developed unexpected leukemias in childhood (Stewart et al., 1958). For years it has been postulated that the use of Thorotrast (radioactive thorium-232), a colloid suspension once used as an alpha-emitting x ray contrast imaging substance, led to an increased incidence of primary liver cancers (Edmonson & Craig, 1987). Follow-up of patients who had received Thorotrast in the past shows a statistically significant increase in the numbers of cancers of the liver, gallbladder, and peritoneum (Anderson & Storm, 1992). The significance of these historical diagnostic studies' findings was that even small doses of radiation could induce cancers.

Radiation carcinogenesis has been heavily studied in animals (Hall, 1994; Upton, 1986). Many of these studies have attempted to correlate the radiation absorbed dose with the occurrence of tumors. Experimental studies on animals have generally shown that the incidence of tumors increases with radiation exposure up to a certain dose but then does not continue to increase indefinitely with increasing total body dose (Hall, 1994).

The Process of Radiation Carcinogenesis

From the studies of radiation-induced cancers in humans and in animals, there is little doubt that ionizing radiation is carcinogenic. Radiation-induced cancers, though, cannot be distinguished from other cancers but are surmised from a statistical excess of tumors based on their expected incidence in a given population (Hall, 1991). Quantifying the incidence of radiation-induced tumors is particularly difficult, especially at low doses (Kathren, 1996).

The process of radiation carcinogenesis is quite complex and raises many questions: What is the biological mechanism for radiation carcinogenesis? What other variables are involved? What sources of radiation induce cancer? Does each type of ionizing radiation induce cancer in the same way? How much radiation exposure can induce cancer? Why are only certain cancers induced by radiation in humans and not others? What factors influence radiation-induced cancers? Why doesn't everyone equally exposed to the same amount of radiation develop cancer? Is ionizing radiation a stronger carcinogen than other agents? How should the benefits of radiation be balanced against its carcinogenic risks and other risks to human beings? Who is most at risk for developing radiation-induced cancers? Oncology nurses often voice two questions: (1) What are the chances that patients treated with radiation therapy will develop a treatment-induced malignancy? and (2) What are the chances that nurses will develop a malignancy from occupational exposure?

Although a great deal of knowledge has been gained from the numerous epidemiological and experimental animal studies, the direct cause-and-effect relationship is difficult to ascertain for many reasons. First, other individual variables (e.g., genetic background, age, geographic location, physical status, and health habits) may contribute to the development of cancer in individuals exposed to ionizing radiation. Individuals need to be closely studied for time periods ranging from decades to a full life span to take into account the latent period between the exposure and the manifestation of many neoplasms. The latent period is the time period between the radiation exposure and the actual appearance of the malignancy. Solid tumors can have latent periods from ten to fifty years, whereas leukemias usually have latent periods of less than ten years (Smith, 1992).

Experimental studies of radiation carcinogenesis in humans are not possible because ethics prohibit using humans in controlled studies to determine the dose-incidence data for specific radiation-induced tumors. In addition, studies that prospectively identify radiation-induced cancers from medical uses of radiation may not take into account other influencing variables such as the individual's underlying disease, medical status, or effects of additional therapies. A person with one cancer may be at an increased risk genetically for another cancer. In addition, the lifestyle that contributed to the occurrence of one cancer may contribute to another type of cancer.

Many persons with cancer, especially children, receive a combination of cancer therapies. This combined approach makes it difficult to ascertain the risk factors for tumor induction from each therapy alone since there may be a synergistic mechanism of induction. Finally, the effects of exposure to high levels of ionizing radiation cannot be extrapolated to the same effect from exposure to low-level ionizing radiation. The sources, amounts, and types of ionizing radiation exposure may lead to quite different effects (National Academy of Sciences, 1990).

Theories of Radiation Carcinogenesis

Radiation carcinogenesis means the induction of cancer by exposure to radiation. The two essential steps for carcinogenesis to occur at the chromosomal molecular level are initiation and promotion (Salvatore et al., 1996). Some type of genetic mutation occurs with initiation while epigenetic changes occur with promotion. The exact biological mechanism of radiation carcinogenesis is unknown but likely is a result of cellular changes that stem from ionizations. These molecular changes may be expressed as damage to the DNA inside the cell's nucleus. DNA damage consists of either structural single-strand or double-strand breaks, the deletion or alteration of a base, or the chemical cross-linking of two DNA strands (see Figure 6-2) (Shields & Harris, 1993). The mechanism that controls and regulates these cellular changes and repair processes is unknown, but several theories exist. Several genetic defects may predispose an individual to develop a radiation-induced cancer (Comings, 1973). Malignant cell transformations are thought to occur when viral-like oncogenes are turned on or stimulated by ionizing radiation exposure. This can occur by either direct activation of oncogenes or by inactivation of antioncogenes (Knudson & Moolgavkar, 1986). Biomedical research suggests that tumorogenesis results from the activation of an oncogene, the loss of a suppressor gene, or a combination of the two (Hall, 1994). Studies have looked specifically at the p53 suppressor gene and cancer induction (Vahakangas et al., 1992). Hall (1994) nicely summarizes the mechanisms of carcinogenesis (see Table 6-1).

Sophisticated studies using microdosimetry approaches have begun to investigate exposure of low doses of radiation. Some of these studies have suggested that low levels of ionizing radiation enhance efforts of cellular repair, resulting in a carcinogenic protective mechanism or radiation hormesis (Cohen, 1994).

Figure 6-2 • Schematic representation of the three ways ionizing radiation damages the DNA molecule. Left to right: double-strand break, deletion of a base, chemical cross-linking of two DNA strands. Adapted from Upton AC. (1982). The biological effects of low-level ionizing radiation. *Scientific American,* 246(2), 42.

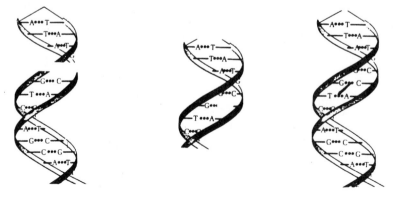

Table 6-1 • Summary of Mechanisms of Carcinogenesis

- Cell proliferation and differentiation is under positive and negative controls.
- Tumorigenesis may result from the activation of an oncogene, the loss of a suppressor gene, or a combination of both.
- Proto-oncogenes are present in every cell and may have been shown to function in regulating cell growth or differentiation.
- Radiation or chemicals may activate a normal proto-oncogene indigenous to the cell. Alternatively a retrovirus may insert an activated oncogene from its own genome into that of the mammalian cell.
- Oncogenes act in a dominant fashion; that is, the presence of a single copy is sufficient to produce the malignant phenotype.
- About 50 oncogenes have been identified so far. Activated *ras* oncogenes have been identified in 10% to 15% of human cancers, but tend to be higher in leukemias and lymphomas and lower in solid tumors.
- Proto-oncogenes can be activated by three mechanisms: (1) a point mutation, (2) a chromosomal rearrangement such as a translocation, and (3) gene amplification.
- Suppressor genes are recessive: that is, both copies must be lost or inactivated for the malignant phenotype to be expressed.
- Retinoblastoma was the first human tumor to be associated with the loss of a suppressor gene.
- At present, there are six principal suppressor genes involved in a wide spectrum of human cancers.
- Mutations in the p53 gene is the most common expression of a suppressor gene.
- In general, two cooperating oncogenes are required to result in the expression of the malignant phenotype. Oncogene products that act in the nucleus (causing immortality) cooperate best with those that act in the cytoplasm (causing loss of contact inhibition). For example, *ras* plus *myc* causes transformation of primary rat fibroblasts, as does *ras* plus an inactivated p53 suppressor gene.
- A number of repair deficient syndromes have been identified in the human: ataxia telangectasia (AT) is the most well known.
- AT homozygotes are sensitive to cell killing by radiation. They also show a very high spontaneous incidence of cancer.
- AT heterozygotes may be, on average, more sensitive to cell killing than normal, but there is too much overlap for persons to be diagnosed on this basis.
- AT heterozygotes show an elevated incidence of spontaneous cancer, particularly breast cancer.
- AT heterozygotes make up only 1% of the population. They may account for 20% of breast cancer, especially in younger women. It has been suggested, but not proven, that AT heterozygotes may be sensitive to radiation-induced cancer. This raises concerns about x ray screening programs such as mammography.

Reprinted with permission from Hall E J. (1994). *Radiobiology for the radiologist* (4th ed.), 346–347. Philadelphia: J. B. Lippincott.

Studies of humans with particular genetic diseases who have inherited susceptibilities to radiation carcinogenesis support the oncogene theories of carcinogenesis. Individuals who have inherited retinoblastoma, xeroderma pigmentosum, ataxia telangiectasia (AT), Bloom's syndrome, and neurofibromatosis appear to have a genetic predisposition for radiation-induced tumors. This genetic predisposition offers some explanation for radiation carcinogenesis, but several mechanisms may be involved.

Overall, there may not be one theory that can totally explain radiation carcinogenesis on a strict biological basis. Several conditions or a combination of heredity and environmental factors may initiate or promote cancer by ionizing radiation. Trosko (1996) offers an explanation of carcinogenesis as a complex, multistep result of a combination of endogenous and exogenous factors. He integrates several carcinogenesis theories and points out that cancer induction cannot be attributed to ionizing radiation alone.

Factors Related to Radiation Carcinogenesis

Information exists concerning factors related to radiation carcinogenesis. Although all types of ionizing radiation damage cells by the processes of excitation and ionization, densely ionizing radiations (alpha particles, neutrons) have an increased biological effectiveness over sparsely ionizing radiations (x rays, gamma rays). Densely ionizing radiations have a high linear energy transfer (LET), whereas sparsely ionizing radiations have a low LET radiation quality. High-LET radiation causes greater biological damage than low-LET radiation. Hence LET is an expression of the relative biological effectiveness (RBE) of ionizing radiation. The RBE of certain ionizing radiation sources might even determine the type of radiation-induced cancer. Follow-up of the Japanese atomic war survivors, for example, showed the number of chronic granulocytic and acute monocytic and undifferentiated leukemias to be four to five times greater in Hiroshima than in Nagasaki. Only Hiroshima's inhabitants received neutron radiation. Survivors of Nagasaki and Hiroshima both had similar incidences of acute lymphocytic and acute granulocytic leukemias (Schull, 1995). This careful analysis was critical in showing a difference between the effects of high-LET and low-LET radiation effects. Equal doses of high-LET and low-LET radiation may not produce the same radiation-induced cancer possibilities.

Dose and dose rate are other factors involved in the development of radiation-induced tumors. Historically, it was believed that the frequency of the occurrence of radiation-induced cancers increased with increasing doses. It was also believed that a threshold dose existed for the induction process. In the 1950s, however, E. B. Lewis proposed that the incidence of cancers increased as a linear, nonthreshold function of the dose of radiation exposure (Upton, 1982). This implication that even low doses of radiation carried a potential carcinogenic risk continues to be controversial among scientists studying the effects of ionizing radiation (Kathren, 1996; National Academy of Sciences, 1996). The simple relationship of dose amount to cancer induction has since been modified by other variables, such as dose rate, fractionation, and type of radiation exposure. These modifications have been based on radiation biology studies of animals extrapolated to humans. Low-LET radiation is less effective in producing supposed aberrant chromosomal changes at low doses than at high doses.

Human studies generally show that the tissues at risk for radiation-induced cancers are those directly exposed to the radiation. Even when total body radiation is given, tumor induction most logically occurs in the tissues that receive and absorb the most radiation dose. With internal radiation emitters, tumors occur in the tissues and organs where the radionuclides selectively concentrate. With medical radiation given externally, tumors occur in tissues and organs located in the radiation field. In addition, specific organs and tissues, including the thyroid, bone marrow, lung, and female breast, are more sensitive to radiation-induced cancer proneness than other tissues (Hall, 1991).

Host factors also contribute to radiation-induced tumors in humans. Children and young adults appear to have a higher risk for certain radiation-induced cancers (leukemias, osteogenic sarcomas, thyroid and breast cancers) than adults. As mentioned previously, individuals who have certain inherited disorders have a heightened sensitivity to radiation and higher incidence of tumors. A host's genetic immune mechanisms may also contribute to the ability to protect against radiation-induced tumors.

Unwanted Health Effects of Ionizing Radiation

The International Council on Radiation Protection (ICRP) classified the unwanted health effects of ionizing radiation into two categories: stochastic and nonstochastic. Stochastic effects are those in which probability or chance of occurrence increases with increasing doses of radiation. The severity of the effect, however, is independent of the dose. Stochastic effects may be either somatic or genetic. Somatic effects are health problems that affect the individual exposed to the radiation, such as radiation-induced cancers. Genetic effects refer to the effects of the radiation manifested in the offspring or future generations of the exposed individuals, i.e., chromosome aberrations in their offspring that may manifest as malignancies. Implied in the definition of stochastic effects is that the induction of cancers is a random process with host factors being equal.

Nonstochastic effects are those health effects in which severity increases with dose and for which a threshold may exist. These effects are also called deterministic effects. Examples of nonstochastic effects are cataracts, growth retardation, sterility, hypothyroidism, and bone marrow depression. A definite dose of radiation can be implicated in the causation of and prediction of these effects. In general, radiation protection measures are intended to avoid nonstochastic effects and minimize the chance for stochastic effects to occur (Hendee, 1993).

Kathren offers the Gompertizian model (see Figure 6-3) as a summary for the existing state of knowledge concerning human radiation response (Kathren, 1996). This model represents both stochastic and deterministic responses and takes threshold doses of radiation and linear, nonthreshold doses into consideration.

Perspective on Radiation Carcinogenesis

Risk Estimates and Risk Assessment

Scientists have attempted to create models for estimating the risks of radiation-induced cancers, but this endeavor remains largely empirical, especially at low doses (Schull, 1992). Moreover, these risk estimates resulted from differing interpretations of the radiation-induced cancer data (Smith, 1992). Several risk models have been offered over the years, each using the available scientific information available at the model's inception. Two models used to predict radiation-induced malignancies are the additive risk model and the multiplicative risk model (Hendee, 1993). The additive risk model, also referred to as the absolute risk model, assumes that radiation can cause cancers over and above the natural incidence of cancers in

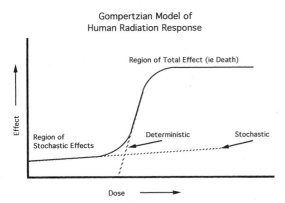

Gompertzian Model of
Human Radiation Response

Figure 6-3 • Schematic of human radiation response. From Kathren RL. (1996). Pathway to a paradigm: The linear non-threshold dose-response model in historical context. *Health Physics, 70*(5), 632.

a given population and that this increased cancer mortality is independent of the host's intrinsic biologic factors. The multiplicative risk model (relative risk model) assumes that the risk of radiation-induced cancers increases with age in conjunction with the natural risk of cancer mortality in a population and that radiation affects the individual's biological factors that promotes carcinogenesis. More recently, this model has been amended as the time-dependent relative risk model to take age of exposure into consideration, based on the most recent assessment of cancer risks of the Japanese atomic bomb survivors (Hall, 1994). It should be kept in mind that traditionally, radiation carcinogenic risk models are based on limited numbers of people who have received large single doses of radiation from atomic weapons and nuclear industry accidents. Models used to predict tumor induction from therapeutic ionizing radiation or low continuous or infrequent radiation exposure must be extrapolated from those high-dose models. Nonetheless, estimates of excess organ-specific cancer mortality risks from ionizing radiation continue to be predicted for the United States' population (Puskin & Nelson, 1995).

Second Malignancies After Radiotherapy

Exposure to therapeutic ionizing radiation or chemotherapy places an individual treated for one tumor at an increased risk for a second, treatment-related malignancy (Mauch, 1995). The current medical literature contains numerous case reports of persons treated with radiation therapy who have

been diagnosed with another cancer (Dodick et al., 1994; Malik et al., 1992; Tamm et al., 1994). Table 6-2 summarizes information regarding second malignancies after cancer therapies in long-term studies of large numbers of patients. The best data concerning second cancers comes from long-term follow-up of patients treated with radiotherapy or chemotherapy for curable tumors, such as Hodgkin's disease (Biti et al., 1994; Hancock et al., 1993; Henry-Amar, 1992; Swerdlow et al., 1992; Tarbell et al., 1993; Tucker, 1993).

Four major carcinogenic risk factors concerning Hodgkin's disease treatment—including extent of initial treatment, female gender (probably related to the female breast sensitivity to cancer induction), use of combined radiation and chemotherapy, and young age at treatment—have been associated with an increased risk of a secondary malignancy (Mauch, 1995). Continued follow-up of long-term survivors may add additional information regarding latency and evolving treatment variable changes. For example, decreasing the dose of radiation for the treatment of Hodgkin's disease may yield different incidences of second malignancies in the future.

With any cancer therapy, the benefit of the treatment should ideally outweigh the risk—especially irreversible, long-term risks. About 5 percent of all patients treated with radiation therapy may develop second malignancies (Hall, 1994). In general, these second malignancies occur in the normal tissues located inside the irradiated field but can also be in tissues remote to the area treated. With increased survivals and cures using modern cancer therapies, there is an estimated increase in the number of treatment-induced second malignancies over the next decades.

Many individuals treated with combination cancer therapies may have a predisposition to development of other cancers based on their genetic makeup, exposure to additional risk factors, or predisposition from natural occurrence in the population. In the case of radiation-induced cancer potential, the choice not to receive radiation based on a small probability of a secondary malignancy may not be a good balance of risk and benefit. However, the risk of second malignancies from radiotherapy should be carefully explained to patients and parents of young patients, and should be clearly stated on the radiation therapy consent form. Modern, highly focused radiotherapy equipment and delivery systems reduce radiation scatter previously found in older equipment on which earlier studies of radiation-induced

Table 6-2 • Studies Reporting Second Malignancies After Radiation Therapy

Reference	Study Type, Location, Time Period	Number of Persons Studied	Results/Conclusions/Comments
Hancock et al. (1993)	Record review Matched case controls Looking specifically for breast cancer incidence Stanford University 1961–1990	2164 total number of patients treated for Hodgkin's disease 885 women survivors	RR of invasive breast cancer 4.1% (95% CI) Young age at time of RT strongly influenced risk for breast cancer In women treated with RT age >30 years, risk not elevated Risk of breast cancer significantly increased with time since treatment Most breast cancers (22 of 26) arose within or close to margin of RT field and were infiltrating ductal carcinomas Addition of chemotherapy drugs increased risk of breast cancer
Boice et al. (1992)	Medical record review of 655 women in whom second breast cancer developed five or more years after initial tumor	Cohort of 41,109 women diagnosed with breast cancer in Connecticut from 1935 to 1982 206 out of 655 received radiotherapy	Increased risk of second contralateral breast cancer in women <35 years old treated with primary RT for breast cancer RR 2.2 (95% CI) age <35 RR 1.46 (95% CI) age 35–44 No increased risk > age 45
van Leeuwan et al. (1994)	Retrospective record review using case controls Assessment of risk of second cancers in Hodgkin's disease patients treated at the Netherlands Cancer Institute and Dr. Daniel den Hoed Cancer Center between 1966 and 1986	1939 total number of Hodgkin's disease patients 146 patients developed a second cancer 552 received RT only	In RT-only group: RR of lung cancer: 4.3 (2.3–7.4 95% CI) 13/3.01 O/E RR of other solid tumors: 1.8 (1.1–2.8 95% CI) 21/11.59 OE RR of non-Hodgkin's lymphoma: 9.9 (2.7–25.4 CI) 4/0.40 O/E Study overall looked at second cancers in patients treated with chemotherapy alone and combination therapies No increased risk of leukemias found in RT alone group
Biti et al. (1994)	Record review of patients treated for Hodgkin's disease at the University of Florence, Arezzo, Italy, between 1960 to 1988 using case controls from Tuscan Tumor Registry	1121 total numbers of Hodgkin's disease patients 745 (67%) treated with RT alone	In RT-only group: Using cumulative 15 year probability (Kaplan-Meier) Overall risk of second tumor: 7.8% Risk of second solid tumor: 7.6% Risk of acute leukemia: 0.2% Second tumors more frequent after CT and increased with CT plus RT
Tucker et al. (1988)	Record review of patients treated for Hodgkin's disease at Stanford University Medical Center from 1965 to 1968 using case controls from the Connecticut Tumor Registry	1507 total patients treated for Hodgkin's disease 714 patients treated with RT alone	In RT-only group: 2 observed cases of leukemia (0.6% actuarial risk at 15 years) 5 observed cases of lymphoma (1.8% actuarial risk at 15 years) 16 observed solid tumors (7.0% actuarial risk at 15 years) Most of solid tumors observed in total number of second tumors were lung cancer All the patients in whom lung cancer developed were smokers and had received radiation therapy

Reference	Study Type, Location, Time Period	Number of Persons Studied	Results/Conclusions/Comments

Chao et al. (1995)	Record review of patients treated for early-stage testicular carcinoma at the Mallinckrodt Institute from 1964 to 1988 using case controls of the Connecticut Tumor Registry	128 patients treated for seminoma	Median follow period of 11.7 years (range 5 to 29 years)
			9 second tumors found
			Actuarial risk of second nontesticular cancer found to be
			   3% at five years
			   5% at 10 years
			   20% at 15 years
			Overall observed incidence of second nontesticular cancers not significantly increased in comparison with expected incidence

Jenkin (1996)	Outcome data for children who received radiation therapy in the management of a brain tumor at the University of Toronto Institutions from 1955 to 1958	Total of 1034 children treated with radiation therapy (87% postoperatively) for various brain tumors	31 patients developed a second tumor
			Cumulative incidence of second tumors:
			   13% at 20 years
			   19% at 30 years
			Most common second tumors:
			glioma (9)
			meningioma (7)
			acute leukemia (5)
			sarcoma (3)
			other tumors (7)

Arai et al. (1991)	Record and tumor registry review of women treated for cancer of the uterine cervix at four major hospitals in Chiba, Tokyo, and Matumo, Japan, from 1961 to 1981	Total of 11,855 women treated for cancer of the cervix 5725 patients treated with RT alone 4161 patients treated with surgery alone 1969 patients treated with post-op RT	O/E ratios of second primary cancers were 0.933 in RT alone 1.074 in post-op RT Significant excess of second primary tumors noted for leukemia and bladder and rectum cancers in the RT-only group
Breslow et al. (1995)	Record review of National Wilm's Tumor Study Group for second malignancies in patients treated at participating institutions from 1969 to 1991 Case controls with national incidence rates to person years classified by age, sex, and calendar year	5,728 total number of patients treated	15 years after the Wilm's tumor diagnosis, cumulative incidence of developing second malignant neoplasm was 1.6% and increasing steadily Abdominal RT as part of initial treatment increased the risk Doxorubicin potentiated the RT effect as highest incidence in second tumors in children who received RT >35Gy with doxorubicin
Bliss et al. (1994)	Record review of patients treated for pituitary tumors in Edinburgh, UK, between 1962 and 1990, compared to age and sex matched population from the Scottish Tumor Registry Sudy specifically looked at incidence of second brain tumors	296 total patients treated with RT	One malignant brain tumor and one meningioma found in survivors of 296 patients Conclusion of researchers was to not alter RT practice for pituitary adenomas based on low incidence of second brain tumor

RT = radiation therapy CT = chemotherapy CI = confidence interval RR = relative risk O/E = observed/expected cancers are based. However, the uncertainty of the risk should be disclosed.

While the potential risk of second malignancies from radiotherapy is small, survivors should continue to get thorough follow-up exams for an indefinite time after primary treatment. It is particularly pertinent for patients with radiation-induced solid tumors that may have a long latency period. Many second malignancies, such as thyroid and breast cancer, are relatively curable in the early stages. Thus early detection is important in improving cures. Children who are cured of one malignancy should be taught to obtain routine medical exams for the rest of their lives. They need to engage in health behaviors that limit risks of the development of other tumors, such as refraining from smoking and following healthy diets as recommended by the American Cancer Society. Nurses must teach the importance of routine follow-up exams and instruct patients in health-promoting behaviors. Young women treated for Hodgkin's disease should be instructed in and encouraged to practice routine breast self-exam. It is advisable for them to begin routine mammographic screening before the age of 35 (Dershaw et al., 1992).

Children treated for early-stage Hodgkin's disease, now receive fewer total doses of both chemotherapy and radiotherapy and may therefore have less risk. The change in reducing the amount and length of both chemotherapy and radiotherapy for certain stages of Wilm's tumor may also lead to a decrease in the amount of treatment-related malignancies.

From an occupational, radiation-protection standpoint, following practices to reduce one's exposure to ionizing radiation while still providing for necessary patient care offers the best safeguard for the prevention of radiation-induced malignancies. Estimates for maximum permissible limits of radiation for occupational and public exposure should be based on the current scientific interpretation of acceptable risks. Nurses need to be aware of their record of radiation exposure.

Combined Effects of Radiation and Other Carcinogens

The interaction of radiation exposure with other agents may play an important role in the carcinogenic induction process. Combined effects may lead to an enhanced, synergistic, or protective response. A better understanding of the molecular and cellular events initiated or promoted by ionizing radiation, alone or in combination with other factors, is needed to clarify the risks of second ma-

lignancies (Schull, 1992). Even though ionizing radiation is a known single agent or complete carcinogen, several other physical or chemical agents may act as cancer promoters. Tobacco smoke is an example. In both human and animal studies, exposure to both radiation and tobacco smoke led to higher incidences of lung cancer than when only radiation exposure was involved (Fry & Ullrich, 1986). Asbestos appears to be another cocarcinogen with radiation in the induction of lung cancer. Chemical carcinogens, such as some chemotherapy drugs, may also promote cancer induction when used with radiation. Patients with Hodgkin's disease who are treated with combined alkylating agent chemotherapy and radiation are thought to have an increased risk of developing treatment-related leukemia, compared with the use of radiation alone (Coleman, 1982). The enhanced carcinogenicity of doxorubicin and abdominal radiation in the treatment of Wilm's tumor has been documented by Breslow et al. (1995).

Radiation Carcinogenesis and Nonionizing Radiation Sources

There have been numerous epidemiologic studies concerning the carcinogenic risks of nonionizing radiation. Heath summarizes 48 epidemiologic observational and case-controlled studies concerning nonionizing radiation and cancer incidences in the United States over the past two decades (Heath, 1996). Human epidemiologic studies looked at rates of cancer among electrical workers, children living in close proximity to electrical power lines, rates of cancers in relation to household appliances, and, most recently, the relationship of electrical appliances and cancer. Experimental studies also investigated the effects of electromagnetic field radiation on cells, tissues, and laboratory animals. To date, no conclusive scientific evidence exists to prove a carcinogenic effect of nonionizing electromagnetic radiation in humans (Heath, 1996; Salvatore & Weitberg, 1996). Some scientists believe that nonionizing electromagnetic radiation sources are not a neoplastic initiator but possibly act as a promotor to human carcinogenesis (Salvatore & Weitberg, 1996).

Summary

Ionizing radiation is a known carcinogen. Most of the evidence in humans that supports this relationship is derived from epidemiological studies of Japanese atomic war survivors and patients treated with radiation therapy for certain benign diseases. The organs that have shown the highest sensitivity for tumor induction by radiation are the thyroid, breast, and bone marrow. A young age at exposure is perhaps the most important factor in humans that influences radiation cancer induction. Radiation's carcinogenic properties should not be the principle concern when people weigh the benefits of radiation therapy for most indicated tumors against the remote risk of a treatment-induced second malignancy. The vast majority of cancers are not radiation induced. Continual efforts should, however, be made to avoid unnecessary radiation exposure. From an occupational exposure standpoint, until exact data are known regarding factors relating to dose and dose rate of ionizing radiation and radiation carcinogenesis, emphasis should remain on keeping levels of ionizing radiation as low as reasonably achievable (ALARA). Continual, in-depth studies of radiation exposure to different populations and the possible interaction with other physical or chemical agents need to be carried out.

Radiation safety practices have greatly improved since the first carcinogenic effects of newly discovered radium and x rays were noted. These safety practices should remain an essential part of any use of radiation in medicine and in industry but should be based on the current scientific data concerning relative risks.

Oncology nurses have a pivotal role in the health education of patients by recommending thorough, long-term follow-up examinations and potential early detection of second malignancies and promoting health habits that may reduce risks for secondary malignancies from other known causes of cancer. Radiation oncology nurses, in particular, must be involved in educating other nurses and health care personnel in good, sound radiation protection practices and balancing concerns about unwanted radiation exposure with necessary patient care.

References

Anderson M & Storm HH. (1992). Cancer incidence among Danish thorotrast exposed patients. *Journal of the National Cancer Institute, 84,* 1318–1325.

Arai T, Nakano T, Fukuhisa K, Kasamatsu T, Tsunematsu R, Masubuchi K, Yamauchi K, Hamada T, Fukuda T, Noguchi H, Murata M. (1991). Second cancer after radiation therapy for cancer of the uterine cervix. *Cancer, 67*(2), 398–405.

Balter M. (1995). Chernobyl's thyroid cancer toll. *Science, 270*(5243), 1757–1758.

Biti G, Cellai E, Magrini SM, Papi MG, Ponticelli P, Boddi V. (1994). Second solid tumors and leukemia after treatment for Hodgkin's disease: an analysis of 1121 patients from a single institution. *International Journal of Radiation Oncology, Biology, Physics, 29,* 25–31.

Bliss P, Kerr GR, Gregor A. (1994). Incidence of second brain tumours after pituitary irradiation in Edinburgh 1962–1990. *Clinical Oncology, 6*(6), 361–363.

Boice JD, Harvey E, Blettner M, Stovall M, Flannery JT. (1992). Cancer in the contralateral breast after radiotherapy for breast cancer. *New England Journal of Medicine, 326,* 781–785.

Boice JD, Preston D, Davis FG, Monson RR. (1991). Frequent chest x-ray fluoroscopy and breast cancer incidence among tuberculosis patients in Massachusetts. *Radiation Research, 125*(2), 214–222.

Breslow NE, Takashima JR, Whitton JA, Moksness J, D'Angio GJ, Green DM. (1995). Second malignant neoplasms following treatment for Wilm's tumor: A report from the national Wilm's tumor study group. *Journal of Clinical Oncology, 13*(8), 1851–1859.

Brown P. (1936). *American martyrs to science through the Roentgen rays.* Springfield, IL: Charles C. Thomas.

Chao CKS, Lai PP, Michalski JM, Perez CA. (1995). Secondary malignancy among seminoma patients treated with adjuvent radiation therapy. *International Journal of Radiation Oncology, Biology, Physics, 33*(4), 831–835.

Cohen BL. (1994). Dose response relationship for radiation carcinogenesis in the low-dose region. *International Archives of Occupational and Environmental Health, 66*(2), 71–75.

Coleman CN. (1982). Secondary neoplasms in patients treated for cancer: Etiology and perspective. *Radiation Research, 92,* 188–200.

Comings DE. (1973). A general theory of carcinogenesis. *Proceedings of the National Academy of Sciences, 70,* 3324–3328.

Conard RA, Paglia D, Larsen P, Sutoe W, Dobyns B, Robbins J, Krotosky W, Field J, Rall J, Wolff J. (1980). *Review of medical findings in a Marshallese population 26 years after accidental exposure to radioactive fallout.* Upton, NY: Brookhaven National Labs.

Court Brown W, Doll R. (1957). Leukemia and aplastic anemia in patients irradiated for ankylosing spondylitis. *Medical Research Council Special Report Series No. 295.* London: 4MSO. HM Stationery Office Special Report Series #295.

Court Brown WM, Doll R. (1965). Mortality from cancer and other causes after radiotherapy for ankylosing spondylitis. *British Medical Journal, 2,* 1327–1332.

Dershaw DD, Yahalom J, Petrek JA. (1992). Breast cancer in women previously treated for Hodgkin's disease: Mammographic evaluation. *Radiology, 184*(2), 421–423.

Dodick DW, Mokri B, Shaw EG, Miller GM, Unni KK. (1994). Sarcomas of calvarial bones: Rare remote effect of radiation therapy for brain tumors. *Neurology, 44*(5), 908–912.

Edmonson HA, Craig IR. (1987). Neoplasms of the liver. In L Schiff & ER Schiff (eds.). *Diseases of the liver,* 1109–1158. Philadelphia: J. B. Lippincott.

Fry RJM, Ullrich RL. (1986). Combined effects of radiation and other agents. In AC Upton, RE Albert, FJ Burns, RE Shore (eds.). *Radiation carcinogenesis,* 437–454. New York: Elsevier Science Publishing.

Hall EJ. (1994). Radiation carcinogenesis. In EJ Hall. *Radiobiology for the radiologist* (4th ed.), 323–350. Philadelphia: J. B. Lippincott.

Hall PF. (1991). Cancer risks after medical radiation. *Medical Oncology and Tumor Pharmacotherapy, 8*(3), 141–145.

Hancock SL, Tucker MA, Hoppe RT. (1993). Breast cancer after treatment of Hodgkin's disease. *Journal of the National Cancer Institute, 85*(1), 25–31.

Heath CW. (1996). Electromagnetic field exposure and cancer: A review of epidemiologic evidence. *CA: A Cancer Journal for Clinicians, 46*(1), 29–44.

Hendee W. (1993). History, current status, and trends of radiation protection standards. *Medical Physics, 20*(5), 1303–1314.

Henry-Amar M. (1992). Second cancer after the treatment for Hodgkin's disease. A report from the International Database on Hodgkin's disease. *Annals of Oncology, 3,* 117–128.

Jenkin D. (1996). Long-term survival of children with brain tumors. *Oncology, 10*(5), 715–719.

Kathren RL. (1996). Pathway to a paradigm: The linear nonthreshold dose response model in historical context: The American Academy of Health Physics 1995 Radiology Centennial Hartman Oration. *Health Physics, 70*(5), 621–635.

Knudson AG, Moolgavkar SH. (1986). Inherited influences on susceptibility to radiation carcinogenesis. In AC Upton, RE Albert, FJ Burns, RE Shore (eds.). *Radiation carcinogenesis,* 401–411. New York: Elsevier Science Publishing.

Looney WB. (1958). Effects of radium in man. *Science, 127* 630–633.

Mabuchi K, Soda M, Ron E, Tokunaga M, Ochikubo S, Sugimoto S, Ikeda T, Terasaki M, Preston DL, Thompson DE. (1994). Cancer incidence in atomic bomb survivors. Part I: Use of the tumor registries in Hiroshima and Nagasaki for incidence studies. *Radiation Research, 137*(2 Suppl), S1–S16.

MacKenzie J. (1965). Breast cancer following multiple fluoroscopies. *British Journal of Cancer, 19,* 1–8.

Malik RK, Fuler GN, Oakes WJ, Tien R, Hockenberger B, Friedman HS, Halperin EC. (1992). Back pain and paraplegia in a fifteen-year-old boy. *Journal of Pediatrics, 121*(4), 652–658.

Martland HS. (1931). The occurrence of malignancy in radioactive persons: A general review of data gathered in the study of radium dial painters with special reference to the occurrence of osteogenic sarcoma and the interrelationship of certain blood diseases. *American Journal of Cancer, 15,* 2435–2516.

Mauch P. (1995). Second malignancies after curative radiation therapy for good prognosis cancers [editorial]. *International Journal of Radiation Oncology, Biology, Physics, 33*(4), 959–960.

National Academy of Sciences/Institute of Medicine. (1996). *Radiation in medicine: a need for regulatory reform.* Washington, DC: National Academy Press.

National Academy of Sciences, National Research Council. (1972). *The effects on populations of exposure to low levels of ionizing radiation.* Report of the Advisory Committee on the Effects of Ionizing Radiation (BEIR I). Washington, DC: National Academy Press.

National Academy of Sciences, National Research Council. (1990). *Health effects of exposure to low levels of ionizing radiation.* Report of the Advisory Committee on the effects of ionizing radiation (BEIR V). Washington, DC: National Academy Press.

Okada S. (1975). *Journal of radiation research: A review of thirty years' study of Hiroshima and Nagasaki atomic bomb survivors.* Chiba, Japan: Japan Research Society.

Preston DL, Kusumi S, Tomonaga M, Izumi S, Ron E, Kuramoto A, Kamada N, Dohy H, Matsuo T, Nonaka H, Thompson DE, Soda M, Mabuchi K. (1994). Cancer incidence in atomic bomb survivors. Part III: Leukemia, lymphoma, and multiple myelomas, 1950–1987. *Radiation Research, 137*(2 Suppl), S68–S97.

Puskin JS, Nelson CB. (1995). Estimates of radiogenic cancer risks. *Health Physics, 69*(1), 93–101.

Salvatore JR, Weitberg AB, Mehta S. (1996). Nonionizing electromagnetic fields and cancer: A review. *Oncology, 10*(4), 563–570.

Schull WJ. (1992). Radiation risk estimation. *Science of the Total Environment, 127*(1–2), 1–8.

Schull WJ. (1995). *Effects of atomic radiation: A half-century of studies from Hiroshima and Nagasaki.* New York: Wiley-Liss.

Shields PG, Harris CC. (1993). Principles of carcinogenesis: Chemical. In VT DeVita et al. (Eds.). Cancer: Principles and practice of oncology (4th ed.), 200–209. Philadelphia: J. B. Lippincott.

Smith H. (1992). The detrimental health effects of ionizing radiation. *Nuclear Medicine Communications, 13*(1), 4–10.

Stewart A, Webb J, Hewitt DA. (1958). A survey of childhood malignancies. *British Medical Journal, 1,* 1495–1508.

Swerdlow A, Douglas A, Hudson G, Bennett M, MacLennan K. (1992). Risk of second primary cancers after Hodgkin's disease by type of treatment: Analysis of 2846 patients in the British national lymphoma investigation. *British Journal of Medicine, 304,* 1137–1148.

Tamm EP, Bluemke DA, Fishman EK. (1994). Renal oncocytoma arising in an irradiated field. *Clinical Imaging, 18*(1), 65–67.

Tarbell N, Gelber R, Weinstein H, Mauch P. (1993). Sex differences in risk of second malignant tumors after Hodgkin's disease. *Lancet, 341,* 1428–1432.

Thompson DE, Mabuchi K, Ron E, Soda M, Tokunaga M, Ochikubo S, Sugimoto S, Ikeda T, Terasaki M, Izumi S, Preston DL. (1994). Cancer incidence in atomic bomb survivors. Part II: Solid tumors, 1958–1987. *Radiation Research 137*(2 Suppl), S17–S67.

Trosko JE. (1996). Role of low-level ionizing radiation in multistep carcinogenic process. *Health Physics, 70*(6), 812–822.

Tucker MA. (1993). Solid second cancers following Hodgkin's disease. *Hematology: Oncology Clinics of North America, 7*(2), 389–400.

Tucker MA, Coleman CN, Cox RS, Varghese A, Rosenberg SA. (1988). Risk of second cancers after treatment for Hodgkin's disease. *New England Journal of Medicine, 318,* 76–81.

Upton AC. (1975). Physical carcinogenesis: Radiation, history, and sources. In FF Becker (ed.). *Cancer: A comprehensive treatise* (vol. 1), 387–403. New York: Plenum Press.

Upton AC. (1982). The biological effects of low level ionizing radiation. *Scientific American, 46,* 41–49.

Upton AC. (1986). Historical perspectives on radiation carcinogenesis. In AC Upton, RE Albert, FJ Burns, RE Shore (eds.). *Radiation carcinogenesis,* 1–10. New York: Elsevier Science Publishing.

Vahakangas KH, Samet JM, Metcalf RA, Welsh JA, Bennett WP, Lane DP, Harris CC. (1992). Mutation of p53 and ras genes in radon associated lung cancer from uranium minors. *Lancet, 339,* 576–580.

van Leeuwen FE, Klokman WJ, Hagenbeek A, van den Belt-Dusebout AW, van Kerkoff EHM, van Heerde P, Somers R. (1994). Second cancer risk following Hodgkin's disease: A 20-year follow-up study. *Journal of Clinical Oncology, 12,* 312–325.

Watanabe KK, Kang HK, Dalager NA. (1995). Cancer mortality risk among military participants of a 1958 atmospheric nuclear weapons test. *American Journal of Public Health, 85*(4), 523–527.

Weiss HA, Darby SC, Doll R. (1994). Cancer mortality following x-ray treatment for ankylosing spondylitis. *International Journal of Cancer 59*(3), 327–338.

Radiation Oncology Research in Clinical Trials

VICKIE K. FIELER

History of Clinical Trials in the United States

Medical research has taken place ever since the practice of medicine was recognized. This research was done by trial and error, with physicians trying new treatments on patients and repeating those treatments on other patients if they appeared to be effective. As medical science developed, the value of medical research became widespread, particularly in the interests of public health. In 1887 the federal government founded the National Institutes of Health (NIH) in order to fund small research programs on the transmission of cholera and other infectious agents (Jenkins & Lake, 1988). Medical research was revolutionized in 1948, when the British Medical Research Council presented the first placebo-controlled, randomized, clinical trial (Jenkins & Hubbard, 1991). Subsequently, the NIH adopted that method as the basis for all medical research.

The National Cancer Institute (NCI) was created in 1937, when President Roosevelt signed the National Cancer Institute Act. The NCI was created to support research, training, and information dissemination related to cancer. President Nixon further expanded the NCI's program of research in 1971 with the National Cancer Act. Also in this legislation, two review boards were created to monitor the NCI's activities. The President's Cancer Panel is an advisory panel of three that reports to the president on the National Cancer Program, and the Cancer Advisory Board consists of twelve scientists or physicians and eight representatives of the general public (Jenkins & Lake, 1988).

The NCI is structured into five divisions, one of which is the Division of Cancer Treatment (DCT). The DCT has five programs, one of which is the Cancer Therapy Evaluation Program (CTEP), which oversees the cooperative group research program (see Figure 7-1). The Radiation Therapy Oncology Group (RTOG) is one of these research programs (Cheson, 1991). See Table 7-1 for a listing of all the groups.

RTOG was organized in 1968 and has about 140 member institutions. The goals of RTOG include these:

1. to increase the survival of patients with local or regional cancer
2. to increase the curative and palliative effects of cancer management
3. to advance knowledge of radiation therapy through clinical trials
4. to reduce morbidity associated with radiation therapy but maintain its efficacy
5. to enhance cooperation between oncology specialists providing multimodality therapy and to evaluate this therapy in clinical trials
6. to translate basic science discoveries into clinical trials
7. to collect data on subjects over time in order to identify factors that might predict treatment results and assist in the design of future clinical trials (Wasserman et al., 1991).

Development of Informed Consent

From 1946 to 1949, the Nuremberg Military Tribunal was held and the Nuremberg Code was developed. This Tribunal investigated war crimes

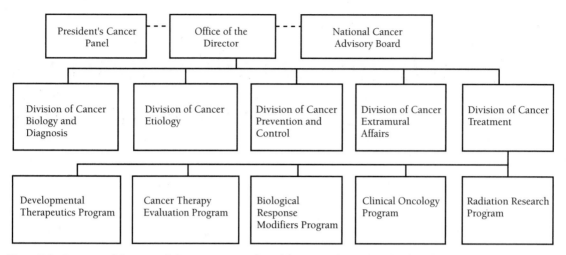

Figure 7-1 • Structure of the National Cancer Institute. Adapted from BD. Cheson (1991). Clinical trials programs. *Seminars in Oncology Nursing, 7,* 237.

that occurred during World War II, which included Nazi human experimentation. The Nuremberg Code specified the basic moral, ethical, and legal concepts related to human experimentation, including the concept of informed, voluntary consent. The Helsinki Declaration followed in 1964 with guidelines for biomedical research using human subjects and was revised in 1975 by the 29th World Medical Assembly (Beauchamp & Walters, 1978). In 1966, the U.S. Office of the Surgeon General issued a regulation that all clinical research be internally reviewed. Prior to this time, there were no specific regulations requiring research review or informed consent. It was generally considered that research related to health care

was good for society and that society's needs were predominant over individual rights.

During the 1960s, there was a shift in public opinion toward individual rights. In 1974, the National Commission for the Protection of Human Subjects of Biomedical and Behavioral Research developed, the Department of Health and Human Services' (DHHS) policy for the protection of human research subjects, which includes the criteria for Institutional Review Boards. In 1979, the same commission published the Belmont Report, which further delineated the ethical principles and guidelines for the protection of human subjects (Jenkins & Hubbard, 1991). The DHHS revised its policy in 1983, mandating that all institutions follow a formally recognized review process for research involving human subjects. These guidelines are mandatory for federally funded research as well as for many other sources of funding (Grady, 1991).

Institutional Review Boards (IRB) require an application, a copy of the proposed research, and a copy of the proposed consent form (if indicated). Three major areas are usually reviewed: protection of subjects' rights, procedures for soliciting subjects, and administrative approval. Many IRBs require an application even if the research involves human subjects indirectly, such as a chart review or a secondary analysis. Written consent forms may not always be required, as in a study using an anonymous, voluntary questionnaire. Subjects must be told about the research either verbally or in writing. As part of the IRB application, the research must state exactly what subjects will be told, when, how, and by whom. Subjects should be given copies of the consent

Table 7-1 • NCI Clinical Cooperative Oncology Groups

CALGB	Cancer and Leukemia Group B
ECOG	Eastern Cooperative Oncology Group
EORTC	European Organization for Research and Treatment of Cancer
NCCTG	North Central Cancer Treatment Group
SWOG	Southwest Oncology Group
CCSG	Children's Cancer Study Group
GOG	Gynecologic Oncology Group
POG	Pediatric Oncology Group
BTCG	Brain Tumor Oncology Group
IRS	Intergroup Rhabdomyosarcoma
NSABP	National Surgical Adjuvant Breast and Bowel Project
NWTS	Wilm's Tumor Study Group
RTOG	Radiation Therapy Oncology Group

Adapted from BD Cheson (1991). Clinical trials programs. *Seminars in Oncology Nursing, 7,* 237.

Table 7-2 • Contents of a Consent Form

- purpose of the research and study questions
- description of design and methods
- what the subject will be expected to do if he/she agrees to participate
- potential benefits, risks, or discomfort
- materials (if subjects wish to see them)
- statement that the investigator is willing to answer questions about the research, including the name and phone number of the investigator
- statement that the subject may refuse to participate or withdraw at any time without jeopardizing his/her regular treatment, and what will happen to the data if the subject decides to withdraw (kept or destroyed)
- if data will be kept for additional research, a statement about how it will be used, whether or not it will be made available to other researchers, and in what form
- what limits will be placed on the use of the data obtained, and the extent to which information concerning individual subjects will be confidential or anonymous
- place for subject's signature, date, and sometimes a witness or guardian

form and any information sheets or letters that are used (University of Rochester, 1993). See Table 7-2 for a listing of the contents of a consent form.

Clinical Trials

Clinical trials are divided into phases based on how "new" is the drug or technology that is under investigation. Phase I trials are generally the first use of the drug or technology in humans. Preclinical work has already been done in laboratories with cultures or in animal studies before human trials begin (see Table 7-3). The goals of phase I research are to determine the maximum tolerated dose in cancer patients using a particular schedule or combination of treatments and to determine the toxicity in normal organ systems. These studies

require very rigorous monitoring. Usually the study begins at a low dose (as determined in animal studies) with three to five patients, and drug doses are increased incrementally until toxicity occurs.

Once the safe dose ranges are established, phase II studies begin. The purpose in phase II is to discover what activity the new drug or technology has in treating different types of cancer. This requires that subjects have measurable disease, relatively normal organ functions, and a life expectancy long enough to allow for monitoring of disease progress.

If a new drug is determined to have a significant effect on a type of cancer, phase III trials are used to compare the new treatment with current standard treatment. Phase III trials have random assignment to treatment conditions. These trials also stratify subjects by variables that may have a significant effect on outcomes such as previous treatments and stage of disease. These studies generally require large numbers of patients in order to determine statistical significance and are most often designed to be multi-institutional (Jenkins & Hubbard, 1991).

After phase III, if the treatment or drug is equal to or more effective than standard treatment, or if it offers additional benefits such as less toxicity, better quality of life, or less expense, it is then submitted to the Food and Drug Administration (FDA). If approved, it becomes available on the market. Because this entire process often takes several years, there are two methods for patients to gain access to investigational drugs or therapies without participating in a clinical trial. The primary method is through "Group C" classification of the drug or therapy. If a patient has a life-threatening disease for which there is not a comparable treatment, a physician may request the treatment

Table 7-3 • Preclinical Animal Studies

Segment I	Reproductive performance	Female and male rats	Effects on gonadal function, estrous cycles, mating behavior, conception rates, early gestation
Segment II	Teratogenesis	Two of three species: mice, rats, rabbits	Drugs given during early pregnancy to evaluate fetal toxicity or teratogenesis
Segment III	Perinatal and postnatal studies	Same	Drugs given during late pregnancy and lactation to evaluate late development, labor and delivery, lactation, neonatal viability, growth

Data from Bush JK. (1994). The industry perspective on the inclusion of women in clinical trials. *Academic Medicine, 69,* 708–715.

outside of the clinical trials. The physician assumes the responsibility for written consent and for monitoring and reporting any adverse effects of the drug. The second method is for a physician to request a "special exception." These are considered individually and the patient must not have any other treatment options. In addition, the treatment must have completed phase I studies (Jenkins & Hubbard, 1991).

An example of phase I research in RTOG is studies using three-dimensional conformal radiation therapy (RT). An example of a phase II research project is hyperfractionation with dose escalation. And finally, an example of a phase III study is comparison of hyperfractionation to standard fractionation.

All studies submitted for clinical trials are structured similarly. The purpose of the research must be clearly identified and supporting background information included of sufficient depth to indicate the importance and rationale of the study. Specific inclusion and exclusion criteria define the study sample, and a plan for how subjects will be recruited is usually included. The study methods section describes the desired sample size, design, procedures, time frames, how outcomes will be measured, and proposed data analysis. Included in studies involving new technology or drugs are pharmaceutical information, toxicity assessment (and treatment, if indicated), patient monitoring, and dose or treatment adjustments. Every study, except one using anonymous questionnaires, requires some type of consent, usually written, and many studies include a section discussing consent procedures. Also included are criteria for study termination, data submission requirements, and references. Many of the clinical trials are accompanied by companion studies, such as a quality of life study (Melink & Whitacre, 1991).

Obstacles in Clinical Trials

Clinical trials have many obstacles. One of the major issues is cost. Typically an individual research grant covers part of the principal investigator's salary, salary for research assistants, direct costs for supplies and equipment, and so on. Federal grants pay an additional amount, referred to as indirect or pooled costs, to help cover expenses such as rent, utilities, and facility maintenance. Currently indirect costs are about 58 percent and can be as high as 75 percent.

Program grants such as ECOG or RTOG are structured differently. They are awarded to an institution or department and provide funds for salaries, supplies, and equipment. Program grants are competitive and are usually awarded for three to five years with an annual review of subject accrual and budget. They do not provide funds for the clinical care that patients receive even if the patient is enrolled in a clinical trial. All of the clinical expenses are billed to the third-party payers or to the patient. This can be justified because it is typical care the patient would receive with standard treatment. Exceptions to this include investigational drugs that are supplied directly from NCI or a pharmaceutical company and are not charged to the patient.

Increasingly, third-party payers are denying payment for "investigational" treatments. A recent example is bone marrow transplants for breast cancer (Johansen et al., 1991). Several insurance companies denied payment for bone marrow transplants for breast cancer because it has not been "proven" to cure disease or prolong survival. The drive to decrease health care costs is forcing both health care providers and patients to scrutinize how health care dollars are being spent. However, without a system to test the efficacy of new treatments, whether paid for by insurers, government, or out-of-pocket, few advances in the treatment of cancer will occur. In the long run, it may be far more expensive for insurers not to pay for clinical trials, if it results in less effective treatments and higher morbidity and mortality (Broder, 1991; Yarbro, 1991).

In addition to the challenges of getting reimbursed for direct care related to research, there will likely be reductions in the amount of research dollars available. In 1995, there was a proposal to cut the NIH budget by 10 percent (Macilwain, 1995) and recommendations to cut the NCI's research budget (Taylor, 1995). The budgets for NIH and NCI were $11.3 billion and $2.1 billion, respectively, in 1995 (Macilwain, 1995; Marshall, 1995). There has also been increasing direction from Congress and from special-interest groups on how research money should be spent. In 1993, President Clinton signed the National Institutes of Health Revitalization Act, which required the NCI to spend a fixed percentage of its budget on cancer control. For 1994, the NCI was to allocate 7 percent to cancer control; in 1995, 9 percent; and in 1996, 10 percent (Duane & Tisevich, 1994).

Another obstacle to clinical trials is patients' refusal to participate. This refusal may be due to inconvenience, cost, fear of "experimenting," and concerns about confidentiality. Participating in a clinical trial may mean agreeing to extra tests and procedures, additional visits to the cancer center, filling out questionnaires, and agreeing to interviews, all at a time when the patient may be adjusting to a diagnosis of cancer and feeling vulnerable (Johansen et al., 1991). Physicians may be reluctant to offer clinical trials as well. Some may believe it conflicts with their role as a care provider, particularly if they believe one treatment to be superior to another. Others may not be willing to do the additional work of entering and caring for patients in clinical trials. Physicians in general practice who are not affiliated with a cancer treatment center may not be aware of what types of clinical trials are available and may not encourage patients to participate (Farrar, 1991; Long, 1991).

Criticisms of the NCI and Clinical Trials

A scathing criticism of the NCI was published in 1993 by Epstein. Among other assertions, Epstein criticized the NCI's leadership and advisory boards for "confusing the public by repeated claims of winning the war against cancer" (Epstein, 1993, p. 109). He presented population-adjusted cancer mortality rates as evidence of losing the war against cancer. In 1980 the mortality rate of cancer was 168 deaths per 100,000 people. In 1984 the rate was 171/100,000 and projected for the year 2000 is 175/100,000. In addition, he presented data that supports an overall increase in cancer rates, not just lung cancer. Epstein describes statistics that indicate that cancer treatment in general has not significantly influenced survival. He also presents a review of the NCI budget, pointing out that little research has been funded on the primary prevention of cancer, the vast majority of sums are spent on cancer treatment, and more specifically, on drug therapy. Billions of dollars have been spent on looking for cures for cancer with minimal success. Epstein questioned why similar amounts of money weren't spent on cancer prevention. This analysis was responsible, in part, for the 1993 National Institutes of Health Revitalization Act, which required increased funding for cancer prevention research.

Other criticisms of the clinical trials program include the historical exclusion of women and minorities. During the early 1800s, oppressed groups such as American slave women were used by physicians who needed to practice surgical techniques (Merkatz & White, 1994). By the turn of the century, it was common practice to use institutionalized populations such as prisoners and those committed to asylums in medical research studies. After World War II and the Nuremburg Trials, standards were set to protect individuals; however, in the United States, the autonomy of individual researchers was generally supported. After the thalidomide disaster, legislation was passed by Congress that gave the FDA power to regulate and approve new drugs. During the late 1960s and early 1970s, several severe abuses of human rights came to light, including the Tuskegee syphilis study, in which almost 400 illiterate black prisoners were not treated for syphilis for a span of 30 years so that researchers could evaluate the natural course of disease (McCarthy, 1994; Merkatz & White, 1994). Through the end of the 1960s and into the 1970s, few people were willing to participate in clinical trials. Clinical trials were seen as dangerous and offering no benefit to the individuals who participated. In 1974, Senator Edward Kennedy pushed the Department of Health, Education, and Welfare (HEW) to develop guidelines for the protection of human subjects. Over the remainder of the decade, these guidelines changed into regulations and included mandatory institutional review boards for the protection of human subjects. The FDA issued a policy in 1977 prohibiting drug companies and others from including pregnant women and women of childbearing potential in studies testing new drugs. The policy was written to exclude women from primarily phase I trials but in practice was very broadly interpreted to exclude women from all drug trials. The reason given for this restriction was protection of the fetus or potential fetus. As McCarthy (1994) pointed out, apparently no thought was given about what would happen if pregnant women took the drugs once they became available on the market.

At no time were any regulations or guidelines issued that prevented minorities from participation in clinical trials; however, with all the abuses that were brought to light, few members of minority groups were willing to participate. In addition, it has been proposed that members of minority groups who fell into low socioeconomic groups had limited access to health care and were rarely offered the opportunity to participate (McCarthy, 1994).

The general view of clinical trials gradually changed during the 1980s from a rather dangerous proposition with little benefits for participants to a way of securing state-of-the-art treatment at a relatively low cost. The general view that women needed protection was changing as early as the 1960s but was not incorporated into bureaucratic thought until the late 1980s and into the 1990s. Because of public pressure, in 1990, the NIH formed the Office of Research on Women's Health. Three goals were identified: (1) to increase research on women's health issues, (2) to ensure adequate representation of women in research, and (3) to increase the number of women in biomedical careers (Pinn, 1994). And finally, in 1993, as part of the NIH Revitalization Act, the FDA lifted the restrictions from the 1977 guidelines. The new guidelines suggest ways to minimize fetal risks (Merkatz & White, 1994). There is concern being expressed by members of the pharmaceutical industry related to legal liability should a woman become pregnant while participating in a drug study. Not only can a woman who became pregnant sue the pharmaceutical company, but 40 states also allow lawsuits to be filed on behalf of the fetus (Bush, 1994).

The 1993 NIH Revitalization Act also addresses the inclusion of minorities in clinical research. This act requires the NIH to include minorities and women in clinical trials unless there is a specific reason not to. These guidelines are vague and there is no specific rules as to sample sizes: "the Director of NIH shall ensure that the trial is designed and carried out in a manner sufficient to provide for a valid analysis of whether the variables being studied in the trial affect women or members of minority groups, as the case may be, differently than other subjects in the trial" (Charrow, 1994, p. 100) Although this act is considered a guideline rather than a regulation, the NIH cannot fund or support research that does not meet these guidelines.

Nurses' Roles in Clinical Trials

Many nursing roles have been identified in the literature related to clinical trials, including clinician, patient advocate, administrator, educator, data manager, and researcher (Engelking, 1991; McEvoy et al., 1991; Wheeler, 1991).

One of the most traditional roles is that of a direct care giver or clinician. In any phase of research, inpatient or outpatient, it is usually the staff nurse that actually administers drug therapy and monitors for patient response to treatment. Nurses assess the toxicities of a new therapy and document patient progress. Nurses are also usually the first-line managers of side effects, assessing the severity of a side effect or toxicity, providing initial treatment, referring/communicating with the physician or investigator, and documenting occurrences (McEvoy et al., 1991).

Advanced-practice nurses (APNs) may provide direct care to patients on clinical trials as well. Nurse practitioners may participate in consult visits, admit patients, write initial orders, and follow patients in the outpatient settings, depending upon practice privileges. Clinical nurse specialists may be trained to provide specific services such as administering tumor vaccines and support staff in providing direct patient care.

Hand in hand with direct care is the educator role. Nurses reinforce the teaching about clinical trials in general, prepare patients for what to expect, and teach self-care management. Randomization into a clinical trial is frequently a difficult concept for patients to understand. Patients may seek out a new treatment to find it is available only in a randomized trial. Patients must accept the risk that they will be randomized into a treatment group that is not receiving the treatment they were seeking. When working with patients in phase I trials, the nurse may not be able to help the patient anticipate what will happen. The side effects and toxicities associated with a new treatment may not be known. The nurse must be alert to the development of unexpected toxicities and be prepared to help patients cope with them (Engelking, 1991). APNs might also be involved in patient education related to clinical trials as well as be responsible for orienting staff nurses to clinical trials and new protocols (Wheeler, 1991).

Nurses serve as patient advocates as part of their direct care role. As an advocate, the nurse works with the patient and family to ensure that they know what the research is about. Nurses can assist patients in decision making by providing information, encouraging questions, and helping patients to identify and prioritize their needs. At times, it may be necessary for a nurse to help a patient withdraw from a study if the patient decides the study is not in his/her best interests (McEvoy et al., 1991).

Many clinical trials can be complex, and nurses are usually very involved in coordination of care and ensuring that all the tests and procedures required for the study are completed. The nurse may be responsible for coordination of the study as well as patient care. Teamwork, collegiality, and communication are essential. APNs may review protocols prior to initiation, in order to evaluate the feasibility of a protocol. The APN would look to see that nursing resources were sufficient to provide safe, high-quality patient care and that the facility has the equipment and backup support to provide emergency as well as routine care.

Nurses also routinely engage in multiple other roles, including counseling, liaison, and supporter. They reassure patients, communicate with family members, communicate between inpatient and outpatient settings, and promote patient autonomy. It would be impossible for clinical research to occur without the contributions of nurses.

Other nursing roles are in the process of evolving. Public education is an area in which nurses could become more active. Nurses could be instrumental in raising public awareness of clinical trials, increasing clinical trial participation, and influencing public policy. Activities as simple as writing letters to the editor of local newspapers can be very effective. Other strategies include writing articles for newspapers and journals, developing information about clinical trials targeted to different cultural backgrounds and languages, writing to legislators, volunteering at health fairs and other public events, and developing programs to educate the public using interactive technology, just to name a few ideas.

Nurses can become more active in developing consulting roles during the development of clinical trials. They can add a holistic view to patient care and incorporate companion studies such as quality of life studies and symptom management studies. Nurses can also be principal investigators, particularly in studies that focus on cancer control, prevention, symptom management, patient education, and quality of life. See Chapter 25 on nursing research.

Participation in clinical trials in radiation therapy can be challenging and complex but also very exciting and rewarding. Nurses are crucial to the success of clinical trials in their current roles of caregiver, educator, and coordinator. Nurses have the opportunity to expand their roles as principal investigators, as public educators, and as informed consumers active in the political process.

References

Beauchamp TL, Walters L. (1978). *Contemporary issues in bioethics.* (pp. 405–407). Belmont, CA: Wadsworth Publishing.

Broder S. (1991). The human costs of cancer and the response of the National Cancer Program. *Cancer, 67*(Supplement), 1716–1717.

Bush JK. (1994). The industry perspective on the inclusion of women in clinical trials. *Academic Medicine, 69*(9), 708–715.

Charrow RP. (1994). Is the NIH Revitalization Act an ethnic-quota law? *Journal of NIH Research, 6*(7), 99–101.

Cheson BD. (1991). Clinical trials programs. *Seminars in Oncology Nursing, 7*(4), 235–242.

Duane B, Tisevich DA. (1994). Congress maintains interest in NIH matters. *Journal of the National Cancer Institute, 86*(5), 337–339.

Engelking C. (1991). Facilitating clinical trials: The expanding role of the nurse. *Cancer, 67*(Supplement), 1793–1797.

Epstein SS. (1993). Evaluation of the National Cancer Program and proposed reforms. *American Journal of Industrial Medicine, 24*, 109–133.

Farrar WB. (1991). Clinical trials: Access and reimbursement. *Cancer, 67*(Supplement), 1779–1782.

Grady C. (1991). Ethical issues in clinical trials. *Seminars in Oncology Nursing, 7*(4), 288–296.

Jenkins J, Hubbard S. (1991). History of clinical trials. *Seminars in Oncology Nursing, 7*(4), 228–234.

Jenkins JF, Lake PC. (1988). Celebration of an era of public service at the National Institutes of Health and the National Cancer Institute. *Cancer Nursing, 11*(1), 58–64.

Johansen MA, Mayer DK, Hoover HC. (1991). Obstacles to implementing cancer clinical trials. *Seminars in Oncology Nursing, 7*(4), 260–267.

Long DG. (1991). Clinical trials: A family physician's perspective. *Cancer, 67*(Supplement), 1798–1799.

Macilwain C. (1995). NIH backers pledge last-ditch stand. *Nature, 375*, 267.

Marshall E. (1995). A new phase in the war on cancer. *Science, 267*(10), 1412–1415.

McCarthy CR. (1994). Historical background of clinical trials involving women and minorities. *Academic Medicine, 69*(9), 695–698.

McEvoy MD, Cannon L, MacDermott ML. (1991). The professional role for nurses in clinical trials. *Seminars in Oncology Nursing, 7*(4), 268–274.

Melink TJ, Whitacre MY. (1991). Planning and implementing clinical trials. *Seminars in Oncology Nursing, 7*(4), 243–251.

Merkatz RB, White S. (1994). Historical background of changes in FDA policy on the study and evaluation of drugs in women. *Academic Medicine, 69*(9), 703–707.

Pinn VW. (1994). The role of the NIH's Office of Research on Women's Health. *Academic Medicine, 69*(9), 698–702.

Taylor R. (1995). Review proposes shift in U.S. cancer funding. *Nature, 375*, 267.

University of Rochester Medical Center, School of Nursing. (1993). *Research Subjects Review Board School of Nursing Subcommittee, Guidelines and Procedures.* Rochester, NY.

Wasserman TH, Phillips TL, Hanks GE, Order SE, Perez CA, Pajak TF, Pakuris E, Brady LW, Leibel SA, Cox JD. (1991). The Radiation Therapy Oncology Group: An update of clinical research activities. *International Journal of Radiation Oncology, Biology, Physics, 20*, 1383–1391.

Wheeler VS. (1991). Preparing nurses for clinical trials: The cancer center approach. *Seminars in Oncology Nursing, 7*(4), 275–279.

Yarbro JW. (1991). Cancer care in the 1990s and the cost. *Cancer, 67*(Supplement), 1718–1727.

II

Treatment of Cancer with Radiation Therapy

Managing Side Effects of Skin Changes and Fatigue

ELLEN SITTON

Symptom distress is multidimensional and may affect physical and psychological feelings of well-being. Side effects of radiation therapy vary with patient and radiation treatment-related factors. The majority of patients undergoing this treatment modality experience skin changes and fatigue. Collaborating with patients to manage these side effects can help alleviate distress caused by these symptoms, minimize them, and improve quality of life during and following radiation therapy.

The first part of this chapter discusses normal skin, skin structural and functional response to irradiation, and factors influencing radiation changes in the skin. The management of both early and late effects of skin irradiation are described. The second part of this chapter discusses fatigue, another symptom experienced by many patients undergoing radiation therapy. Acute and chronic fatigue, studies of fatigue in radiation oncology, factors contributing to fatigue, and fatigue assessment and management are presented.

History of Skin Irradiation

Fletcher (1985) described the history of the earliest effects of radiation on the skin after the discovery of x rays in 1895. Severe dermatitis was noted in a medical student who checked the x ray tubes by taking frequent x rays of his hand. Soon thereafter, x rays were used to treat breast cancer with the belief that if x rays could kill skin cells, they could kill cancer cells. Methods of measuring doses of radiation were unknown and treatments were not initially fractionated. The term, Haut (skin) erythema dose (HED), was used from 1900 until the 1920s to describe the dose required to produce a brisk skin reaction. In the 1930s, Baclesse treated breast cancer with very large total doses of radiation given in multiple fractions over a period of 12 to 16 weeks. Early effects of erythema were reduced by this method, but late effects were significant and severe. These effects included fibrosis with skin retraction, changes in pigmentation, and pain. In the 1950s to 1960s, inoperable breast cancer was treated by some investigators with 25 Gray (Gy) for two doses in two consecutive days or over one week. This resulted in severe fibrosis in irradiated fields and caused severe complications of frozen shoulder, lymphedema, radiation pneumonitis, and pulmonary fibrosis. The importance of fractionation of the total dose and its early and late effects on skin and other tissues is much better understood today. However, research continues to evaluate the most effective methods of radiation dose delivery.

Skin: Anatomy and Physiology

Skin serves as a physical barrier to the environment, to protect the body against infection. It also protects the body from fluid and electrolyte loss and has sensory and immune functions. Skin is composed of the epidermis and dermis covering the subcutaneous tissues, and skin appendages formed by the infolding of the epidermis (see Figure 8–1).

Epidermis

The epidermis varies in thickness from 30 to 300 μm and is connected to the dermis by the

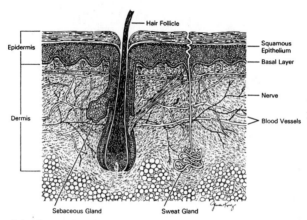

Figure 8-1 • Normal anatomy of the skin. With permission from Woodburn R (1983). *Essentials of Human Anatomy,* (7th ed.). New York: Oxford University Press.

basement membrane. A single layer of cells makes up the lowest layer, the basal layer, which proliferates to maintain a constant population with cell loss equal to cell growth. Cells, keratinocytes, gradually move from the basal layer through the nondividing malpighian layer to the stratum corneum, a layer of dead cells that slough from the skin surface. The minimum time for a basal cell to pass from the basal layer through the malpighian layer is 13 days, with approximately another 13 days to pass through the stratum corneum (Archambeau et al., 1995). The epidermis contains no blood vessels or nerves.

Melanocytes are located in the epidermis and are nonepithelial in origin. Melanocytes are located at the junction of the basal layer of the epidermis with the dermis and are the pigment-producing cells of the skin. Pigmentation of the skin is related to activation of existing melanin and increased melanin production.

Many growth factors are believed to have a role in wound healing. Epidermal growth factor (EGF) and transforming-growth-factor-α (TGF-α) stimulate epidermal cell growth and differentiation (Ebling et al., 1992). EGF promotes wound healing in experimental ulcers and animal models. TGF-α is produced by and stimulates growth in keratinocytes. Growth factors and other immunological cytokines (e.g., interleukin-1, interleukin 3), Langerhans cells, and T-cells also have a role in the skin immune functions.

Dermis

Beneath the basal layer of the epidermis is the dermis, which is 1–3 mm thick and is composed largely of collagen fibers produced by fibroblasts. The dermis contains the blood vessels, which supply nutrients to the epidermis, lymph vessels, and nerves. The lower dermis contains connective tissue stroma with collagen bundles, scattered fibroblasts, and small blood vessels. Skin appendages include hair follicles and glands (sebaceous and sweat). The epidermis invaginates into hair follicles and sweat gland ducts. Sebaceous glands, which are associated with hair follicles, are found throughout the skin with the exception of the palms of the hands and soles of the feet. They are most prevalent on the face and upper back and chest. Sweat glands are found throughout the skin except for nailbeds. A subcutaneous fat layer, which may be up to several centimeters thick, is bonded to the dermis.

Normal Skin Response to Irradiation

Archambeau and associates (1995) described the smallest unit of skin structure as a microvessel and associated epidermis and dermis. Skin response to irradiation is dependent upon dose and reflects changes in the cellular components of the epidermis, dermis, and vasculature. Both early and late changes that occur are indicative of an ongoing restructuring of these populations. Following irradiation, there is a dose-dependent loss of cells in the epidermis, dermis, and microvasculature endothelium. Dose above the tolerance of the tissue results in necrosis.

Radiation fractionation generally consists of daily fractions of 1.8 to 2.0 Gy (Gray) Monday through Friday until the prescribed dose of radiation is reached. Archambeau and colleagues (1995) delivered a dose of 60 Gy in 2.0 Gy fractions with no treatment on weekends (Table 8–1). Basal cell loss occurred after doses of 20 to 25 Gy

Table 8-1 • Changes in Basal Cell Population with 60 Gy Delivered in 2 Gy Fractions Over 42 Days

Change	Dose	Effect
Basal cell density	20–25 Gy	Decrease in density of basal cells begins (basal cell loss)
	50 Gy	Nadir of basal cell loss
	60 Gy	Basal cell number close to beginning level due to repopulation during irradiation
Mitotic index	40 Gy	Increase in mitotic index (cell division) through the end of the course of radiation therapy
Microvasculature	0–60 Gy	No change found *during* treatment

Data reprinted by permission of the publisher from Archambeau JO, Pezner R, Wasserman T (1995). Pathophysiology of irradiated skin and breast. *International Journal of Radiation Oncology, Biology, Physics, 31,* 1171–1185. Copyright 1995 by Elsevier Science Inc.

with the lowest number observed after 50 Gy. At 60 Gy the number of basal cells had increased to original levels due to an increase in proliferation of basal cells (repopulation).

Telangiectasia are dilated vascular channels, which appear as red, prominent, thin-walled blood vessels frequently seen within one to two years after irradiation. Telangiectasia are often used as an endpoint to measure late effects of radiation. Skin dose that produces a 10 percent incidence of telangiectasia at 5 years is 50 Gy and the dose that produces a 3 percent incidence of necrosis is 69 Gy (Archambeau et al., 1995). Higher doses will increase the incidence of late changes.

Normal skin response to radiation depends on numerous patient and treatment-related factors. Radiation factors include the use of electron beam, tissue equivalent (bolus) material on the skin surface, accelerated fractionation, and large treatment fields. Patient factors include skin folds in irradiated volume, tangential fields, poor nutritional status, and the use of irritants to irradiated skin (Sitton, 1992a). Intercurrent disease such as ataxia-telangiectasia, differences between radiosensitivity of individuals, and combined radiation with chemotherapy and hyperthermia can also influence response to irradiation. Further discussion of these factors follows.

Radiation Factors

Beam Type and Energy

Prior to the 1960s, orthovoltage machines used in radiation therapy delivered 100% of the dose to the skin. Subsequently, skin reaction frequently limited the dose that could be delivered to the tumor. With the use of megavoltage machines, high-energy gamma rays (cobalt-60) and x rays (betatron, linear accelerator) deliver only 20 to 30 percent of the given dose to the skin. With some treatments, there may be no visible skin changes even at the completion of radiation therapy. When the skin or tissues directly beneath the skin need

treatment, higher skin doses (approximately 85 to 98 percent) can be delivered using electron beam energies. Placing 1 to 2 cm of tissue-equivalent material (bolus) to the treatment field surface during irradiation increases the skin dose. This technique is important if the skin or structures near the surface require higher doses than those delivered without the bolus.

Fractionation

Fractionation of dose generally spares acute reactions in skin due to proliferation of the epithelium during treatment. However, the severity of early effects of radiation on the skin do not predict for late effects (Panizzon & Goldschmidt, 1991; Perez & Brady, 1992). Total dose and dose per fraction are important in determining late effects of radiation. Large doses per fraction result in more severe late reactions.

Fractionation schedules are prescribed on the basis of the tumor cell growth, histologic type, and location of tumor. Accelerated radiation therapy with multiple daily fractions can increase local control in rapidly growing tumors. Research suggests that a minimum of 4 and possibly 6 or 8 hours should be allowed between fractions to allow maximum repair of normal tissues (Perez & Brady, 1992).

Nyman and Turesson (1995) compared early and late skin reactions with 4, 8, and 24 hours between radiation fractions. Two fractions per day were given with the 4- and 8-hour schedules. Acute and late reactions for the 4- and 8-hour groups were comparable. Indicators of acute reactions were erythema and desquamation; indicator of late reaction was telangiectasia. Postmastectomy parasternal fields were irradiated using different intervals between fractions of 2 to 2.25 Gy for each of the two fields. Total dose for all fractionation schedules was 50 Gy. Significantly less total intensity of erythema was found in the 4- and 8- hour compared with the 24-hour fractionation schedules. Erythema peaked one week earlier in the 4- and 8-hour schedules than in the 24-hour fractionation schedules. Late reactions as measured by telangiectasia were significantly increased with the 8-hour fractionation schedule compared with the 24-hour schedule. The investigators concluded that 4- and 8-hour intervals between fractions were not enough time for complete repair of sublethal damage for late-reacting tissues in skin using telangiectasia as the endpoint.

Volume of Skin Irradiated

As the volume of tissue irradiated with a specified dose is increased, the tolerance of the normal tissue is reduced (Perez & Brady, 1992). When the total skin surface is treated with electron beam irradiation for cutaneous T-cell lymphoma, the total dose of 36 Gy is administered over approximately 8 weeks. In contrast, a head and neck tumor covering a much smaller volume of skin may be treated to more than 70 Gy in a period of approximately 7 weeks, a dose that the entire skin surface could not tolerate.

Patient Factors

Skin Folds

When skin folds are included in the treatment field, there is a higher risk of skin reaction and breakdown. Examples of such areas are the axilla, inframammary region, groin, and perineum. Skin folds create an uneven distribution of radiation dose, because they provide an environment in which there is increased moisture, friction, and warmth.

Tangential Radiation Fields

In tangential radiation fields, or in fields where a sloping skin surface occurs at the edge of the field, a higher dose is delivered to the sloping skin. If the field is uneven in thickness, as in the example of breast tangential fields, the exit dose from the radiation beam will be higher in the thinner area near the nipple resulting in higher doses to the skin. This problem may be corrected with the use of wedges that compensate for the uneven dose distribution.

Nutrition

Normal tissue healing occurs during and after radiation treatment. Much of the repair from radiation injury occurs in the first four to six hours after a dose of radiation. For optimal healing to occur, adequate nutrients such as proteins and vitamins must be available for repair of damaged tissue. Patients are generally encouraged to avoid weight loss during radiation therapy and to eat a balanced diet.

Intercurrent Disease

In patients with ataxia-telangiectasia (AT), clinical and cellular abnormalities occur with radiation therapy (Shore, 1990). Irradiated AT cultured fibroblasts show DNA repair and replication abnormalities (Malkinson, 1993). Some patients demonstrate high sensitivity to radiation therapy with a high incidence of skin necrosis. Other genetic disorders (e.g., Gardner's syndrome, Fanconi's anemia, Bloom's syndrome, familial dysplastic nevus syndrome) have an increased sensitivity in cultured cells to ionizing radiation or increased risk of development of multiple cutaneous carcinomas (e.g., nevoid basal cell carcinoma syndrome) (Malkinson, 1993).

Individual Differences

Clinical and in vitro studies demonstrate individual differences in response to radiation. This variation in radiosensitivity may influence the level of reactions to irradiation that develop (Russell et al., 1994). Other factors such as age can influence response to treatment. For example, dry skin is common in elderly patients and can be compounded at the treatment site by irradiation.

Treatment Factors

Chemotherapy

When patients with cancer are treated with chemotherapy combined with radiation therapy, either sequentially or concurrently, an additive effect between the treatment modalities may be expected and tolerance to a given dose of radiation may be decreased. Radiation recall of erythematous reaction in the irradiated area may occur when patients who have received radiation therapy are subsequently given adriamycin, actinomycin D, methotrexate, bleomycin, or 5-FU (Archambeau et al., 1995; Madhu & Rochford, 1993; Yokel & Hood, 1993). Adriamycin and actinomycin D are associated with both radiation enhancement (an increase in skin reaction) and radiation recall reactions (Yokel & Hood, 1993).

Radiation enhancement occurs when the intensity of the skin reaction to simultaneous administration of chemotherapy and radiation therapy is greater than that expected with radiation therapy alone. Skin effects with adriamycin may include erythema, vesiculation, desquamation, and hyperpigmentation. Radiation recall may occur in the treatment site with administration of actinomycin D many months after completion of radiation therapy and possibly years after administration of adriamycin (Yokel & Hood, 1993).

Administration of methotrexate within three weeks after radiation therapy may result in erythema and ulceration in the treatment field. Bleomycin or 5-FU after radiation therapy may result in an erythematous radiation recall reaction in the treatment portal. Recently there have been reports in the literature of radiation recall effects with paclitaxel (Phillips et al., 1995; Raghavan et al., 1993; Shenkier & Gelmon, 1994). Madhu and Rochford (1993) described "reverse recall" in which patients experience more severe skin reactions in the irradiated field 30 days or more after administration of busulphan.

Increased subcutaneous fibrosis was reported in patients who received cyclophosphamide, methotrexate, and 5-fluorouracil (CMF) chemotherapy after irradiation of the chest wall (Bentzen et al., 1990). Telangiectasia, used as the endpoint for late reactions, continued to progress after 10 years.

Hyperthermia

Hyperthermia is the therapeutic use of heat in the treatment of disease. Heat is cytotoxic at temperatures greater than 42.5°C (108°F). Hyperthermia is generally used in combination with another treatment modality such as radiation therapy or chemotherapy and is rarely used alone. Cell kill due to hyperthermia can be synergistically enhanced by radiation therapy and some chemotherapeutic agents. Hyperthermia is believed to inhibit repair of radiation injury. Well-vascularized tissue is sensitive to radiation therapy and relatively resistant to hyperthermia (Overgaard, 1989).

When combined radiation therapy and hyperthermia (thermoradiotherapy) are given immediately following one another, the risk of normal tissue damage increases if critical normal tissue has been heated (Overgaard, 1989). The extent that late radiation damage is enhanced is unclear. Thermoradiotherapy currently may be used in palliative treatment, particularly in previously irradiated sites with recurrent tumor. It may also have a role in improving local control of locally advanced tumors.

Engin and colleagues (1995) studied 126 patients undergoing thermoradiotherapy to determine factors that would predict for skin reactions.

Skin reactions of erythema and thermal blisters were influenced by previous radiation therapy, previous radiation therapy dose, concurrent radiation therapy dose, and number of hyperthermia treatments. Patients were less likely to exhibit skin reactions if they had previous radiation therapy and higher, rather than lower, previous radiation doses. Patients were more likely to exhibit skin reactions with higher doses of radiation and concurrent hyperthermia, and with higher total number of hyperthermia treatments. Enhanced skin reactions did not pose a clinical problem. Hyperthermia is discussed in further detail in Chapter 4.

Early Effects of Irradiation

The use of high-energy x rays to irradiate patients with cancer reduces the dose at the skin surface compared to early machines that delivered surface doses of 100%. Skin effects are easy to follow during the treatment course, and knowledge of potential changes allows the nurse to work with the patient to manage early side effects of radiation on the skin. Clinical experience and research data identify time–dose schedules appropriate to achieve local control and an acceptable cosmetic result (Archambeau et al., 1995).

Radiation-induced early changes are a result of injury to the skin and its appendages, and to reduced basal-layer proliferation. Early changes include erythema, pigmentation, epilation, dry desquamation, and moist desquamation. Healing should occur by 50 days after radiation therapy is completed (Archambeau et al., 1995). Grading systems for early and late effects of radiation on the skin have been developed by the Radiation Therapy Oncology Group (RTOG) and the European Oncology Radiation Therapy Cooperative group (EORTC) (see Table 8–2).

Erythema is related to an increase in blood volume in the vascular plexus beneath the epidermis (see Figure 8–2 and Color Plate 1). Radiation-induced erythema may be due to an inflammatory response to the death of basal cells in the epidermis. However, the pathophysiologic mechanism is not clear (Hopewell, 1990; Panizzon & Goldschmidt, 1991; Russell et al., 1994). A very mild erythema occasionally may be observed in the first week of treatment and as early as 24 hours after the first treatment. More pronounced erythema with inflammation and dry desquamation may occur after 2 to 3 weeks of radiation therapy (see Figure 8–3 and Color

Table 8-2 • Acute Radiation Morbidity Scoring Criteria (RTOG) and Late Radiation Morbidity Scoring Scheme (RTOG, EORTC) for Skin

0	Grade 1	Grade 2	Grade 3	Grade 4	Grade 5
ACUTE MORBIDITY					
No change over baseline	Follicular, faint or dull erythema, epilation, dry desquamation, decreased sweating	Tender or bright erythema, patchy moist desquamation, moderate edema	Confluent, moist desquamation, other than skin folds, pitting edema	Ulceration, hemorrhage, necrosis	
LATE MORBIDITY					
None	Slight atrophy, pigmentation change, some hair loss	Patchy atrophy, moderate telangiectasia, total hair loss	Marked atrophy, gross telangiectasia	Ulceration	Death directly related to radiation late effect

Plate 2). Dry desquamation results from the inability of the basal layer to proliferate sufficiently to replace the epidermal surface cells. With an additional 1 to 2 weeks of treatment, epilation (hair loss within the treatment field) and reduced function of sebaceous and sweat glands occurs.

Moist desquamation with denuded areas exposing the dermis and serosanguinous oozing peaks after 4 to 6 weeks of irradiation. This reaction generally reepithelializes within 1 to 2 months after the course of radiation treatment (see Figure 8–4 and Color Plate 3). Pain occurs when sensitive nerve endings are exposed due to loss of epidermis. Moist desquamation is more

likely to occur in areas of friction and moisture (e.g., inframammary fold, axilla, groin). On occasion, a break in treatment is necessary to allow the skin to recover. However, treatment breaks may also allow repopulation of tumor cells and are to be avoided when possible. Skin reaction at the end

Figure 8-3 • Increased pigmentation and dry desquamation secondary to breast irradiation.

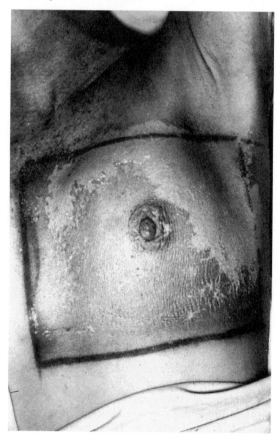

Figure 8-2 • Erythema secondary to breast irradiation.

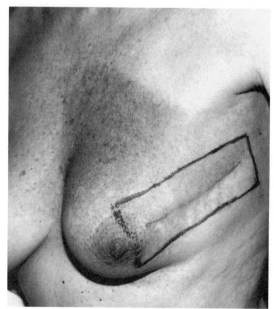

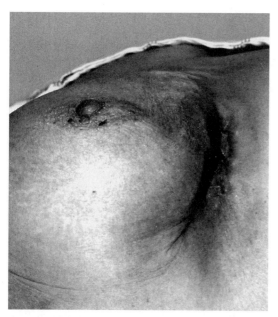

Figure 8-4 • Moist desquamation secondary to breast irradiation. Note increased skin reaction in skin fold in inframammary region.

of the course of radiation therapy may progress for approximately 1 week and then begin to heal relatively quickly over the next 3 to 6 weeks (Malkinson, 1993). After healing, irradiated skin may appear normal for many years.

Irradiation of melanocytes results in an increased production of melanin. This increases pigmentation of the skin, which may be observed during radiation and will most often fade within 6 months. Increased pigmentation, however, may persist for months after the course of treatment.

Epilation in the irradiated volume can be permanent with very high doses of radiation. However, regrowth of hair after 2 to 3 months generally occurs. Some changes in characteristics of the hair may be evident such as slower growth rate, more sparse hair, and change in hair color or appearance.

Management of Early Effects

Management of early skin changes related to radiation therapy is being researched. Goals of management include minimizing symptoms, promoting healing, and preventing infection. Recommendations are frequently made to minimize irritants to irradiated skin including sun exposure, and mechanical, chemical, and thermal irritants

(Sitton, 1992b) (see Table 8–3 and Table 8–4). Mild soap such as Dove (Lever Brothers, New York, NY) (Frosch & Kligman, 1979) and mild shampoos (e.g., baby shampoo) with gentle washing may be recommended while the skin is dry and intact. Soaps are generally alkaline (pH 9–10) and may irritate damaged skin. Cleansers and soaps with a pH closer to that of skin (pH 6.8) may be less irritating, but soaps and cleansers should not be used on badly irritated skin (Arndt, 1995).

Erythema and dry desquamation may be treated with topical applications of lotions or creams (Malkinson, 1993). Ointments are better tolerated on inflamed skin than are creams, lotions, or gels (Arndt, 1995). Some believe that topical corticosteroids have little effect on acute radiation dermatitis (Malkinson, 1993). Others recommend 1 percent hydrocortisone ointment two to three times per day for erythema (Madhu & Rochford, 1993; Panizzon & Goldschmidt, 1991). Topical steroids may mask superficial

Table 8-3 • Recommendations for Reducing Irritants to Irradiated Skin

SUN EXPOSURE

Protect from direct sun exposure: Cover or shade area. After healing, use sunscreen with 15 or greater sun protection factor (SPF).

MECHANICAL IRRITANTS

Minimize friction: Wash area with hands, not with a washcloth; pat dry with soft, clean towel or blow dry with hair dryer on cool setting: wear loose-fitting, soft clothing.

Shave with electric shaver, not blade razor.

Avoid scratching.

Avoid rubbing vigorously and massaging.

Avoid use of tape.

CHEMICAL IRRITANTS

Use only mild soap and rinse thoroughly.

Apply only recommended substances.

Avoid use of deodorants.

Use mild detergent to wash clothing.

THERMAL IRRITANTS

Use tepid water.

Avoid exposure to temperature extremes.

Avoid application of ice packs or heat (e.g., heating pad, hot water bottle, sun lamp).

OTHER

Keep skin folds dry.

Wear cotton clothing (absorbent; allows evaporation of moisture).

Prevent infection.

Adapted with permission from Sitton E (1992b). Early and late radiation-induced skin alterations. Part II: Nursing care of irradiated skin. *Oncology Nursing Forum 19*, 911.

Table 8-4 • Recommendations for Skin Care

Recommendation	Source
ERYTHEMA	
Skin care lotions, creams, gels, or ointments without alcohol, menthol, and other chemical irritants.	Dunne-Daly, 1995; Malkinson, 1993; Sitton, 1992b
1% hydrocortisone ointment.	Madhu & Rochford, 1993; Panizzon & Goldschmidt, 1991; Solan, et al., 1992
DRY DESQUAMATION	
Same as for erythema.	Same as for erythema
Cornstarch in dry areas only.	Dunne-Daly, 1995; Farley, 1991
MOIST DESQUAMATION	
Dressings (e.g., hydrogel, hydrocolloid, polyurethane film)	Dunne-Daly, 1995; Gallagher, 1995; Roof, 1991; Shimm & Cassidy, 1994; Shell, Stanutz, & Grimm, 1986; Sitton, 1992b, Strunk & Maher, 1993
Cleanse with 1/3 strength hydrogen peroxide, normal saline, or a wound cleanser.	Dunne-Daly, 1995; Gallagher, 1995; Sitton, 1992b, Solan, et al., 1992; Strunk & Maher, 1993
Silver sulfadiazine	Shimm & Cassidy, 1994; Solan, et al., 1992

infections. Hydrophilic topical ointments such as Aquaphor (Beiersdorf, Inc., Norwalk, CT), Eucerin (Beiersdorf, Inc.), and Lubriderm (Warner-Lambert Company, Morris Plains, NJ) are soothing, relieve dryness, and are frequently recommended for dry desquamation.

Cornstarch may be recommended for dry desquamation and erythema but should not be used in areas of moist desquamation. A moist environment provides an opportunity for the cornstarch to ferment, producing glucose, and promote fungal growth. Cornstarch is absorbent and must be thoroughly removed before reapplication in order to prevent abrasive conglomerates.

Areas of moist desquamation should be kept clean and free of crusts in order for reepithelialization to occur (Madhu & Rochford, 1993). Reepithelialization starts from the periphery of the moist desquamation area and from surviving cells within the treated area. Astringents and antiseptics such as hydrogen peroxide, hypochlorite (Dakin's solution), aluminum acetate solutions [e.g., Domeboro (Miles, Inc., West Haven, CT)], or iodine solutions have been recommended to cleanse the area. However, these agents interfere

with fibroblast migration and epithelial proliferation and do not promote effective wound healing, which is promoted by autolytic debriding hydrogels (Shimm & Cassady, 1994).

A moist wound environment facilitates healing by enhancing the rate of reepithelialization (Arndt, 1995). Occlusive dressings prevent the wound from drying, protect it from trauma, help promote healing, and promote comfort. Wound fluid contains both inflammatory cells that aid in digestion of necrotic debris and helps prevent infection, and growth factors that can affect epidermal migration (Arndt, 1995). Hydrogels such as Vigilon (Bard Home Health Division, Murray Hill, NJ) are frequently recommended for moist desquamation because they absorb wound exudate, are nonadherent, and can easily be removed for the radiation treatment (Dunne-Daly, 1995; Gallagher, 1995; Roof, 1991; Shimm & Cassidy, 1994; Sitton, 1992b; Strunk & Maher, 1993). Hydrocolloids such as Duoderm (E.R. Squibb & Sons, Inc., Princeton, NJ) quickly absorb fluid from the surface of the skin thus reducing the potential for maceration, but are more difficult to remove for treatment.

Moisture-vapor-permeable (MVP) dressings such as Tegaderm (3M Health Care, St. Paul, MN) were found to be effective in patients with moderate to severe radiation effects (Shell et al., 1986). However, these dressings are nonabsorbent and fluid accumulation in moist desquamation under the dressing may cause maceration of the tissues. They also adhere to the skin and may strip new epithelium when removed. An advantage of MVP dressings is that they are not thick enough to act as bolus material and do not need to be removed prior to treatment. Silver sulfadiazine (Silvadene) has broad antibacterial action and may be prescribed twice daily for moist desquamation.

Ascorbic acid is an antioxidant and has been shown to radioprotect nonmalignant tissue. Halperin and associates (1993) evaluated the effectiveness of topical ascorbic acid in prevention of radiation dermatitis. Percutaneous absorption studies demonstrated that 12 percent of the ascorbic acid solution (10 percent solution) traversed the stratum corneum in 72 hours. However, no significant difference in skin reaction was found between the ascorbic acid solution and placebo.

Sucralfate cream has antiinflammatory properties and stimulates cell growth. This cream was evaluated in a randomized, double-blind study of 44 patients receiving electron beam to the chest wall postmastectomy (Maiche et al., 1994). Patients served as their own controls using sucralfate cream to one side of the scar and a placebo on the other side twice daily during and for 2 weeks after treatment. The investigators found that sucralfate had a protective effect on the skin during irradiation. Skin areas to which sucralfate cream was applied had significantly less skin reaction and faster recovery after completion of treatment.

Dini and colleagues (1993) conducted a phase I study of Bioshield (Farmitalia Carlo Erba, Milan, Italy), a nonpharmacological topical product with a mixture of hydrophobic (stearic acid) and hydrophilic (propylene glycol, glycerol, and polyunsaturated alcohols) substances in a foam emulsion. The product, which is only available in Italy, was tested for its tolerability and effectiveness in treatment of early skin reactions to radiation. The product was well-tolerated and results of the study were encouraging, with disappearance of symptoms in 58 percent of patients.

Late Effects of Irradiation

Late radiation changes are progressive and may begin to appear 10 weeks after irradiation (Archambeau et al., 1995; Panizzon & Goldschmidt, 1991). Late effects may not be evident for years after treatment. They include atrophy, fibrosis, xerosis (dry skin), hypo- or hyperpigmentation, telangiectasia, and necrosis. The skin becomes thinned and dry. Atrophy and fibrosis in the dermis and subcutaneous tissue are due to response of dermal fibrocytes to irradiation (see Figure 8–5 and Color Plate 4) (Archambeau et al., 1995; Martin et al., 1993). Atrophy may be due to fibrocyte loss and reabsorption of collagen. Fibrosis may be a proliferative response of surviving fibrocytes to abnormal amounts of growth factors from injured tissues. This response reflects local repair and consolidation of inflammatory changes (Archambeau et al., 1995; Martin et al., 1993). Mechanisms of fibrosis and its progressive nature are not clear. Fibrosis is characterized by progressive induration, edema, and thickening of the dermis and subcutaneous tissues (Fajardo, 1982) and may cause limitation of motion or nerve entrapment.

A thinned epidermis, and atrophy and fibrosis of the dermis and skin appendages, result from irradiation. Reduced function of sebaceous glands contributes to skin dryness and fragility. Sweat glands are often markedly reduced in number and may show atrophic changes. Xerosis (dry skin) may cause pruritus. Scratching or rubbing the area increases irritation and itching. The aim of thera-

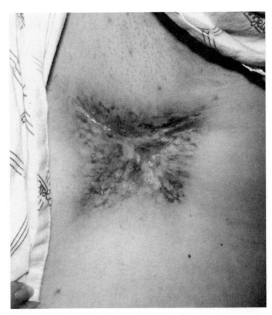

Figure 8-5 • Late skin changes including fibrosis, pigmentation changes, telangiectasia, and retraction in the axilla approximately 2 years after 45 Gy (5Gy × 9 in 4½ weeks) plus hyperthermia for recurrent melanoma.

peutic measures is to keep the skin moist and prevent further drying. Mild soaps or non-soap cleansers and warm rather than hot water may be recommended. Frequent use of lubricating agents is encouraged. These are best applied when the skin is moist, for example, immediately after bathing. The elderly who often have increased problems with dry skin may be more affected by xerosis.

Hypopigmentation indicating skin atrophy and loss of melanocytes may occur after 1 to 5 years in some individuals, especially those with dark skin (Shimm & Cassady, 1994). Endothelial cells of small arteries, capillaries, and sinusoids are vulnerable to the effects of radiation (Fajardo & Berthrong, 1988). Fibrosis in small arteries within the irradiated volume of tissue results in narrowing or obliteration. Upper dermal capillaries, venules, and lymphatics frequently become dilated (Malkinson, 1993). Telangiectasia (dilated vascular channels) appear as red, prominent, thin-walled blood vessels, often within 1 to 2 years after irradiation (see Figure 8–6 and Color Plate 5). Reduction of blood flow reduces the availability of oxygen and nutrients to area tissues. Minor trauma to the atrophic irradiated skin may result in ulceration and necrosis. Necrosis is related to vascular insufficiency (Hopewell, 1990).

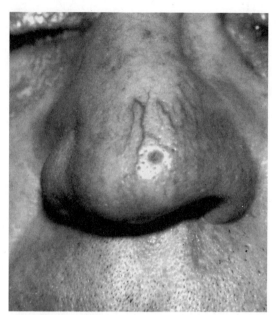

Figure 8-6 • Late skin changes of telangiectasia approximately 2 years after interstitial implant for squamous cell carcinoma of the nasal vestibule.

Carcinogenesis

Historically, a number of benign disorders were treated with ionizing radiation including ringworm of the scalp, acne of the face, hyperthyroidosis, eczema, and tuberculous lymphadenitis. In addition, people with tuberculosis often had multiple fluoroscopies. Many cases of chronic radiodermatitis and skin cancer have been reported from these uses. Ionizing radiation exposure has been associated with an increased risk of development of secondary skin cancer especially in areas associated with higher radiation dose, larger skin volume irradiated, individuals with less melanin pigmentation, and postradiation chronic exposure to sun (Malkinson, 1993; Modan et al., 1993; Panizzon & Goldschmidt, 1991; Shore, 1990). Secondary radiation-induced malignancies in the treated field generally occur after a latent period of 10 to 15 years (Shimm & Cassady, 1994) and can range from 4 to 40 years with a median of 24.5 years (Panizzon & Goldschmidt, 1991). Multiple lesions can develop, particularly in areas of chronic radiodermatitis. The skin is much less likely to develop potentially fatal radiation-induced cancers than are other tissues. For example, lesions are more easily detected early than tumors deeper within the body. Secondary malignancies reported include basal cell carcinoma (BCC) (most frequent), squamous cell carcinoma (SCC), and infrequently, fibrosarcoma. Sarcoma of the scalp has been reported years after cranial irradiation (Chang et al., 1995).

Management of Late Effects

Because late effects of radiation therapy cannot be altered once the lesion is present, nursing management is aimed at symptom relief, prevention of injury and infection, and promotion of healing.

Topical application of oil-in-water emulsions reduces dryness, and occasional use of topical corticosteroids may reduce inflammation and pruritus (Malkinson, 1993).

Late ulcerations and necrosis (extremely rare) of irradiated skin may occur years after treatment with high doses of radiation. Precipitating factors include trauma, chronic friction or pressure, local infection, sun exposure, and progressive atrophy with deep blood vessel occlusion. Ulcerations are generally painful, slow to heal, and persistent. Chronic ulcerations must be differentiated from carcinoma. Management includes prevention of infection as in moist desquamation reactions. Surgical management is sometimes required with skin graft after excision using wide and deep margins to ensure relatively healthy tissue to allow engraftment.

Summary

The response of skin to irradiation is highly complex and is dependent upon many radiation-related, patient-related, and treatment-related factors. No standardized treatment of skin reactions related to radiation therapy exists at this time. There are numerous recommendations in the literature but a paucity of research. Patient education regarding care of early and late manifestations of radiation skin effects is an essential part of the nursing management of the patient undergoing radiation therapy. In addition to avoiding irritants and applying only recommended products, likely effects of irradiation must be explained to the patient in order to prevent unnecessary alarm.

Fatigue

Fatigue has been described as the most frequently reported symptom of cancer and cancer treatment (Nail & Jones, 1995; Oberst et al., 1991; Smets et al., 1993; Winningham et al., 1994). Fatigue has been reported in 65 to 100 percent of patients undergoing radiation therapy (Blesch et al., 1991; Fobair et al., 1986; Nail & Jones, 1995). The pathophysiology of fatigue is unknown. Fatigue may affect quality of life, overall level of comfort, physical functioning, concentration, and social activities. Understanding the nature of fatigue and working with patients to adapt to it is an important aspect in the effective management of the patient undergoing radiation therapy.

Historically, fatigue in the cancer patient received little attention and few published studies examined this phenomenon. Smets and associates (1993) performed a Medline literature search for the years 1980 to 1991 with the parameters of fatigue (included in the title) and cancer (either in the title, a keyword, or in the abstract). Eight of the nine references found in this search were in the nursing literature. Recently, more emphasis has been placed on this very prevalent symptom experienced by cancer patients. Since Haylock and Hart (1979) published their article on radiation and fatigue, numerous studies and observations in radiation oncology have addressed fatigue as an effect related to radiation therapy.

Fatigue and Cancer

Patients with cancer have many factors influencing fatigue including the disease process, other concomitant diseases, and treatment and psychological issues of dealing with the diagnosis and treatment of cancer. Irvine and associates (1991) listed possible correlates of fatigue in patients with cancer as sleep/rest patterns, psychological distress, anemia, weight loss, and functional performance. Fatigue related to cancer treatment may have a profound effect on quality of life (Nail & Jones, 1995). Noyes and associates (1990) measured the physical and emotional distress related to the disease in 400 patients with cancer. They found that physical manifestations of cancer were the greatest overall source of distress, and that loss of energy and pain were ranked as most distressing.

Piper and associates (1987) and Varricchio (1995) differentiated acute and chronic fatigue (see Table 8–5). Acute fatigue serves a protective function and is characterized by localized intermittent symptoms, rapid onset, and short duration. It is generally perceived as an expected tiredness. Chronic fatigue has no known function and is characterized by constant or recurrent tiredness lasting a minimum of a month, insidious onset, and cumulative effects. Chronic fatigue is perceived as abnormal or excessive generalized tired-

Table 8-5 • Acute and Chronic Fatigue

ACUTE FATIGUE
Protective purpose
May result from work performed exceeding available energy resources
Rapid onset
Intermittent, short duration
Expected tiredness
Adequate rest may be effective in management

CHRONIC FATIGUE
Unknown purpose
Insidious onset, cumulative effect
Constant or recurrent tiredness (≥ 1 month)
Perceived as abnormal, excessive, generalized
May involve both somatic and psychological factors
Rest alone is generally not effective in relieving fatigue

Data from Piper BF, Lindsey AM, and Dodd MJ (1987). Fatigue mechanisms in cancer patients: Developing nursing theory. *Oncology Nursing Forum, 14,* 17–23 and Varricchio CG (1995). Measurement issues in fatigue. *Quality of Life—A Nursing Challenge, 4,* 20–24.

ness. Patients with cancer may experience both acute and chronic fatigue.

Early research on fatigue focused on

1. physical performance,
2. efforts to understand fatigue related to a reduction in performance, and
3. methods of improving performance.

This early research was most often conducted in the industrial environment and on athletes. A more subjective view of fatigue in which the patients' responses to fatigue are based on their perceptions and not an objective performance test is appropriate when caring for patients with cancer (Nail & Winningham, 1993; Piper et al., 1987; Varricchio, 1995). Fatigue can be considered a subjective phenomenon described by many terms including tiredness, weakness, exhaustion, lack of energy, lack of purpose, lethargy, sleepiness, malaise, generalized lassitude, changes in ability to concentrate, impaired mobility, increased discomfort and decreased functional status related to a decrease in energy, increased discomfort and decreased efficiency, and generalized weariness. Nail and Winningham (1995) have written an excellent review comparing fatigue and weakness in the cancer patient. They describe weakness as a decrease in muscle strength or endurance compared with a baseline level. Many definitions of fatigue appear in the literature (see Table 8–6). Most often, fatigue is considered a multidimensional, subjective phenomenon.

In addition to physical descriptions of fatigue, difficulty in thinking, forgetfulness, and inability to concentrate are cognitive impairments associated with fatigue in patients with cancer (Cimprich, 1993; Cimprich, 1995; Haylock & Hart, 1979; Rhodes et al., 1988). Psychological factors also influence fatigue in the cancer patient. Depression is frequently associated with fatigue, and fatigue has been found to be significantly related to mood and intensity of pain (Blesch et al., 1991). Patients treated for Hodgkin's disease who continued to experience low energy levels were found to have higher depression scores (Fobair et al., 1986). Depression may be not only a cause but also a result of persistent feelings of tiredness (Smets et al., 1993).

No universal research-based definition of fatigue has been accepted, which makes fatigue research and measurement difficult. A major difficulty is differentiating causes, indicators, and effects of fatigue (Rhodes & McDaniel, 1995; Winningham et al., 1994). Mechanisms of fatigue are unclear, and measurement of this subjective symptom is difficult.

Models of Fatigue in Cancer

Models of fatigue in cancer make an attempt to link concepts of fatigue with contributing factors and manifestations (Aistars, 1987). The Integrated Fatigue Model (IFM) includes indicators of fatigue that are subjective (perceptual) and objective (physiological, biochemical, and behavioral) (see Figure 8–7) (Piper et al., 1987). Mechanisms considered most likely to influence fatigue were:

accumulation of metabolites, changes in energy and energy substrate patterns (possibly due to conditions such as cachexia, anorexia, infection), activity/rest patterns, sleep/wake patterns, disease patterns, treatment patterns, symptom patterns, psychological patterns, oxygenation patterns, changes in regulation/transmission patterns, and other related patterns. No attempt is made in this model to identify which, if any, variables are more important than others. This model, though, may guide the assessment of possible etiologies of fatigue in order to select appropriate interventions.

Winningham's psychobiologic-entropy model associates fatigue, disease, treatment, activity, symptoms, energy, and functional status (Winningham et al., 1994) (see Figure 8–8). Fatigue may be a primary symptom related to preexisting conditions, disease, and treatment, or a secondary symptom related to the patient's response to other symptoms (Nail & Winningham, 1993). In this model, fatigue is defined as an energy deficit, and fatigue and other symptoms are related to the patient's activity and functional status. Balance between activity and rest is an important concept. Nursing management of fatigue may be based on this model. Winningham (1995a) includes five propositions central to relating activity and rest, symptom management, and fatigue in cancer. At the 1995 Oncology Nursing Society Fatigue Initiative through Research and Education (FIRE) Conference, Winningham expanded these to ten propositions (Winningham, 1995b) (see Table 8–7).

Table 8-6 • Definitions of Fatigue

Definition	Resource
A subjective self-evaluation of sensations associated with discomfort, decrease in motor and mental skill, and increased task aversion.	Haylock & Hart, 1979
A subjective feeling of tiredness that is influenced by circadian rhythm.	Piper, Lindsey, & Dodd, 1987
A condition characterized by subjective feelings of generalized weariness, weakness, exhaustion, and lack of energy resulting from prolonged stress that is directly or indirectly attributable to the disease process.	Aistars, 1987
A condition characterized by the subjective feeling of increased discomfort and decreased functional status related to decreased energy.	Pickard-Holley, 1991
A multidimensional concept with several modes of expression: physical, cognitive, in activity or in motivation, acute or chronic.	Smets et al., 1993
An energy deficit related to concepts of disease, treatment, activity, rest, symptom perception, and functional status.	Winningham et al., 1994
A subjective feeling of tiredness that is affected by circadian rhythm and that can change in unpleasantness, variation, intensity, and the amount of distress it causes.	Rhodes & McDaniel, 1995

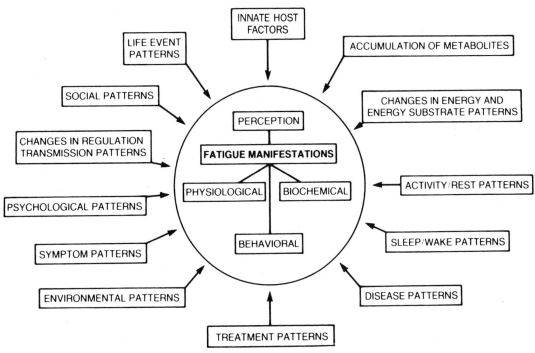

Figure 8-7 • Piper's Integrated Fatigue Model. Reproduced with permission from Piper BF, Lindsey AM, & Dodd MJ (1987). Fatigue mechanisms in cancer patients: Developing nursing theory. *Oncology Nursing Forum, 14,* 19.

Quality of Life

The patient with cancer is often confronted with increased psychosocial and physical demands of the cancer diagnosis and treatment. Fatigue affects many dimensions of the cancer patient's life and may result in impairment of function interfering with quality of life (see Table 8–8).

Donnelly and Walsh (1995) reported a prospective study of prevalence and severity of symptoms in 1000 patients with advanced cancer. Three of the six most frequent clinically important symptoms related to concepts often associated with fatigue are easy fatigue (67 percent), weakness (64 percent), and lack of energy (59 percent). More than 75 percent of the patients who reported these symptoms rated them as moderate to severe.

Fatigue, pain, decrease in appetite, and insomnia were the most important symptoms described in 56 patients with newly diagnosed lung cancer in a study by McCorkle and Quint-Benoliel (1983). Mood disturbances were also reported by these cancer patients.

Measurement of Fatigue

Measurement of the multidimensional experience of fatigue is difficult and may be influenced by a number of factors including timing of assessment, the patient's culture, the patient's developmental stage, and medications. Self-report instruments are frequently used to measure fatigue as a subjective phenomenon. This symptom has most often been measured by single items in general symptom lists such as the Symptom Distress Scale (McCorkle & Young, 1978), the Symptom Profile (King et al., 1985), or the fatigue subscale of the Profile of Mood States (POMS) (Spiegel et al., 1981). A number of scales have been used to measure fatigue in patients with cancer including the Rhoten Fatigue Scale (Rhoten, 1982), Fatigue Feeling Checklist (Pearson & Byers, 1956), Fatigue Symptom Checklist (Kogi, et al., 1970), and Piper Fatigue Self-Report Scale (Piper et al., 1989a) (see Table 8–9). A new instrument, the Multidimensional Fatigue Inventory (MFI) has recently been developed to measure fatigue (Smets et al., 1995). Patients with cancer receiving radiation therapy were one of seven groups used to test the MFI.

Fatigue in Radiation Oncology

Fatigue experienced by the patient undergoing radiation therapy has been documented in numerous

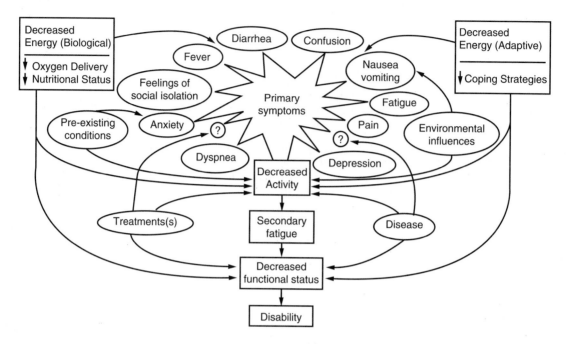

Figure 8-8 • The Psychobiological-Entropy Model of Functioning. Copyright © 1995 by Maryl L. Winningham. All rights reserved. Used with written consent of the author.

publications. Although the etiology is unclear, this symptom increases over the course of treatment (Graydon et al., 1995; Haylock & Hart, 1979; King et al., 1985; Kobashi-Schoot et al., 1985). In their early study of fatigue, Haylock and Hart (1979) used a 30-question checklist describing the experience of fatigue. Thirty patients undergoing external beam irradiation to localized fields completed this checklist daily throughout the course of radiation therapy. Fatigue feeling scores were found to be significantly lower on Sundays. This correlates with the weekend break from treatment that is characteristic of most regimens. This weekend effect has not been found in other studies (Greenberg et al., 1992; Kobashi-Schoot et al., 1985). A statistically significant increase in mean fatigue scores from the beginning of treatment to the end was found.

King and associates (1985) interviewed 96 subjects weekly during the radiation therapy course and then monthly for 3 months afterward using the Symptom Profile developed for the study. Fatigue was reported in patients with chest (93 percent), head and neck (68 percent), prostate and bladder (65 percent), and gynecologic (72 percent) irradiation. Peak incidence of fatigue occurred in most groups from the third week through the end of treatment and was reported as

continuous during the last 2 weeks. Subjects described fatigue as worse in the afternoon and reported that resting or sleeping at that time helped reduce fatigue. Fatigue persisted through the third month after treatment in a substantial number of patients. Greenberg and colleagues (1992) also found fatigue in patients being irradiated to most likely occur in the late afternoon and early evening.

Kobashi-Schoot and colleagues (1985) developed four scales: physical fatigue scale, mental fatigue scale, malaise scale, and psychological complaint scale. Over the course of the radiation treatments, physical fatigue (especially in the third week of treatment) and malaise were found to increase significantly. Two thirds of patients reported feelings of mental fatigue. Patients with malignant lymphoma and uterine cancer described significant decrease in malaise after the weekend compared to no significant decrease in patients with breast or bladder cancer irradiation.

Seventy-five of 76 patients (99 percent) receiving either radiation therapy or chemotherapy for breast or lung cancer experienced fatigue (Blesch et al., 1991). Two-thirds of these patients described their fatigue as moderate to severe. Fatigue intensity was significantly correlated with pain severity and psychological variables of the

Table 8-7 • Ten Propositions Explaining Fatigue in Cancer

1. Too much rest as well as too little rest contributes to increased feelings of fatigue.
2. Too little activity as well as too much activity contributes to increased feelings of fatigue.
3. A relative balance between activity and rest promotes restoration—an imbalance promotes fatigue and deconditioning.
4. Deconditioning is the adaptive energetic response whereby an organism's biological work potential is decreased over time.
5. Everyday energy expenditure in activity is the most potent known regulator of the body's energy systems. ("Use it or lose it.")
6. Any symptom/condition that contributes to decreased activity will lead to deconditioning, increased fatigue, and decreased functional status.
7. Any intervention that provides relief of a symptom/condition which contributes to decreased activity may simultaneously serve to mitigate fatigue and promote functioning providing that intervention does not have a sedating or catabolic effect.
8. The experience of fatigue potentiates distress associated with other symptoms/conditions.
9. The experience of other symptoms/conditions potentiates feelings of fatigue.
10. Deconditioning and perceived fatigue interact to make every aspect of life more stressful and negatively impact quality of life, thus contributing to increased suffering.

Profile of Mood States (POMS) (fatigue-inertia, tension-anxiety, depression-dejection, anger-hostility, and confssion-bewilderment subscales).

Faithfull (1991) reported that 100 percent of patients receiving cranial irradiation reported a "somnolence syndrome," which is excessive sleepiness, drowsiness, lethargy, and anorexia. Six weeks of data collection began after completion of radiation therapy and no pretreatment data were collected in patients with brain tumors. The sample size included only seven patients who completed the study.

Greenberg and associates (1992) studied 15 women undergoing breast irradiation who completed three daily measures of fatigue. They reported mild fatigue with no reduction on weekends, with a decrease over the first three weeks posttreatment. Patients with lung cancer treated with radiation therapy reported fatigue and skin problems as the most frequent side effects (Larson et al., 1993).

Fobair and colleagues (1986) used a questionnaire to survey 403 long-term survivors of Hodgkin's disease to determine type and frequency of problems. Radiation therapy was used either alone or in combination with chemotherapy in 95 percent of subjects. Median time since treatment was 9 years. Ninety percent of patients reported energy loss during treatment. Satisfactory energy levels had not returned in 37 percent of patients and the remaining 63 percent indicated that 12 to 16 months or more were required for normal energy levels to return after treatment. Longer intervals for energy return were related to age over 30 years and combined therapy for advanced stage disease. Patients with energy loss were also more likely to be depressed.

After completion of a course of radiation therapy, fatigue may persist for a period of time (Fobair et al., 1986; Graydon, 1994; King et al., 1985; Nail, 1993). This phenomenon is not well understood. King and colleagues (1985) studied the onset, frequency, duration, and severity of radiation side effects, including fatigue. Study subjects were being treated to chest, head and neck, genitourinary, and gynecological sites. Weekly interviews during treatment and monthly interviews after completion for 3 months were done using a symptom checklist that included a single fatigue item. All

Table 8-8 • Impact of Fatigue

Dimension	Potential Impact
Emotional	Mood alteration (e.g., depression, irritability, decreased patience); decreased coping ability; decreased motivation
Cognitive	Decreased directed attention; impaired thinking, attention, and concentration; impaired ability to make treatment decisions; decreased ability to learn information related to cancer and its treatment
Activities	Impaired performance; reduced ability to set goals, plan, initiate, or persist in activity requiring effort; decreased activity; decreased movement; low energy levels; other physical distress; rest/sleep increase; impaired performance
Family	Parenting; relationships; sexuality; role changes
Social/Cultural	Decreased social functioning; social withdrawal; changes in nature of interactions; cultural expectations; withdrawal; isolation; dependence on others
Occupational/Role	Absenteeism; lack of concentration; financial impact; health insurance issues
Symptoms	Adherence to treatment regimen
Spiritual	Quality of life; meaning; suffering

Table 8-9 • Measurement of Fatigue

Measurement	Source	Description
Symptom Distress Scale	McCorkle & Young, 1978	General symptom checklist
Symptom Profile	King et al., 1985	General symptom 15-item checklist and Likert-type scale for severity rating
Profile of Mood States (POMS)	Spiegel et al., 1981	General 65-word symptom checklist. Most frequently used fatigue measure in cancer research. Developed as a mood scale. Validity established.
Rhoten Fatigue Scale	Rhoten, 1982	Cancer symptom checklist. Visual analog scale and rating scale, 4 general categories for subjective responses and objective checklist.
Fatigue Feeling Checklist	Pearson & Byars, 1956	Ten-item checklist. Measure of subject's level of fatigue.
Fatigue Symptom Checklist	Kogi, 1970	Written to assess fatigue in work situations. Thirty symptoms in 3 subscales: general feelings of sleepiness, mental feelings of fatigue, and physical sensations
Piper Fatigue Self-Report Scale	Piper et al., 1989a	Four dimensions of fatigue: temporal, intensity, affective, and sensory. 41 visual analog scales
Multidimensional Fatigue Inventory (MFI)	Smets et al., 1995	20-item self-report to assess fatigue in 4 dimensions: general fatigue, physical fatigue, mental fatigue, reduced motivation, and reduced activity

groups identified fatigue as a predominant side effect during treatment. The majority reported that their most pronounced period of fatigue occurred in the afternoon, and a substantial number reported a gradual decline but persistence of fatigue into the third month following treatment.

Fifty-three women who had radiation therapy after breast-conserving surgery for cancer were interviewed a mean of 7 weeks after completion of the course of radiation therapy. Results indicated little change in their usual functioning and level of emotional distress and very few symptoms following irradiation (Graydon, 1994). Fatigue was reported by patients and was correlated with a poorer level of functioning. Problems related to insomnia and fatigue were the most often reported symptoms in this study. Results also indicated that fatigue was still present in some women 4 to 12 weeks after completion of radiation therapy.

Nail (1993) described the nature and severity of side effects, level of negative mood, level of disruption in usual activities, and use of coping strategies of 30 women undergoing intracavitary irradiation for gynecological cancer. The highest level of fatigue (reported on the POMS) was on the day after treatment as compared to before, during, and one to two weeks after treatment. Patients were on complete bed rest during the brachytherapy procedure, a factor that may also contribute to fatigue. Fatigue level continued to remain higher than the pretreatment level 1 to 2 weeks after completion of treatment. Persistent fatigue has

implications for planning of patient care. This information should be included in preprocedure patient education and guide nursing management after treatment.

Factors Contributing to Fatigue

Exact mechanisms causing fatigue are unknown. Fatigue may be related to both the disease process and treatments including surgery, radiation therapy, chemotherapy, and biotherapy. Treatment factors may play a significant role in the incidence of fatigue. For the patient with cancer receiving radiation therapy, certain factors may be present that can be identified as actual or potential causes of fatigue. These factors include:

- *Destruction of cells by radiation therapy*. Haylock and Hart (1979) discussed radiation-related cellular breakdown with accumulation of by-products as a possible cause of fatigue. This hypothesis has not yet been tested.
- *Decreased nutrition*. Several symptoms related to radiation therapy of specific sites may contribute to decreased nutrition (less than body requirements). These include mucositis, xerostomia, nausea, vomiting, esophagitis, gastritis, and diarrhea. Decreased intake, depletion of protein stores, anorexia, and metabolic changes may contribute to lack of energy and fatigue. Haylock and Hart (1979) described a positive relationship between fatigue and weight loss in 30 patients receiving radiation therapy. Abnormal muscle function due to

imbalance of metabolites and possible loss of muscle mass may result from malnutrition.

- *Anemia.* In the patient undergoing radiation therapy, anemia can result when large areas of active bone marrow are treated. Anemia reduces the oxygen-carrying ability of the blood and may contribute to fatigue.

- *Combination therapy.* With combined modality therapy more patients experience either previous or concomitant chemotherapy, which may increase fatigue during radiation therapy. Recent surgery may also contribute to increased levels of fatigue during radiation.

- *Drugs used for symptom control.* Medications with sedative effects used to control a variety of symptoms associated with the disease or side effects of treatment may have an effect on fatigue. These include analgesics, antiemetics, some antidepressants, anticonvulsants, and hypnotics. Insomnia has been identified as a problem in the patient with cancer and can contribute to the patient's tiredness (McCorkle & Quint, 1983). Drugs used to control these and other symptoms can also contribute to fatigue.

- *Pain.* Blesch and associates (1991) found a correlation between the severity of pain and intensity of fatigue.

- *Psychologic factors.* Anxiety related to undergoing a course of radiation therapy may adversely affect fatigue levels. Education of patients concerning the treatment modality may reduce anxiety. Fatigue may also accompany depression in cancer patients (Blesch et al., 1991; Fobair et al., 1986; Smets et al., 1993).

- *Role performance.* Many patients continue to maintain as normal as possible daily routines and activities during the weeks of their radiation therapy course. Treatment related symptom distress can affect their ability to function. Daily trips to the radiation therapy treatment center can be physical and emotional factors in increasing the patient's fatigue. In a study by Oberst et al. (1991) fatigue was found to be the most prevalent and distressing symptom in 72 patients undergoing radiation therapy, and traveling every day for treatment was the most demanding self-care task.

Assessment and Management of Fatigue

Fatigue assessment methods in clinical practice may be similar to those used for pain. The patient's own description of fatigue and possibly a 1 to 10 scale with 1 being no fatigue and 10 being the most fatigue possible may be used (Winningham et al., 1994). Assessment should include information concerning patterns of fatigue, effects on mood and ability to concentrate, nutrition, sleep/rest/activity patterns, factors that increase and relieve fatigue, effect of fatigue on daily life, the meaning of fatigue to the patient, and expression of fatigue within the patient's culture.

Few comprehensive patient education materials are currently available (Skalla & Lacasse, 1992b). Skalla and Lacasse (1992a) developed a patient education tool for management of fatigue using rest, naps, efficient planning, reading, walk/exercise, distraction, sleep, balanced diet, comfort, social activities, and symptom relief. The American College of Physicians (1994) included a chapter on tiredness and fatigue in their book written for patients and families about caring at home for the patient with cancer. The chapter includes an overview of the home-care plan for tiredness and fatigue, which addresses the following topics: understanding the problem, when to get professional help, what you can do to help, possible obstacles, and carrying out and adjusting your plan. Recommendations include suggestions for assisting the patient to get the most out of the day by planning, prioritizing, balancing activity and rest, and relaxing. Possible obstacles and adjusting the plan of care are addressed.

Fatigue can have a profound effect on the patient treated for cancer affecting many dimensions of the individual's life. Although recommendations are frequently made for management of fatigue by health care professionals, research-based interventions for fatigue in oncology have not generally been investigated scientifically. Because the underlying etiology of fatigue in the patient with cancer is unknown, interventions are directed toward symptom management, energy (conservation and restoration), and emotional support. Nursing management of fatigue should include collaboration with the patient to achieve the highest possible quality of life. Few research studies have addressed management of fatigue in the radiation therapy setting in spite of reports of fatigue in a large percentage of patients.

Symptom Management

Many factors contribute to the level of fatigue experienced by patients with cancer. Treatment-related fatigue is an expected, transient side effect. Fatigue directly related to radiation therapy is usually self-limiting (King et al., 1985). However, several months may be required for patients to recover completely from radiation-induced fatigue. This is an important factor to include in patient education. While the severity and duration of fatigue are not always predictable, the radiation oncology nurse can offer guidelines in addition to adequate rest to the patients for anticipating and managing fatigue and utilizing their energy most effectively.

Specific symptoms experienced by the patient treated with radiation therapy should be addressed. Careful monitoring of blood counts, with blood transfusions and/or recombinant erythropoietin when indicated can help relieve anemia. Side effects of treatment that contribute to fatigue such as pain, nausea, vomiting, and diarrhea should be kept to a minimum with drug and nondrug interventions. Adequate nutrition, hydration, and electrolyte balance may contribute to the patient's feelings of well-being.

Strategies to Reduce Fatigue

Graydon and associates (1995) studied strategies that patients used to reduce fatigue while undergoing chemotherapy or radiation therapy. Strategies were categorized in four dimensions: (a) reducing or ceasing activity (lie down, nap, sit, sleep, stop what one's doing), (b) increasing physical or social activity (exercise, socialize, walk), (c) distraction (listen to music, read, watch TV), and (d) other (ask for help, do something different, eat or drink, work). Effective strategies among 54 women receiving radiation therapy were found to include sleeping, exercise, doing something different, and talking to friends. Patients can be encouraged to anticipate a decrease in their fatigue level during the weekend, as found by Haylock and Hart (1979).

It is not uncommon for patients with cancer to be advised to rest. However, too much rest and too little activity may result in physiologic deterioration, fatigue, and reduced functional status (Winningham, 1995a; Winningham et al., 1994). Rest alone is frequently not effective in patients with multiple factors influencing fatigue, especially if the patient is experiencing chronic fatigue. Understanding factors that contribute to fatigue is essential for development of interventions to reduce or prevent fatigue. The nurse can work with patients to conserve energy and develop activity/rest patterns based on assessment of the fatigue.

Functional capacity and independence can be impaired by side effects of cancer treatment and resulting inactivity (Wells, 1990). Beneficial effects of exercise have been studied in cancer patients. Exercise training in individuals with cancer has been shown to significantly improve functional capacity (MacVicar et al., 1989). In a study of women with breast cancer, the women who exercised had a significantly higher quality of life compared to nonexercisers (Young-McCaughan & Sexton, 1991). Women with breast cancer receiving chemotherapy had physical and psychosocial benefits from a modest walking exercise program and support group (Mock et al., 1994). All subjects in both groups reported fatigue at some time during treatment. However, those in the experimental group were able to consistently and progressively increase physical activity levels over the course of chemotherapy, whereas the standard care group experienced a progressive decrease in activity with comparable chemotherapy. Lower levels of fatigue and nausea were also found in the group of exercising women.

Patients with cancer must be carefully evaluated prior to beginning any program involving exercise. For example, weight-bearing exercise may be contraindicated in patients with bone metastases. Cachectic patients may not be able to participate in exercise programs.

Patients who have been treated for cancer are likely to be more sedentary after treatment than prediagnosis. Bloom et al. (1990) found that among 85 men who had been treated for Hodgkin's disease, more sedentary activities were correlated with higher scores on the Fatigue subscale of the POMS and more active patterns were correlated with higher scores on the Vigor subscale of the POMS and self-reports of higher energy and health status.

Piper et al. (1989b) described three strategies useful for effective management of fatigue: energy conservation, effective energy utilization, and energy restoration. Recommendations to limit expenditure of energy may be made. Rest helps conserve energy. Reducing nonessential activities will also conserve energy. Asking or allowing others to help with home activities such as cleaning, cooking, shopping, transportation, and care of children will also contribute to conservation of energy. Prioritizing, careful planning, and scheduling of activities can be effective in efficient use of available energy. Maintenance of normal night-time sleep patterns and good nutrition may contribute to energy restoration. Resting or napping during the day may also be helpful. Additional restorative activities may include relaxation or diversion such as social visits, reading, watching television or movies, listening to music, and participating in enjoyable hobbies or activities (Piper et al., 1989b; Skalla & Rieger, 1995).

Cimprich (1993, p.83) defines directed attention as "the capacity to inhibit or block competing stimuli or distractions during purposeful activity." Directed attention is necessary to process information concerning diagnosis and treatment of cancer. Patients with cancer are at risk for developing attentional fatigue with decreased ability to concentrate and direct attention. This fatigue is generally due to high demands made on attentional capacity. Thirty-two women with early breast cancer participated in a study to determine whether an intervention could maintain or restore directed attention (Cimprich, 1993). Restorative activities most frequently selected by participants included walking or sitting in a park, bird watching, or tending flowers or plants. Participants in the intervention group had significant improvement in attentional capacity with three attention-restoring activities for 20 to 30 minutes per week for 3 months.

Two nursing interventions for managing loss of concentration in patients with cancer are recommended by Cimprich (1995). The first intervention is to conserve attentional capacity by decreasing environmental demands that cause attentional fatigue. Environmental demands may be reduced by improving patient education interventions, modifying the health environment to reduce attentional demands, and teaching patients and families strategies to minimize activities requiring attention. The second recommendation is to control the overall level of attentional fatigue by promoting adequate rest and recovery of directed attention.

Emotional Support

Spiegel and associates (1981) conducted a one-year study of the effects of weekly support group meetings for women with metastatic breast cancer. Eighty-six women were randomly assigned to the one-year support group program or control group. All women received psychological tests every four months. Those attending support groups had more vigor and less fatigue. A trend toward decreased depression was shown but was not statistically significant. Management of depression may affect the level of fatigue experienced. In weekly group psychotherapy for cancer patients undergoing radiation therapy, Forester and colleagues (1993) found reduced emotional and physical distress (including fatigue) in those having psychotherapy compared to the control group.

Eighty-two outpatients undergoing radiation therapy were randomly assigned to a relaxation training group or a control group (Decker et al., 1992). The treatment group had reductions in tension, depression, anger, and fatigue. Relaxation training may substantially improve several parameters related to quality of life.

Conclusion

Research related to fatigue in the patient with cancer and particularly in the patient undergoing radiation therapy is in the early stages. Fatigue is an area that provides an opportunity for clinical nursing research and the potential to influence the individual's quality of life. The lack of a clear, accepted definition of fatigue increases the difficulty in measuring this symptom. Research is also hampered by the multiple factors contributing to fatigue in the patient with cancer. Methodology for good measurement and determining the correlates of fatigue may assist in determining effective research-based interventions. Results of the few studies available in radiation therapy-related fatigue can be used to guide nursing assessment, prepare patients for expected side effects during and following radiation therapy, management of fatigue, and evaluation of effectiveness of nursing interventions.

Patient education regarding expectations of experiencing treatment-related fatigue may increase the patient's ability to cope with and manage this symptom. In addition, patient education may reduce anxiety related to what could feel to the patient like an unexpected reduction in energy, which may cause fear that tumor progression is the cause of the fatigue. Nursing research in patients with cancer related to assessment and intervention for fatigue should consider the impact on quality of life in the efforts to guide clinical practice. Results of studies in fatigue can be used to guide nursing assessment, prepare patients for expected side effects during and following radiation therapy, manage fatigue, and evaluate the effectiveness of nursing interventions. Providing patients with information about available support services may assist the patient in managing daily activities and responsibilities.

Summary

Radiation therapy is a major treatment modality in cancer management. Patients undergoing irradiation experience treatment-related side effects that vary in intensity based on many factors. Skin changes and fatigue occur in many patients and must be addressed in patient care management. Skin changes can often be seen and are "concrete" while fatigue is subjective and may not be visible to others. Both generally appear gradually as the radiation dose accumulates. It is important for the patient, family, and significant others to have information about management of these often-distressing side effects in order to minimize their impact on the patient during and following irradiation. Nursing research regarding effective management of both of these side effects is very much needed.

References

Aistars J (1987). Fatigue in the cancer patient: A conceptual approach to a clinical problem. *Oncology Nursing Forum, 14*, 25–30.

American College of Physicians. (1994). Tiredness and fatigue. In PS Houts, AM Nezu, CM Nezu, JA Bucher, A Lipton, & CA Bean (Eds.), *American College of Physicians Home Care Guide for Cancer: How to Care for Family and Friends at Home*, (pp. 33–40).

Archambeau JO, Pezner R, & Wasserman T (1995). Pathophysiology of irradiated skin and breast. *International Journal of Radiation Oncology, Biology, Physics, 31*, 1171–1185.

Arndt KA (1995). Formulary. In KA Arndt (Ed.), *Manual of Dermatologic Therapeutics with Essentials of Diagnosis*, (5th ed., pp. 253–352). Boston: Little, Brown.

Bentzen SM, Turesson I, & Thames HD (1990). Fractionation sensitivity and latency of telangiectasia after postmastectomy radiotherapy: A graded-response analysis. *Radiotherapy and Oncology, 18*, 95–106.

Blesch KS, Paice JA, Wickham R, Harte N, Schnoor DK, Purl S, Rehwalt M, Kopp PL, Manson S, Coveny SB, McHale M, & Cahill M (1991). Correlates of fatigue in people with breast or lung cancer. *Oncology Nursing Forum, 18*, 81–87.

Bloom JR, Gorsky RD, Fobair P, Hoppe R, Cox RS, Varghese A, & Spiegel D (1990). Physical performance at work and at leisure: Validation of a measure of biological energy in survivors of Hodgkin's Disease. *Journal of Psychosocial Oncology, 8*, 49–63.

Chang SM, Barker FG, Larson DA, Bollen AW, & Prados MD (1995). Sarcomas subsequent to cranial irradiation. *Neurosurgery, 36*, 685–690.

Cimprich B. (1993). Development of an intervention to restore attention in cancer patients. *Cancer Nursing, 16*, 83–92.

Cimprich B. (1995). Symptom management: Loss of concentration. *Seminars in Oncology Nursing, 11*, 279–288.

Decker TW, Cline-Elsen J, & Gallagher M (1992). Relaxation therapy as an adjunct in radiation oncology. *Journal of Clinical Psychology, 48*, 388–393.

Dini D, Macchia R, Gozza A, Bertelli G, Forno GG, Guenzi M, Bacigalupo A, Scolaro T, & Vitale V (1993). Management of acute radiodermatitis: Pharmacological or nonpharmacological remedies? *Cancer Nursing, 16*, 366–370.

Donnelly S, & Walsh D (1995). The symptoms of advanced cancer. *Seminars in Oncology, 22*, 67–72.

Dunne-Daly CF (1995). Skin and wound care in radiation oncology. *Cancer Nursing, 18*, 144–162.

Ebling FJ, Eady RA, & Leigh IM (1992). Anatomy and organization of human skin. In RH Champion, JL Burton, & FJ Ebling (Eds.), *Textbook of Dermatology* (5th ed., pp. 49–123). Oxford, England: Blackwell Scientific.

Engin K, Tupchong L, Waterman FM, McFarlane JD, Hoh LL, & Leeper DB (1995). Predictive factors for skin reactions in patients treated with thermoradiotherapy. *International Journal of Hyperthermia, 11*, 357–364.

Faithfull S (1991). Patients' experience following cranial radiotherapy: A study of the somnolence syndrome. *Journal of Advanced Nursing, 16*, 939–946.

Fajardo LF (1982). Skin. In L. Fajardo (Ed.), *Pathology of Radiation Injury*, (pp. 186–199). New York: Masson.

Fajardo LF, & Berthrong M. (1988). Vascular lesions following radiation. *Pathology Annual, 23*, 297–330.

Farley KM (1991). Cornstarch as a treatment for dry desquamation. *Oncology Nursing Forum, 18*, 134.

Fletcher GH (1985). History of irradiation in the primary management of apparently regionally confined breast cancer. *International Journal of Radiation Oncology, Biology, Physics, 11*, 2133–2142.

Fobair P, Hoppe RT, Bloom J, Cox R, Varghese A, & Spiegel D (1986). Psychosocial problems among survivors of Hodgkin's disease. *Journal of Clinical Oncology, 4*, 805–814.

Forester B, Kornfeld DS, Fleiss JL, & Thompson S (1993). Group psychotherapy during radiotherapy: Effects on emotional and physical distress. *American Journal of Psychiatry, 150*, 1700–1706.

Frosch P, & Kligman A (1979). The soap chamber: A new method for assessing the irritancy of soaps. *Journal of the American Academy of Dermatology, 1*, 35–41.

Gallagher, J. (1995). Management of cutaneous symptoms. *Seminars in Oncology Nursing, 11*, 239–247.

Graydon JE (1994). Women with breast cancer: Their quality of life following a course of radiation therapy. *Journal of Advanced Nursing, 19*, 617–622.

Graydon JE, Bubela N, Irvine D, & Vincent L (1995). Fatigue-reducing strategies used by patients receiving treatment for cancer. *Cancer Nursing, 18*, 23–28.

Greenberg D, Sawicka J, Eisenthal S, & Ross D (1992). Fatigue syndrome due to localized radiation. *Journal of Pain and Symptom Management, 7*, 38–45.

Halperin EC, Gaspar L, George S, Darr D, & Pinnell S (1993). A double-blind, randomized, prospective trial to evaluate topical vitamin C solution for the prevention of radiation dermatitis. *International Journal of Radiation Oncology, Biology, Physics, 26*, 413–416.

Haylock PJ, & Hart LK (1979). Fatigue in patients receiving localized radiation. *Cancer Nursing, 2*, 461–467.

Hopewell, JW (1990). The skin: Its structure and response to ionizing radiation. *International Journal of Radiation Biology, 57*, 751–773.

Irvine DM, Vincent L, Bubela N, Thompson L, & Graydon J (1991). A critical appraisal of the research literature investigating fatigue in the individual with cancer. *Cancer Nursing, 14*, 188–199.

King KB, Nail LM, Kreamer K, Strohl RA, & Johnson JE (1985). Patients' descriptions of the experience of receiving radiation therapy. *Oncology Nursing Forum, 12*, 55–61.

Kobashi-Schoot JA, Hanewald GJ, Van Dam FS, & Bruning PF (1985). Assessment of malaise in cancer patients treated with radiotherapy. *Cancer Nursing, 8*, 306–313.

Kogi K, Saito Y, & Mitsuhashi T (1970). Validity of three components of subjective fatigue feelings. *Journal of Scientific Labour, 46*, 251–270.

Larson PJ, Lindsey AM, Dodd MJ, Brecht ML, & Packer A (1993). Influence of age on problems experienced by patients with lung cancer undergoing radiation therapy. *Oncology Nursing Forum, 20*, 473–480.

MacVicar MG, Winningham ML, & Nickel JL (1989). Effects of aerobic interval training on cancer patients' functional capacity. *Nursing Research, 38*, 348–351.

Madhu JJ, & Rochford R (1993). Skin and soft tissue toxicity. In M John, M Flam, S Legha, and T Phillips (Eds.), *Chemoradiation: An Integrated Approach to Cancer Treatment*, (pp. 502–510). Philadelphia: Lea and Febiger.

Maiche A, Isokangas OP, & Grohn P (1994). Skin protection by sucralfate cream during electron beam therapy. *Acta Oncologia, 33*, 201–203.

Malkinson FD (1993). Radiobiology of the skin. In TB Fitzpatrick, AZ Eisen, K Wolff, IM Freedberg, & KF Austen (Eds.), *Dermatology in General Medicine, Volume I*, (4th ed., pp. 1598–1608). New York: McGraw-Hill.

Martin M, Lefaix JL, Pinton P, Crechet F, & Daburon F (1993). Temporal modulation of TGF-β1 and β-actin gene expression in pig skin and muscular fibrosis after ionizing radiation. *Radiation Research, 134*, 63–70.

McCorkle R, & Quint-Benoliel J (1983). Symptom distress, current concerns and mood disturbance after diagnosis of life-threatening disease. *Social Science and Medicine, 17*, 431–438.

McCorkle R, & Young K (1978). Development of a symptom distress scale. *Cancer Nursing, 1*, 373–378.

Mock V, Burke MB, Sheehan P, Creaton EM, Winningham ML, McKenney-Tedder S, Schwager LP, & Liebman M (1994). A nursing rehabilitation program for women with breast cancer receiving adjuvant chemotherapy. *Oncology Nursing Forum, 21*, 899–908.

Modan B, Alfandary E, Shapiro D, Lusky A, Chetrit A, Shewach-Millet M, & Movshovitz M (1993). Factors affecting the development of skin cancer after scalp irradiation. *Radiation Research, 134*, 125–128.

Nail LM (1993). Coping with intracavitary radiation treatment for gynecologic cancer. *Cancer Practice, 1*, 218–224.

Nail LM, & Jones LS (1995). Fatigue as a side effect of cancer treatment: Impact on quality of life. *Quality of Life—A Nursing Challenge, 4*, 8–13.

Nail LM, & Winningham ML (1993). Fatigue. In SL Groenwald, M Goodman, MH Frogge, and CH Yarbro (Eds.), *Cancer Nursing: Principles and Practice*, (3rd ed.), (pp. 608–619). Boston: Jones and Bartlett.

Nail LM, & Winningham ML (1995). Fatigue and weakness in cancer patients: The symptom experience. *Seminars in Oncology Nursing, 11*, 272–278.

Noyes R, Kathol RG, Debelius-Enemark P, Williams J, Mutgi A, Suelzer MT, & Clamon GH (1990). Distress associated with cancer as measured by the illness distress scale. *Psychosomatics, 31*, 321–330.

Nyman J, & Turesson I (1995). Does the interval between fractions matter in the range of 4–8 h in radiotherapy? A study of acute and late human skin reactions. *Radiotherapy and Oncology, 34*, 171–178.

Oberst MT, Hughes SH, Chang AS, & McCubbin MA (1991). Self-care burden, stress appraisal, and mood among persons receiving radiotherapy. *Cancer Nursing, 14*, 71–78.

Overgaard J (1989). The current and potential role of hyperthermia in radiotherapy. *International Journal of Radiation Oncology, Biology, Physics, 16*, 535–549.

Panizzon RG, & Goldschmidt H (1991). Radiation reactions and sequelae. In H Goldschmidt & RG Panizzon (Eds.), *Modern Dermatologic Radiation Therapy*, (pp. 25–36). New York: Springer-Verlag.

Pearson RG, & Byers GE (1956). *The Development and Validation of a Checklist for Measuring Subjective Fatigue*. (Report No. 56–115). Randolph AFB, Texas: School of Aviation, USAF.

Perez CA, & Brady LW (1992). Overview. In CA Perez & LW Brady (Eds.), *Principles and Practice of Radiation Oncology*, (2nd ed., pp. 1–64). Philadelphia: JB Lippincott.

Phillips KA, Urch M, & Bishop JF (1995). Radiation-recall dermatitis in a patient treated with paclitaxel [letter]. *Journal of Clinical Oncology, 13*, 305.

Pickard-Holley S (1991). Fatigue in cancer patients: A descriptive study. *Cancer Nursing, 14*, 13–19.

Piper BF, Lindsey AM, & Dodd MJ (1987). Fatigue mechanisms in cancer patients: Developing nursing theory. *Oncology Nursing Forum, 14*, 17–23.

Piper BF, Lindsey AM, & Dodd MJ (1989a). Development of an instrument to measure the subjective dimension of fatigue. In SG Funk, EM Tournquist, MT Champagne, LA Copp, RA Wiese (Eds.), *Key Aspects of Comfort: Management of Pain, Fatigue and Nausea*, (pp. 199–208). New York: Springer-Verlag.

Piper BF, Rieger PT, Brophy L, Haeuber D, Hood LE, Lyver A, & Sharp E (1989b). Recent advances in the management of biotherapy-related side effects: Fatigue. *Oncology Nursing Forum, 16*, 27–34.

Raghavan VT, Bloomer WD, & Merkel DE (1993). Taxol and radiation-recall dermatitis [letter]. *Lancet, 341*, 1354.

Rhodes VA, & McDaniel RW (1995). Fatigue and advanced illness. *Quality of Life—A Nursing Challenge, 4*, 14–19.

Rhodes VA, Watson PM, & Hanson BM (1988). Patients' descriptions of the influence of tiredness and weakness on self-care abilities. *Cancer Nursing, 11*, 186–194.

Rhoten D (1982). Fatigue and the postsurgical patient. In CM Norris (Ed.), *Concept Clarification in Nursing*, (pp. 277–300). Rockville, MD: Aspen.

Roof LM (1991). The use of Vigilon primary wound dressing in the treatment of radiation dermatitis. *Oncology Nursing Forum, 18*, 133–134.

Russell NS, Knaken H, Bruinvis IA, Hart AA, Begg AC, & Lebesque JV (1994). Quantification of patient to patient variation of skin erythema developing as a response to radiotherapy. *Radiotherapy and Oncology, 30*, 213–221.

Shell JA, Stanutz F, & Grimm J (1986). Comparison of moisture vapor permeable (MVP) dressings to conventional dressings for management of radiation skin reactions. *Oncology Nursing Forum, 13*, 11–16.

Shenkier T, & Gelmon K (1994). Paclitaxel and radiation-recall dermatitis [letter]. *Journal of Clinical Oncology, 12*, 439.

Shimm DS, & Cassady JR (1994). The Skin. In JD Cox (Ed.), *Moss' Radiation Oncology: Rationale, Technique, Results*, (7th ed.), (pp. 99–118). St. Louis, MO: Mosby.

Shore RE (1990). Overview of radiation-induced skin cancer in humans. *International Journal of Radiation Oncology, Biology, Physics, 57*, 809–827.

Sitton E (1992a). Early and late radiation-induced skin alterations part I: Mechanisms of skin changes. *Oncology Nursing Forum, 19*, 801–807.

Sitton E (1992b). Early and late radiation-induced skin alterations part II: Nursing care of irradiated skin. *Oncology Nursing Forum, 19*, 907–912.

Skalla KA, & Lacasse C (1992a). Fatigue and the patient with cancer: What is it and what can I do about it? *Oncology Nursing Forum, 19*, 1540–1541.

Skalla KA, & Lacasse C (1992b). Patient education for fatigue. *Oncology Nursing Forum, 19*, 1537–1539.

Skalla KA, & Rieger PT (1995). Fatigue. In PT Rieger (Ed.), *Biotherapy: A Comprehensive Overview*, (pp. 221–242). Boston: Jones and Bartlett.

Smets EM, Garssen B, Bonke B, & DeHaes JC (1995). The multidimensional fatigue inventory (MFI) psychometric qualities of an instrument to assess fatigue. *Journal of Psychosomatic Research, 39*, 315–325.

Smets EM, Garssen B, Schuster-Uitterhoeve AL, & de Haes JC (1993). Fatigue in cancer patients. *British Journal of Cancer, 68*, 220–224.

Solan MJ, Brady LW, Binnick SA, & Fitzpatrick PJ (1992). In CA Perez & LW Brady (Eds.), *Principles and Practice of Radiation Oncology* (2nd ed., pp. 479–495.). Philadelphia: JB Lippincott.

Spiegel D, Bloom JR, & Yalom I (1981). Group support for patients with metastatic disease. *Archives of General Psychiatry, 38*, 527–533.

Strunk B, & Maher K (1993). Collaborative nurse management of multifactorial moist desquamation in a patient undergoing radiotherapy. *Journal of Enterostomal Therapy Nursing, 21*, 152–157.

Varricchio CG (1995). Measurement issues in fatigue. *Quality of Life—A Nursing Challenge, 4*, 20–24.

Wells R (1990). Rehabilitation: Making the most of time. *Oncology Nursing Forum, 17*, 503–507.

Winningham ML (1995a). Fatigue: The missing link to quality of life. *Quality of Life—A Nursing Challenge, 4*, 2–7.

Winningham ML (1995b). *Ten Propositions Explaining Fatigue in Cancer*. Paper presented at the meeting of the Oncology Nursing Society Fatigue Initiative through Research and Education, Phoenix, AZ.

Winningham ML, Nail LM, Burke MB, Brophy L, Cimprich B, Jones LS, Pickard-Holley S, Rhodes V, St.Pierre B, Beck S, Glass EC, Mock VL, Mooney KH, & Piper B (1994). Fatigue and the cancer experience: The state of the knowledge. *Oncology Nursing Forum, 21*, 23–36.

Woodburn RT (1983). *Essentials of Human Anatomy*, (7th ed.). New York: Oxford University Press.

Yokel BK, & Hood AF (1993). Mucocutaneous complications of antineoplastic therapy. In TB Fitzpatrick, AZ Eisen, K Wolff, IM Freedberg, & KF Austen (Eds.), *Dermatology in General Medicine, Vol. I*, (4th ed., pp. 1795–1806). New York: McGraw-Hill.

Young-McCaughan S, & Sexton DL (1991). A retrospective investigation of the relationship between aerobic exercise and quality of life in women with breast cancer. *Oncology Nursing Forum, 18*, 751–757.

Breast Cancer

SUSAN R. MAZANEC

The spectrum of breast cancer, from early diagnosis to local recurrence to metastatic disease, has overwhelming statistics. In the United States, breast cancer is the most common malignancy in women with an overall lifetime risk of developing the disease as 1 in 8 (Wingo, et al., 1995). The incidence of breast cancer continues to increase. It is estimated that 1.5 million women will be diagnosed with breast cancer during this decade (National Institute of Health (NIH) Consensus Statement, 1990). In 1996, approximately 180,200 women were diagnosed with breast cancer with 44,000 estimated deaths from the disease (Parker et al., 1997). Many women will encounter radiation therapy as part of their treatment regimen.

Radiation therapy plays a key role in breast cancer treatment. With the refinement of treatment planning and improved techniques in delivery, women with early stage breast cancer have an alternative to mastectomy. Radiation therapy also continues to be an integral part of the treatment of women with a local recurrence or metastatic disease.

This chapter will review the use of radiation therapy in the treatment of breast cancer, including the indications for treatment, goals, and technical considerations. Acute and late side effects will be outlined. The nursing role in symptom management, patient education, and supportive care will be discussed.

An Overview of Breast Cancer

To have a better understanding of the role of radiation in the treatment of breast cancer, it is essential to have a general knowledge of breast anatomy, cancer development, and the staging of breast cancer. The breasts or mammary glands are located between the third and sixth or seventh rib and extend from the edge of the sternum to the axilla. They are composed of 15 to 20 lobes, connective tissue, blood vessels, nerves, and lymphatic vessels. Epithelium-lined ducts extend from the numerous saclike, milk secreting structures of the lobes called the alveoli and terminate at the nipple. Just below the nipple and areola, which is the dark skin around the nipple, the ducts dilate and form sinuses, from which many small ducts extend out through the nipple. The glandular and ductal structures of the breast are surrounded by fatty tissue and ligaments that support the breast and attach it to the chest wall and skin.

The superficial lymphatics of the breast are continuous with the skin over the chest wall, abdomen, and neck. These lymphatics end in the subareolar network and eventually drain primarily through the axillary lymph nodes. The deeper lymphatics of the breast drain through three pathways: the axillary, internal mammary, and transpectoral routes. The principal pathway for most of the breast, especially the upper and lower quadrants of the lateral breast, is through the axilla (Wang, 1988). Lymph vessels from the medial and central portion of the breast drain into the internal mammary lymph nodes. The transpectoral route runs through the pectoralis muscles to the ipsilateral supraclavicular lymph node group (Wang, 1988) (Figure 9–1).

The natural history of breast cancer may be variable and unpredictable with periods of indolent activity or aggressive growth and metastasis (Harris et al., 1993). Recent scientific advances have led to a greater understanding of the biology of breast cancer. Hormone sensitivity, measurement of tumor cell kinetics, oncogenes, growth factors, and tumor suppressor genes are areas of study that may enhance the ability to predict tumor behavior, prognosis, and optimal treatment for breast cancer patients. They may also aid the

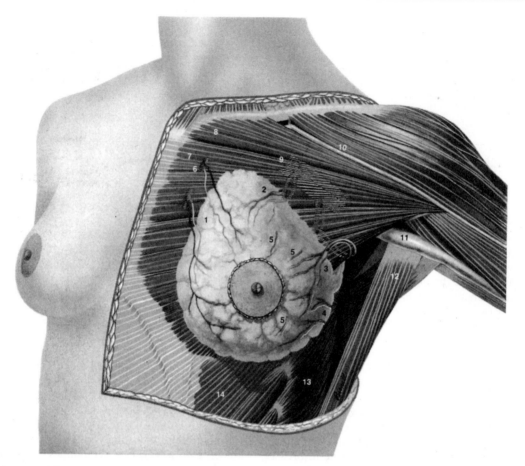

Figure 9-1 • The lymphatic drainage of the breast showing lymph node groups and levels. From Osborne MP (1987). Breast development and anatomy. In JR Harris, S Hellman, IC Henderson, and DW Kinne (Eds.), *Breast Diseases* (pp.1–14). Philadelphia: Lippincott-Raven. Reprinted with permission.

1. Internal mammary artery and vein
2. Substernal cross drainage to contralateral internal mammary lymphatic chain
3. Subclavius muscle and Halsted's ligament
4. Lateral pectoral nerve (from the lateral cord)
5. Pectoral branch from thoracoacromial vein
6. Pectoralis minor muscle
7. Pectoralis major muscle
8. Lateral thoracic vein
9. Medial pectoral nerve (from the medial cord)
10. Pectoralis minor muscle
11. Median nerve
12. Subscapular vein
13. Thoracodorsal vein

A. Internal mammary lymph nodes
B. Apical lymph nodes
C. Interpectoral (Rotter's) lymph nodes
D. Axillary vein lymph nodes
E. Central lymph nodes
F. Scapular lymph nodes
G. External mammary lymph nodes

Level I lymph nodes: lateral to lateral border of pectoralis minor muscle
Level II lymph nodes: behind pectoralis minor muscle
Level III lymph nodes: medial to medial border of pectoralis minor muscle

development of new therapies and preventive measures (Davidson, 1991).

Risk Factors

Risk factors are variables that may be associated to some degree with increased potential for disease development (Morra & Blumberg, 1991). Risk factors may be genetic or environmental. Female gender, advancing age, family history of breast cancer, and history of cancer in the other breast are relevant risk factors (Fleming & Fleming, 1994). Although other risk factors for the development of breast cancer have been identified, age is considered the most significant (Scanlon,

1991). Between the ages of 60 and 79 a woman has a 1 in 14 probability of developing invasive breast cancer, as compared to a 1 in 26 chance between the ages of 40 and 59 (Parker et al., 1996).

Ten to 15 percent of breast cancers occur in patients with a family history (Hulka & Stark, 1995). A family history of breast cancer is a complex risk factor and may vary with the proximity of the relative, the relative's age at diagnosis, and whether the disease was bilateral. A one and one-half to twofold increased risk is associated with an affected first-degree (maternal or paternal) relative. The risk may further increase if the relative's cancer was bilateral and if the diagnosis was made before the age of 40 (Harris et al., 1992). About one-half of familial-related breast cancers are related to a susceptibility gene for breast cancer, called BRCA1, which in a mutant form fails to suppress breast tumor development (Hulka & Stark, 1995). This gene is particularly associated with breast cancer occurring in young women before age 40.

Risk factors that are related to women's reproductive history are based on the belief that endogenous hormones play a role in breast cancer development. Established risk factors associated with a slight increase in risk include: early menarche (less than 12 years), late age at menopause (over 55 years), nulliparity, and more than 30 years old at first full-term pregnancy (Harris et al., 1992, Pt. I). Bilateral oophorectomy, without exogenous estrogen replacement, appears to confer a protective effect in young women (Hulka & Stark, 1995).

The issue of whether the use of exogenous hormones increases one's risk for breast cancer development remains unclear. There is evidence that the use of estrogen supplements in post-menopausal women is associated with a 40 percent increased risk during the period of use and a slight increase in risk after the supplement is stopped, particularly after prolonged use (Harris et al., 1992, Pt. I). When progesterone is combined with estrogen, there is no reduction in risk (Hulka & Stark, 1995). Although there is no firm evidence to link short- or long-term use of oral contraceptives with breast cancer development, the issue remains controversial (Harris et al., 1993).

Benign breast disease refers to a heterogeneous group of disorders including fibrocystic disease, cystic disease, chronic cystic mastitis, and mammary dysplasia. These conditions are generally not associated with an increased risk for breast cancer (Morra & Blumberg, 1991). More specifically, only those conditions with proliferative epithelial changes or atypical hyperplasia have a twofold or fourfold increased risk, respectively (Harris et al., 1992, Pt. I).

Numerous environmental factors have been cited as potential risk factors. Exposure of the breast to therapeutic doses of ionizing radiation at a young age is a significant risk factor. For example, mantle irradiation for Hodgkin's disease may increase the risk of breast cancer (Hancock, 1993). Dietary intake of fat has not been conclusively correlated with an increased risk, and the finding that vitamin A intake may have a protective effect has not been substantiated (Hulka & Stark, 1995). Excessive use of alcohol (more than 2 to 3 drinks per day) is associated with an increased risk (Harris et al., 1993). The benefits of exercise, particularly during adolescence and young adulthood, in reducing the risk for breast cancer later in life has been suggested but not thoroughly investigated (Hulka & Stark, 1995). Obesity is not strongly linked to an increased risk for breast cancer development, but is strongly associated with decreased survival once breast cancer occurs (Harris et al., 1992, Pt. I). The association between cigarette smoking and risk for breast cancer has not been confirmed (Lichter et al., 1992). A summary of factors and their relative risk for the development of breast cancer can be found in Table 9–1.

Breast Cancer Detection

Early detection of breast cancer is critical for assuring the most favorable prognosis. Detection of breast abnormalities is achieved by breast self-examination (BSE), physical examination by a health professional, and mammography (Table 9–2). Although the role of BSE in reducing breast cancer mortality rates has not been established, it is strongly recommended as part of the process of early detection (Goodman & Harte, 1990). It is estimated that 90 percent of palpable breast cancers are found through BSE (Scanlon, 1991). Annual examinations by a health care professional should be performed with careful attention to the patient's risk factors for breast cancer including her menstrual, reproductive, and family history. Both BSE and clinical examinations should be done a few days after menstruation is complete, when tenderness and nodularity are minimal. Clinical indications for further evaluation and/or a biopsy include: a persistent breast mass, a serous or bloody nipple discharge, skin dimpling, a peau d'orange appearance, and breast inflammation or pain (Dow, 1991; Harris et al., 1993).

Table 9-1 • Risk Factors for Breast Cancer

Factor	High-risk Group	Low-risk Group
	RR >4·0	
Age	Old	Young
Country of birth	North America Northern Europe	Asia, Africa
Two first degree relatives with breast cancer diagnosed at an early age	Yes	No
History of cancer in one breast	Yes	No
	RR 2·1—4·0	
Nodular densities on mammogram (postmenopausal)	Densities occupy >75% of breast volume	Parenchyma composed entirely of fat
One first-degree relative with breast cancer	Yes	No
Biopsy-confirmed atypical hyperplasia	Yes	No
High-dose radiation to chest	Yes	No
Oophorectomy before age 35	No	Yes
DEMOGRAPHIC	RR 1·1—2·0	
Socioeconomic status	High	Low
Place of residence	Urban	Rural
Race/ethnicity		
Breast cancer at >40 yr	Caucasian	Asian
Breast cancer at <40 yr	Black	Asian
Religion	Jewish	Seventh-day Adventist, Mormon
HORMONAL		
Age at first full-term pregnancy	≥30 yr	<20 yr
Age at menarche	<12 yr	>14 yr
Age at menopause	≥55 yr	<45 yr
Obesity (postmenopausal)	Obese	Thin
Parity (postmenopausal)	Nulliparous	Multiparous
Breast feeding (premenopausal)	None	Several years
Hormonal contraceptives		
Breast cancer at <45 years	Yes	No
Hormone replacement therapy	Yes	No
OTHER		
Height	Tall	Short
History of primary cancer in endo-metrium, ovary, or colon	Yes	No
Alcohol consumption	Yes	No

From Stark AT (1995). Breast cancer: Cause and prevention. *Lancet, 346,* 883–887. Reprinted with permission.

Mammography is used with clinical examination both as a screening tool for breast cancer and as a diagnostic tool to gain more information when suspicion for breast cancer is high. An irregular or stellate mass, tissue retraction, clustered microcalcifications, and breast edema are mammographic signs of malignancy (Lichter et al., 1992). The benefits of mammography are well established. Modern mammography may detect 95 percent of all breast cancers and, when used as a screening tool, may reduce mortality rates by 40 percent especially in women greater than 50 years of age (Blamey et al., 1994). The relationship between mammography and a reduction of mortality rates in younger women between the ages of 40 and 49 has not been established (Harris et al., 1992, Pt. I). The improved imaging techniques with mammography allow for visualization of clinically undetected microcalcifications and thus, have led to an increase in the number of women diagnosed with preinvasive lesions (Hetelekidis et al., 1995). Bilateral mammograms are done prior to the biopsy with magnification views of any microcalcifications. However, a breast ultrasound may be indicated instead of a mammogram to confirm a cystic lesion or fibroadenoma in young women less than 30 years of age (Lichter et al., 1992). New techniques for imaging the breast are under investigation and include magnetic resonance imaging, digital mammography, computer-aided diagnosis, and positron emission tomography (Adler & Wahl, 1995).

Biopsy Techniques

Several biopsy techniques may be used to obtain tissue for diagnosis when a palpable breast mass is present. These include: excisional biopsy, incisional biopsy, fine-needle aspiration, and core needle biopsy. Excisional biopsy, or complete removal of the mass, is an operative procedure that may be undertaken as a definitive treatment for women undergoing breast conservation treatment. Incisional biopsy is usually reserved for women with locally advanced disease that cannot be completely excised. Fine-needle aspiration is a cost effective, outpatient technique that involves placing a needle in the breast mass to obtain cytologic material for analysis. A core needle biopsy is another simple procedure that uses a needle to obtain a core of tissue for histologic analysis. There are advantages and disadvantages to each of these techniques. The physician will consider the patient's age, menopausal status, mammographic changes, and history to assess the risk for malignancy and to select the appropriate biopsy technique.

The surgical biopsy of nonpalpable breast abnormalities requires specific localization techniques with mammography to accurately locate the suspicious area, minimize the amount of breast tissue removed, and assure good cosmetic results (Harris et al., 1993). With mammographic guidance, a wire is placed into the breast along a needle track in close proximity to the lesion. The wire is left in place to serve as a reference point for locating the breast lesion on mammography and then guiding the excision of the appropriate area of breast tissue (Dow, 1991). Mammograms are taken of the biopsy specimen to ensure that the target lesion or calcifications were completely excised.

Stereotactic breast biopsy may be employed to diagnose nonpalpable, mammographically detected breast lesions. This technique offers several advantages over standard surgical biopsy practice, including decreased cost, minimal complications, negligible disfigurement, lack of postbiopsy changes on mammography, and increased availability and efficiency (Schmidt, 1994). During a stereotactic biopsy, the patient is placed prone on a special x ray table with a circular opening through which the breast is positioned and stabilized. Stereotactic x rays, a reference grid, and computer are used to accurately pinpoint needle placement under local anesthesia. The procedure takes approximately one hour and is generally well tolerated by the patient. Mild breast discomfort, tenderness, or bruising at the biopsy site are potential side effects.

Stereotactic breast biopsy may apply either fine-needle aspiration or core biopsy techniques. Stereotactic fine-needle aspiration (SFNA) may be used to evaluate mammographic abnormalities that are not highly suspicious for breast cancer (Schmidt, 1994). Limitations of SFNA are its inability to identify invasion, a high rate of obtaining insufficient tissue for diagnosis, and its reliance on the cytopathologist's expertise (Parker et al., 1991; Schmidt, 1994). More recently, stereotactic core needle biopsy (SCNB) has gained acceptance as an alternative to an open surgical biopsy. Histologic examination of a core of tissue, which is obtained through a 14-gauge needle using a biopsy gun, usually provides a definitive diagnosis and an assessment of invasion if the lesion is malignant (Parker et al., 1991). Additional benefits of SCNB are that surgical procedures are avoided with a benign diagnosis and that information about a malignant lesion may help tailor the surgical treatment (Parker et al., 1990).

Staging of Breast Cancer

Staging of breast cancer is helpful in predicting prognosis, selecting treatment, and facilitating comparisons between treatment regimens. The TNM staging system by the American Joint Committee on Cancer is a clinical staging system based on physical examination, radiologic evaluation, and surgical staging procedures (Table 9–3). Other information, which is part of the pretreatment evaluation, includes a chest x ray, complete blood count, and liver chemistries. Further pathologic data, including histologic examination of the axillary specimen, is used for pathologic staging. Pathologic staging is important because it provides a histologic confirmation of axillary lymph node status and thus, is a more accurate prediction of prognosis than clinical staging (Harris et al., 1992, Pt. II).

Prognostic Factors

Several established prognostic factors are used to predict an individual's risk for recurrence or death from their disease. Prognostic factors may also be helpful in therapeutic decisions by identifying those groups of patients who may benefit from adjuvant therapy. The most significant prognostic factor in breast cancer is the presence of axillary node metastasis (Elledge et al., 1992). Tumor size is another established prognostic factor and is often included with lymph node involvement as part of the TNM staging system. Both increased lymph node involvement and increased tumor size have independent negative effects on survival (Carter et al., 1989). For example, if the extent of axillary lymph node involvement is greater than four lymph nodes, the prognosis is poor despite the tumor size (Carter et al., 1989).

The histopathological analysis of the tumor also offers prognostic information. Types of breast cancer associated with a good prognosis when axillary lymph nodes are not involved include: ductal carcinoma in situ, pure tubular cancer, papillary cancer, and medullary cancer (McGuire & Clark, 1992). Another histopathologic feature used as a prognostic indicator is nuclear grade. The Bloom and Richardson grading system is a commonly used scheme that assesses the degree of duct formation, the characteristics of the nuclei, and the number of mitoses (Simpson & Page, 1992). This information will determine the degree of differentiation of the tumor and is expressed as a classification of Grade I, well-differentiated; Grade II, moderately differentiated; and Grade III, poorly differentiated. Tumor grade can correlate independently with overall prognosis. The prognosis associated with Grade I tumors is better than that with Grade III tumors (Elledge et al., 1992).

Analysis of steroid hormone receptors, including the estrogen receptor (ER) and progesterone receptor (PR), is used in conjunction with other indicators to predict prognosis. In general, studies indicate that the prognosis is more favorable with ER-positive tumors than ER-negative tumors (Elledge et al., 1992). The primary use of steroid hormone receptor assays, in addition to prognostic indications, is to identify those patients who might benefit from adjuvant hormonal manipulation (McGuire & Clark, 1992).

DNA flow cytometry provides information about tumor cell growth by estimating the percentage of cells dividing (S-phase fraction) and the amount of DNA in each cell (ploidy). Studies have shown that the S-phase fraction is a good prognostic indicator regardless of the ploidy status of the tumor, with high S-phase fraction indicating a poor prognosis (Elledge et al., 1992). Tumors with abnormal amounts of DNA (aneuploid) are associated with a poor prognosis (McGuire & Clark, 1992). More recently, other factors are being evaluated for their prognostic significance. These include: the HER-2/neu oncogene; the enzyme cathepsin D; epidermal growth factor receptor; a protein called pS2; and several others. Their role in breast cancer management is yet to be determined.

Types of Breast Cancer

Histopathologic types of breast cancer are classified as either ductal or lobular (Table 9–4). In situ carcinomas have malignant changes within the ducts or lobules and no invasion through the basement membrane into the surrounding tissue (Hetelekidis et al., 1995). Invasive breast cancer refers to a heterogeneous group of tumors that arise in either the ducts or lobules and extend through the basement membrane into the adjacent tissue. Tumors may be of mixed histology. For example, a tumor that is predominantly invasive breast cancer may have a component of in situ carcinoma as well.

There has been a dramatic increase in the frequency of diagnosed cases of ductal carcinoma in situ (DCIS) because of mammographic screening and the detection of clinically occult microcalcifications (Harris et al., 1992, Pt. II). DCIS, which is a preinvasive lesion, is also referred to as intraductal carcinoma and may be classified into several subtypes, based on histologic morphology: comedo, cribiform, papillary, micropapillary, and solid. Some lesions may exhibit a mixture of these subtypes. Characteristics that differentiate each

Table 9-3 • 1992 AJCC Classification System for Cancer of the Breast

PRIMARY TUMOR (T)

Definitions for classifying the primary tumor (T) are the same for clinical and for pathological classification. The telescoping method of classification can be applied. If the measurement is made by physical examination, the examiner will use the major headings (T1, T2, or T3). If other measurements, such as mammographic or pathologic, are used, the examiner can use the telescoped subsets of T1.

TX	Primary tumor cannot be assessed	
T0	No evidence of primary tumor	
Tis	Carcinoma in situ: intraductal carcinoma, lobular carcinoma in situ, or Paget's disease of the nipple with no tumor	
T1	Tumor 2 cm or less in greatest dimension	
	T1a	0.5 cm or less in greatest dimension
	T1b	More than 0.5 cm but not more than 1 cm in greatest dimension
	T1c	More than 1 cm but not more than 2 cm in greatest dimension
T2	Tumor more than 2 cm but not more than 5 cm in greatest dimension	
T3	Tumor more than 5 cm in greatest dimension	
T4	Tumor of any size with direct extension to chest wall or skin	
	T4a	Extension to chest wall
	T4b	Edema (including peau d'orange) or ulceration of the skin of the breast or satellite skin nodules confined to the same breast
	T4c	Both (T4a and T4b)
	T4d	Inflammatory carcinoma (See the definition of inflammatory carcinoma below)

Note: Paget's disease associated with a tumor is classified according to the size of the tumor.

REGIONAL LYMPH NODES (N)

NX	Regional lymph nodes cannot be assessed (e.g., previously removed)
N0	No regional lymph node metastases
N1	Metastases of movable ipsilateral axillary lymph node(s)
N2	Metastases to ipsilateral axillary lymph node(s) fixed to one another or to other structures
N3	Metastases to ipsilateral internal mammary lymph node(s)

PATHOLOGIC CLASSIFICATION (pN)

pNX	Regional lymph nodes cannot be assessed (e.g., previously removed, or not removed for pathologic study)	
pN0	No regional lymph node metastasis	
pN1	Metastasis to movable ipsilateral axillary lymph node(s)	
	pN1a	Only micrometastasis (none larger than 0.2 cm)
	pN1b	Metastasis to lymph node(s), any larger than 0.2 cm
		pN1bi Metastasis in one to three lymph nodes, any more than 0.2 cm and all less than 2 cm in greatest dimension
		pN1bii Metastasis to four or more lymph nodes, any more than 0.2 cm and all less than 2 cm in greatest dimension
		pN1biii Extension of tumor beyond the capsule of a lymph node metastasis less than 2 cm in greatest dimension
		pN1biv Metastasis to a lymph node 2 cm or more in greatest dimension
pN2	Metastasis to ipsilateral axillary lymph nodes that are fixed to one another or to other structures	
pN3	Metastasis to ipsilateral internal mammary lymph node(s)	

DISTANT METASTASIS

MX	Presence of distant metastasis cannot be assessed
M0	No distant metastasis
M1	Distant metastasis (includes metastasis to ipsilateral supraclavicular lymph node(s))

STAGE GROUPING

Stage 0	Tis	N0	M0
Stage I	T1	N0	M0
Stage IIA	T0	N1	M0
	T1	N1*	M0
	T2	N0	M0
Stage IIB	T2	N1	M0
	T3	N0	M0
Stage IIIA	T0	N2	M0
	T1	N2	M0
	T2	N2	M0
	T3	N1	M0
	T3	N2	M0

Table continued on following page

Table 9-3 • 1992 AJCC Classification System for Cancer of the Breast *(Continued)*

Stage IIIB	T4	Any N	M0
	Any T	N3	M0
Stage IV	Any T	Any N	M1

INFLAMMATORY CARCINOMA

Inflammatory carcinoma is a clinicopathologic entity characterized by diffuse brawny induration of the skin of the breast with an erysipeloid edge, usually without an underlying palpable mass. Radiologically, there may be a detectable mass and characteristic thickening of the skin over the breast. This clinical presentation is due to tumor embolization of dermal lymphatics. The tumor of inflammatory carcinoma is classified as T4d.

---

* Note: The prognosis of patients with N1a is similar to that of patients with pN0.

From American Joint Committee on Cancer (1992). *Manual for Staging of Cancer* (4th ed.). Philadelphia: Lippincott-Raven. Reprinted with permission.

subtype include: the appearance of the nuclei (pleomorphic vs. monomorphic), the proliferation rate, the presence of necrosis, the overexpression of the HER-2/*neu* (c-*erb*B-2) oncogene, the extent of microinvasion, and the mammographic appearance (Harris et al., 1992, Pt, II). DCIS may be a multicentric disease, but rather typically involves a segment of the breast (Hetelekidis et al., 1995). Axillary lymph node metastasis is rare with DCIS, which may eliminate the need for an axillary dissection in a patient with this diagnosis (Lichter et al., 1992). The natural history of DCIS, and whether DCIS has the potential to progress to invasive cancer if left untreated, are issues that are not resolved (Harris et al., 1992. Pt. II).

Lobular carcinoma in situ (LCIS) is rarely palpable and is not usually observed with mammography. It is typically found incidentally during microscopic review of a biopsy for a benign breast problem and is characterized by proliferation of malignant cells within the lobules. LCIS occurs more frequently in premenopausal women, has a tendency to be multicentric, and is also likely to be found in the contralateral breast (Lichter et al., 1992). LCIS does not evolve into an invasive cancer, but rather is a marker for the potential development of invasive cancer (Harris et al., 1992, Pt. II). Women with LCIS have an increased risk for the development of invasive cancer in both breasts, and consequently need to be followed closely (Scanlon, 1991).

Approximately 75 percent of all invasive breast cancers are infiltrating ductal carcinoma (Pierson & Wilkinson, 1991). This tumor commonly appears as a hard, fibrous lump. Infiltrating ductal carcinoma does not have any specific histologic features and is referred to as "adenocarcinoma of the breast–not otherwise specified (NOS)" (Scanlon, 1991). In contrast, infiltrating lobular carcinoma is more rare, accounting for 5

to 10 percent of breast cancers, and is palpated as a diffuse thickening in the breast (Harris et al., 1992, Pt. II). Infiltrating ductal carcinoma and infiltrating lobular carcinoma are similar in that they both can be associated with axillary lymph node involvement or distant metastasis.

Tubular carcinoma accounts for approximately two percent of all breast cancers (Pierson & Wilkinson, 1991). This tumor is well-differentiated, with characteristic tubular structures noted microscopically. The prognosis is good with low potential for axillary metastases (Simpson & Page, 1992).

Mucinous (colloid) carcinoma comprises approximately two percent of all breast cancers and typically presents as a palpable mass in older women (Pierson & Wilkinson, 1991). Abundant extracellular mucin surrounding tumor cells is the characteristic microscopic finding for this tumor (Rosen, 1991).

Medullary carcinoma accounts for five to nine percent of breast cancers and occurs most often in women less than 50 years of age (Rosen, 1991). Clinical features may include a large tumor size, circumscription, cystic changes, and rapid tumor growth (Pierson & Wilkinson, 1991). Medullary carcinoma is often associated with bilateral breast cancer (Rosen, 1991). Papillary, adenoid cystic, apocrine, metaplastic, and secretory are more rare forms of invasive breast cancer.

Inflammatory breast carcinoma accounts for one to four percent of all breast cancers (Swain & Lippman, 1991). It is a distinct clinical entity, characterized by features of: skin erythema, which may vary from pink to a purplish discoloration; increased warmth of the skin; edema, which may appear as peau d'orange; and induration of the skin (Parker et al., 1991). These findings are related to the involvement of the dermal lymphatics with malignant cells. A detectable mass is evident in approximately half of patients with inflamma-

Table 9-4 • Pathologic Types of Breast Cancer

NONINVASIVE (OR IN SITU OR PRECANCER)
Confined to its site
Lacks potential to spread to other parts of the body

DUCTAL (OR INTRADUCTAL, DCIS)
Malignant cells of ductal origin that are contained in the duct
Often presents as microcalcifications on mammogram, or with bloody nipple discharge
Rarely presents as a lump

LOBULAR (LCIS)
Abnormal cells of lobular origin that are contained within the lobule of the breast
Usually bilateral or multicentric
Not visible on mammogram, and does not present as a palpable mass
Often diagnosed incidentally at the time of a biopsy for other reasons

INVASIVE (OR INFILTRATING)
Invasive capacity outside cells of origin
Potential to spread from the breast through the blood vessels (primarily) and lymphatics to other organs
General category of breast cancer is adenocarcinoma
Specific types are:

DUCTAL
Malignant cells of breast duct origin have broken through the walls of the duct and are now found in the surrounding breast tissue and fat
Most common type of invasive breast cancer (about 70% to 80% of all breast cancer)
Usually presents as a solid mass, may have a spiculated (star-shaped) appearance on mammogram

LOBULAR
Malignant cells of breast lobule origin are now invading into the surrounding breast tissue and fat
Comprises about 5% of breast cancer
May present as a large, lumpy area, a thickening, or with a large lump

COMBINATIONS
Often combinations of cell types (invasive, both ductal and lobular, as well as noninvasive) present in the breast tumor
Less common types of breast cancer include medullary, mucinous, tubular, papillary and inflammatory

SPECIAL CASES
Inflammatory
Uncommon
Often mistaken for cellulitis or lactational mastitis

From C Engelking, BH Kalinowski (eds). (1995). *A comprehensive guide to breast cancer treatment: Current issues and controversies.* New York: Triclinica Communications Inc. Reprinted with permission.

tory breast cancer and axillary nodal involvement is common (Swain & Lippman, 1991). The clinical course of inflammatory breast cancer is associated with rapid tumor progression over a brief time (Parker et al., 1991). Although inflammatory breast cancer has been associated with a very poor prognosis, recent therapeutic approaches utilizing combined modality treatment have improved disease-free and overall survival rates (Jaiyesimi et al., 1992).

One to four percent of women with breast cancer will have Paget's disease of the nipple (Blakeley, et al., 1994). The clinical presentation of Paget's disease is a persistent, scaly, erythematous lesion of the nipple and areola. In a review of 214 cases of Paget's disease by Ashikari and colleagues (1970), approximately 50 percent had underlying palpable breast masses most of which were infiltrating carcinoma. The prognosis for Paget's disease is based on the associated type of breast cancer and the extent of axillary node involvement. Patients with Paget's disease without an underlying mass have an excellent prognosis if treated appropriately (Blakeley et al., 1994).

Breast Cancer in Men

Male breast cancer occurs rarely and accounts for fewer than one percent of all breast cancers

(Donegan, 1991). It is estimated that in 1996 there will be 1,400 new cases of male breast cancer in the United States (Parker et al., 1996). Several groups have been associated with an increased incidence of breast cancer including: Jewish males, men with Klinefelter's syndrome, and men who have had the mumps infection after the age of 20 (Wilhelm & Wanebo, 1991). Gynecomastia is not linked to breast cancer (Monyak & Levitt, 1992). Men with breast cancer may typically present with a firm mass in the subareolar area, nipple discharge or ulceration, and axillary adenopathy (Donegan, 1991). The histologic types of male breast cancer are similar to those in women, with the exception that lobular carcinoma is rare (Wilhelm & Wanebo, 1991). Diagnostic and therapeutic techniques are comparable to those used for breast cancer in women.

The Role of Radiation Therapy in the Treatment of Primary Breast Cancer

Breast Conservation Treatment

In 1990, a consensus development panel of the National Institutes of Health concluded that "breast conservation treatment (BCT) is an appropriate method of primary therapy for the majority of women with stage I and II breast cancer and is preferable because it provides survival equivalent to total mastectomy and axillary dissection while preserving the breast" (NIH Consensus Statement, 1990). Fisher et al. (1989) describe a five-year disease-free survival rate of 77 percent for women with stage I or II node-negative breast cancer treated with lumpectomy and irradiation as compared with 75 percent for similar women who underwent mastectomy. Breast conservation treatment consists of complete excision of the gross tumor, followed by radiation therapy to the breast. The goals of BCT are to achieve local tumor control with minimal cosmetic deformity.

Indications

Multiple factors are considered when selecting a patient for BCT. These include: mammographic evaluation, histologic assessment of the tumor, and the patient's expectations and preferences (Cox & Winchester, 1992). Mammographic evidence of a large tumor size in relation to the breast, two separate malignant lesions in the same breast, and extensive malignant microcalcifica-

tions are relative contraindications for BCT (Recht & Harris, 1990). These patients require more extensive resections, compromising cosmetic outcomes. There is controversy as to whether the location of the tumor may preclude breast conservation. Patients who present with a nipple discharge or who have a tumor in the subareolar area, generally require resection of the nipple areolar complex, which may result in poor cosmesis (Pierce & Harris, 1992). However, Fisher (1995) describes potential for an excellent cosmetic result despite removal of the nipple areolar complex.

Histologic assessment of the tumor is also considered in the selection of patients for BCT. Of primary importance is a microscopic examination of the presence or absence of tumor at the surgical margins. Close or involved margins is a prognostic indicator for risk of local failure after BCT (Wazer, 1994). Treatment decisions to minimize local recurrence risk may include reexcision of the tumor bed prior to breast irradiation or boost irradiation to the area of concern.

Another histologic feature associated with an increased risk of recurrence is an extensive intraductal component (EIC) (Yarnold, 1991). Patients with tumors having an EIC generally have more residual tumor after resection than other patients and require reexcision to achieve clear microscopic margins prior to BCT (Recht & Harris, 1990).

Although mastectomy has been the traditional treatment approach to ductal carcinoma in situ (DCIS), there is increasing evidence to support the use of BCT in the treatment of DCIS. Fisher et al. (1993) found that 5-year event-free survival with breast irradiation after lumpectomy was 84.4 percent, as compared to 73.8 percent in women treated with lumpectomy alone. In this same study by Fisher et al. (1993), the investigators concluded that radical treatment of DCIS with mastectomy is not justified considering the significantly reduced incidence of ipsilateral tumors after BCT. Women with DCIS may be candidates for BCT if they have limited extent of disease, negative microscopic margins of resection, and no remaining evidence of microcalcifications on mammography after the biopsy (Hetelekidis et al., 1995).

The patient's own viewpoint toward treatment, potential for recurrence, sexuality, physical functioning, and quality of life are essential considerations in selection for BCT (Cox & Winchester, 1992). A patient's preference for mastectomy may reflect concerns about radiotherapy side effects, inconvenience, and efficacy (Ward et al.,

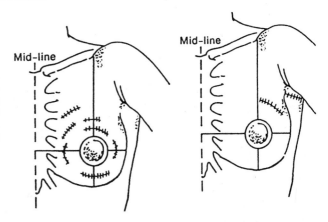

Figure 9-2 • Recommended incisions for lumpectomy. From Fisher B (1991). Lumpectomy (segmental mastectomy) and axillary dissection. In KI Bland & EM Copeland III (Eds.), *The Breast: Comprehensive Management of Benign and Malignant Diseases* (pp. 634–652). Philadelphia: WB Saunders. Reprinted with permission.

1989). The patient's expectations for cosmetic outcome with BCT must also be thoroughly explored. Poor cosmetic outcomes are associated with a large tumor size, small breast size, and treatment factors including excessive surgical resection, high radiation doses, and poor dosimetry (Yarnold, 1991). Women with large breasts are not excluded from BCT, but require extra care in surgical and radiation techniques to achieve a good cosmetic outcome (Gray et al., 1991). In general, good to excellent cosmetic outcomes are achieved in 80 to 90 percent of all women receiving BCT (Moffat, 1994). Other patient-related factors that are contraindications for BCT are pregnancy during irradiation, a history of prior irradiation in the breast area, and a history of collagen vascular disease (Cox & Winchester, 1992).

Surgical Techniques

The surgical technique used on the breast during a diagnostic biopsy or definitive local excision is very important to the cosmetic result. Although various surgical procedures may be used, such as partial mastectomy, wide local excision (tylec-tomy), or lumpectomy, the overall surgical goal is to completely remove the breast mass with a small margin of normal breast tissue and not deform the breast. Recommendations for optimal cosmesis include: placement of a curvilinear skin incision over the tumor; avoidance of skin retraction or "tunneling;" preservation of the fat layer overlying breast tissue; meticulous hemostasis; and avoidance of drains (Cox & Winchester, 1992). Recommended and nonrecommended incisions are illustrated in Figures 9–2 and 9–3. At the time of the surgical procedure, metallic clips may be placed at the tumor site to aid in radiation therapy planning.

Axillary lymph node dissection helps to determine prognosis and aids in selecting patients for systemic treatment. A separate incision is often used for the axillary dissection. Levels of dissection are described as I, II, and III, meaning below, behind, and above the pectoralis minor muscle (Falk, 1994). The level of dissection may vary according to the size and histology of the tumor (Cox & Winchester, 1992). It is recommended that a level I and II dissection is done for invasive

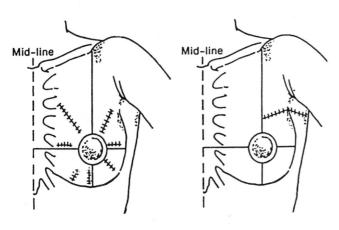

Figure 9-3 • Nonrecommended incisions for lumpectomy. From Fisher B (1991). Lumpectomy (segmental mastectomy) and axillary dissection. In KI Bland & EM Copeland III (Eds.), *The Breast: Comprehensive Management of Benign and Malignant Diseases* (pp. 634–652). Philadelphia: WB Saunders. Reprinted with permission.

tumors that are less than 2 cm in diameter. A level III dissection is advised for larger tumors or for any patient with palpable axillary lymph nodes (Moore & Kinne, 1995). Axillary dissections are not routinely performed in patients with DCIS (Hetelekidis et al., 1995). After axillary dissection, range of motion exercises to preserve shoulder mobility should begin early in the postoperative period.

Radiation Therapy Techniques

Radiation therapy is usually begun 2 to 4 weeks after surgery. During simulation and treatment the patient is positioned supine with one or both arms abducted over her head. This position moves the arm out of the radiation beam, as well as flattens the breast, removing skin folds. Immobilization casts are used to aid in daily replication of the treatment set-up, as well as to provide support for the arm. Maintaining this position during simulation and treatment may be difficult for women with limited shoulder range of motion. Adequate

patient preparation as well as analgesics and a review of range of motion exercises will promote comfort.

The entire breast is treated through medial and lateral tangential fields that are directed obliquely to the chest wall (Figure 9–4, Fields A and B). Yarnold (1991) describes the borders of these fields as extending from the level of the suprasternal notch to the inframammary fold. The anterior midline marks the medial border and the midaxillary line is the lateral border. The irradiated field includes a 1 cm margin above the nipple and the posterior margin encompasses 1 to 2 cm of underlying lung tissue (Yarnold, 1991). Computerized treatment planning is used to select treatment angles as well as appropriate wedges and beam blocks. The goals of treatment planning are to achieve a homogenous dose of radiation to the entire breast, minimize lung exposure, and optimize cosmesis.

The borders of the tangential fields may need to be matched carefully to other fields when treat-

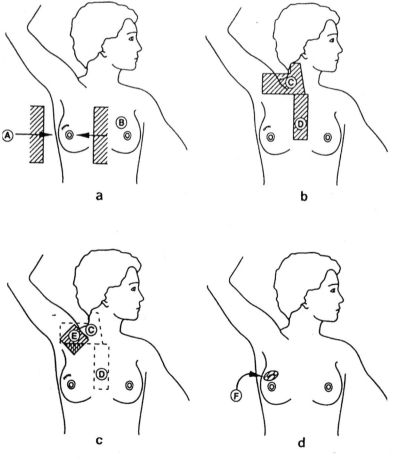

a

b

c

d

Figure 9-4 • Fields A and B = tangential. C = supraclavicular. D = internal mammary. E = posterior axillary. F = boost field. From Mansfield CM, Krishnan L, Komarnicky LT, et al. (1991). A review of the role of radiation therapy in the treatment of patients with breast cancer. *Seminars in Oncology, 18,* 525–535. Reprinted with permission.

ment to the axilla or supraclavicular area is indicated (Figure 9–4, Fields C and E). Overlap between adjacent fields is associated with increased risk of skin reactions and fibrosis, and will compromise the cosmetic outcome of BCT. It is recommended that if the axilla has been surgically dissected, axillary nodal irradiation is not indicated (NIH Consensus Statement, 1990). Whenever possible, radiation to the axilla after dissection is avoided because of the increased morbidity rate and risk for lymphedema and brachial plexus neuropathy (Falk, 1994). However, some clinicians will irradiate the axilla and supraclavicular nodes if four or more axillary lymph nodes are positive or if there is extranodal extension of the malignancy (Lichter et al., 1992). Radiation to the internal mammary nodes is given in a very select group of patients and care must be taken to reduce exposure to the heart, esophagus, and thoracic vertebral bone marrow (Moffat, 1994). The internal mammary treatment field is illustrated in Figure 9–4, Field D.

The radiation dose to the whole breast is 4500 to 5500 cGy given 5 days a week in daily fractions of 180 to 200 cGy. A course of treatment lasts 4½ to 6 weeks. The beam energy used is 4 to 8 MeV photons or cobalt-60. Controversy exists as to whether a boost dose to the tumor bed is needed in addition to whole-breast irradiation. Proponents for giving a boost feel that local control will be improved without risk to cosmesis. However, a study from the National Surgical Adjuvant Breast and Bowel Project (NSABP) found that the local recurrence rate was 10 percent in their group of patients who did not receive boost irradiation to the tumor bed (Fisher et al., 1989). This recurrence rate is similar to the rate described in other trials in which patients received boost treatments. Unlike the NSABP group, the patients in the comparison trials did not have consistently negative surgical margins (Wilson & Cox, 1995). Although indications for adding a boost treatment are unclear, current recommendations advocate its use, especially when margins are close or involved (Moffat, 1994). The boost dose may be omitted in patients who have had very wide local excisions with negative margins (Cox & Winchester, 1992).

Boost irradiation can be delivered by electrons or brachytherapy (Figure 9–4, Field F). The boost dose is 1000 to 1500 cGy at 200 cGy fractions. The electron boost treatments are often carefully planned with computed tomography scanning, to identify the limited field encompassing the tumor bed and surgical scar (Mansfield et al., 1991). Brachytherapy boost treatments use interstitial implantation of 192 iridium strands. As described by Mast and Mood (1990), treatment is usually initiated 7 to 14 days after completion of the external beam photon treatment and requires a surgical procedure for insertion of after-loading catheters. With the catheters in place, simulation films are taken to aid in treatment planning. The volume of tissue to be treated and the length and strength of radioactive material needed in each catheter are determined. The patient remains in the hospital for 2 to 3 days. (See Chapter 3 for further information on brachytherapy.)

Adjuvant Chemotherapy

Adjuvant systemic therapies are now commonly offered to select groups of women after conservative surgery. Clinicians are confronted with the challenge of integrating radiation therapy and chemotherapy, while working to achieve common goals of high rate of survival, low rate of local recurrence, few complications, and good cosmetic results (Harris & Recht, 1993). There are no guidelines regarding optimal sequencing of chemotherapy and radiation therapy (NIH Consensus Statement, 1990). Enhanced acute skin reactions are common with concurrent chemotherapy, especially when the daily radiation dose fraction exceeds 200 cGy (Mansfield, et al., 1991). Another concern is the potential for enhanced late reactions, which has led some clinicians to reduce the daily dose fraction to 180 cGy (Yarnold, 1991). An alternate strategy is to sequence therapy, often delaying radiation until adjuvant chemotherapy is complete. However, this strategy may not be optimal due to the increased risk of local recurrence when radiation is delayed (Harris & Recht, 1993).

Follow-Up Care

Women who have completed BCT should receive a physical examination every 3 to 6 months for the first 3 years and then on a biannual basis. A mammogram is recommended at six-month intervals during the first year after treatment and then annually (Cox & Winchester, 1992). During physical examination and mammography, close attention is given to the primary tumor site and incision, where most recurrences are located (Pierce & Harris, 1992). Unlike recurrence after mastectomy, local relapse after BCT is not associated with a poor prognosis and is usually treated with mastectomy (Lichter et al., 1992).

Assessment of the overall cosmetic result should occur at each follow-up visit. Postradiation normal tissue changes may continue to occur in the treated breast for 3 years after BCT (Moffat, 1994). Although these changes are subtle and uncommon, they may include breast swelling, fibrosis, and retraction (Pierce & Harris, 1992). Cutaneous telangiectasia may also evolve (Moffat, 1994). Haffty (1992) contends that, although a patient's physical exam tends to stabilize 1 year after therapy, frequent follow-up visits are necessary to distinguish between evolving posttreatment tissue changes and early local recurrences.

Generally, evaluation of the cosmetic result is subjective in nature and is accomplished by physician and patient assessment. A 4-point scoring system of breast cosmesis has been recommended by the American College of Radiology, the American College of Surgeons, the College of American Pathologists, and the Society of Surgical Oncology (Cox & Winchester, 1992). The ratings are defined in Table 9–5. More recently, Sacchini (1995) employed a more objective approach to measuring cosmetic outcome after BCT. Using computerized video filming, they found that radiation therapy does not influence breast symmetry and cosmetic results when compared to a similar group of patients who did not receive radiation.

Postmastectomy Radiation

The goal of postmastectomy radiation therapy is to eradicate any tumor cells remaining in the chest wall, peripheral lymph nodes, or the surgical scar. Studies have clearly demonstrated that post mastectomy radiotherapy decreases the rate of local-regional failure in high-risk patients (Pierce & Glatstein, 1994). Patients at high risk include those with large primary tumors, tumors that are fixed to the skin or ulcerated, four or more positive nodes, and positive surgical margins or fixation of the primary tumor to the chest wall (Wilson, 1994). Whether there is a reduction in distant metastasis and a survival benefit with postmastectomy radiation is uncertain. Studies suggest that there may be a very select subgroup of

patients who may benefit in terms of survival from postmastectomy radiation therapy. Advocates of the use of postmastectomy radiation to improve survival challenge the assumption that breast cancer is a systemic disease in all patients (Uematsu et al., 1993).

When radiation therapy is combined with chemotherapy, local-regional control and disease-free survival are enhanced especially in high-risk patients (Levitt, 1994). Again, the issue of how best to integrate the chemotherapy and radiation therapy is unclear. Radiation treatment to the internal mammary nodes may impact the ability to give chemotherapy because the bone marrow and mediastinal structures are affected (Pierce & Glatstein, 1994).

Women undergoing mastectomy may choose to have immediate or delayed reconstruction using one of various methods. These may include use of an implant, tissue expander, or a transfer of the patient's own tissue from the latissimus dorsi muscle, gluteal muscle, or transverse rectus abdominis muscle. Optimally, the need for postmastectomy radiation should be anticipated and reconstruction should be performed after the patient has completed the course of irradiation. Radiation therapy immediately after breast reconstruction is feasible, but is associated with a poor cosmetic outcome and an increased incidence of complications (Kuske et al., 1991). Halpern and colleagues (1990) followed 11 patients with subcutaneous breast implants for more than six years after breast irradiation. Because 9 patients had bilateral reconstruction, the contralateral, nonirradiated breast served as control for assessing cosmetic changes. They found that fibrotic changes occurred in both breasts, but evolved more slowly in the nonirradiated breast. To achieve optimal cosmetic results, the investigators recommend lower radiation doses (4500 cGy in 5 weeks) and avoidance of radiation therapy immediately after reconstructive surgery.

Postmastectomy Radiation Therapy Techniques

Postmastectomy radiation therapy may consist of several fields including the chest wall and peripheral lymphatic regions. Careful matching of the borders of the different fields is necessary to avoid excessive dose at junctions. McNeese et al. (1992) describe the borders of the chest wall field as being contiguous with the internal mammary field and supraclavicular field, extending down to the level of the xiphoid and laterally to the midaxillary line. Additional lateral fields may be necessary if the scar extends beyond the midaxillary line. The

Table 9-5 • 4-Point Scoring System of Breast Cosmesis

Excellent (9-10)	Treated breast is almost identical to untreated breast
Good (7-8)	Minimal difference between the treated and untreated breast
Fair (5-6)	Obvious difference between the treated and untreated breast
Poor (1-4)	Major functional and aesthetic sequelae in the treated breast

From DP Winchester, JD Cox. (1992). Standards for breast conservation. *Ca-A Cancer Journal for Clinicians* 42(3), 134-162. Reprinted with permission.

chest wall may be treated using 6 to 9 MeV electrons to a dose of 5000 cGy over 5 weeks. When photons are used to treat the chest wall, tangential fields are set up. Because of the skin-sparing capacity of photons and high-energy electrons, bolus material may be placed over the chest wall for all or a portion of the treatments. The bolus acts to increase the dose of radiation at the skin surface.

The internal mammary lymph nodes are usually treated with electrons to reduce exposure to the underlying structures of the lung and heart. The field extends from the head of the clavicle to the lower border of the chest wall field and is approximately 7 cm wide (McNeese et al., 1992). The dose prescribed is usually 4500 to 5000 cGy in 6 weeks (Wang, 1988). Because of the depth of the internal mammary nodes, electron energies of 12 to 13 MeV are recommended (McNeese et al., 1992). Various techniques may be used to treat the supraclavicular and axillary areas. An anterior supraclavicular-axillary field may extend 1 cm across the midline of the neck and laterally to the acromial process with an inferior border at the level of the second intercostal space (McNeese et al., 1992). The radiation beam may be angled slightly to reduce irradiation of the trachea, esophagus, and cervical spinal cord and custom blocks are designed to protect the head of the humerus (Wilson, 1994). In addition, a posterior axillary boost field may be given to increase the dose to the midaxillary area (Wang, 1988). The anterior supraclavicular-axillary field is treated with photons to a dose of 5000 cGy in 5 weeks (McNeese et al., 1992).

Preoperative Radiation Therapy

The theoretical goal of preoperative radiation is to reduce tumor bulk so that a more limited surgery may be performed. However, preoperative radiation is seldom used in the care of patients with breast cancer except in situations where an inoperable tumor may be rendered operable by preoperative radiation (Wilson, 1994). This therapeutic approach has been used by some investigators who gave preoperative radiation therapy to women with large breast tumors and achieved tumor regression to allow for breast conservation therapy (Calitchi, 1991).

Radiation Therapy for Local-Regional Recurrence

Women with uncontrolled local-regional recurrence after mastectomy often confront distressing symptoms such as pain, tumor ulceration, and bleeding. Radiation therapy is an effective means to prevent these unpleasant symptoms and im-prove the patient's quality of life. One-fourth of these women with local-regional recurrences will survive more than 10 years despite the fact that recurrence of breast cancer after mastectomy usually is associated with systemic metastasis (Wilson & Cox, 1995).

Most local-regional recurrences involve the chest wall and present as a single nodule in or around the mastectomy scar (Schwaibold, 1991). The supraclavicular fossa is another common site of recurrence. An aggressive local treatment approach to eradicate all local-regional disease is advocated and results in a local-regional control rate of approximately 70 percent (Bedwinek, 1990). In addition, Halverson et al. (1990) suggest that for some patients with local-regional recurrences, radiation therapy can be a curative treatment.

When possible, surgical removal of any accessible chest wall nodules should be done prior to radiation to enhance local control (Wilson, 1994). After excision, radiation therapy is given to encompass the entire chest wall (Schwaibold, et al., 1991). Controversy exists as to whether elective or prophylactic irradiation should be given to uninvolved nodal sites. Several investigators support elective irradiation of the supraclavicular fossa to improve local-regional control (Bedwinek, 1990; Schwaibold, et al., 1991). Elective treatment to the internal mammary and axillary regions is not advocated because of the low frequency of recurrence in these areas and also because of the increased potential complications with treatment (Halverson et al., 1990). If the local-regional recurrence is located in a lymph node site, elective irradiation is usually given to the chest wall (Bedwinek, 1990).

Dose recommendations to achieve local-regional control are based on tumor size. After excision, 5000 cGy is the minimum dose required to the chest wall (Schwaibold et al., 1991). However, if gross disease is present and less than 3 cm in dimension, at least 6000 cGy is recommended (Halverson et al., 1990). Higher doses, up to 7000 cGy, are advocated by Bedwinek (1990) as part of an aggressive approach to achieve local-regional control. The dose recommendation for elective irradiation to uninvolved sites is 4500 to 5000 cGy (Schwaibold et al., 1991).

Radiation Therapy for Locally Advanced Breast Cancer

There are many different clinical presentations of locally advanced breast cancer, including a primary tumor larger than 5 cm; large, fixed axillary lymph nodes; and lymphedema (Wang, 1988).

Occult, distant metastases are also usually associated with locally advanced breast cancer (Wilson & Cox, 1995). A combined modality approach including radiation therapy, mastectomy, and chemotherapy offer the best chance for local-regional control and disease-free survival (Graham et al., 1991). The aim of radiation therapy as part of this approach is to control the tumor locally without causing excessive treatment-related morbidity (Wilson, 1994).

Optimal sequencing of the various therapies remains undetermined. One approach is to administer multiagent chemotherapy prior to radiation therapy or mastectomy. This neoadjuvant chemotherapy reduces the primary tumor and provides early treatment to micrometastases (Graham et al., 1991). Large, inoperable tumors may be converted to a resectable status by neoadjuvant chemotherapy (Wilson, 1994). If the tumor remains inoperable after chemotherapy, external radiation therapy or brachytherapy may be considered (Wang, 1988). Radiation doses near 7000 cGy are required to treat bulky, unresectable disease (greater than 5 cm in diameter) and are associated with severe complications including fibrosis and tissue necrosis (Wilson, 1994). More standard doses are used as an adjuvant after chemotherapy and mastectomy.

An aggressive, multimodality approach to treatment of locally advanced breast cancer has an increased risk for both acute and late complications (Graham et al., 1991). Acute effects may include enhanced skin reactions, pulmonary toxicity, nausea, vomiting, and neutropenia. Late effects include arm edema, brachial plexus injury, lung fibrosis, rib fractures, and cardiomyopathy (Graham et al, 1991).

Radiation Therapy for Metastatic Disease

Radiation therapy is very effective in alleviating the distressing symptoms of metastatic breast cancer. The overall goal of palliative radiation is to improve the patient's quality of life by relieving symptoms with a brief, effective treatment course with few side effects.

Central Nervous System Metastases

Breast cancer is the second most common malignancy associated with brain metastases (Coia, 1992). Most often, patients with brain metastases present with complaints of headache, but other symptoms may include: motor weakness, impaired mentation, behavioral changes, increased intracranial pressure, sensory loss, and lethargy (Borgelt et al., 1980). Treatment with whole-brain irradiation will relieve symptoms in 70 to 90 percent of patients (Coia, 1992).

The diagnosis of brain metastasis is made with magnetic resonance imaging (MRI) or computed tomography (CT) scan. Treatment typically involves administration of corticosteroids to rapidly improve neurological symptoms, followed by a course of whole-brain irradiation. The Radiation Therapy Oncology Group (RTOG) has undertaken several studies to determine optimal dose fractionation for palliation of brain metastases. The results of these studies show that short treatment schedules (20 Gy in 1 week) are equally as effective in palliation and survival as longer courses (30 Gy in 2 weeks) (Coia, 1992). Generally, a more protracted course of radiation therapy may be given to patients with favorable prognostic characteristics. These characteristics were described for all types of patients with brain metastasis by Diener-West et al. (1989). They included: a Karnofsky performance status greater than 70, an absent or controlled primary tumor, age less than 60 years, and metastatic spread only to the brain. The investigators were able to predict probability of survival based on the number of favorable characteristics a patient possessed. For example, patients with all four favorable characteristics had a predicted 200-day survival of 52 percent; whereas those who possessed none of the favorable characteristics had an 8 percent predicted probability of surviving more than 200 days.

Other treatment options may include surgery. Patients with a solitary brain metastasis and no other evidence of metastatic disease may undergo surgical resection followed by adjuvant radiation therapy (Smalley et al., 1987). Stereotactic radiosurgery is an option for the treatment of solitary brain metastasis as well as recurrent brain metastasis after standard radiation therapy (Loeffler et al., 1990).

Patients with breast cancer may confront other problems related to central nervous system metastasis. Fifteen to 25 percent of all cases of spinal cord compression are related to a diagnosis of metastatic breast cancer (Mendenhall, 1991). Most often, the compression associated with metastatic breast cancer is secondary to vertebral collapse or soft-tissue extension from a vertebral body (Mendenhall, 1991). The patient with spinal cord compression often presents with back pain with or without neurologic symptoms. Early diagnosis with the use of MRI and prompt treatment with corticosteroids and surgery or radiation is critical to neurological stabilization and recovery (Bates, 1992). Patients who are candidates for treatment with radiation therapy include those with gradual onset of symptoms, minimal structural compression or spinal instability, multiple levels of compression, tumors of the cauda equina, and poor surgical qualifications (Bates, 1992). The radiation dose is generally 30 Gy delivered in daily fractions of 3 Gy (Mendenhall, 1991).

Although rare, breast cancer is the most common cancer associated with choroidal metastases, an intraocular lesion with complications of blindness and glaucoma (Mendenhall, 1991). Radiation therapy is the primary treatment for choroid metastasis and is effective in improving visual symptoms (Harris et al., 1993). The prescribed radiation dose may range from 30 to 40 Gy in 10 to 20 daily fractions, respectively (Mendenhall, 1991).

Carcinomatous meningitis is another complication that may occur in the patient with metastatic breast cancer. Generally, this condition is treated with intrathecal chemotherapy, but cranial or cranial-spinal radiation may be given if the patient has symptoms of cranial nerve palsies (Wilson et al., 1995).

Bone Metastases

Painful skeletal metastases may develop in a significant percentage of patients with metastatic breast cancer. It is estimated that 40 to 60 percent of all patients with bone metastases have a primary diagnosis of breast cancer (Mendenhall, 1991). Patients with metastatic breast cancer confined to the skeleton may survive for a long period of time, and thus, may benefit greatly from palliative radiation therapy (Springfield, 1991). Early treatment with radiation will provide pain relief in approximately 80 percent of patients (Bates, 1992). Skeletal metastases associated with breast cancer are osteolytic or osteoblastic, causing bone destruction and weakening of the bone matrix (Springfield, 1991). The osteolytic process places the patient at risk for pathologic fractures, especially when weight-bearing bones are involved and more than 50 percent of the cortex has been destroyed (Bates, 1992).

Various dose-fraction schedules may be employed. Single or parallel opposed fields to the involved, symptomatic bone may be treated in 300 cGy fractions for 10 days, to reach a total dose of 3000 cGy. Shorter or more protracted courses of treatment may be indicated in special situations. For example, a single-dose fraction of 600 or 800 cGy may provide rapid pain relief in patients with a short life expectancy (Bates, 1992). Single-dose hemibody irradiation may be offered when there are multiple, symptomatic skeletal metastases. Poulter et al. (1992) conclude that hemibody irradiation, when added to local-field irradiation, offers safe, effective pain relief and also delays the development of new metastases and reduces the need for retreatment. Hemibody treatment is delivered through anterior and posterior fields with a dose of 600 cGy to the upper hemibody and 800 cGy to the lower hemibody (Mendenhall, 1991). An impending or pathologic fracture is treated with surgical fixation followed by postoperative radiation therapy. Again, various dose schemes may be used to control tumor growth and promote bone repair, ranging from 2000 cGy in 5 daily fractions to 3500 cGy in 10 daily fractions (Springfield, 1991).

Strontium-89, a systemic radiopharmaceutical, may also be employed to manage bone pain especially in patients with multiple bone metastases who have failed standard treatments. In a review of recent clinical trials, Robinson et al. (1993) report that 80 percent of patients with bone metastases from breast or prostate cancer experience pain relief after outpatient, intravenous therapy with strontium-89. Strontium-89 mimics calcium and is absorbed by bone, particularly in areas of bone metastases (Robinson et al., 1993). Continued use of analgesics is necessary because pain relief is usually delayed, beginning 7 to 21 days following treatment. The duration of response may last 3 to 6 months and treatments may be repeated every 3 months (Robinson et al., 1993). The primary side effect is bone marrow suppression.

Liver Metastases

Palliative radiation therapy may be used to relieve abdominal pain from hepatomegaly associated with hepatic metastases. The recommended radiation dose is 2100 to 3000 cGy in 300 cGy fractions through anterior and posterior portals (Mendenhall, 1991).

Acute Side Effects of Radiation Therapy

The primary side effect that develops during treatment is a skin reaction. The skin in the treatment field gradually becomes erythematous and/or hyperpigmented. For many women, the skin color changes are subtle and are not evident until the third week of treatment or a dose of 3000 cGy is reached with standard fractions. Pruritus and dry desquamation may occur near the end of the treatment course. Occasionally, patients may experience a moist desquamation in skin folds or regions of friction such as the inframammary or infraaxillary areas. Earlier, more intense skin reactions may be seen in patients who have recently completed chemotherapy or who are receiving concurrent chemotherapy. Agents that are likely to potentiate skin effects are actinomycin D, bleomycin sulfate, doxorubicin HCl (Adriamycin), hydroxyurea, 5-fluouracil, and methotrexate (Mc Donald, 1992). Acute skin reactions are self-limiting and usually resolve in 10 to 14 days after treatment.

Other acute effects, associated with whole-breast irradiation, include transient pain or discomfort in the breast; nipple tenderness or sensitivity; and mild breast edema. Breast edema may take up to 18 months to resolve (Wazer, 1994). Hair loss will occur in the treated area.

Late Effects and Complications with Radiation Therapy

Late complications following radiation therapy to the breast itself are rare, but may be associated with the treatment technique used, the addition of chemotherapy, and the radiation dose given (Pierce & Harris, 1992). More significant late complications are associated with treatment to regional lymph node areas of the axilla, supraclavicular fossae, and the internal mammary areas. The lung, mediastinum, heart, ribs, shoulder joint, and brachial plexus are vital structures in close proximity to these lymph node areas and are thus at risk for development of late radiation effects.

Skin Late Effects

For several years after radiation therapy, the normal breast tissue will continue to change. Subtle reactions may be reported by the patient, including increased swelling, firmness, and shrinkage of the breast. Hypochromia, atrophy, and telangiectasia are late skin sequelae that may occur especially in boost areas, where the skin receives high doses of radiation (Wilson & Cox, 1995).

Brachial Plexopathy

The brachial plexus is a network of lower cervical and first dorsal nerves and extends from the lower lateral neck area to the axilla. The numerous branches of the brachial plexus supply the arm, forearm, and hand. Brachial plexopathy may be caused by tumor infiltration or by fibrosis secondary to radiation and/or surgery (McGrath,

1992a). Although brachial plexopathy may initially present as tingling and numbness of the fingers and weakness of the hand and arm, pain and disabling paralysis may occur late in the clinical course (Killer & Hess, 1990). The clinical course may be either transient or more progressive and irreversible (McGrath, 1992a). The focus of treatment is pain control and arm mobilization.

Brachial plexopathy after radiation therapy is considered an unusual complication and is associated with high doses of radiation to the axilla (Salner et al., 1981). In one series, symptoms of reversible brachial plexopathy were noted in less than 2 percent of 565 patients who received definitive radiation for breast cancer (Salner et al., 1981). In this report, the onset of mild paresthesias and occasional weakness and pain occurred 4.5 months after treatment. Most patients had complete resolution of symptoms. The researchers did find a significant incidence of reversible brachial plexopathy in those patients who had received adjuvant chemotherapy in addition to the radiation. Some studies suggest a higher incidence of brachial plexopathy in patients treated by axillary dissection and less conventional doses of radiation therapy (Olsen et al., 1990).

Bone Necrosis

A small portion of the chest wall is included in the treatment volume during tangential beam irradiation of the breast. Late effects include rib fractures, which may occur in 1 to 2 percent of patients and localized fat necrosis, which is seen in 1 to 8 percent of treated patients (Kurtz & Miralbell, 1992). Rib fractures generally heal without treatment.

Lymphedema

Lymphedema is the accumulation of lymph fluid in the subcutaneous interstitial tissues, caused by a disruption in the lymphatic system. Normally, the protein-rich lymph fluid has a unidirectional flow from the distal to the proximal portion of the extremity through thin-walled lymph vessels that parallel the course of the circulatory system. The primary, superficial lymphatics form a permeable, capillary-like network that facilitates the movement of fluid and protein from the interstitial space into larger secondary channels that have valves (Horsley & Styblo, 1991). The lymph fluid then filters through lymph nodes and eventually empties into large lymphatic ducts, which return the fluid to the venous circulation. Lymph drainage from the arm flows through the lymph nodes of the axilla to the right lymphatic duct and into the subclavian vein.

Lymph flow is slow and is dependent on external factors such as gravity, the contraction of muscles through which the lymph flows, and changes in intrathoracic pressures during respiration. The multiple valves in the lymph vessels also facilitate unidirectional flow.

When the movement of lymph is disrupted, proteins accumulate in the interstitial spaces, which causes an increase in osmotic pressure and the drawing of more water into the tissue, creating edema (McGrath, 1992b). In the woman with breast cancer, lymphedema may be caused by surgical removal of lymph nodes, radiation therapy to the axilla, infection, or recurrent tumor. This is referred to as secondary lymphedema. Lymphedema may be more transient immediately after surgery and the patient's swelling of the fingers, hand, or arm will subside once collateral lymphatic circulation develops. This type of postoperative lymphedema is thought to be secondary to surgical trauma as the lymph nodes are dissected (Horsley & Styblo, 1991). A more chronic type of lymphedema may develop months to years after initial treatment for breast cancer. With chronic lymphedema, arm swelling may stabilize or progress to extensive pitting edema, which may interfere with mobility of the arm and shoulder.

Radiation therapy may cause lymphedema because it causes fibrosis of the lymph nodes, leading to lymphatic obstruction. The addition of postmastectomy adjuvant radiotherapy to the axilla greatly increases the incidence of lymphedema. Ryttov and colleagues (1988) measured arm edema in three groups of patients who had undergone mastectomy and partial axillary dissection. Forty-six percent of the patients who received adjuvant radiotherapy developed lymphedema as compared to 11 percent of the patients who underwent surgery alone and 6 percent of the patients who received only adjuvant chemotherapy.

Larson et al. (1986) related the risk of lymphedema to the extent of axillary dissection. They reviewed the records of 475 women with breast cancer, of which 91 percent received axillary irradiation. Overall, the risk for edema was 13 percent at 6 years for those patients who had axillary surgery and 4 percent for those patients who did not have surgery. The researchers found a higher risk for edema in those patients who had a full dissection (37 percent risk) as compared to those who had a lower dissection (8 percent risk) and those who had an axillary sampling (4 percent risk). There was not an increased risk associated with radiotherapy after limited dissection, but the risk of

lymphedema after full dissection and axillary irradiation was 36 percent. The patients in this study were treated between 1968 and 1980 when the use of postoperative full axillary irradiation was common. More recently, the incidence of lymphedema has decreased as a result of more conservative surgical procedures and the trend to avoid axillary irradiation after dissection (Horsley & Styblo, 1991).

Taking measures to reduce the risk of developing lymphedema must be a lifelong practice for the patient. Proper shoulder and arm exercises, avoidance of trauma or excessive pressure on the arm, and early recognition of infection are critical to preventing lymphedema. Early detection facilitates successful treatment of lymphedema with conservative measures such as arm elevation, custom-fitted graded-pressure garments, isometric exercises, weight control, and analgesics. Antibiotics are used to treat cellulitis of the extremity. Intermittent pneumatic pressure is used to manage moderate lymphedema and involves placing the arm into a cuff that inflates and deflates sequentially according to a prescribed time schedule (McGrath, 1992b). An Ace bandage is wrapped around the extremity after each session of pneumatic compression. Manual lymph drainage (MLD) is also used to treat moderate lymphedema and employs a unique method of massage to redirect lymph fluid into functioning lymphatic channels (Lamontanaro, 1995). MLD is followed by wrapping the arm with foam, cotton padding, and elastic wrap.

Cardiac Effects

Historically, postmastectomy treatment of the internal mammary lymph nodes and ipsilateral supraclavicular nodes was routinely accomplished with a single photon field to the anterior chest, referred to as the "hockey stick" portal. This technique, which is no longer advocated today, is associated with cardiac complications including accelerated coronary atherosclerosis and myocardial infarction (Harris & Hellman, 1988). Current treatment techniques minimize cardiac exposure with the use of tangential fields or electrons to treat internal mammary nodes. Generally, the volume of heart exposed during tangential breast irradiation is 12 percent with left-breast treatment and zero exposure with right-breast treatment (Shapiro & Recht, 1994).

Second Malignancies

The potential for radiation-induced second malignancies is a serious concern because a growing proportion of women undergoing breast conservation irradiation have a long life expectancy after treatment (Lavey et al., 1990). Most of the rare occurrences of radiation-induced sarcomas in breast cancer patients are associated with outdated treatment techniques employing postmastectomy orthovoltage irradiation to multiple fields including the regional lymph nodes (Shapiro & Recht, 1994). The incidence of radiation-induced sarcoma is low with modern treatment techniques and is described as a 0.2 percent risk per decade after treatment (Lavey et al., 1990).

Kurtz and colleagues (1987) reviewed records of 300 patients with stage I and II breast cancer who were 10 years posttreatment. The treatment had consisted of tumor excision and megavoltage irradiation delivering a total dose of 4500 to 6000 cGy to the breast and 6000 to 8000 cGy to the primary tumor area. Regional lymph node areas were also treated. One chest wall sarcoma was reported among the 300 patients.

The risk for the development of contralateral breast cancer is another concern for women undergoing breast irradiation. This risk is associated with many factors including a histology of invasive or in situ lobular cancer, a young age at diagnosis, and a family history of breast cancer (Shapiro & Recht, 1994). During breast or chest wall irradiation, the contralateral breast may be exposed to 5 to 10 percent of the dose prescribed (Lavey et al., 1990). Radiation-induced breast cancer has a latency period of approximately 10 years as is evident from patients treated with mantle irradiation (Shapiro & Recht, 1994). The question of whether radiation to the breast increases one's risk for the development of contralateral breast cancer is unanswered because most studies analyzing this issue have too short follow-up, small numbers of patients, or too few patients under age 45 (Moffat, 1994; Shapiro & Recht, 1994). In the above-mentioned study by Kurtz and associates (1987), an increased incidence of contralateral breast cancer in the patients treated with radiation after surgery was not identified in the second decade posttreatment. Although most studies report very little or no increased risk for subsequent contralateral breast cancer, a study by Boice et al. (1992) found a significant, small, increased risk for women less than 45 years of age at treatment.

Nursing Care

Nursing care of the woman with breast cancer is complex and multidimensional, with a focus on meeting physical, emotional, and informational needs. These needs vary as the patient moves through the treatment process. The following is a review of nursing care and issues pertinent to the pre-, peri- and postradiation treatment periods. Patient assessment, teaching, management of side effects, psychosocial issues, sexual implications, and follow-up care are addressed.

Pretreatment Care of the Patient: Decision-Making Issues

Often the radiation oncology nurse's first contact with the patient is during the consultation visit, when the patient is gathering information to select treatment. Today, women with early-stage breast cancer confront multiple treatment choices and play an active role in the decision-making process. For many women, this period of diagnosis and treatment decision-making is a time of crisis with intense emotions, fears, and misconceptions. Rowland & Holland (1989) describe the shift in decision-making concerns as a result of changes in medicine and society over the past two decades (Table 9–6). Several studies have focused on the decision-making process, describing the emotional impact as well as the factors that influence a woman's decision about primary breast cancer treatment.

Ward and colleagues (1989) explored the decision-making process in 22 women one to two weeks after undergoing a modified radical mas-

Table 9-6 • Changes in the Psychological Issues in Primary Breast Cancer Treatment: Past and Present

15–20 years ago	The present
Fears of breast cancer and mastectomy	Fears of breast cancer and choice of treatment options
One stage biopsy with or without mastectomy under anesthesia	Knowledge of two stage procedure and two treatment options (mandated by law in some states)
Little participation in treatment decision	Full participation in care and choices made by patient
Little or no discussion of survival or prognosis	Full disclosure of survival prognosis
Full reassurance about future; minimal follow-up	Limited emphasis on reassurance about future; emphasis on frequent and long-term observation
Minimal social support or special rehabilitative programs	Access to self-help and support groups; availability of reconstruction; information that node-negative women should receive chemo or hormone therapy

From JH Rowland & JC Holland. (1989). Breast Cancer. In JC Holland & JH Rowland (Eds.), *Handbook of Psychooncology*, (pp. 188-207). New York: Oxford University Press. Copyright 1989 by Oxford University Press. Reprinted with permission.

tectomy (MRM) or breast-conserving therapy (BCT). Although the women in both groups were demographically similar, women choosing BCT were significantly younger than those who underwent a MRM. The MRM group expressed concerns about the radiotherapy, including side effects, inconvenience, and efficacy. The BCT group identified concerns about the impact of loss of a breast on body integrity. The researchers also found that all the women wished to participate to some degree in the decision-making process, and that they identified the physician as the most important source of information. Women in the BCT group viewed the nurse as the second most important source of information. The significance of personal interaction in the decision-making process highlights the need for nurses to be accessible to the patient and her family. Answering questions, discussing options, and reviewing side effects are interventions that facilitate and support the decision-making process.

An exploratory study about the role of information in the decision-making process was undertaken by Hughes (1993). Using an observer checklist, she reviewed the amount and nature of information given to 71 women with stage I or II breast cancer who were in the treatment decision-making process. The subjects' recall of information given during the consent process was also evaluated 6 to 8 weeks after surgery. Unlike the finding by Ward et al. (1989), older women in this study were more likely to choose lumpectomy than younger women. Income was related to treatment selection, with lower-income patients favoring mastectomy. The amount of information and the manner in which it was presented were found to have little impact on treatment decisions, but rather, informal sources of information given prior to the clinic visit were considered important by women selecting mastectomy. Recall of information given during the diagnostic period was very poor. Hughes (1993) concludes that nurses and physicians must be aware that factors other than information provided in the clinic influence a patient's treatment decision. These factors may include: the media, information from family or significant others, and a previous negative experience with breast cancer. Assessment of these factors prior to the consultation may help clarify misconceptions and tailor the education process to the individual.

Personality profiles of patients selecting MRM or BCT have been described by Wolberg and colleagues (1987). Preoperative psychosexual assessment of 110 women who were choosing between MRM and BCT resulted in identification of distinct personality characteristics between the two groups. Women choosing mastectomy were found to be more anxious, more distressed, and more likely to avoid stress rather than confront it. They also reported more sexual relationship problems than the women choosing BCT. Psychological traits reflecting the importance of physical appearance, self-interest, and body image were more apparent in women electing BCT. Age was not found to be a factor in treatment choice. Although posttreatment follow-up was not done in this study, the researchers suggest that the personality characteristics may correlate with psychosocial adjustment after treatment and that further studies are needed in this area.

Pretreatment Assessment and Teaching

Once the patient has made the decision to proceed with radiation therapy, her needs may shift to include more detailed information about self-care during treatment and the actual simulation and treatment process. Patient assessment and teaching are ongoing throughout the entire treatment course and are a multidisciplinary effort. A carepath or critical pathway may be used to map the care of the patient against a timeline. Focus areas of the carepath include assessment, teaching, and discharge planning, as well as documentation of patient outcomes (Table 9–7). The radiation oncology nurse may formally begin this process at a scheduled presimulation visit with the patient.

Initial assessment of the woman with breast cancer should include an appraisal of the woman's perception of the impact of the diagnosis on her life. Sinsheimer and Holland (1987) identify three key factors that will influence a woman's psychological adaptation to breast cancer: the age of the woman, her usual coping strategies, and her social supports. Young women, who are facing the developmental tasks of intimacy and childbearing, react to the threat of breast cancer on their body image and sexuality, whereas older women may perceive the cancer as more of a threat to life (Sinsheimer & Holland, 1987). Effective coping strategies in previous life crises and available social supports, including her spouse, family, and friends, facilitate the adaptation process. Early assessment of these factors will help to identify women who are particularly vulnerable to distress and who may benefit from counseling during the treatment period.

Pretreatment anxiety as measured by a trait anxiety scale was found to be an indicator of those patients who were likely to experience psychological distress during radiation therapy for early breast cancer (Wallace et al., 1993). Patients with high trait anxiety scores were noted to have more symptoms during treatment, more emotional disruption, and more changes in quality of life (Wallace et al., 1993). Although measurement of trait anxiety scores may not be feasible in many radiation oncology clinics, the nurse's assessment of the patient's level of anxiety pretreatment may help target those patients who may require more frequent assessments or counseling during treatment.

Physical assessment during this initial contact with the patient should include range-of-motion of the ipsilateral upper extremity as well as the patient's ability to lie comfortably in the treatment position. If lymphedema is present, a baseline assessment should include measurements of the circumference of the upper and lower arm of both extremities at specified reference points, strength and mobility of the arm, color, turgor, pulses, and any signs of infection (McGrath, 1992b). Physical examination of the breast prior to treatment is essential, particularly in women who have had postoperative complications, such as seroma or hematoma formation, infection, or delayed wound healing. Assessment of a tumor wound or skin nodules should include the size and distribution, odor, drainage, signs of infection, pain, and morphological characteristics such as scales, fissures, crusts, or erosion (Stair, 1985).

Pretreatment patient education should provide cognitive information, specifically the who, what, when, why, where, and how of a situation (Dodd & Ahmed, 1987). For the woman with breast cancer, information before the simulation about positioning, disrobing, measurements, markings, and photographs may help to lessen feelings of vulnerability. The patient must be assured that the staff will attend to comfort and privacy needs whenever possible. Pretreatment discussion about skin assessment and self-care during treatment will help the patient anticipate side effects and gain an understanding of how to deal with them. Hopefully, this information will promote a feeling of control and facilitate coping.

Nursing Management of Acute Side Effects

The predominant side effect that a patient undergoing breast irradiation will experience is a skin reaction. Identification of patients who are at risk for the development of skin problems, including intense erythema and moist desquamation in the inframammary fold or axillary area, will allow for early intervention to prevent or mitigate the reaction when possible. Risk factors for increased skin reaction include: 1) large breasts, 2) skinfolds in the infra-axillary area, 3) prior or concurrent chemotherapy, 4) presence of a tumor wound, 5) use of a bolus material during treatment, and 6) history of sensitive skin. At the minimum, weekly assessment of the patient is necessary to monitor the skin reaction and to offer guidance about skin care. Measures to promote maintenance of skin integrity during treatment may vary according to institutional practice, but in general focus on gentle cleansing, reducing friction on the skin, increasing aeration to skin folds, minimizing chemicals on the skin, and applying lotions or creams to moisturize the skin. Instructions about use of deodorant or lotion during treatment and recommendations about wearing a bra should be tailored to the needs of the patient. A thorough discussion of management of skin reactions, including dry and moist desquamation, may be found in Chapter 8.

Fatigue, another common side effect during radiation therapy, has been studied in women undergoing treatment for breast cancer. Greenberg and colleagues (1992) describe the fatigue experienced by 15 women with early-stage, node-negative breast cancer who were undergoing radiation therapy after lumpectomy. The women had no other medical problems, were not receiving chemotherapy, and had a mean age of 46 years. The researchers found that the level of fatigue was mild and that it peaked during the fourth week of treatment, plateaued thereafter, and resolved in three weeks after treatment. The pattern of fatigue did not correlate with clinical depression, sleep patterns, exercise performance, or select biological markers, such as orthostatic vital signs, mean thyroid hormone, hematocrit, weight loss, or serum albumin. The researchers also found that patients continued to feel fatigued on weekends and that the electron-boost period was associated with the same degree of fatigue.

Another study by Graydon (1994) found that fatigue was persistent after radiation therapy. She assessed quality of life in 53 women who had undergone breast conservation surgery and radiation by exploring their ability to perform activities of daily living, their emotional distress, and their symptoms. The investigator found that there was minimal negative impact on quality of life; the women were functioning well, they were not distressed, and had few symptoms. Fatigue was the

Table 9-7 • Breast Simulation Education and Breast Treatment Carepath

Focus	First Visit Date:	Pre-simulation Nursing Visit Date:	Simulation Tech Visit Date:	Post-simulation Date:
CONSULTATION	MD: History and Physical MD: Simulation request form MD: Diagnosis MD: Treatment consent form MD: Photo consent ×3 MD/RN: Assessment of arm ROM and need for instruction MD/RN: Instructional video ☐ SEC: ID Photo ☐ SEC: Schedule simulation ☐ SEC: Schedule RN visit ☐ SEC: Order outside pathology report ☐ SEC: Release of information form signed ☐ SEC: UHC chart ordered	RN: History and physical RN: Instructional sheet RN: NCI booklet RN: Referrals as needed to: ☐ Social Work ☐ Dietitian ☐ University Home Care ☐ Other (describe)	☐ RTT: Assess mobility of pt. on transfer ☐ RTT: Assess arm ROM ☐ RTT: Assess patient comfort ☐ RTT: Check for patient photo consent. Reinforce previous teaching	MD: Prescription written and signed MD: Films outlined for block cutting
TEACHING RE: DEPT. ROUTINE	☐ SEC: Parking pass ordered ☐ SEC: Address transportation and wheelchair needs with pt. ☐ SEC: Explain check-in routine MD: Willoughby office	RN: Availability of RN, SW, MD RN: Weekly treatment visit RN: Weekly weight RN: On-call routine		☐ RTT: Explanation of next two appts.: • First treatment is lengthy • Routine treatment ☐ RTT: Schedule next appt. ☐ RTT: Explain pt. satisfaction survey

Table continued on following page

Outcomes	Met	Not Met	Comments	Date/Initials
1. Patient views instructional video prior to simulation.				
2. Patient meets with RN prior to simulation.				
3. Patient verbalizes understanding of procedure prior to simulation.				
4. Patient states understanding of potential acute side effects.				
5. Patient is able to describe skin care measures.				
6. Patient states understanding of importance of skin marking preservation.				

Table 9-7 • Breast Simulation Education and Breast Treatment Carepath (*Continued*)

Focus	First Visit Date:	Pre-simulation Nursing Visit Date:	Simulation Tech Visit Date:	Post-simulation Date:
PRE-SIMULATION TEACHING	RN: Written instructional folder MD: Verbal Instructions: • What is simulation? • Multiple people in simulation room • Room environment • Hard table • Two-hour duration • Breast exposure • Alpha cradle • Wire contour • Photo explanation and photo consent • Simulation films • Markings on breasts • Tattoos • CT, if necessary	RN: Assess patient knowledge needs and reinforce previous teaching: • What is simulation? • Multiple people in simulation room • Room environment • Hard table • Two-hour duration • Breast exposure • Alpha cradle • Wire contour • Photo explanation • Simulation films • Markings on breasts • Tattoos • CT, if necessary	☐ RTT: Verbal instructions to patient: ☐ Alpha Cradle • purpose • construction • warm ☐ Exposure of both breasts ☐ Simulation process • time involved • immobility • limited conversation • breathe normally • lights go on and off • machine rotates • people come in and out of room ☐ Measurements ☐ Markings on breasts and waist ☐ Simulation films ☐ Wire contour ☐ Positioning photo purpose ☐ Treatment field photo ☐ Tattoos	☐ RTT: CT, for treatment planning if necessary ☐ RTT: Tattoos ☐ RTT: Explain importance of reproduction: • Call attention to arm position and back position ☐ RTT: Pre-treatment planning blocks cut ☐ RTT: Physics calculated and computer plan made
SKIN CARE INSTRUCTIONS	MD: Describe skin changes: • hyperpigmentation • erythema • pruritis • dry desquamation • moist desquamation	RN: Describe skin changes RN: Describe skin care measures RN: Discuss bathing RN: Describe appropriate clothing RN: Discuss preservation of skin markings	☐ RTT: Review importance of skin markings ☐ RTT: Review preservation of skin markings	
SIDE EFFECTS INSTRUCTIONS	MD: Describe acute and chronic side effects: • skin reaction • fatigue • breast swelling • fibrosis • telangiectasia • rib fractures • lung changes • arm edema	RN: Review recommendations: • activity • nutrition RN: Review self-care measures		

Focus	First Rx Day Date:	Weekly Visit	Last Treatment	First F/U Visit
TEACHING	☐ RTT: Review Dept. Routine ☐ RTT: Review Rx procedure: • cameras • intercoms • noise, time, lights • port films • measurements • positioning • math calculation check • actual treatment ☐ RTT: Review tattoo procedure:	RN/MD: Review Skin Care RN/MD: Indicate skin care interventions: ☐ cornstarch_____ ☐ cream _____ ☐ lotion_____ ☐ topical steroid_____ ☐ gel_____ ☐ dressing_____ ☐ analgesic_____ ☐ other_____ ☐ none_____	RN: Post-treatment skin care RN: Breast self-exam RN: Lymphedema prevention RN/MD: Interventions ☐ cornstarch_____ ☐ cream _____ ☐ lotion_____ ☐ topical steroid_____ ☐ gel_____ ☐ dressing_____ ☐ analgesic_____ ☐ other_____ ☐ none_____	RN/MD: Review Skin Care RN/MD: Interventions ☐ cornstarch_____ ☐ cream _____ ☐ lotion_____ ☐ topical steroid_____ ☐ gel_____ ☐ dressing_____ ☐ analgesic_____ ☐ other_____ ☐ none_____
PHYSICAL ASSESSMENT		RN/MD: Assess Skin Integrity: 0—No change 1—Faint erythema/dry desquamation 2—Tender, bright erythema/patchy moist desquamation moderate edema 3—Confluent moist desquamation (other than skin folds) 4—Ulceration, hemorrhage, necrosis (RTOG Scoring Criteria) RN/MD: Assess Comfort: 0. No change 1. Itching 2. Discomfort/tenderness 3. Pain 4. Fatigue RN/MD: Assess Weight. RN/MD: Assess CBC	RN/MD: Assess Skin Integrity: ☐ 0 ☐ 1 ☐ 2 ☐ 3 ☐ 4 RN/MD: Assess Comfort: 0. No change 1. Itching 2. Discomfort/tenderness 3. Pain 4. Fatigue RN/MD: Assess Weight RN/MD: Assess CBC	RN/MD: Assess Skin Integrity: ☐ 0 ☐ 1 ☐ 2 ☐ 3 ☐ 4 RN/MD: Assess Comfort: 0. No change 1. Itching 2. Discomfort/tenderness 3. Pain 4. Fatigue RN/MD: Assess Weight RN/MD: Assess CBC
DISCHARGE PLANNING	☐ RTT: Schedule Treatment Appointment	RN/MD: Referral to SW/Support Group PRN	RN/RTT: Inform pt. of follow-up appt. RN/MD: Referral to SW/Support Group PRN	RN/MD: Referral to SW/Support Group PRN
OUTCOMES		1. Patient is able to verbalize self-care measures to control symptoms.	1. Patient sees RN on last visit day. 2. Patient explains post-treatment skin care. 3. Patient describes symptoms which require calling the MD/RN prior to the F/U visit. 4. Patient has F/U visit scheduled.	1. Patient is able to verbalize self-care measures to control symptoms. 2. Patient understands F/U schedule and routine.

most common symptom reported and was significantly related to the reported level of functioning and the extent of symptoms. That is, women with more fatigue had more disruption with functioning and more symptoms, such as insomnia, decreased mobility, and pain. Graydon (1994) stresses that the duration of fatigue may extend to 12 weeks after radiation therapy.

These studies have implications for nurses. First, assessment of fatigue and its impact on the patient's lifestyle should continue throughout the treatment and follow-up periods. The nurse must help the patient to understand that fatigue is an expected side effect from the therapy, to recognize the pattern of fatigue, and to modify behaviors or activities that might offset the fatigue. Ongoing assessment of the patient will promote early identification of other reversible factors that may cause fatigue, such as poor nutritional intake, dehydration, and electrolyte imbalance (Nail & Winningham, 1995). Lastly, the nurse must be aware that women with intense or prolonged fatigue may have more disruptions in their functional status and more symptoms. Interventions may be required to manage symptoms, mobilize supports, and conserve energy. Referrals to a social worker, community agencies, or support group may also be appropriate.

The impact of comorbidity and functional status in older adults with cancer has also been studied. Forty percent of all women with invasive breast cancer are more than 65 years old and most of these women will have one or more comorbid conditions (Satariano, 1992). Lindsey et al. (1994) assessed the variables of weight, functional status, comorbidity, nutritional intake, side effects, and social support in 45 cancer patients undergoing lung or breast irradiation. The mean age of the patients was 69.8 years and most of them had at least one comorbid condition such as arthritis, hypertension, or heart disease. The researchers found that the patients tolerated the treatment well and that there were no significant differences in the measured variables between patients with a comorbid condition and those without one. However, they did find that the caloric intake of this elderly sample was not adequate to meet activity requirements throughout the treatment period and at the three month follow-up period. The researchers recommend that nurses closely monitor the older patient's intake, offer suggestions to increase intake, and help them to modify activities during the treatment period.

Unlike the results in the study by Lindsey et al. (1994), a report from Satariano et al. (1990) found that women with breast cancer, aged 65 to 74, experienced functional disability, particularly with tasks involving upper-body strength, for more than a year after diagnosis. Younger women, aged 55 to 64, also reported more difficulty with physical tasks, but unlike the older group, were able to return to normal functioning within 12 months. The researchers propose that the development of rehabilitative services for breast cancer patients must reflect the prevalence and variation of functional disability in different age groups.

Quality of Life and Psychosocial Issues During Primary Treatment

Many of the studies addressing psychosocial issues focus on adaptation during primary treatment, comparing groups of patients selecting breast conservation treatment (BCT) versus mastectomy. Levy and colleagues (1989) found that patients undergoing BCT were significantly more depressed and distressed at three months posttreatment than those women undergoing mastectomy. The researchers postulate that the emotional distress may be related to the patient confronting a treatment choice without enough information about BCT. Lack of social support was also identified as a factor contributing to higher levels of distress.

A study by Ganz et al. (1992) also found that BCT did not protect the women from psychological distress or disruption in quality of life. The researchers prospectively evaluated quality of life, performance status, and psychological adjustment in 57 women who had a modified radical mastectomy and 52 who had breast conservation surgery and radiation therapy. There were no significant differences in any of these areas between the two groups except in the area of body image and clothing problems, with women in the BCT group having a better outcome. Of interest in this study is a nonstatistical trend for women in the BCT group to have an increase in distress at one month after surgery, during the radiation period. The level of distress declined markedly at 4 months after surgery for the BCT group and at 6 months for the mastectomy group. The authors conclude that the findings suggest that women undergoing BCT need more short-term, intensive counseling during the period of radiation therapy and that patients undergoing mastectomy may require long-term psychosocial interventions, with particular attention to needs regarding body image and clothing. Other studies also support these findings of better body image after BCT (Mock, 1993; Noguchi et al., 1993; Schain et al., 1994).

Fears about possible recurrence of cancer in the breast may also contribute to psychological distress in women undergoing BCT. Noguchi et al. (1993) found that fears of cancer recurrence were reported by 95 percent of women undergoing BCT, a result similar to that of the group which underwent mastectomy with immediate breast reconstruction. Stefanek (1992) also concluded that there was no difference in fears of cancer recurrence between BCT and mastectomy groups. These findings highlight the need for nurses to recognize that women with early breast cancer have fears and concerns, regardless of the type of treatment.

Psychosocial Adaptation—Age Related Differences

There are few studies that have explored age-related differences in psychosocial adjustment. Vinokur and colleagues (1990) assessed physical and mental health functioning in 274 women with breast cancer throughout the first year after diagnosis. The average age of the participants was 58.8 years. Sixty-three percent had undergone a total or modified radical mastectomy. The percentage of patients receiving radiation therapy was not assessed. Although physical functioning improved throughout the year, mental health did not. Younger patients with advanced disease or physical impairments were more psychologically distressed than older patients with similar problems. Younger patients perceived the breast cancer as a greater threat, resulting in psychologic distress. Older patients were found to be more impaired physically or functionally.

Age-related differences were also noted by Mor et al. (1994), who analyzed physical and psychosocial quality of life in 262 women with breast cancer. Again, radiation therapy was not assessed as part of the treatment characteristics of the sample. Chemotherapy was given to 80 percent of the younger women (ages 24 to 54) and 67 percent of the older women (more than 55 years). Although the younger women had greater social and financial resources, the researchers found that this group reported higher levels of emotional distress, more financial problems, more difficulty maintaining daily activities, and more unmet needs for assistance than their older counterparts. Mor and colleagues (1994) propose that the results relate to the women's perceived threat of the illness to their social roles of provider and caregiver for the family. They also assert that older women and

their families may view the breast cancer as an expectation of the aging process.

Nurses may draw several implications from these studies. First, psychological recovery after the diagnosis of breast cancer is a process that may persist for years after treatment, even when physical recovery has occurred. Second, throughout the treatment and follow-up period, the nurse should explore patients' perception of the impact of their illness on their lives. Lastly, the nurse must be aware that the issues that women confront and the needs that they express may differ as a result of their ages, life stages, and the roles that they have assumed. Young women with breast cancer may require more emotional support, whereas older women may need assistance with house work, shopping, personal care, and other daily needs.

Psychosocial Impact of Recurrent Disease

Although studies report conflicting results as to whether the psychological impact of recurrence is more stressful than the initial diagnosis, it is recognized that psychosocial issues at the time of breast cancer recurrence change to predominantly existential and health concerns (Mahon et al., 1990; Worden, 1989). Factors that may be associated with increased stress during this period include: multiple physical problems and limitations; limited social supports; presence of other social, family, work, or financial concerns; and young age at recurrence (Worden, 1989). Nurses can target their interventions to minimize these factors by alleviating physical symptoms, enhancing supports, and addressing other concerns.

A descriptive study by Lewis and Deal (1995) explored the experience of breast cancer recurrence with married couples. Fifteen women, aged 32 to 54 years, and their husbands were interviewed at an average time of 12.7 months after diagnosis of the recurrence. The authors found that the couples worked actively to "balance" the impact of the cancer recurrence with other aspects of their lives. The couples used avoidant strategies to accomplish this "balance." These strategies included focusing on the treatment and not the actual meaning of the cancer recurrence and limiting discussions about sensitive issues regarding the recurrence. Lewis and Deal (1995) offer three recommendations for nurses. First, nurses should gently support the couple's "illusions" or beliefs by encouraging discussion and listening to their experience, without aggressive questioning or confrontations. Second, couples may need help to recognize and express their sad feelings, rather than suppress them. Third, the nurse must realize that some emotional distress and marital tension may be unrelated to the recurrence and that a referral to a counselor may be necessary.

Psychosocial Impact on the Family

Most studies of the psychological impact of breast cancer on the spouse demonstrate that the spouse also experiences some degree of emotional distress (Northouse et al., 1991). An earlier study by Wellisch et al. (1978) discovered that sleeping problems, decreased appetite, and work disruption were common reactions among men whose partners had had mastectomies. In a longitudinal study by Northouse (1990), psychosocial adjustment was assessed in 41 patients and their husbands up to 18 months after mastectomy. She found that both patients and their husbands had mild to moderate distress that persisted 18 months after the postoperative period. In addition, younger husbands reported less positive mood states than older husbands.

Ongoing emotional distress was also identified in a study of the effect of treatment on psychosocial adjustment among husbands by Omne-Ponten et al. (1993). Although almost 50 percent of the sample expressed persistent emotional distress, the researchers did not find a statistical difference in degree of emotional disturbance between husbands of women who underwent BCT and those who had a mastectomy. They also noted that there was not an identified subgroup of husbands who were more vulnerable to distress, there were few reported work disturbances, and there were anecdotal reports of the husband's perception of not being included by the medical staff in clinical discussions. Northouse et al. (1991) identify three factors that may place a husband at risk for increased psychologic distress. These include a perception of little social support, increased demands as a result of the type of disease and intensity of the treatment, and limited information from health care professionals.

The impact of breast cancer on children has been studied by Lewis (1990). Interviews were conducted with young school-aged children (7 to 10 years), older school-aged children (10 to 13 years), and adolescents (14 through 19 years). Children were asked to express their feelings or concerns about their mother's illness. The young school-aged children expressed feelings of sadness, fear, and loneliness and were worried about the near future and maintaining an intact family unit. The older school-aged children voiced concern about how the mother's illness changed their own life, including disruption of activities and more household responsibilities. They also indicated a need for more information about cancer and the treatments. The adolescents expressed conflict between their desire for independence from the family and the family's need to remain cohesive and interdependent.

Nurses must be aware that the impact of breast cancer is felt by the entire family and that assessments of the family's response and interventions to mitigate their stress should be ongoing and extend into the posttreatment period. Interventions that are family-focused have been outlined by Lewis (1990).

Sexuality Issues

The impact of the diagnosis of breast cancer and therapy on sexuality is another area of comparison between women undergoing BCT and mastectomy. Schain et al. (1994) found that at six months after treatment, women who had undergone mastectomy had significantly increased distress with sexual relations. This level of subjective sexual difficulties lessened over time, and at 12 and 24 months after treatment was equal to the distress that women undergoing BCT reported. The researchers postulate that the sexual distress associated with BCT may be due to posttreatment changes in the breast, concurrent medical or psychological problems, or other noncancer-related issues.

McCormick and colleagues (1989) also explored sexual satisfaction in women one to eight years after completing BCT. Overall, a high level of satisfaction was reported by the women who were sexually active. However, specific problems during sexual activity such as an awareness of numbness in the breast, increased breast discomfort, less nipple sensation, and avoidance of the breast were noted in 41, 48, 33, and 39 percent of the women, respectively.

Women with breast cancer undergoing chemotherapy or hormonal therapy, in addition to radiation therapy, may have more significant disruption of sexual functioning, related to menopausal and treatment symptoms. Vaginal dryness and thinning, decreased libido, hot flashes, alopecia, weight gain, nausea, fatigue, and other symptoms will affect sexual functioning and expression. The sexual functioning of women with advanced or metastatic breast cancer may be influenced by fatigue, pain, visible wounds, and other physical symptoms.

It is imperative that sexuality be addressed with every women with breast cancer, regardless of the type of treatment. Discussions about sexuality and the impact of the treatment should be introduced by the nurse at diagnosis, throughout treatment, and into the follow-up period (Lamb 1995). Bellettieri (1993) suggests two questions that may be explored by the health care professional: "Since your diagnosis, have you noticed any changes in the way you think or feel about yourself physically or sexually?" and "Since diagnosis or treatment, have you noticed any changes in sexual activity, such as the desire to engage in sexual activity or the physical response while engaged in it?" These questions and subsequent discussions may help to identify concerns, clarify information, and screen women who may need further counseling. Schover (1991) identifies patients at risk for sexual problems, including young women, women without a supportive partner, single women, women who wish to conceive another child, and those with a history of sexual problems or trauma.

The nurse may help to manage side effects that impact sexual functioning or offer specific suggestions to resolve problems and enhance sexuality. Interventions may include a discussion of strategies to alleviate fatigue, use of a breast prosthesis or lingerie during sexual activity, alternate sexual positions to avoid an uncomfortable breast or arm, alternate pleasurable activities to offset changes in breast sensation, use of vaginal lubricants and dilators, and ways to promote verbal and nonverbal communication (Schover, 1991). Whenever possible, the partner should be encouraged to express concerns and to participate in mutual problem-solving.

Survivorship Issues

Survivorship, which has been defined as "living through and beyond a diagnosis of cancer," has associated biomedical, psychosocial, economic legal, and spiritual/existential effects (Leigh, 1992). The survivor of breast cancer will encounter challenges related to each of these effects. Included in the biomedical aspects of survivorship are issues related to follow-up care. At each follow-up visit, the nurse or physician should assess the patient's understanding of the need for regular physical examinations, mammograms, blood work, and other tests. The practice of breast self-examination (BSE) should be reviewed with the patient, with particular attention given to the patient's concerns about changes in the irradiated breast or chest wall.

Often, gentle encouragement may be needed to help the woman resume the practice of BSE after treatment.

Education of the patient regarding lymphedema prevention is another aspect of follow-up care for those patients who are at risk for its development. Providing the patient with a list of do's and dont's related to use of the arm, the signs and symptoms of lymphedema, actions to take if a problem occurs, and arm exercises to promote lymph drainage will enhance self-care activities. Pictorial descriptions of postaxillary dissection exercises are provided by Brown, Eyles and Bland (1991). Humble (1995) offers an excellent review of the nursing role in the management of a patient with lymphedema (Table 9–8).

Pregnancy after breast irradiation is another survivorship issue. Dow and colleagues (1994) explored the effect of pregnancy on treatment outcome and quality of life among 23 women who had children after breast-conserving surgery and radiation therapy. The subjects were young with a mean age of 30.4 years at diagnosis and had either stage I or II breast cancer. Eighteen percent had received adjuvant chemotherapy. Comparison of the subjects to a case-matched sample revealed that there were no increased risks for recurrence or survival disadvantage for women with pregnancies after breast conservation treatment. Children and family concerns were identified by the mothers as having great impact on their perception of quality of life. Although Dow et al. (1994) recognize several design problems with the study, they suggest that generally, patients delay pregnancy for 1 year after treatment and that health care providers tailor their recommendations to the patient's clinical situation and personal preferences, which include quality of life issues.

Lactation may also be influenced by breast irradiation. Women contemplating pregnancy after breast cancer treatment should be aware of their limited lactation potential in the irradiated breast. Postradiation fibrosis, ductal shrinkage, and atrophy of the lobules will generally inhibit the irradiated breast from undergoing changes during pregnancy and will diminish or prevent lactation after delivery (Niefert, 1992). However, offering reassurance about the safety of breast feeding with the nontreated breast will help to alleviate concerns and promote a satisfying breast feeding experience.

Psychosocial aspects of survivorship among women treated for breast cancer were qualitatively described by Carter (1993). She described various

Table 9-8 • Patient Education for Lymphedema Prevention

NURSING DIAGNOSIS
Knowledge deficit regarding potential development of lymphedema

NURSING INTERVENTIONS
Provide a peaceful, relaxed atmosphere to facilitate the educational process.

Review the definition, risk factors, and etiology of lymphedema.

Review signs and symptoms.
a. Heaviness or fullness of extremity
b. Increase in size of extremity compared to opposite extremity as evidenced by increasing tightness of clothes, shoes, or jewelry on the affected side
c. Weakness
d. Limited range of motion
e. Stiffness
f. Numbness
g. Redness
h. Warmth

Teach prevention measures.
a. Avoid constricting clothing such as tight sleeves or jewelry and stockings that constrict.
b. Avoid carrying a purse or heavy object on extremity at risk.
c. Protect extremity at risk from trauma (e.g., venipunctures, fingersticks, IVs, blood pressure checks); wear gloves if working in garden, cutting meat, or washing dishes with detergents; wear a thimble if sewing; wear shoes to protect lower extremities; avoid cuticle damage; use electrical razor when shaving axilla or legs.
d. Keep skin well-lubricated to prevent dryness and cracking.
e. Avoid sunburns and exposure to temperature extremes.
   Use sunscreens.
   Use oven mitts.
   Avoid use of icepacks and heating pads on extremity at risk.
f. Avoid prolonged dependency of extremity; support extremity so that distal end is higher than proximal end when engaging in sedentary activities.
g. List medications that patient is currently taking or foods high in fat or salt that may influence fluid retention and weight gain.
h. Have patient identify resources in the community to contact for more information.

Describe appropriate action if injury occurs.
a. Wash with soap and water and cover.
b. Call health care provider if redness, warmth, or swelling occur.

Demonstrate exercises to promote lymph drainage.

Provide a copy of *Lymphedema: An Informational Booklet,* from the National Lymphedema Network.

Refer to community resources.
a. National Lymphedema Network (800–541–3259)
b. Susan G. Komen Breast Cancer Foundation (800–462–9273)
c. American Cancer Society (800–227–2345)
d. National Cancer Institute (800–4–CANCER)

From Humble CA (1995). Lymphedema: Incidence, pathophysiology, management, and nursing care. *Oncology Nursing Forum, 22,* 1503–1509. Reprinted with permission of the publisher, Oncology Nursing Press, Inc.

phases that the women moved through during the survival process. These included interpreting the diagnosis within the context of their own lives; confronting their mortality; reprioritizing their activities, lifestyles, and goals; accepting and integrating the experience of cancer into their lives; proceeding with life by putting the cancer experience behind them; and lastly, preserving the capacity to relive and reintegrate former experiences in an effort to give meaning to the past, present, or future. Women were found to move in and out of these phases in a nonlinear, often simultaneous manner. The author concludes that psychologic adaptation along the "survival trajectory" is often complex and intense, and that

trained professionals, community resources, and support groups should consider in their interventions the uniqueness of the individual's experience with survival.

Numerous national and local organizations are available to offer information, advocacy, and support to the woman with breast cancer. A detailed listing of breast cancer resources may be obtained from the National Alliance of Breast Cancer Organizations (NABCO; 800-719-9154). Other resources include: The Susan G. Komen Foundation (800-IM-AWARE), The National Breast Cancer Coalition (202-296-7477), The American Cancer Society (800-ACS-2345), The Cancer Information Service of the National Cancer Institute

(800-4-CANCER), and The National Coalition for Cancer Survivorship (301-650-8868).

Summary

Breast cancer is the most common malignancy in women in the United States and poses significant health issues related to prevention, detection, treatment, and survivorship. Throughout the spectrum of breast cancer, radiation therapy plays a key role in the health care management of the patient. Breast conservation treatment achieves local tumor control with minimal cosmetic deformity and has been designated by the National Institutes of Health as an alternative to a mastectomy for selected breast cancer patients. Radiation therapy is used to decrease local-regional recurrences after mastectomy in high-risk patients. Symptoms associated with local-regional recurrences and locally advanced breast cancer may be controlled with radiation therapy. Radiation therapy remains the mainstay of treatment for metastatic breast cancer with the overall goal of improving the patient's quality of life by relieving symptoms. The most common acute side effect associated with breast or chest wall irradiation is a skin reaction, which may become intensified with concurrent chemotherapy. Late effects and complications of radiation therapy to the breast and lymph node areas are related to the treatment technique used, the addition of chemotherapy, and the radiation dose given.

Nursing care of the woman with breast cancer is complex and multidimensional, with a focus on meeting physical, emotional, and informational needs. During the pretreatment phase, decision-making issues and informational needs must be addressed. Patient assessment and teaching are ongoing throughout the entire treatment course and are a multidisciplinary effort. Nursing management of skin reactions should focus on early intervention to prevent or mitigate the reaction when possible. Assessment of fatigue and its impact on the patient's lifestyle is imperative. The need for ongoing assessment of the patient's and family's psychological recovery is supported by numerous studies, which have focused on quality of life and psychosocial issues throughout the breast cancer trajectory. Discussions related to sexuality should be introduced early so that the nurse may identify concerns, clarify information, and screen women who may need further counseling. Survivors of breast cancer will encounter challenges related to follow-up care, prevention of complications, pregnancy options, and psychological adaptation as they integrate the experience of cancer into their lives.

References

Adler DD & Wahl, RL (1995). New findings for imaging the breast: Techniques, findings, and potential. *American Journal Roentgenology, 164,* 19–30.

American Cancer Society, Recommendations for the early detection of breast cancer. American Cancer Society, Cuyahoga County Unit. American Joint Committee on Cancer (1992). 1992 AJCC Classification System for Cancer of the Breast. From *Manual for Staging of Cancer* (4th ed.), Philadelphia: Lippincott-Raven.

Ashikari R, Park K, Huvos AG, & Urban JA (1970). Paget's disease of the breast. *Cancer, 26,* 680–685.

Bates T (1992). A review of local radiotherapy in the treatment of bone metastases and cord compression. *International Journal of Radiation Oncology, Biology, Physics, 23,* 217–221.

Bedwinek J (1990). Radiation therapy of isolated local-regional recurrence of breast cancer: Decisions regarding dose, field size, and elective irradiation of involved sites. *International Journal of Radiation Oncology, Biology, Physics, 19* (4), 1093–1095.

Bellettieri RJ (1993). Quality of life—before, during, and after treatment. *Annals of New York Academy of Sciences, 698,* 372–377.

Blakeley S, Fornage BD, Rapini RP & Duvic M (1994). Ductal carcinoma after conservative management of Paget's disease of the breast: A case report. *Breast Disease, 7,* 361–366.

Blamey RW, Wilson ARM, Patnick J, & Dixon JM (1994). Screening for breast cancer. *British Medical Journal, 309,* 1076–1079.

Boice JD, Harvey EB, Blettner M, Stovall M & Flannery JT (1992). Cancer in the contralateral breast after radiotherapy for breast cancer. *New England Journal of Medicine, 326,* 781–785.

Borgelt BB, Gelber R, Kramer S, Brady LW, Chang CH, Davis LW, et al. (1980). The palliation of brain metastases: Final results of the first two studies by the Radiation Therapy Oncology Group. *International Journal of Radiation Oncology, Biology, Physics, 6,* 1–9.

Brown M, Eyles H, & Bland KI (1991). Nursing care for the patient with breast cancer. In KI Bland & EM Copeland III (Eds.), *The Breast: Comprehensive Management of Benign and Malignant Diseases* (pp. 1053–1080). Philadelphia: WB Saunders.

Calitchi E, Otmezguine Y, Feuilhade F, Piedbois P, Pavlovitch JM, Brun B, et al. (1991). External irradiation prior to conservative surgery for breast cancer treatment. *International Journal of Radiation Oncology, Biology, Physics, 21,* 325–329.

Carter BJ, (1993). Long-term survivors of breast cancer: A qualitative descriptive study. *Cancer Nursing, 16,* 354–361.

Carter CL, Allen C, & Henson DE (1989). Relation of tumor size, lymph node status, and survival in 24,740 breast cancer cases. *Cancer, 63,* 181–187.

Coia LR (1992). The role of radiation therapy in the treatment of brain metastases. *International Journal of Radiation Oncology, Biology, Physics, 23,* 229–238.

Cox JD & Winchester DP (1992). Standards for breast-conservation treatment. *CA-A Cancer Journal for Clinicians, 42,* 134–162.

Davidson N (1991). Biology of breast cancer. *Current Opinion in Oncology, 3,* 988–994.

Diener-West M, Dobbins TW, Phillips TL, & Nelson DF (1989). Identification of an optimal subgroup for treatment evaluation of patients with brain metastases using RTOG study 7916. *International Journal of Radiation Oncology, Biology, Physics, 16,* 669–673.

Dodd MJ & Ahmed N (1987). Preference for type of information in cancer patients receiving radiation therapy. *Cancer Nursing, 10,* 244–251.

Donegan WL (1991). Cancer of the breast in men. *CA-A Cancer Journal for Clinicians, 41,* 339–354.

Dow KH (1991). Newer developments in the diagnosis and staging of breast cancer. *Seminars in Oncology Nursing, 7,* 166–174.

Dow KH, Harris JR, & Roy C (1994). Pregnancy after breast-conserving surgery and radiation therapy for breast cancer. *Journal of the National Cancer Institute Monographs, 16,* 131–137.

Elledge RM, McGuire WL & Osborne CK (1992). Prognostic factors in breast cancer. *Seminars in Oncology, 19,* 244–253.

Falk SJ (1994). Radiotherapy and the management of the axilla in early breast cancer. *British Journal of Surgery, 81,* 1277–1281.

Fisher B (1991). Lumpectomy (segmental mastectomy) and axillary dissection. In KI Bland & EM Copeland III (Eds.), *The Breast: Comprehensive Management of Benign and Malignant Diseases.* (pp. 634–652). Philadelphia: WB Saunders.

Fisher B (1995). Breast-conserving surgery in the treatment of invasive breast cancer: Its validity and outstanding issues. *Breast Journal, 1,* 380–385.

Fisher B, Costantino J, Redmond C, Fisher E, Margolese R, Dimitrov N, et al. (1993). Lumpectomy compared with lumpectomy and radiation therapy for the treatment of intraductal breast cancer. *New England Journal of Medicine, 328,* 1581–1586.

Fisher B, Redmond C, Poisson R, Margolese R, Wolmark N, Wickerham L, et al. (1989). Eight-year results of a randomized clinical trial comparing total mastectomy and lumpectomy with or without irradiation in the treatment of breast cancer. *New England Journal of Medicine, 320,* 822–828.

Fleming ID & Fleming MD (1994). Breast cancer in elderly women. *Cancer Supplement, 74,* 2160–2164.

Ganz PA, Coscarelli Schag CA, Lee JJ, Polinsky ML, & Tan SJ (1992). Breast conservation versus mastectomy: Is there a difference in psychological adjustment or quality of life in the year after surgery? *Cancer, 69,* 1729–1738.

Goodman M & Harte N (1990). Breast cancer. In S Groenwald, MH Frogge, M Goodman, & CH Yarbro (Eds.), *Cancer Nursing Principles and Practice* (pp. 722–750). Boston: Jones and Bartlett.

Graham MV, Perez CA, Kuske RR, Garcia DM & Fineberg B (1991). Locally advanced (noninflammatory) carcinoma of the breast: results and comparison of various treatment modalities. *International Journal of Radiation Oncology, Biology, Physics, 21,* 311–318.

Gray JR, McCormick B, Cox L & Yahalom J (1991). Primary breast irradiation in large-breasted or heavy women: analysis of cosmetic outcome. *International Journal of Radiation Oncology, Biology, Physics, 21,* 347–354.

Graydon JE (1994). Women with breast cancer: Their quality of life following a course of radiation therapy. *Journal of Advanced Nursing, 19,* 617–622.

Greenberg DB, Sawicka J, Eisinthal S, & Ross D (1992). Fatigue syndrome due to localized radiation. *Journal of Pain Symptom Management, 7,* 38–45.

Haffty BG (1992). Follow-up and salvage therapy for the conservatively treated breast cancer patient. *Seminars in Radiation Oncology, 2,* 132–139.

Halpern J, McNeese MD, Kroll SS, & Ellerbroek N (1990). Irradiation of prosthetically augmented breasts: A retrospective study on toxicity and cosmetic results. *International Journal of Radiation Oncology, Biology, Physics, 18,* 189–191.

Halverson KJ, Perez CA, Kuske RR, Garcia DM, Simpson JR, & Fineberg B (1990). Isolated local-regional recurrence of breast cancer following mastectomy: Radiotherapeutic management. *International Journal of Radiation Oncology, Biology, Physics, 19,* 851–858.

Hancock SL, Tucker MA & Hoppe RT (1993). Breast cancer after treatment of Hodgkin's disease. *Journal of the National Cancer Institute, 85,* 25–31.

Harris JR & Hellman S (1988). Put the "hockey stick" on ice. *International Journal of Radiation Oncology, Biology, Physics, 15,* 497–499.

Harris JR, Lippman ME, Veronesi U, & Willett W (1992). Breast cancer (First of three parts). *New England Journal of Medicine, 327,* 319–326.

Harris JR, Lippman ME, Veronesi U & Willett W (1992). Breast cancer (Second of three parts). *New England Journal of Medicine, 327,* 390–397.

Harris JR, Morrow M, & Bonadonna G (1993). Cancer of the breast. In VT DeVita, Jr., S Hellman, & S Rosenberg (Eds.), *Cancer: Principles and Practice of Oncology* (4th ed., pp. 1264–1332). Philadelphia: JB Lippincott.

Harris JR & Recht A (1993). How to combine adjuvant chemotherapy and radiation therapy. *Recent Results in Cancer Research, 127,* 129–136.

Hetelekidis S, Schnitt SJ, Morrow M, & Harris JR (1995). Management of ductal carcinoma in situ. *CA-A Cancer Journal for Clinicians, 45,* 244–253.

Horsley JS, III & Styblo T (1991). Lymphedema in the postmastectomy patient. In K Bland & E Copeland III (Eds.), *The breast: Comprehensive Management of Benign and Malignant Diseases.* (pp. 701–706). Philadelphia: WB Saunders.

Hughes KK (1993). Decision making by patients with breast cancer: The role of information in treatment selection. *Oncology Nursing Forum, 20,* 623–628.

Hulka BS & Stark AT (1995). Breast cancer: cause and prevention. *Lancet, 346,* 883–887.

Humble CA (1995). Lymphedema: Incidence, pathophysiology, management, and nursing care. *Oncology Nursing Forum, 22,* 1503–1509.

Jaiyesimi IA, Buzdar AU, & Hortobagyi G (1992). Inflammatory breast cancer: A review. *Journal of Clinical Oncology, 10,* 1014–1024.

Killer HE & Hess K (1990). Natural history of radiation-induced brachial plexopathy compared with surgically treated patients. *Journal of Neurology, 237,* 247–250.

Kurtz JM, Amalric R, Delouche G, Pierquin B, Roth J & Spitalier JM (1987). The second ten years: Long-term risks of breast conservation in early breast cancer. *International Journal of Radiation Oncology, Biology, Physics, 13,* 1327–1332.

Kurtz JM & Miralbell R (1992). Radiation therapy and breast conservation: cosmetic results and complications. *Seminars in Radiation Oncology, 2,* 125–131.

Kuske RR, Schuster R, Klein E, Young L, Perez CA & Fineberg B (1991). Radiotherapy and breast reconstruction: Clinical results and dosimetry. *International Journal of Radiation Oncology, Biology, Physics, 21*, 339–346.

Lamb MA (1995). Effects of cancer on the sexuality and fertility of women. *Seminars in Oncology Nursing, 11*, 120–127.

Lamontanaro C (1995). Handling lymphedema. *PT Today, 3*, 14–22.

Larson D, Weinstein M, Goldberg I, Silver B, Recht A, Cady B, et al. (1986). Edema of the arm as a function of the extent of axillary surgery in patients with stage I-II carcinoma of the breast treated with primary radiotherapy. *International Journal of Radiation Oncology, Biology, Physics, 12*, 1575–1582.

Lavey RS, Eby NL & Prosnitz LR (1990). Impact of radiation therapy and/or chemotherapy on the risk for a second malignancy after breast cancer. *Cancer, 66*, 874–881.

Leigh S (1992). Cancer survivorship issues. In JC Clark & RF McGee (Eds.) *Core Curriculum for Oncology Nursing* (2nd ed., pp. 257–262). Philadelphia: WB Saunders.

Levitt SH (1994). The importance of locoregional control in the treatment of breast cancer and its impact on survival. *Cancer, 74*, 1840–1846.

Levy SM, Herberman RB, Lee JK, Lippman ME & d'Angelo T (1989). Breast conservation versus mastectomy: Distress sequelae as a function of choice. *Journal of Clinical Oncology, 7*, 367–375.

Lewis FM (1990). Strengthening family supports: cancer and the family. *Cancer, 65*, 752–759.

Lewis FM & Deal LW (1995). Balancing our lives: A study of the married couple's experience with breast cancer recurrence. *Oncology Nursing Forum, 22*, 943–953.

Lichter AS, Adler DD, August DA, Honig SF, Lippman ME, & Schottenfeld DA (1992). Breast cancer. In WJ Hoskins, CA Perez, & RC Young (Eds.), *Principles and Practice of Gynecologic Oncology* (pp. 827–889). Philadelphia: JB Lippincott.

Lindsey AM, Larson PJ, Dodd MJ, & Brecht ML (1994). Comorbidity, nutritional intake, social support, weight, and functional status over time in older cancer patients receiving radiotherapy. *Cancer Nursing, 17*, 113–124.

Loeffler JS, Kooy HM, Wen PY, Fine HA, Cheng CW, Mannarino EG, et al. (1990). The treatment of recurrent brain metastases with stereotactic radiosurgery. *Journal of Clinical Oncology, 8*, 576–582.

Mahon SM, Cella DF, & Donovan MI (1990). Psychosocial adjustment to recurrent cancer. *Oncology Nursing Forum, 17*, 47–54.

Mansfield CM, Krishnan L, Komarnicky LT, Ayyangar KM & Kramer CA (1991). A review of the role of radiation therapy in the treatment of patients with breast cancer. *Seminars in Oncology, 18*, 525–535.

Mast DE & Mood DW (1990). Preparing patients with breast cancer for brachytherapy. *Oncology Nursing Forum, 17*, 267–270.

McCormick B, Yahalom J, Cox L, Shank B & Massie MJ (1989). The patient's perception of her breast following radiation and limited surgery. *International Journal of Radiation Oncology, Biology, Physics, 17*, 1299–1302.

McDonald A (1992). Altered protective mechanisms. In KH Dow & LJ Hilderly (Eds.), *Nursing Care in Radiation Oncology* (pp. 96–125). Philadelphia: WB Saunders.

McGrath EB (1992a). Myelopathy, brachial plexopathy, and osteoradionecrosis. In KH Dow & LJ Hilderly (Eds.), *Nursing care in radiation oncology* (pp. 334–341). Philadelphia: WB Saunders.

McGrath EB (1992b). Lymphedema. In KH Dow & LJ Hilderly (Eds.), *Nursing Care in Radiation Oncology* (pp. 323–333). Philadelphia: WB Saunders.

McGuire WL & Clark GM (1992). Prognostic factors and treatment decisions in axillary-node–negative breast cancer. *New England Journal of Medicine 326*, 1756–1760.

McNeese MD, Fletcher GH, Levitt SH, & Khan FM (1992). Breast cancer. In SH Levitt, FM Khan, & RA Potish (Eds.), *Levitt and Tapley's Technological Basis of Radiation Therapy: Practical Clinical Applications* (pp. 232–247). Philadelphia: Lea & Febiger.

Mendenhall NP (1991). Palliative radiation therapy for disseminated breast cancer. In K Bland & E Copeland III (Eds.), *The Breast: Comprehensive Management of Benign and Malignant Diseases* (pp. 957–973). Philadelphia: WB Saunders.

Mock V (1993). Body image in women treated for breast cancer. *Nursing Research, 42*, 153–157.

Moffat F (1994). *Locoregional treatment considerations in early breast cancer*. Austin: RG Landes.

Monyak D & Levitt SH (1992). Breast: Locally advanced (T3 and T4) and recurrent tumors. In CA Perez & LW Brady (Eds.), *Principles and Practice of Radiation Oncology* (2nd ed., pp. 948–969). Philadelphia: JB Lippincott.

Moore MP & Kinne DW (1995). The surgical management of primary invasive breast cancer. *CA-A Cancer Journal for Clinicians, 45*, 279–288.

Mor V, Malin M, & Allen S (1994). Age differences in the psychosocial problems encountered by breast cancer patients. *Journal of the National Cancer Institute Monographs, 16*, 191–197.

Morra ME & Blumberg BD (1991). Women's perceptions of early detection in breast tumor: How are we doing? *Seminars in Oncology Nursing, 7*, 151–160.

Nail LM & Winningham ML (1995). Fatigue and weakness in cancer patients: The symptom experience. *Seminars in Oncology Nursing, 11*, 272–278.

National Alliance of Breast Cancer Organizations. New York, NY.

National Institute of Health. (1990). Treatment of early breast cancer. *NIH Consensus Development Conference Consensus Statement 1990 June 18–21, 8*, 1–19.

Neifert M (1992). Breastfeeding after breast surgical procedure or breast cancer. *NAACOG's Clinical Issues in Perinatal & Women's Health Nursing, 3*, 673–682.

Noguchi M, Kitagawa H, Kinoshita K, Earashi M, Miyazaki I, Tatsukuchi S, et al. (1993). Psychologic and cosmetic self-assessments of breast conserving therapy compared with mastectomy and immediate breast reconstruction. *Journal of Surgical Oncology, 54*, 260–266.

Northouse L (1990). A longitudinal study of the adjustment of patients and husbands to breast cancer. *Oncology Nursing Forum, 17*, 39–45.

Northouse L, Cracchiolo-Caraway A, & Appel CP (1991). Psychologic consequences of breast cancer on partner and family. *Seminars in Oncology Nursing, 7*, 216–223.

Olsen NK, Pfeiffer P, Mondrup K & Rose C. (1990). Radiation-induced brachial plexus neuropathy in breast cancer patients. *Acta Oncologica, 29*, 885-890.

Omne-Ponten M, Holmberg L, Bergstrom R, Sjoden PO, & Burns T (1993). Psychosocial adjustment among husbands of women treated for breast cancer; mastectomy vs. breast-conserving surgery. *European Journal of Cancer, 29A*, 1393–1397.

Parker LM, Boyages J & Eberlein TJ (1991). Inflammatory carcinoma of the breast. In JR Harris, S Hellman, IC Henderson & DW Kinne (Eds.) *Breast Diseases* (2nd ed., pp. 775–782). Philadelphia: JB Lippincott.

Parker SH, Lovin JD, Jobe WE, Luethke JM, Hopper KD, Yakes WF, et al. (1990). Stereotactic breast biopsy with a biopsy gun. *Radiology, 176*, 741–747.

Parker SH, Lovin JD, Jobe WE, Burke BJ, Hopper KD, & Yakes WF. (1991). Nonpalpable breast lesions: Stereotactic automated large-core biopsies. *Radiology, 180,* 403–407.

Parker SL, Tong T, Bolden S, & Wingo PA (1997). Cancer statistics, 1996. *CA-A Cancer Journal for Clinicians, 47,* 5–27.

Pierce LG & Glatstein E (1994). Postmastectomy radiotherapy in the management of operable breast cancer. *Cancer Supplement, 74,* 477–485.

Pierce SM & Harris JR (1992). Radiation therapy to the breast: practical aspects. *Journal of the American Medical Women's Association, 47,* 174–187.

Pierson KK & Wilkinson EJ (1991). Malignant neoplasia of the breast: Infiltrating carcinomas. In KI Bland & EM Copeland III (Eds.), *The Breast: Comprehensive Management of Benign and Malignant Diseases* (pp. 193–209). Philadelphia: WB Saunders.

Poulter CA, Cosmatos D, Rubin P, Urtasun R, Cooper JS, Kuske RR, et al. (1992). A report of RTOG 8206: A phase III study of whether the addition of single dose hemibody irradiation to standard fractionated local field irradiation is more effective than local field irradiation alone in the treatment of symptomatic osseous metastases. *International Journal of Radiation Oncology, Biology, Physics, 23,* 207–214.

Recht A & Harris JR (1990). Selection of patients with early-stage breast cancer for conservative surgery and radiation. *Oncology, 4,* 23–30.

Robinson R, Preston DF, Baxter KG, Dusing RW, & Spicer JA (1993). Clinical experience with strontium-89 in prostatic and breast cancer patients. *Seminars in Oncology, 20,* Suppl 2, 44–48.

Rosen PP (1991). The pathology of invasive breast carcinoma. In JR Harris, S Hellman, IC Henderson & DW Kinne (Eds.), *Breast Diseases* (2nd ed., pp. 245–296). Philadelphia: JB Lippincott.

Rowland JH & Holland JC (1989). Breast cancer. In JC Holland & JH Rowland (Eds.), *Handbook of Psychooncology: Psychological Care of the Patient with Cancer* (pp. 188–207). New York: Oxford University Press.

Ryttov N, Holm NV, Qvist N, & Blichert-Toft M (1988). Influence of adjuvant irradiation on the development of late arm lymphedema and impaired shoulder mobility after mastectomy for carcinoma of the breast. *Acta Oncologica, 27,* 667–670.

Sacchini V, Luini A, Agresti R, Greco M, Manzari A, Mariani L, et al. (1995). The influence of radiotherapy on cosmetic outcome after breast conservative surgery. *International Journal of Radiation Oncology, Biology, Physics, 33,* 59–64.

Salner AL, Botnick LE, Herzog AG, Goldstein MA, Harris JR, Levene MB, et al. (1981). Reversible brachial plexopathy following primary radiation therapy for breast cancer. *Cancer Treatment Reports, 65,* 797–802.

Satariano W (1992). Comorbidity and functional status in older women with breast cancer: Implications for screening, treatment, and prognosis. *Journal of Gerontology, 47* (special issue), 24–31.

Satariano WA, Ragheb NE, Branch LG & Swanson GM (1990). Difficulties in physical functioning reported by middle-aged and elderly women with breast cancer: A case-control comparison. *Journal of Gerontology: Medical Sciences, 45,* M3–11.

Scanlon EF (1991). Breast cancer. In AI Holleb, DJ Fink, & GP Murphy (Eds.), *Textbook of Clinical Oncology* (pp. 177–193). Atlanta: American Cancer Society.

Schain WS, d'Angelo TM, Dunn ME, Lichter AS, & Pierce LJ (1994). Mastectomy versus conservative surgery and radiation therapy: Psychosocial consequences. *Cancer, 73,* 1221–1228.

Schmidt RA (1994). Stereotactic breast biopsy. *CA-A Cancer Journal for Clinicians, 44,* 172–191.

Schover LR (1991). The impact of breast cancer on sexuality, body image, and intimate relationships. *CA-A Cancer Journal for Clinicians, 41,* 112–120.

Schwaibold F, Fowble BL, Solin LJ, Schultz DJ & Goodman RL (1991). The results of radiation therapy for isolated local regional recurrence after mastectomy. *International Journal of Radiation Oncology, Biology, Physics, 21,* 299–310.

Shapiro CL & Recht A (1994). Late effects of adjuvant therapy for breast cancer. *Journal of the National Cancer Institute Monographs, 16,* 101–112.

Simpson JF & Page DL (1992). Prognostic value of histopathology in the breast. *Seminars in Oncology, 19,* 254–262.

Sinsheimer LM & Holland JC (1987). Psychological issues in breast cancer. *Seminars in Oncology, 14,* 75–82.

Smalley SR, Schray MF, Laws ER, Jr., & O'Fallon JR. (1987). Adjuvant radiation therapy after surgical resection of solitary brain metastasis: Association with pattern of failure and survival. *International Journal of Radiation Oncology, Biology, Physics, 13,* 1611–1616.

Springfield DS (1991). Management of osseous metastases and impending pathological fractures. In K Bland & E Copeland III (Eds.), *The Breast: Comprehensive Management of Benign and Malignant Diseases* (pp. 974–981). Philadelphia: WB Saunders.

Stair JC (1985). Skin integrity, impairment of: Related to malignant skin lesions. In JC McNally, JC Stair, & ET Somerville (Eds.), *Guidelines for Cancer Nursing Practice* (pp. 170–174). Orlando: Grune & Stratton.

Stark AT (1995). Breast Cancer: Cause and prevention. *Lancet, 346,* 883–887.

Stefanek ME (1992). Psychosocial aspects of breast cancer. *Current Opinion in Oncology, 4,* 1055–1060.

Swain SM & Lippman ME (1991). Locally advanced breast cancer. In KI Bland & EM Copeland III (Eds.), *The Breast: Comprehensive Management of Benign and Malignant Diseases* (pp. 843–862). Philadelphia: WB Saunders.

Uematsu M, Bornstein B, Recht A, Abner A, Come SE, Shulman LN. (1993). Long-term results of post-operative radiation therapy following mastectomy with or without chemotherapy in stage I-III breast cancer. *International Journal of Radiation Oncology, Biology, Physics, 25,* 765–770.

Vinokur AD, Threatt BA, Vinokur-Kaplan D, & Satariano WA (1990). The process of recovery from breast cancer for younger and older patients: Changes during the first year. *Cancer, 65,* 1242–1254.

Wallace LM, Priestman SG, Dunn JA, & Priestman TJ (1993). The quality of life of early breast cancer patients treated by two different radiotherapy regimens. *Clinical Oncology, 5,* 228–233.

Wallgren A (1992). Late effects of radiotherapy in the treatment of breast cancer. *Acta Oncologica, 31,* 237–242.

Wang CC (1988). Cancer of the breast. In CC Wang (Ed.), *Clinical Radiation Oncology: Indications, Techniques, and Results* (pp. 180–195). Littleton: PSG.

Ward S, Heidrich S, & Wolberg W (1989). Factors women take into account when deciding upon type of surgery for breast cancer. *Cancer Nursing, 12,* 344–351.

Wazer DE (1994). The role of radiation in breast conserving therapy. *Obstetrics and Gynecology Clinics of North America, 21,* 681–691.

Wellisch DK, Jamison KR, & Pasnau, RO (1978). Psychosocial aspects of mastectomy: II. The man's perspective. *American Journal of Psychiatry, 135,* 543–546.

Wilhelm MC & Wanebo HJ (1991). Cancer of the male breast. In K Bland & EM Copeland III (Eds.), *The Breast: Comprehensive Management of Benign and Malignant Diseases* (pp. 1030–1033). Philadelphia: WB Saunders.

Wilson JF (1994). The breast. In JD Cox (Ed.), *Moss' Radiation Oncology: Rationale, Technique, Results* (pp. 355–401). St. Louis: Mosby.

Wilson JF & Cox JD (1995). Definitive, adjuvant, and palliative radiation therapy for mammary cancer. In W L Done-gan & J S Spratt (Eds.), *Cancer of the breast* (pp. 505–518). Philadelphia: WB Saunders.

Wingo PA, Tong T, & Bolden S (1995). Cancer statistics, 1995. *CA-A Cancer Journal for Clinicians, 45,* 8–30.

Wolberg WH, Tanner MA, Romsaas EP, Trump DL, & Malec JF (1987). Factors influencing options in primary breast cancer treatment. *Journal of Clinical Oncology, 5,* 68–74.

Worden JW (1989). The experience of recurrent cancer. *CA-A Cancer Journal for Clinicians, 39,* 305–310.

Yarnold JR (1991). Early stage breast cancer: treatment options and results. *British Medical Bulletin, 47,* 372–387.

Central Nervous System Tumors

JENNIFER DUNN BUCHOLTZ

Central nervous system tumors have been treated with radiation therapy for decades. The modern treatment of these tumors highlights several of the recent advances in delivering radiation therapy with added precision and sparing of normal brain cells. This chapter presents an overview of central nervous system tumors including their incidence and prevalence, diagnosis, and treatment. The use of radiation therapy, including the newer techniques of radiosurgery and particle therapy and the management of radiotherapy side effects, are discussed. Quality of life issues unique to patients with central nervous system tumors and their treatment are also presented.

Incidence and Prevalence

Central nervous system (CNS) tumors can be either primary or metastatic in origin. More than 100,000 people in the United States develop brain metastasis each year (Lesser & Grossman, 1993). Primary CNS tumors occur much less frequently. In 1996, the number of new cases of primary cancers of the brain and central nervous system, excluding pituitary tumors, was estimated at 17,600 (10,100 in men and 7,500 in women) (Parker et al., 1997). Estimated deaths in 1997 from these cancers was 13,200 (7,200 in men and 6,000 in women) (Parker et al., 1996). Although these latter numbers remain high, over the past thirty years survival rates have somewhat improved for persons with primary CNS cancers (Parker et al., 1997). Overall, CNS tumors represent only 1.3 percent of all diagnosed cancers and 2 percent of all cancer deaths. Only in white American males do CNS cancers appear (in last place) on the list of the top ten malignancies for cancer deaths (Parker et al., 1996).

Although primary brain tumors can occur at any age, there are two peak incidences: in children less than age twelve and adults over age 55 (Newton, 1994). (See Chapter 17 for pediatric brain tumors.) The location of tumors in the brain differs in adults than in children, with most adult brain tumors occurring supratentorially in the cortical, subcortical, and basal ganglia regions.

Etiology

Dominant risk factors for primary brain tumors are not well known. There is some evidence that genetic disorders, such as neurofibromatosis, Li-Fraumeni syndrome, Turcot's syndrome, and von Hippel-Lindau disease predispose individuals to the development of certain types of brain tumors (Black, 1991). Environmental factors are inconclusive. A few studies have linked industrial chemicals, pesticides, and even hair dyes to primary malignant brain tumors, but their findings have not been significant (Wrensch et al., 1993). To date, no conclusive evidence exists correlating either head trauma or low frequency electromagnetic radiation, including the use of cellular phones, with the induction of brain tumors (Heath, 1996; Wrensch et al., 1993). There is some epidemiologic evidence that exposure to cranial irradiation increases the risk for astrocytomas and meningiomas (Schoenberg, 1991). Viruses, such as the human immunodeficiency virus (HIV) and the Epstein-Barr virus, have been implicated in the cause of primary brain lymphomas (Levine, 1990). Similar to many cancers, a combination of genetics and environmental risk factors may be involved. In recent years, the National Familial Brain Tumor Registry has begun to keep records concerning familial and environmental factors identified in patients diagnosed with a primary brain tumor (Grossman et al., 1995). Molecular research involving protooncogenes, tumor suppressor genes, and angiogenesis may explain the development of brain tumors in the future (Black, 1991; Lubbe et al., 1995).

Classification

Several classification systems exist for primary CNS tumors. These include the Kernohan system, in use since 1949 (Kernohan et al., 1949), and the World Health Organization (WHO) system of 1979 (Zulch, 1979). The current system used by many clinicians is the revised WHO classification system (Kleihues et al., 1993). In general, brain tumors are classified based on the phenotype of their cell of origin and degree of differentiation. The major tissues of origin and resultant tumor type are glial cells (astrocytomas and oligodendrogliomas); meninges (meningiomas); cranial nerves (schwannomas); pituitary gland (pituitary adenomas); and blood vessels (hemangiomas). The names of brain tumors based on their histology are often long and confusing to patients and families. Moreover, there is added confusion regarding the terms benign versus malignant and low versus high grade. Some believe that even histologically benign brain tumors should be regarded as locally malignant due to their volume restrictions on spread within the cranium (Karlsson et al., 1992). Since the exact histology of the tumor dictates the type of recommended treatment, it is not unusual for institutions to obtain a second opinion about the pathological specimen. This waiting time can add more stress for the patient and family during the diagnostic period.

Primary brain tumors have a spectrum of aggressiveness. Tumors such as meningiomas and pituitary adenomas may take several years to grow, whereas high-grade astrocytomas may double their cell volume in as short as twenty days (Yamashita & Kuwabara, 1983).

In general, primary brain tumors rarely metastasize outside of the brain or cranial spinal access (Karlsson et al., 1992). This, in part, is due to a lack of a lymphatic drainage system within the brain. Some high-grade brain tumors can spread into the central nervous system through seeding into the subarachnoid space or ventricles. Tumors more likely to do so are those located close to the cerebral spinal fluid channels (Karlsson et al., 1992).

Clinical Presentation

Central nervous system tumors present with generalized signs and symptoms due to cerebral edema or focal signs and symptoms caused by an expanding tumor exerting compression of brain tissue. Specific signs and symptoms from these are listed in Table 10–1. Brain edema stems from alteration of the blood–brain barrier. The types of brain tumors that have the most associated brain edema at presentation include brain metastases, astrocytomas, meningiomas, and oligodendrogliomas (Karlsson et al., 1992). Focal signs and symptoms, such as paresis, aphasia, olfactory hallucinations, and short-term memory problems can help implicate the location of the tumor inside the brain. Figure 10–1 displays the cerebral hemispheres of the brain and their related functions. Specific endocrine problems can suggest pituitary tumor. Common signs and symptoms of various brain tumors are listed in Table 10–2.

Diagnostic Work-Up

The diagnostic work-up for central nervous system tumors includes a careful history and physical with a thorough neurological examination. Oftentimes, it is important to query family members or significant others concerning the patient's signs and symptoms, as subtle changes in memory, speech, and other cognitive functions may not be apparent to the patient.

Advances in radiologic neuroimaging have dramatically improved the diagnosis of central nervous system tumors (Ramsey, 1994). Computerized tomography (CT) and magnetic resonance imaging (MRI) are commonly employed if central nervous system disease is expected. These tests have virtually eliminated the need for patients to receive more invasive procedures, such as

Table 10-1 • Signs and Symptoms of Brain Tumors

Generalized Signs and Symptoms	Focal Symptoms
Headache	Focal motor or sensory seizures
Nausea/vomiting	
Generalized seizure activity	Personality or cognitive changes
Cognitive and personality changes	
	Limb weakness
Alteration in consciousness	Speech disturbances
Double vision	Visual field changes
	Limb uncoordination

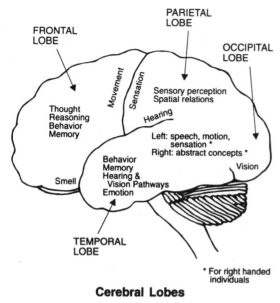

Cerebral Lobes

Figure 10-1 • Functions of the cerebral hemispheres. (From: The American Brain Tumor Association *A Primer of Brain Tumors*, 6th ed., 1996, p. 18. Used with permission.)

myelography and routine lumbar punctures. In both CT and MRI scans, the use of their respective contrast agents greatly improves tumor enhancement, as tumors that alter the normal blood–brain barrier allow contrast agents to permeate brain tumor vasculature. Specific information about radiologic neurodiagnostic tests, including positron emission tomography (PET) and single photon emission computerized tomography (SPECT) are given in Table 10–3.

Treatment

Surgery

Surgery remains the most important treatment for most CNS tumors. When possible, complete surgical resection of the tumor is attempted, since this offers the best chance for cure, especially when employed for histologically benign tumors. Factors that determine the ease of complete surgical resection include the tumor location, size, consistency, infiltrative nature, vascular components, and the overall medical status of the patient. When complete surgical resection is not possible, surgical debulking can be performed, which can not only establish a tissue diagnosis, but often improve the patient's symptoms caused by tumor compression. The advent of stereotactic brain biopsy has dramatically improved the sampling of

tumor tissue. Stereotactic brain biopsies are extremely useful when surgical resection is not possible or does not offer a therapeutic advantage. Besides the advent of stereotactic biopsy, other technical improvements in neurosurgery include more precision-guided surgical systems, such as the operating microscope, lasers, ultrasonic applicators, and improved electrophysiologic monitoring techniques (Laws & Thapar, 1993). For vascular tumors, preoperative embolization may be done to reduce total blood loss during surgery, shorten the operative time, and offer better protection of the normal brain tissue from surgical trauma (Rodesch & Lasjaunais, 1991). Surgical mortality from brain surgery is relatively low in the arena of experienced neurosurgeons (Black, 1991; Wilson, 1994). The technical advances previously mentioned have made it possible for neurosurgeons to reach tumors at the base of the skull that were unapproachable before the mid-1980s (Akeyson & McCutcheon, 1996).

Potential risks from the actual tumor resection include hemorrhage, brain injury, and herniation. Potential postoperative complications include pulmonary embolism, hematomas, wound flap infection, deep vein thrombosis, and meningitis (Wilson, 1994). Preoperative, intraoperative, and postoperative nursing care of patients undergoing neurosurgical procedures are thoroughly reviewed by Hickey (1992).

Radiation Therapy

Radiation therapy has played a major role in the treatment of primary brain tumors for decades. Alone or in combination with surgery, it can be given for curative intent, control of tumor growth, or palliation of neurologic complications from an expanding tumor. Radiotherapy may be highly successful in preventing certain tumors, such as pituitary adenomas and meningiomas, from growing back after incomplete surgical resection. In patients with higher-grade astrocytomas, radiation has been shown to prolong survival in randomized trials (Kristiansen et al., 1981; Karlsson et al., 1992). There is an absence of randomized, controlled trials in the use of radiation therapy for low-grade astrocytomas. Thus, controversy exists regarding radiation. (Cairncross & Laperriere, 1989; Wharam, 1993). Finally, the use of radiation in the palliation of brain metastasis is widely accepted (DeAngelis, 1994).

The dose of radiation used and technical aspects of treatment will depend upon the tumor histology, location, grade, radioresponsiveness, intent of therapy, and patient status. Table 10–4 gives a detailed overview of the technical aspects

Table 10-2 • Symptoms, Signs, and Diagnostic Characteristics of Various Intracranial Tumors

Tumor	Common Symptoms	Common Signs	Diagnostic Characteristics*
PRIMARY			
Malignant astrocytoma	Headache, seizure, unilateral weakness, mental changes	Focal presentation related to tumor location	Enhancing CT lesion, tumor blush on angiography
Glioblastoma multiforme (GM)			Hypodense interior of enhanced CT lesion
Astrocytoma with anaplastic foci (AAF)			No hypodense interior portion of enhanced CT lesion
Brain stem or thalamus	Nausea, vomiting, ataxia	Increased intracranial pressure (papilledema), abducens and oculomotor nerve defects	May not enhance on CT scan; biopsy may not be appropriate
Meningioma (B, M)	Localized headache, seizure	Focal presentation related to tumor location	Enhancing CT lesion associated with dura
Astrocytoma (B, M)	Headache, seizure, unilateral weakness, mental changes	Focal presentation related to tumor location	May not enhance on CT
Cerebral	Headache, seizure, unilateral weakness, mental changes	Focal presentation related to tumor location	
Cerebellar	Occipital headache	Increased intracranial pressure (papilledema), abducens and oculomotor nerve defects; coordination	
Brain stem or thalamus	Nausea, vomiting, ataxia	Increased intracranial pressure (papilledema), abducens and oculomotor nerve defects; coordination	May be seen only on MR imaging; biopsy may not be appropriate
Optic nerve	Ocular changes	Ocular changes	Detailed CT scan
Pituitary (B, M)	Vertex headache, ocular changes	Ocular, endocrine abnormalities	Hormone analysis; resection gives histopathology
Medulloblastoma (M)	Morning headaches, nausea, vomiting	Coordination, increased intracranial pressure (papilledema), abducens and oculomotor nerve defects	CT scan, careful lumbar puncture recommended
Ependymoma (B, M)	Morning headaches, nausea, vomiting	Coordination, increased intracranial pressure (papilledema), abducens and oculomotor nerve defects	CT scan, careful lumbar puncture recommended
Hemangioma, arteriovenous malformation (B, M)	"Migrainous" headache	Focal presentation related to tumor location	Angiography; biopsy may not be appropriate
Neurilemoma, schwannoma neurinoma (B, M)	Unilateral deafness, vertigo	Ipsilateral acoustic and facial or trigeminal nerve defects	CT scan; resection gives histopathology
Oligodendroglioma (B, M)	Insidious headache, mental changes	Focal presentation related to tumor location	Radiographic calcification
Sarcoma (M), neurofibroma (B)	Focal presentation related to tumor location	Focal presentation related to tumor location	
Pinealoma (B, M), dysgerminoma	Various (ocular, vestibular, endocrine)	Parinaud's syndrome, endocrine changes, ocular changes. Increased intracranial pressure (papilledema), abducens, and oculomotor nerve defects	Biopsy or resection may not be obtained; markers in CSF may be informative

Table continued on following page

Table 10-2 • Symptoms, Signs, and Diagnostic Characteristics of Various Intracranial Tumors *(Continued)*

Tumor	Common Symptoms	Common Signs	Diagnostic Characteristics*
Lymphoma (M), reticulum cell sarcoma, microglioma	Focal presentation related to tumor location	Focal presentation related to tumor location	"Soft" CT enhancement
Unspecified (B, M)	Focal presentation related to tumor location	Focal presentation related to tumor location	
OTHER			
Craniopharyngioma	Headache, mental changes, hemiplegia, seizure, vomiting (and ocular changes)	Cranial nerve defects (II–VII)	Bone erosion, mass effect from base of skull
Syringomyelia, syringobulbia	Pain, weakness	Sensory level, paresis	MR imaging, CT scan; myelogram; biopsy not appropriate
Midline granuloma syndrome, lymphoid granulomatosis	Various (ocular, vestibular, endocrine)	Various (ocular, vestibular, endocrine)	Diagnosis presumed
Arachnoiditis		Fasciculations	

* Unless noted, biopsy is assumed.
B: benign; M: malignant; CT: computed tomography; MR: magnetic resonance.
From Karlsson UL , Leibel SA, Wallner K & Davis LW (1992). Brain. In: CA Perez & LW Brady (Eds.), *Principles and Practice of Radiation Oncology*. (2nd ed., p. 516). Philadelphia: Lippincott-Raven. Used with permission of the publisher.

of treatment for many primary brain tumors. In general, histologically benign tumors with discrete borders are treated with narrow margins of radiotherapy beams, while infiltrative, high-grade tumors require larger radiotherapy field sizes to encompass surrounding areas of edema. For high-grade tumors with edema, radiotherapy portals are usually planned based on the patient's preoperative MRI scan. Whole-brain radiation therapy is no longer recommended for high-grade astrocytoma because it adds to morbidity but not survival (Leibel & Sheline, 1987).

Treatment Planning for Brain Radiotherapy

Along with the many technological improvements in neurosurgery, there have been significant advances in the planning and delivery of therapeutic radiation to the brain. These advances have generally centered on improving the precision of the radiation beam delivery and sparing of normal brain tissues. Head immobilization devices, CT-based simulation, three-dimensional computer planning, the use of multileaf collimators, stereotactic radiotherapy delivery, and additional newer modalities have all been used in CNS irradiation. These newer approaches have offered additional challenges to nurses caring for patients. Specific head immobilization devices are used not only to reproduce the treatment position for accuracy, but also to allow the radiotherapy treatment marks to be placed on the mask versus on the patient's scalp or face. Although this offers many advantages for treatment set-ups, the patient may need to be screened for the ability to wear a mask and instructed in how to release the mask should untoward problems, such as vomiting, occur. Often the mask may be made more comfortable by slight modifications, like cutting out holes in the eyes, nares, and mouth area. Head immobilization masks can be made in under ten minutes and are made directly before the simulation x ray pictures are taken.

The use of the CT scanner in treatment planning (Figure 10–2) has added responsibilities for the nurse in radiation oncology. For example, the nurse may need to establish IV access for the administration of intravenous contrast agents, if used for visualizing the patient's brain tumor. A written procedure for IV access as well as management of IV contrast reactions is warranted. Patients need to be screened for any possible past allergic reactions to contrast and assessed as to their kidney status, since the contrast material is excreted by the kidneys. A recent serum blood urea nitrogen (BUN) and serum creatinine are good screening tools to assess kidney function. Contrast agents can be in either iodinated form or non-iodinated form. Although fewer allergic reactions occur with the non-iodinated form, anaphylaxis can still occur with this agent. A discussion of contrast reactions and their management is provided by the American College of Radiology (1991).

In general, most brain radiation therapy simulation procedures are accomplished in under one hour. The exception to this would be a possible three-hour planning time required for cran-

Table 10-3 • Information Regarding Neurodiagnostic Tests for CNS Tumors

Test	Purpose	Patient Experience	Approximate Time Required	Potential Risks	Comments
Computerized tomography (CT)	Detect brain, spine abnormalities, including masses, edema	Lie on narrow table, head inside large donut-shaped ring; IV contrast usually given	30 minutes (brain) 45 minutes (spine)	Allergic reaction to IV contrast agent	Uses ionizing radiation; Useful in evaluating bony abnormalities of skull; IV contrast reactions can be mild to severe, including anaphylaxis; requires informed consent; 3-D pictures using special computers
Magnetic resonance imaging (MRI)	Detect brain, spine abnormalities, including edema, and nature/extent of tumor blood flow	Lie on thin table inside large magnet; claustrophobic feeling; loud noises from magnet, sounds like galloping, drilling; some scanners play music, videotapes; IV contrast usually given	45–60 minutes (brain) 2–3 hours (total spine)	Anxiety, claustrophobia	Preferred method of neuroimaging; More expensive than CT; Sedation/antianxiety medicines may be required; Does not use ionizing radiation; Reactions to IV contrast gadolinium rare; Not used for patients with metal foreign bodies, pacemakers; More sensitive than CT for detecting multiple brain mets, posterior fossa and spinal lesions; Open scanners may give lower quality images; Patient weight limit 300 lbs for most scanners; MR angiography fast replacing need for traditional invasive angiogram
Positron emission tomography (PET)	Measures regional brain metabolism, and cerebral blood flow; may show difference between radiation necrosis and recurrent tumors	Lie on narrow table; patient wears customized mask; head in special holder; IV and/or arterial line required	2 hours	Arterial line complications	Limited availability; Uses positron-emitting radionuclides; thymidine and glucose common radiotracers; Insurance reimbursement a problem
Single photon emission computed tomography (SPECT)	Attempts to show difference between radiation necrosis and recurrent tumors; differentiate lymphoma from nonneoplastic masses in AIDS patients	IV radionuclide used; patient scanned on traditional nuclear medicine-like table	May be scanned at set time after radionuclide given, similar to bone scan		Uses conventional radiotracers; More available and less expensive than PET

(From: Sheidler, VR & Bucholtz JD: Central nervous system tumors. In McCorkle R et al. (eds.): *Cancer nursing: A comprehensive textbook,* W.B. Saunders, 1996, p 830. With permission from the publisher.)

Table 10-4 • Suggested Photon Irradiation Technique and Doses (1 MV–10 MV)* for Various CNS Tumors

Tumor	Large fields	Small fields	Technical Aspects
PRIMARY			
High-grade astrocytoma			
Glioblastoma multiforme	about 4000	about 2000–3000 BO	Tolerance 5000–6000 cGy/5–7 weeks; often large fields lateral opposing or "whole brain"; smaller fields depend on location of tumor margin, usually ≥2 cm from tumor or edema; dose fraction ≤200 cGy
Astrocytoma with anaplastic foci	about 4000	about 2000–3000 BO	Tolerance 5000–6000 cGy/5–7 weeks; often large fields lateral opposing or "whole brain"; smaller fields depend on location of tumor margin, usually ≥3 cm from tumor or edema; dose fraction ≤200 cGy
Brain stem or thalamus		5500	Usually lateral parallel opposing fields, sometimes with PA field
Meningioma (B, M)		5500	Field size dependent on tumor size, location, and histology; tangential parallel opposed or perpendicular oblique beams may be used for peripheral lesions
Astrocytoma (B, M) Cerebral	5500		Generous margins, commonly through lateral and AP beams if lesion is frontal, lateral parallel opposed or perpendicular oblique beams if parietal and lateral, and PA beams if the lesion is occipital
Cerebellar		5500	Usually lateral parallel opposed beams, but three fields or arc desirable
Brain stem or thalamus		5500	Lateral parallel opposed and PA beams
Optic nerve		5000	Lateral, 15-degree oblique parallel opposed beams
Pituitary (B, M)		5000	Lateral parallel opposed beams *or* 360-degree rotation *or* 220-degree rotation arcs with reversed wedges
Medulloblastoma (B, M) or high-grade intracranial ependymoma		1000 BO	Lateral parallel opposed and wedged or perpendicular wedged beams to remaining tumor location at 200 cGy per fraction *and*
	4500		lateral parallel opposed helmet fields, 180 cGy fractions *and*
	<4000		PA beam(s) to spinal axis with 150 cGy fractions *and* moving gap junctions *and*
		1000 BO	to gross remaining tumor *or* if patient is <3 years old
	3500		to cranial contents *and*
	<3000		to spinal canal *and*
		1000 BO	to gross remaining tumor
Low-grade ependymoma		5500	Small fields for low-grade tumor
Hemangioma, arteriovenous malformation (B, M)		5000	Small fields with preferentially multibeam geometry
Neurilemoma, schwannoma, neurinoma (B, M)		5000	Small fields with preferentially multibeam geometry
Oligodendroglioma (B, M)		5500	AP and lateral beams if lesion is frontal
Sarcoma (M)	5000	1000 BO	If malignant, neuraxis irradiation may be necessary (as for medulloblastoma above)
Neurofibroma (B)	5000 or	5000	Large field if multiple; small field if solitary
Pinealoma, dysgerminoma, embryonal carcinoma		2000	AP–PA parallel opposed beams, *then* CT scan; *add*
		3500	three-beam "box" technique if unchanged or benign histology
	3500		*or* if decreased on CT or malignant histopathology *add* lateral parallel opposed helmet fields *plus*
	3500		PA beam(s) to spinal axis with gapped and moving junctions (as for medulloblastoma above)
Lymphoma (M), reticulum cell sarcoma, microglioma	5000		Lateral parallel opposing helmet beams
Unspecified (B, M)	Variable		Beam geometry depends on tumor location

Table 10-4 • Suggested Photon Irradiation Technique and Doses (1 MV–10 MV)* for Various CNS Tumors (*Continued*)

| Tumor | Dose (cGy) | | Technical Aspects |
	Large fields	Small fields	
OTHER			
Craniopharyngioma		5000	"Large" local field, often lateral parallel opposing beams
		1000–	*and* small multibeam *or* rotation ports
		2000 BO	*except* in children, multibeam
		5500	
Syringomyelia, syringobulbia	2000		PA narrow beams or perpendicular oblique PA beams
Midline granuloma syndrome, lymphoid granulomatosis		5000	Lateral parallel opposing helmet fields
Arachnoiditis	2000		Smallest possible fields encompassing involved areas

* 80–100 cm SSD (source-skin distance) or SAD (source-axis distance), 100 to 300 cGy/minute, 180–200 cGy/fraction, 5 times/week unless otherwise noted.
AP: arteroposterior beam direction; B: benign; BO: boost; M: malignant; PA: posteroanterior beam direction.
(From Karlsson UL, Leibel SA, Wallner K & Davis LW (1992). Brain. In: Perez CA, Brady LW (Eds.): *Principles and practice of radiation oncology*, Lippincott-Raven Publishers, 1992, pp 534–535. With permission from the publisher.)

iospinal radiation therapy using a standard fluoroscopic simulator, as adjacent cervical spine and lateral brain radiation fields must be carefully matched to avoid either overdosing or underdosing the cervical spine (Digel et al., 1994). Use of the newer CT scan for simulation can accomplish this needed planning in half the time of the fluoroscopic planning.

Side Effects of Brain Radiation

Since the normal cells of the adult brain are not actively dividing cells, in general, these tissues well tolerate the standard radiotherapy. Conventional fraction doses of 180 to 200 centiGray (cGy), administered five days per week to a total dose of 6,000 cGy, will not produce significant morbidity in most patients receiving involved field brain radiotherapy (Levin et al., 1993). Some clinical cen-

ters may treat high-grade astrocytomas with a split-course treatment plan, administering 300 cGy fractions in seventeen treatments, with a two-week treatment break after 3000 cGy. The potential acute, acute-delayed, and long-term side effects of brain radiation are listed in Table 10–5.

Acute reactions include cerebral edema, fatigue, hair loss, and scalp reactions. Radiation-induced brain edema is usually not a problem if the patient is already taking an adequate dose of dexamethasone. Patients who are not on this steroid at the initial occurrence of signs and symptoms of edema may be placed on dexamethasone and should be given information relating to the many potential side effects of steroid use. Since these side effects can be difficult for patients, occasionally symptomatic measures that deal with headaches and nausea caused by brain edema may be

Figure 10-2 • Photographs of ACQSIM CT simulation system. (Courtesy of Picker International, Highland Heights, OH).

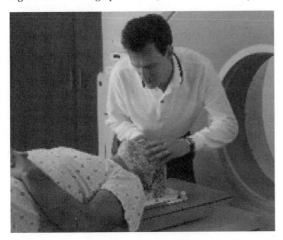
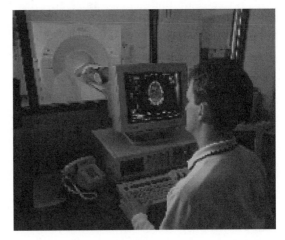

Table 10-5 • Side Effects of Radiation Therapy to the Brain

Side Effect	Comments
ACUTE	
Cerebral edema	May occur early in course of treatment; headache, nausea, vomiting, neurologic changes
	Treated with glucocorticoids, usually dexamethasone
Fatigue	Variable amount; increased if patients receiving concomitant chemotherapy
Alopecia	Hair loss limited to areas transited by beam
	May take 3–6 months after treatment to regrow
	No known preventative measure once threshold dose received
Skin reactions—scalp	Erythema, dry desquamation common; moist desquamation rare
	Symptoms more pronounced at skin folds (behind ears, forehead)
	May be more enhanced by chemotherapy and head immobilization devices
SUBACUTE	
Radiation somnolence syndrome	Can occur 6–12 weeks after treatment; lasts up to 2 weeks
	Symptoms—excessive sleepiness, lethargy, exacerbation of previous neurologic deficits
	Possible etiology—temporary demyelination of certain brain cells or radiation changes in capillary permeability
	Can be symptomatically treated with glucocorticoids
LONG TERM	
Radiation necrosis	Occurs in 4–9% of patients
	Increased incidence with high doses
	Difficult to distinguish from recurrent tumor on CT/MRI
	May require surgical treatment
White matter changes	Present on CT/MRI, but patient asymptomatic
Cognitive changes	Evidence for cognitive changes in young children treated during brain development
	Few prospective studies
	Data show both normal cognitive function and cognitive decline
	Cognitive function assessment should use neuropsychologic instruments, in addition to Karnofsky and IQ
	Cognitive change in adults—memory deficits most often reported
	Tumor, surgery, and chemotherapy may also be responsible for cognitive changes
Decreased hormone production	Occurs in 40–50% of patients treated for pituitary tumors
	Develops slowly over several years
	Requires follow-up with endocrinologist
	All hormones replaceable with medications
Radiation-induced neoplasms	Rare; may take years to develop

(Data from Hoffman, Levin, and Wilson, 1979; Delattre et al., 1988; Levin et al., 1993; Moore et al., 1991; Meadows et al., 1981; Imperato, Paleologos, and Vick, 1990; Maire et al., 1987; Hochberg and Slotnick, 1980; Kleinberg, Wallner, and Malkin, 1993; Armstrong et al., 1993; Archibald et al., 1994; Blevins and Wand, 1993; Bucholtz, 1992.)
(From: Sheidler VR and Bucholtz JD: Central nervous system tumors. In McCorkle R et al. (eds.): *Cancer nursing: A comprehensive textbook,* W.B. Saunders, 1996, p 835. Reprinted with permission.)

managed with analgesics and antiemetic medications before instituting steroids. Table 10–6 lists many of the potential side effects of dexamethasone. Significant nursing time and responsibility are given to assist patients who require long-term steroid use to cope with the many side effects. Of the many medications patients with a brain tumor may need to take, long-term use of steroids appears to most adversely affect the patient's quality of life.

The amount of radiation-induced fatigue during and after brain radiation therapy varies per patient. Patients treated with very small radiation therapy fields, such as for pituitary adenomas, may not experience the same degree of fatigue as those patients treated with whole-brain radiotherapy for brain metastases. Patients may find it necessary to take a nap after receiving treatment.

Radiation-induced alopecia is limited to the exact radiotherapy portals and begins after threshold dose. It may take three to six months for the hair to regrow. Regrown hair may have both a different color and consistency. Depending on both the total dose of radiation given, and individual sensitivity of the hair follicles to radiation, some patients may experience permanent hair loss or thinning in the radiotherapy fields. Permanent hair loss is not common under a total dose of 5500 cGy. Delivery of the radiotherapy beams with higher-energy machines may offer some protection from permanent hair loss, with the scalp receiving less of the total dose than is given on lower-energy machines.

Skin reactions are usually not severe from radiation therapy to the scalp but may be more pro-

Table 10-6 • Possible Side Effects of Dexamethasone

Body System	Effect
Gastrointestinal system	Increased appetite
	Gastric irritation
	Nausea
	Diarrhea or constipation
	Abdominal distension
	Gastrointestinal hemorrhage
Endocrine system	Hyperglycemia
	Cushingoid state
	Menstrual irregularities
	Secondary adrenal insufficiency (with abrupt steroid with-drawal)
Neurologic system	Mood swings
	Restlessness
	Insomnia
	Vertigo
	Psychoses
Dermatologic system	Acne
	Impaired wound healing
	Skin thinning/atrophy
	Petechiae/ecchymosis
	Hirsutism
Musculoskeletal system	Myopathies of long muscles
	Osteoporosis
Circulatory system	Sodium retention
	Potassium loss
	Hypertension
Immune system	Increased susceptibility to infection (especially candida)

nounced in areas of skin folds, such as behind the ears. Friction to the skin caused by the arms of a patient's glasses may irritate the skin reaction further. The use of a bolus and certain head immobilization devices may also add to the scalp reaction. Erythema and dry desquamation can be managed with standard skin products used for radiation skin reaction. Moist desquamation is rarely seen with conventional fractionation and standard treatment to the scalp.

A possible acute-delayed reaction to brain radiotherapy is "radiation somnolence syndrome," which can occur six to twelve weeks following the completion of therapy. This syndrome, characterized by excessive sleepiness, lethargy, or an exacerbation of previous neurologic signs and symptoms, is thought to be due to a temporary demyelination of certain brain cells or radiation changes in capillary permeability (Delattre et al., 1988; Hoffman et al., 1979). Although this syndrome causes great alarm in patients and their families, it is usually self-limiting and does not cause irreversible problems. Some patients with neurologic compromise need to reinstitute steroid treatment or have their tapering dose of steroids increased.

Possible late effects of brain radiotherapy include radiation necrosis, asymptomatic white matter changes, cognitive changes, decreased production of hormones, and rare occurrences of secondary brain malignancies. Clinically evident radiation necrosis occurs in approximately 4 to 9 percent of patients treated for brain tumors and is directly related to dose, with an increased incidence seen in patients treated with higher doses to the brain (Levin et al., 1993). Unfortunately, radiation necrosis can lead to similar neurologic deficits as brain tumors. Moreover, it is difficult to distinguish radiation necrosis from growing brain tumor using head CT or MRI. Radiation necrosis may require tissue confirmation and surgical intervention. Newer radiologic techniques like PET and SPECT scans attempt to distinguish necrosis from active brain tumor tissue.

White matter changes from radiation seen on follow-up head scans may be focal or diffuse, depending on the volume and areas of the brain treated. Often, these white matter changes are asymptomatic.

There is lack of conclusive information regarding the extent of potential cognitive changes as a result of late radiation injury in adults. Few prospective studies have been done to study the occurrence and extent of cognitive problems contributed to brain irradiation. More literature exists concerning this effect in children treated with brain radiation therapy for CNS primary tumors and leukemia (Meadows et al., 1991; Moore et al., 1991). Some studies have shown cognitive decline (Hochberg & Slotnick, 1980; Imperato et al., 1990; Maire et al., 1987), while others have not shown a progressive decline in neuropsychologic function after completion of cranial irradiation (Kleinberg et al., 1993). Memory deficits appear to be the most often-seen cognitive change. Similar to any long-term radiation effects, a combination of variables may contribute to a decline in certain cognitive functions, including injury to the brain by the tumor itself, enhanced effects of surgery, chemotherapy, antiseizure medications, and/or other brain-aging phenomena. Certain researchers suggest that systematic studies of neuropsychological function should include not only Karnofsky performance and IQ testing but also more sophisticated neuropsychological instruments that are better equipped to identify and quantify neuropsychologic changes (Archibald et al., 1994; Armstrong et al., 1993). Referral to a specialist in neurocognitive assessment and subsequent treatment may assist some patients to cope better with cognitive changes such as memory deficits.

Partial or complete hypopituitarism may develop in persons who receive radiation therapy to the hypothalamus. This effect occurs in 40 to 50 percent of patients receiving this therapy and develops insidiously over several years after radiotherapy is completed (Blevins & Wand, 1993). Certain hormones, such as growth hormone, are affected more than others. Patients treated with radiation therapy for hypothalamic or pituitary region tumors should be closely followed by an endocrinologist or physician who can monitor hormone levels and production. Fortunately, affected hormones can be easily replaced by prescription hormone medicines. It is not yet clear if growth hormone needs to be given to adults.

Specialized Brain Radiotherapy Delivery Techniques

STEREOTACTIC RADIOSURGERY

Stereotactic radiosurgery (SRS) involves the precise delivery of radiation to a small, well-defined intracranial lesion. It delivers this precise treatment while normal adjacent brain tissues only millimeters away are spared from the dose. There are three currently used delivery machines or techniques to deliver radiosurgery:

1. the gamma knife, or Leskell Gamma Unit, first developed by Swedish neurosurgeon Dr. Lars Leskell, which contains 201 separate sources of cobalt-60 arranged 1 millimeter apart in a large helmet structure;
2. the modified linear accelerator, which uses four or five noncoplanar arcs to deliver precise photon beams, or dedicated linear accelerator built for radiosurgery; and
3. charged particle beams of either protons, helium ions, or carbon ions (Flickinger, et al., 1994).

All of these technologies require extensive treatment planning, rigid head immobilization, sophisticated computer planning, and the joint skills of neurosurgeons, radiation oncologists, radiation physicists, and therapists to plan for and deliver the precision required for radiosurgery treatment.

Stereotactic radiosurgery involves the delivery of one to a few large fractions of high-dose radiation to intracranial tumors with discrete borders. Radiosurgery is indicated for patients who have small tumors or arteriovenous malformations when surgical resection is not possible, or the risk of embolizations of these lesions is too great (Flickinger et al., 1994). The most common brain lesions treated with stereotactic radiosurgery are arteriovenous malformations (AVMs), acoustic neuromas, meningiomas, and pituitary

adenomas. Solitary brain metastases are also treated with radiosurgery, sometimes avoiding neurosurgical resection, for a boost dose after conventional whole-brain radiotherapy.

STEREOTACTIC RADIOTHERAPY

Stereotactic radiotherapy (SRT) uses the computer planning, precise delivery of the radiation, and adapted head immobilization devices to deliver fractionated radiation therapy to brain tumors in needed doses while more effectively sparing normal brain tissues from potential radiation damage. SRT is most often used for

1. small volume, well-defined brain tumors;
2. inoperable brain tumors due to a deep, central location in the brain or location near critical brain structures;
3. recurrent tumors in prior irradiated areas;
4. histologically known tumors that respond well to conventional RT; and
5. pediatric brain tumors in order to decrease possibility of late tissue effects (Dunbar & Loeffler, 1994).

Examples of the above tumors include pituitary adenomas, meningiomas, craniopharyngiomas, low-grade astrocytomas, optic pathway gliomas, retinoblastomas, and acoustic neuromas.

Due to the fractionation schedule of SRT, head immobilization is not fixated with screws into the skull as it is with radiosurgery, but is accomplished by a rigid, relocatable head immobilization device. There are several of these in use, some designed by individual institutions. The most common frames are the Gill Thomas II and the Laitinen frames. The frame chosen must allow for a precise reproduction of the patient's head position for each fractionated treatment.

Due to the technology involved, patients undergoing SRT require both longer planning and treatment times than are needed for conventional treatment. A patient receiving standard, fractionated involved-field radiation therapy might be on the treatment table an average of fifteen minutes per day, whereas SRT may require up to one hour per day depending on the specific treatment. Some patients may require analgesics if the head immobilization device or treatment position is uncomfortable.

SIDE EFFECTS OF SRS AND SRT

There are usually few acute side effects of radiosurgery since treatment volumes of normal brain structures are minimized (Krause et al., 1991).

Patients may, however, experience discomfort from the invasive, fixated head frame or an infection at the pin sites. The hair does not need to be shaved for the pin site placement for SRS. In addition, hair loss may not be experienced for either SRS or SRT, unless the brain lesion treated is close to the scalp. Long term effects of SRS may include brain edema, damage to cranial nerves, and brain necrosis. It may also take two years time before an arteriovenous malformation (AVM) is obliterated by SRS (Flickinger et al., 1994).

STEREOTACTIC BRACHYTHERAPY

Temporary stereotactic placement (or brachytherapy) of iridium-192 or iodine-125 has been most often used in patients who have high-grade astrocytomas in order to deliver a focal dose of radiation and avoid further treatment dose to already irradiated normal brain tissues (Shreive et al., 1994). Brachytherapy is generally administered as part of a clinical trial, and not considered standard treatment. The major side effect of stereotactic brachytherapy is brain necrosis, which may require surgical resection. Protection measures with iodine-125 and iridium-192 are presented in Chapter 3.

PARTICLE THERAPY

Particle therapy employs specialized equipment for the delivery of subatomic particles, such as protons, neutrons, and helium ions. These beams of radiation, available only in a select few institutions in the United States, offer distinct advantages for the treatment of certain brain and spinal cord tumors based on several factors:

1. accurate shaping of the beam, offering better dose localization to the tumor;
2. an improved biologic effect on tumor cell kill than obtained with standard radiation photons due to the high linear energy transfer (LET) properties of charged particles, and
3. a decreased dose to normal cells since the charged particles are delivered in a finite path to the desired depth into the tumor, and do not exit through normal cells (Laperriere & Bernstein, 1994; Munzenrider & Crowell, 1994).

Tumors that require a higher dose than can be safely administered to normal brain tumor cells with conventional photon radiation may be more safely treated with particle beams that can better conform to the tumor, thereby sparing normal cells.

Examples of CNS tumors treated with the proton beam include skull based tumors, such as chordomas and chondrosarcomas, uveal melanomas, meningiomas, craniopharyngiomas, and arteriovenous malformations. At present, the two proton beam facilities in the United States are at the Harvard Cyclotron Laboratory in Massachusetts and at Loma Linda University Medical Center in California. The Loma Linda facility is the first configured synchrotron developed for clinical treatment use for patients. Other facilities have used particle accelerators designed originally for physics research and adapted to treat patients. Several institutions are in the development stages of designing clinical proton beam facilities (Munzenrider & Crowell, 1994).

Patient preparation for proton beam therapy is more time consuming than conventional photon beam preparation, involving detailed CT and three-dimensional, "beam's eye view" treatment planning. Radiographic port filming verification is done before each treatment. Similar to radiosurgery planning, head immobilization is crucial. Patients may also require additional surgical tumor localization with possible tumor resection before starting proton beam therapy. Metallic markers surgically implanted into the skull for use during treatment planning and treatment positioning may also be done (Munzenrider & Crowell, 1994). Some patients may receive a combination of external beam radiation with conventional photons and proton beam therapy for fractionated treatment.

CNS tumors treated with the neutron beam in the past were high-grade astrocytomas. Unfortunately no survival rate improvements were seen in patients treated with the neutron beam versus the conventional photon beam in a randomized Radiation Therapy Oncology Group (RTOG) study (Laramore et al., 1988). A renewed interest in the use of neutrons has occurred in the past few years with a resurgence of boron neutron capture therapy (BNCT). With this therapy, patients are administered a boron-containing compound that is meant to be preferentially taken up by brain tumor cells as opposed to normal brain cells. When then administered thermal neutrons, the brain tumor cells containing the boron compound are selectively flooded with the neutrons allowing a higher radiation dose to the tumor cells than to the normal cells. The boron compounds used for BCNT, as early as 1954 and through the 1960s in the United States, were found to be too concentrated in blood vessels (excess normal toxicity) causing brain swelling, cerebral necrosis, and perivascular fibrosis (Laperriere & Thapar, 1994). Newer boron compounds are thought to be more selective to tumor cells, and research efforts are aimed at developing boron compounds attached to monoclonal antibodies for even better tumor cell selectivity (Wazer et al., 1994). Treatment centers in the United States that clinically use BNCT are Brookhaven National Laboratory/State University of New York at Stony Brook, and the New England Medical Center/Massachusetts Institute of Technology.

Chemotherapy

In the past, chemotherapy has had a very limited role in the treatment of CNS tumors. In general, earlier chemotherapeutic agents did not penetrate the blood–brain barrier and did not offer improved survival in patients with high-grade malignancies. Most known chemotherapeutic agents have been evaluated in the treatment of CNS tumors (Lesser & Grossman, 1993b; Mahaley, 1991) but only a few agents have shown to be of clinical use in high-grade astrocytomas. In the evaluation of chemotherapeutic agents, there have been limited controlled, prospective trials (Fine, 1994).

Chemotherapeutic drugs that cross the blood–brain barrier, such as the nitrosureas, cisplatin, and procarbazine, are the most commonly used drugs for malignant astrocytomas. Only the nitrosurea drug, BCNU, given in combination with radiation therapy, is considered standard treatment for high-grade astrocytomas with reported response rates of 10 to 40 percent (Fine et al., 1993). Although BCNU has been delivered by various routes in different clinical trials (intraarterially and inside implanted polymers in the brain at the time of surgery), the intravenous route of 240 mg/m^2 every six weeks is the standard method of administration (Sheidler & Bucholtz, 1996; Brem et al., 1995; Walker et al., 1980). Toxicity includes bone marrow depression and gastrointestinal irritation. More recently, a combination of procarbazine, lomustine (CCNU) and vincristine has been used to treat anaplastic astrocytomas following radiation therapy (Lesser & Grossman, 1993b). This drug combination has also shown some activity in the treatment of oligodendrogliomas.

CNS lymphomas and leptomeningeal disease are more routinely treated with chemotherapeutic agents. Because tumor cells disseminate throughout the entire neurospinal axis, intrathecal delivery of chemotherapy is needed in leptomeningeal disease. Methotrexate, thiotepa, and cytarabine are the agents given in treating neoplastic meningitis either by lumbar puncture or through an Ommaya reservoir (Lesser & Grossman, 1993a). In general, leptomeningeal disease or neoplastic meningitis carries a poor prognosis, but patients who have a good performance status with few neurologic deficits and a primary tumor that is slowly progressive, may benefit the most from intrathecal chemotherapy and radiation therapy (Lesser & Grossman, 1993a).

Brain Metastases

Brain metastases, the most common neurologic complication of cancer, occur in 24 percent of all patients with systemic cancers (DeAngelis, 1994; Patchell, 1991). Tumors of the lung, breast, kidney (renal cell), colon, and skin (melanoma) are the most common primary cancers that spread to the brain. The vast majority of brain metastases occur in the cerebral hemispheres (80 percent), with 17 percent in the cerebellum and 3 percent in the basal ganglia or brainstem (Lesser & Grossman, 1993b). Brain metastases are believed to arrive from hematogenous spread from primary or metastatic foci in the lungs.

Brain metastases may be single or multiple in number. About 50 percent of all brain metastases present with solitary lesions (DeAngelis, 1994). Presenting signs and symptoms of brain metastases are similar to those of primary brain tumors and are due to edema or focal pressure signs.

Radiation Therapy

The standard treatment of brain metastases includes a combination of whole-brain radiation therapy and steroids. This combination achieves symptomatic relief of neurologic signs and symptoms in 70 to 90 percent of patients (Coia, 1992). Steroids (the usual dose is 4 mg of dexamethasone every 6 hours) can dramatically improve neurologic symptoms from brain metastases within 24 to 48 hours. Depending on individual patient status, radiation therapy can be delivered in ten, 300 cGy fractions to a total of 3000 cGy for patients with an expected prognosis of less than one year, or in smaller 180 to 200 cGy fractions to a higher total dose for patients with a better prognosis (Buckner, 1992). Different fractionation schemes and total doses have also been studied (Buckner, 1992).

Head MRI scans are more sensitive than head CT scans for detecting small brain metastases, but are also more costly. A radiographic finding of a solitary brain metastasis is significant, as the radiation therapy treatment plan may be different than whole-brain radiotherapy. First, pathologic confirmation may be suggested, as the possibility of a second primary brain tumor must be ruled out. A prospective study of 54 patients with radiographic confirmation of a suspected solitary brain metastasis, underwent histological confirmation of the lesion and 11 percent of patients were found to have a glioma or nonneoplastic diagnosis (DeAngelis, 1994). In addition, surgical removal of the solitary lesion followed by a higher dose of radiation to the solitary lesion site, delivered after whole-brain irradiation, has been shown to improve patient survival (Wharam, 1993). Patients who present with solitary brain metastasis and an unknown primary tumor may also have a better overall survival than those patients who have multiple brain metastases. Most patients with brain metastases die within four to six months from progressive, systemic disease (DeAngelis, 1994).

The treatment set-up to deliver whole-brain therapy is, perhaps, one of the simplest radiation therapy delivery techniques. Simulation is not required, as the treatment can be set up clinically on the treatment machine with opposed lateral whole-brain treatment fields. Recurrent focal brain metastasis that occurs after standard cranial radiation therapy can be retreated with radiosurgery or brachytherapy.

Chemotherapy

In general, chemotherapy has a limited role in the treatment of brain metastases, but may be used for individuals who have chemotherapy-sensitive primary tumors, such as choriocarcinoma. Unfortunately, many chemotherapy drugs used for drug-sensitive tumors may not adequately cross the blood–brain barrier and reach microscopic disease in the brain.

Nursing Care of Patients Receiving CNS Irradiation

The nursing care of patients with CNS tumors involves not only the usual activities of patient/family teaching, assistance in management of side effects, and psychological support and counseling, but also special attention to other quality of life issues unique for patients with brain tumors. Nursing interventions also are aimed at helping patients and their families cope with the common, additive side effects of other medications commonly required, such as antiseizure drugs and steroids; teaching patients to help prevent or promptly detect common problems associated with brain tumors, such as deep vein thromboses (DVT); and assisting patients with crucial rehabilitation and quality of life issues raised by the diagnosis of a brain tumor.

The nurse in radiation oncology must monitor the many side effects of the drugs commonly used by patients with brain tumors, and help patients to understand that many of the functional problems they encounter can be attributed to steroids and antiseizure medications. Prompt recognition of potentially serious side effects, such as Stevens-Johnson syndrome, attributed to phenytoin sensitivity, is crucial in preventing serious patient morbidity. There is an increased incidence of this syndrome in patients on phenytoin who are receiving whole-brain radiation therapy (Stein & Chamberlain, 1991). Stein and Chamberlain (1991) provide an excellent reference on the management of seizures in the patient with cancer. In addition, since serum levels of antiseizure medications can be altered by tapering doses of steroids and certain chemotherapy drugs, monitoring of antiseizure serum levels is important (Grossman et al., 1989; Schwandt, 1994).

Thromboembolic disease is associated with brain tumors (Norris & Grossman, 1994). There is some controversy regarding the use of anticoagulant therapy for patients with DVTs or pulmonary embolisms, out of fear of possible brain hemorrhage, especially if the patient is thrombocytopenic from chemotherapy. With careful monitoring, anticoagulants have been shown to be safely administered to these patients (Norris & Grossman, 1994).

The functional losses attributed to brain tumors and their treatments, including loss of mobility and cognitive impairments, create numerous challenges for patients and their families. Proximal myopathy from long-term steroid use is devastating for many patients, often affecting simple tasks such as stair climbing and getting up from a chair. The added weight gain and body image changes produced by long-term steroid use also create several real and potential coping problems. Some patients with tremendous weight gain cannot safely fit on the MRI table. After long-term steroid use, patients are eager to discontinue their steroids, but require careful tapering to avoid steroid withdrawal crisis. Even with careful steroid tapering, patients may have a return of edema and need to resume higher doses of dexamethasone. Emotionally, this can be very difficult for patients and families. They should be warned that steroid tapering cannot always be successful.

An additional stressful time for patients with high-grade astrocytoma centers around follow-up head scan tests. Patients and families need to understand that the interpretation of MRI and CT scans can be difficult because images are affected by postirradiation changes and adjustment in steroid doses. Since the brain does not have a mechanism to promptly rid itself of dead tumor cells, patients and families should be taught that even if the treatment has been successful, the brain may not appear completely normal on the scan.

Patients presenting with seizures may not be allowed to drive for legal reasons for a specified amount of time, despite having well-controlled seizures. These restrictions depend on the regulations of their state's Motor Vehicle Department. The Epilepsy Foundation of America has published regulations and recommendations concerning seizures and driving by state location (Epilepsy Foundation of America, 1992).

The supportive care of patients with CNS tumors has been described by Wegmann (1991), Amato (1991), and Newton and Mateo (1994). One organization that offers both support and free, published materials on CNS tumors for patients and families is the American Brain Tumor Association, 2720 River Road, Des Plaines, IL 60018, 1-800-886-2282.

References

Akeyson EW & McCutcheon IE (1996). Management of benign and aggressive intracranial meningiomas. *Oncology, 10,* 747–756.

Amato CA (1991). Malignant gliomas: Coping with a devastating illness. *Journal of Neuroscience Nursing, 23,* 20–22.

American College of Radiology (1991). *Manual on iodinated contrast media.* Reston, VA: American College of Radiology.

Archibald YM, Lunn D, Ruttan LA, McDonald MD, DelMaestro F, Barr HWK, Pexman JH, Fisher BJ, Gaspar LE & Cairncross JG (1994). Cognitive functioning in long term survivors of high grade glioma. *Journal of Neurosurgery, 80,* 247–253.

Armstrong C, Mollman J, Corn BW, Alavi J & Grossman M (1993). Effects of radiation therapy on adult brain behavior: Evidence for a rebound phenomenon in a phase I trial. *Neurology, 43,* 1961–1965.

Black P (1991). Brain tumors (Parts I & II). *New England Journal of Medicine, 32,* 1471–1475, 1555–1564.

Blevins LS & Wand GS (1993). Pituitary adenomas. In: RT Johnson, JW Griffin & BC Decker (Eds.), *Current Therapy in Neurologic Disease* (pp. 231–235). St. Louis: Mosby Year Book.

Brem H, Piantadosi S, Burger PC, Walker M, Selker R, Vick NA, Black K, Sisti M, Brem S, Mohn G, Muller P, Morawetz R & Schold SC for the Polymer Brain Tumor Treatment Group (1995). Intraoperative controlled delivery of chemotherapy by biodegradable polymers: Safety and effectiveness for recurrent gliomas evaluated by a perspective, multi-institutional, placebo-controlled clinical trial. *Lancet, 345* (8956), 1008–1012.

Bucholtz JD (1992). Radiation carcinogenesis. In KH Dow & LJ Hilderley (Eds.), *Nursing Care in Radiation Oncology* (pp. 342–357). Philadelphia: WB Saunders.

Buckner J (1992). Surgery, radiation therapy and chemotherapy for metastatic tumors of the brain. *Current Opinion in Oncology, 4,* 518–524.

Cairncross JG & Laperriere NJ (1989). Low grade glioma: To treat or not to treat? *Archives of Neurology, 46,* 1238–1239.

Coia LR (1992). The role of radiation therapy in the treatment of brain metastases. *International Journal of Radiation Oncology, Biology, Physics, 23,* 229–238.

DeAngelis LM (1994). Management of brain metastases. *Cancer Investigation, 12,* 156–165.

Delattre JY, Rosenblum MK, Thaler HT, Mandell L, Shapiro WR & Posner JB (1988). A model of radiation myelography in the rat: Pathology, regional permeability changes and treatment with dexamethasone. *Brain, 111,* 1319–1336.

Digel CA, Mayer R, Latronico D, Jackson J & Wharam MD (1994). Dosimetric comparison of five craniospinal therapy techniques. *Radiation Therapist, 3,* 95–102.

Dunbar SF & Loeffler JS (1994). Stereotactic radiation therapy. In: PM Mauch & JS Loeffler (Eds.), *Radiation Oncology: Technology and Biology* (pp 237–251). Philadelphia: WB Saunders.

Epilepsy Foundation of America (1992). *Driving and Epilepsy.* Landover, Maryland.

Fine, HA (1994). The basis for current treatment recommendations for malignant gliomas. *Journal of Neuro-Oncology, 20,* 111–120.

Fine HA, Dear KBG, Loeffler JS, Black PM & Canellos GP (1993). Meta-analysis of radiation therapy with and without adjuvant chemotherapy for malignant gliomas in adults. *Cancer, 71,* 2585–2597.

Flickinger JC, Lunsford LD & Kondziolka D (1994). Radiosurgery. In: PM Mauch & JS Loeffler. *Radiation Oncology: Technology and Biology* (pp. 198–215). Philadelphia: WB Saunders.

Grossman SA, Osman M, Hruban RH & Piantadosi S. (1995). Familial gliomas: The potential role for environmental exposures. *Proceedings of the American Society of Clinical Oncology, 14,* 149.

Grossman SA, Sheidler VR & Gilbert MR. (1989). Decreased phenytoin levels in patients receiving chemotherapy. *American Journal of Medicine, 87,* 505–510.

Heath CW (1996). Electromagnetic field exposure and cancer: A review of epidemiologic evidence. *Ca-A Cancer Journal for Clinicians, 46,* 29–44.

Hickey JV (1992). *Neurological and neurosurgical nursing* (3rd ed., pp. 299–324), Philadelphia: JB Lippincott.

Hochberg FH & Slotnick B (1980). Neuropsychologic impairment in astrocytoma survivors. *Neurology, 30,* 172–177.

Hoffman WF, Levin VA & Wilson CB (1979). Evaluation of malignant glioma patients during the post-irradiation period. *Journal of Neurosurgery, 50,* 624–628.

Imperato JP, Paleologos NA & Vick NA (1990). Effects of treatment on long term survivors with malignant astrocytomas. *Annals of Neurology, 28,* 818–822.

Karlsson UL, Leibel SA, Wallner K & Davis LW (1992). Brain. In: CA Perez & LW Brady (Eds.), *Principles and Practice of Radiation Oncology* (2nd ed., pp. 515–552). Philadelphia: JB Lippincott.

Kernohan JW, Mabon RF, Svien HJ & Adson AW (1949). A simplified classification of gliomas. *Proceedings Staff Meetings of Mayo Clinic, 24,* 71–75.

Kleihues P, Burger PC & Scheithauer BW (1993). Histological Typing of Tumours of the Central Nervous System. (2nd ed., p. 51). Berlin: Springer-Verlag, World Health Organization.

Kleinberg L, Wallner K & Malkin MK (1993). Good performance status of long-term disease free survivors of intracranial gliomas. *International Journal of Radiation Oncology, Biology, Physics, 26,* 129–133.

Krause EA, Lamb S, Ham B, Larson DA & Gutin PH (1991). Radiosurgery: A nursing perspective. *Journal of Neuroscience Nursing, 23*, 24–27.

Kristiansen K, Hagan S, Kollevold T, Torvik A, Holme I, Nesbakken R, Hatlevoll R, Lindgren M, Brun A, Lindgen S, Notter G, Anderson AP & Elgen K (1981). Combined modality therapy of operative astrocytomas grade III and IV: Confirmation of the value of post-operative irradiation and lack of potentiation of bleomycin on survival time. A prospective multicenter trial of the Scandinavian Glioblastoma Study Group. *Cancer, 47*, 649–652.

Laperriere NJ & Bernstein M (1994). Radiotherapy for brain tumors. *Ca-A Cancer Journal for Clinicians, 44*, 96–108.

Laramore GE, Diener-West M, Griffin TW, Nelson JS, Griem ML, Thomas FJ, Hendrickson FR, Griffin BR, Myrianthopoulous LC, Saxon J. (1988). Randomized neuron dose searching study for malignant gliomas of the brain: Results of an RTOG study. *International Journal of Radiation Oncology, Biology, Physics, 14*, 1093–1102.

Laws ER & Thapar K (1993). Brain tumors. *Ca-A Cancer Journal for Clinicians, 43*, 263–271.

Leibel SA & Sheline GE (1987). Radiation therapy for neoplasms of the brain. *Journal of Neurology, 66*, 1–22.

Lesser GJ & Grossman SA (1993a). Metastatic cancer to the brain and spinal cord. In: JE Niederhuber (Ed.), *Current Therapy in Oncology* (pp. 224–230), St. Louis: Mosby-Year Book, Inc.

Lesser GJ & Grossman SA (1993b). The chemotherapy of adult primary brain tumors. *Cancer Treatment Reviews, 19*, 261–281.

Levin VA, Gutin PH & Leibel SA (1993). Neoplasms of the central nervous system. In: VT DeVita, S Hellman & SA Rosenberg (Eds.), *Cancer: Principles and Practice* (pp. 1679–1737). Philadelphia: JB Lippincott.

Levine AM (1990). Lymphoma in acquired immunodeficiency syndrome. *Seminars in Oncology, 17*, 104–112.

Lubbe J, vonAmmon K, Watanabe K, Hegi ME & Kleihues P (1995). Familial brain tumor syndrome associated with a p53 germline deletion of codan 236. *Brain Pathology, 5*, 15–23.

Mahaley MS (1991). Neuro-oncology index and review. *Journal of Neuro-Oncology, 11*, 85–147.

Maire JPL, Coudin P, Geurin J & Caudry M (1987). Neuropsychologic impairment in adults with brain tumors. *American Journal of Clinical Oncology, 10*, 156–162.

Meadows AT, Gordon J, Massari DJ, Littman P, Fergusson J & Moss K (1981). Declines in IQ scores and cognitive dysfunction in children with acute lymphocytic leukaemia treated with cranial irradiation. *Lancet, 2*, 1015–1018.

Moore IM, Kramer JH, Wara W, Halberg F & Ablin AR (1991). Cognitive function in children with leukemia. *Cancer, 68*, 1913–1917.

Munzenrider JE & Crowell C (1994). Charged particles. In PM Mauch & JS Loeffler (Eds.), *Radiation Oncology: Technology and Biology* (pp. 34–55). Philadelphia: WB Saunders.

Newton HB & Mateo MA (1994). Uncertainty: Strategies for patients with brain tumor and their families. *Cancer Nursing, 17*, 137–140.

Newton HB (1994). Primary brain tumors: Review of etiology, diagnosis and treatment. *American Family Physician, 49*, 787–797.

Norris LK & Grossman SA (1994). Treatment of thromboembolitic complications in patients with brain tumors. *Journal of Neuro-Oncology, 22*, 127–137.

Parker SL, Tong T, Bolden S & Wingo PA (1997). Cancer statistics. *Ca-A Cancer Journal for Clinicians, 47*, 5–27.

Patchell RA (1991). Brain metastases. *Neurology Clinics, 9*, 817–824.

Ramsey RG (1994). The order of neurodiagnostic procedures. In RA Ramsey (Ed.), *Neuroradiology* (pp. 1–19). Philadelphia: WB Saunders.

Rodesch G & Lasjaunais P (1991). Embolization and meningiomas. In O Al-Mefty (Ed.), *Meningiomas* (pp. 285–297). New York: Raven Press.

Schoenberg BS (1991). Epidemiology of primary intracranial neoplasms: Disease distribution and risk factors. In M Salcman (Ed.), *Neurobiology of Brain Tumors* (pp. 3–18). Baltimore: Williams & Wilkins.

Schwandt RE (1994). Selected aspects of phenytoin therapy in oncology practice. *Cancer Control: Journal of the Moffatt Cancer Center, 1*, 150–155.

Sheidler VR & Bucholtz JD (1996). Nervous system tumors. In R McCorkle, M Grant, M Frank-Stromborg, S Baird (Eds). *Cancer Nursing: A Comprehensive Textbook* (2nd ed.), Philadelphia: Saunders.

Shreive DC, Gutin PH & Larson DA (1994). Brachytherapy. In PM Mauch & JS Loeffler (Eds.), *Radiation Oncology: Technology and Biology*, Philadelphia: WB Saunders.

Stein DA & Chamberlain MC (1991). Evaluation and management of seizures in the patient with cancer. *Oncology, 5*, 33–40.

Walker MD, Green SB, Byar DP, Alexander E Jr, Batzdorf U, Brooks WH, Hunt WE, McCarty CS, Mahaley MS Jr, Mealey J Jr, Owens G, Ransohoff J II, Robertson JT, Shapiro WR, Smith KR Jr, Wilson CB & Strike TA (1980). Randomized comparison of radiotherapy and nitrosureas for the treatment of malignant glioma after surgery. *New England Journal of Medicine, 303*, 1323–1329.

Wazer DE, Zamenhoff RG, Harling OK & Madoc-Jones H (1994). Boron neutron capture therapy. In PM Mauch & JS Loeffler (Eds.), *Radiation Oncology: Technology and Biology* (pp. 167–191). Philadelphia: WB Saunders.

Wegman J (1991). CNS tumors: Supportive management of the patient and family. *Oncology, 5*, 109–113.

Wharam MD (1993). Brain tumors: Radiation therapy. In JE Niederhuber (Ed.), *Current Therapy in Oncology* (pp. 542–550). St. Louis: Mosby-Year Book.

Wilson CB (1994). Generalized considerations. In MLJ Apuzzo (Ed.), *Brain Surgery: Complication Avoidance and Management* (pp. 177–185). New York: Churchill Livingstone.

Wrensch M, Bondy MI, Wrencke J & Yost M (1993). Environmental risk factors for primary brain tumors: A review. *Journal of Neuro-Oncology, 17*, 47–64.

Yamashita T & Kuwabara T (1983). Estimation of rate of growth of malignant brain tumors by computed tomography scanning. *Surgical Neurology, 20*, 464–468.

Zulch KJ (1979). Histological typing of tumors of the central nervous system. Geneva: World Health Organization.

Gastrointestinal Cancers

JOANNE FRANKEL KELVIN

Cancers of the gastrointestinal (GI) tract are responsible for almost 25 percent of all deaths from cancer in the United States. In 1996, there were an estimated 225,900 new GI cancer diagnoses and 127,070 deaths (Parker et al., 1997). The incidence and mortality of specific GI cancers are listed in Table 11–1.

Anatomy and Physiology

The gastrointestinal tract (Figure 11–1) is essentially a hollow muscular tube extending from the mouth through the esophagus, stomach, small intestine, colon, rectum, and anus. The accessory gastrointestinal organs are the liver, gallbladder, and pancreas. The major functions of the GI tract include the mechanical and chemical breakdown of food and the absorption of digested nutrients, water, and electrolytes (Guyton, 1991; McCance & Huether, 1994).

The esophagus is approximately 25 cm long and conducts food substances from the pharynx to the stomach through peristalsis. Although there are no distinct anatomic regions, the esophagus is described as having four segments: cervical, upper thoracic, midthoracic, and lower thoracic. At its distal end is the esophageal sphincter, which prevents reflux of gastric contents.

The stomach is delineated into three sections: the upper fundus, the middle body or corpus, and the lower antrum. The stomach secretes digestive juices, mixes ingested food with these juices to begin digestion and converts food to semifluid chyme, and then stores the chyme until it can be accommodated by the duodenum. The stomach is bordered below by the pylorus, which regulates emptying of chyme into the small intestine.

The small intestine is 5 to 7 meters long and is divided into three segments: the duodenum, the jejunum, and the ileum. The proximal portion of the small intestine secretes some digestive enzymes, and with pancreatic enzymes and bile salts, continues food digestion initiated in the stomach. Peristaltic movements push the chyme through the remainder of the small intestine, which absorbs nutrients, water, and electrolytes. The ileocecal valve regulates the emptying of chyme from the small intestine into the large bowel.

The large bowel is about 1.5 meters long. The colon lies within the peritoneal cavity, above the peritoneal reflection, and includes the cecum and the ascending, transverse, descending, and sigmoid regions. The rectum comprises the lower 12 to 15 cm of the large bowel and is located at and below the peritoneal reflection and thus is extraperitoneal.

The function of the proximal portion of the large bowel is to absorb water and electrolytes from the chyme and transform chyme into solid feces. The distal portion of the large bowel stores fecal matter until defecation occurs.

The anal canal is about three to four centimeters long and extends from the lower border of the rectum to the anal verge. The perianal skin below the anal verge is referred to as the anal margin. The muscles that comprise the internal and external anal sphincters control defecation.

The liver, gallbladder, and pancreas are accessory organs of the GI tract. The pancreas is 20 cm long, with the head lying in the curve of the duodenum, the body positioned behind the stomach, and the tail extending to the spleen. It secretes enzymes necessary for digestion of carbohydrates, proteins, and fats. The pancreas also has an endocrine function; it secretes insulin and glucagon. The liver is located under the right diaphragm and is divided into right and left lobes. It produces bile, which is necessary for fat digestion and absorption. Bile is stored in the gallbladder, a

Table 11-1 • GI Cancers: Estimated United States Incidence and Mortality Rates, 1997

Site	Incidence % of all cancers	Incidence	Mortality
Esophagus	0.9	12,500	11,500
Stomach	1.6	22,400	14,000
Small intestine	0.4	4,900	1,140
Large intestine	6.8	94,100	46,600
Rectum	2.7	37,100	8,300
Anus, anal canal and anorectum	0.3	3,400	410
Liver and intra- hepatic bile duct	1.0	13,600	12,400
Gallbladder and other biliary	0.5	6,900	3,500
Pancreas	2.0	27,600	28,100
Other and unspecified	0.2	3,400	1,120
Total		225,900	127,070

Data from Parker SL, Tong T, Bolden S, & Wingo PA. (1997). Cancer statistics: 1997. *Ca-A Cancer Journal for Clinicians, 47,* 5-27.

saclike structure that lies inferior to the liver. The liver is also involved in the metabolism of nutrients absorbed from the GI tract. A series of connecting ducts from the liver, gallbladder, and pancreas provide passage of secretions needed for digestion and absorption into the duodenum.

The wall of the GI tract is organized into four concentric layers as shown in Figure 11–2 (Guy-

ton, 1991; McCance & Huether, 1994). The innermost layer is the *mucosa*, a mucous membrane with a lining layer of epithelial tissue. The entire epithelial population is replaced regularly as the cells are sloughed off into the intestinal lumen. Mucus glands produce secretions that facilitate passage of food substances through the GI tract and provide protection to the epithelial lining against mechanical or chemical damage. The *submucosa* is a layer of connective tissue containing blood vessels, lymphatics, and nerves. The submucosal nerve plexus controls GI secretion and local blood flow. The *muscularis* contains longitudinal and circular layers of smooth muscle with the myenteric nerve plexus between them. This nerve plexus controls GI motility, which is the result of mixing and propulsive peristaltic muscle movements. In general, parasympathetic innervation increases GI tract secretion and motility, and sympathetic innervation inhibits it. The outermost layer of the wall is the *serosa*, a serous membrane with an outer layer of squamous epithelium.

Pathophysiology

GI tract cancers generally arise within the mucosa, and most are *adenocarcinomas.* The tumor may grow as a mass projecting into the lumen or can infiltrate the wall, often circumferentially,

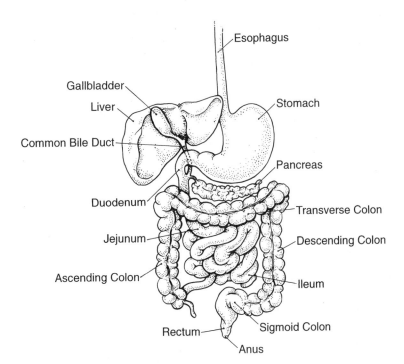

Figure 11-1 • The gastrointestinal tract.

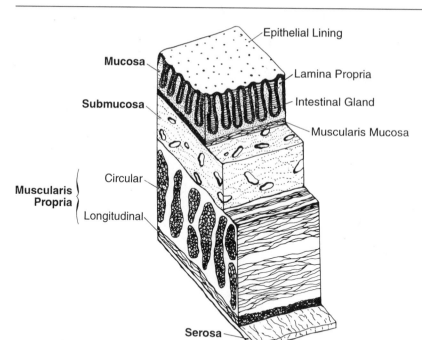

Mucosa

Submucosa

Muscularis Propria { Circular

Longitudinal

Epithelial Lining

Lamina Propria

Intestinal Gland

Muscularis Mucosa

Serosa

Figure 11-2 • Cross section of the gastrointestinal tract wall.

encircling and narrowing it. As the tumor grows, obstruction or bleeding can develop. The tumor *spreads locally* by extension through the concentric layers of the GI tract wall and invasion of adjacent structures. This can lead to fistula formation or perforation. The tumor *spreads regionally* through the lymphatic system and *spreads distantly* by hematogenous dissemination, most commonly to the liver, lung, and bones. The tumor also spreads by peritoneal seeding within the abdominal and pelvic cavities.

GI cancers progress insidiously during the early stages of tumor growth. Signs and symptoms are often vague and nonspecific, initially resembling more common benign GI disorders. As a result, patients do not generally seek medical treatment early and often present with advanced disease.

Principles of Diagnosis and Staging

Accurate diagnosis and staging of GI cancers is essential to assure that appropriate decisions are made regarding treatment. Although a variety of different staging systems have been used in the past, the *TNM Staging System* of the American Joint Committee on Cancer (AJCC) is now generally recommended. This involves a scoring of the extent of local tumor growth (T), the status of regional and distant lymph nodes (N), and the presence of distant metastasis (M). Together these determine the stage of disease (I through IV). Hill, Roberts, and Schwab (1992) describe a variety of diagnostic techniques used in the staging of patients with GI cancers.

Diagnostic imaging techniques include plain x rays, barium studies, and computerized tomography (CT) scans. Plain abdominal films can provide evidence of liver enlargement, soft tissue masses, ascites, or bowel obstruction (i.e., dilated loops of bowel and air-fluid levels). Chest x rays can establish the presence of metastatic disease of the lung (i.e., pulmonary nodules or pleural effusion). Double-contrast barium studies can detect the presence and location of mucosal irregularities, but may not differentiate benign from malignant lesions and do not provide information on the depth of tumor extension. CT scans of the abdomen, with oral contrast, examine the body from the lung bases to the iliac crests. If sigmoid or rectal lesions are suspected, the pelvis is included, with rectal contrast. Although magnetic resonance imaging of the abdomen or pelvis is being used more frequently, it does not provide a clear advantage over CT except for the diagnosis of liver metastasis (Hill et al., 1992). Additional diagnostic imaging studies that may be performed include nuclear scans of the liver and bones to determine if there is metastatic disease in these sites.

Endoscopy is an essential part of the staging workup of patients with GI cancers. Flexible fiberoptic instruments can be used in both the upper tract (to the distal duodenum) and the lower tract (to the cecum). Endoscopy enables the physician to directly visualize the tumor and obtain brushings for cytology and tissue samples for biopsy. *Endoscopic ultrasound*, a relatively new tool that enables visualization of a depth of up to 8 cm, provides information regarding the size of the tumor, the depth of invasion through the GI tract wall, and the presence of lymphadenopathy.

Laparoscopy may be included in the staging workup of patients, most commonly with upper GI cancers. It can be effective in detecting peritoneal tumor implants and liver metastasis.

A number of laboratory studies are also obtained during the patient's workup. Liver function tests can indicate liver metastasis, and a complete blood count can indicate anemia secondary to acute or occult blood loss. Relevant serum tumor markers, such as CEA (carcinoembryonic antigen) and CA 19-9 (carbohydrate antigen), although not specific enough to be used in screening or diagnosing particular GI cancers, are obtained prior to initiating treatment. These markers are useful when repeated at intervals to monitor the patient's response to treatment.

The specific diagnostic tests most commonly used in the staging of particular GI cancers are listed in Table 11–2.

Table 11-2 • GI Cancers: Diagnostic Tests

Diagnostic Test	Esophagus	Stomach	Pancreas	Colorectal	Anal
RADIOLOGY					
Chest x ray	X	X	X	X	X
Contrast study	Barium swallow (esophogram)	Upper GI		Barium enema	
CT scan	Chest and upper abdomen	Abdomen and pelvis	Abdomen	Abdomen and pelvis	Pelvis
Other			Percutaneous transhepatic cholangiography Angiography		
ENDOSCOPIC EXAM	Esophagoscopy	Gastroscopy	Endoscopic retrograde cholangiography	Proctosigmoidoscopy Colonoscopy	Anoscopy Proctoscopy
	Ultrasound	Ultrasound		Ultrasound Rectal: MRI	Ultrasound
LABORATORY STUDIES					
CBC		X		X	
Chemistry		Liver function tests	Pancreatic function tests	Liver function tests	
Tumor markers		CEA, CA 19-9	CEA, CA 19-9, and POA	CEA	
OTHER TESTS					
To detect local invasion	Upper and mid thoracic lesions: bronchoscopy and thoracoscopy				
For palpable lymph nodes	Cervical or supraclavicular LN biopsy				Inguinal LN biopsy
To detect peritoneal implants	Lower lesions: laparoscopy		Laparoscopy		

Data from Hill MC, Roberts IM, and Schwab F (1992). Imaging techniques in the diagnosis and staging of gastrointestinal cancer. In J Ahlgren and J Macdonald (Eds.), *Gastrointestinal Oncology,* (pp. 13–18). Philadelphia: JB Lippincott.

Principles of Treatment

GI cancers are treated most frequently with surgery when the goal of treatment is cure. The likelihood of prolonged disease-free survival after surgical resection alone depends on the site and stage of disease, but generally is poor for most GI cancers as illustrated in Table 11–3 (Wanebo & Turk, 1992). All have a significant risk of local recurrence and distant metastasis after surgery. As a result, postoperative *adjuvant* therapy has been widely used. Adjuvant therapy may include radiation therapy to improve local control, chemotherapy to prevent metastatic disease, or combined modality therapy with both radiation and chemotherapy. More recently, the use of preoperative *neoadjuvant* therapy has been recommended for selected patients. Treatment is with radiation therapy, chemotherapy, or a combination of these therapies. Specific advantages of neoadjuvant therapy include improved local tumor control, improved tumor resectability, use of conservative organ-sparing surgical procedures, and early administration of systemic therapy for cancers at high risk of metastatic spread (Kelsen, 1993). In fact, based on the effectiveness of neoadjuvant therapy in cancers of the esophagus and anus, combined modality therapy is now used as an alternative to surgery for cure in many patients with these cancers.

Surgery

Curative surgical resection is the treatment of choice for most early stage GI cancers when complete tumor resection is possible and there are no medical contraindications. The procedure generally begins with an exploration of the abdomen to determine if there is lymphadenopathy, liver metastasis, peritoneal seeding, or ascites. The structures adjacent to the tumor are examined to determine if there is tumor adherence or invasion and to evaluate if the tumor can be completely resected. The resection is then performed, removing the primary tumor and adherent adjacent structures, with adequate margins. The surrounding lymph node-bearing tissue is also removed (Wanebo & Turk, 1992). The extent of resection required for many tumors is controversial.

Surgery can also play a role in treatment if curative resection is not possible. Aggressive palliative surgery may improve the quality of life for selected patients with locally advanced or metastatic GI cancers. Depending on the site, the tumor may be resected or bypassed to prevent or treat complications of obstruction, bleeding, and pain.

Radiation Therapy

Radiation therapy is used in the treatment of patients with GI cancers both with curative intent and for palliation of symptoms. It can be used alone, as the primary treatment, or in combination with chemotherapy. It can be administered preoperatively, in an attempt to reduce tumor bulk and improve resectability, or postoperatively, in an attempt to eradicate residual gross or microscopic tumor cells. The challenge in administering radiation therapy is to direct a high enough dose to the tumor to eradicate the disease, while assuring that the surrounding normal tissues receive doses below those that would cause significant toxicity. This is particularly difficult when treating GI cancers because the mucosa throughout the GI tract is extremely sensitive to the effects of ionizing radiation.

There are several methods of administering radiation therapy to patients with GI cancers. *Fractionated external beam radiation therapy* provides a deeply penetrating homogeneous dose distribution. *Brachytherapy* allows the delivery of a high dose of radiation to a small localized area, and *intraoperative radiation therapy* involves the delivery of radiation directly to the tumor or tumor bed during a surgical procedure. The tumor may be surgically resected, leaving residual gross or microscopic disease, or may be unresectable. The surrounding normal structures, particularly the radiosensitive small intestine, are manually displaced from the treatment field during the procedure, the site to be treated is directly visualized, and the target area is treated with a single high dose of 1000 to 2000 cGy. Intraoperative radiation therapy can be delivered in two ways: (1) external beam treatment with electrons from a linear ac-

Table 11-3 • GI Cancers: 5-Year Survival Rates After Surgical Resection

Site	5-Year Survival Rate (%)
Esophagus	10–20
Stomach (Proximal)	15
Stomach (Distal)	30
Pancreas	15
Colon	40–85
Rectum	40–90

Adapted with permission from Wanebo HJ and Turk PS (1992). General surgical principles in gastrointestinal cancer. In J Ahlgren and J Macdonald (Eds.), *Gastrointestinal Oncology* (pp. 19–28). Philadelphia: JB Lippincott.

celerator, using a cone to direct the beam to the target, or (2) high-dose rate brachytherapy, using a flexible multichannel applicator placed on the tumor bed and loaded with iridium-192. The linear accelerator cone or brachytherapy applicator and sources are removed after treatment is delivered, and the surgery is completed.

The method of treatment most commonly used in the treatment of patients with GI cancers is fractionated external beam radiation therapy. The treatment position and technique are determined by the location of the tumor and the total dose to be delivered. Treatment planning is essential before beginning treatment to localize the target area and minimize dose to the surrounding normal tissue. Localization techniques include simulation x rays and CT scans. To assure accurate visualization of structures in the field, patients are often given oral contrast solution before x rays or CT are performed (e.g., Polibar, a barium sulfate suspension used if no CT is involved; Gastrografin, used with CT). If a CT scan is not available for treatment planning, an intravenous contrast (e.g., Reno-60) is administered in some instances to visualize the kidneys (Caudry, 1992; Minsky, 1996). Blocks are designed to size and shape the beams. Multiple field techniques, generally with three fields (anterior–posterior [AP] or posterior–anterior [PA], and laterals or obliques) or four fields (AP, PA, and laterals), and shrinking fields with reduction in target volume (i.e., come down) are used to ensure that normal tissues do not receive excessive doses of radiation. An additional strategy to minimize dose to normal tissue is the use of a boost to the primary site, administered by interstitial or intraluminal brachytherapy or by intraoperative radiation therapy.

Chemotherapy

GI cancers have a wide range of sensitivity to chemotherapy, but generally respond in 10 to 25 percent of patients. Historically, chemotherapy was used primarily for palliation of locally advanced or metastatic disease. However, new chemotherapeutic approaches, often in combination with radiation therapy, have led to the increasing use of chemotherapy in the curative treatment of many GI cancers.

The use of combined modality therapy allows for the simultaneous delivery of local and systemic therapy, with two potential benefits: (1) increased cell-kill in the treatment field, reducing local failure and (2) treatment of disease outside of the treatment field, reducing distant metastasis (Raef-

sky & Wasserman, 1992). However, the use of combined modality therapy not only has the potential to improve therapeutic results, but may also lead to increased toxicity.

A variety of sequences (e.g., concurrent, sequential, alternating), methods of chemotherapy administration (e.g., bolus, continuous infusion), and methods of radiation therapy delivery (e.g., external beam, brachytherapy) have been used in combined modality therapy (Raefsky & Wasserman, 1992). The optimal approach for most cancers has not yet been determined.

The major chemotherapeutic agent used in the treatment of GI cancers is the fluoropyrimidine 5-fluorouracil (5-FU). The primary mechanism of action is inhibition of the enzyme thymidylate synthase, preventing the cell from synthesizing thymine needed for DNA replication. Cell death occurs in the S phase of the cell cycle. Additional cytotoxic activity results from incorporation of 5-FU into RNA and DNA (Ahlgren, 1992). A number of different drugs have been used to enhance or modulate the effects of 5-FU, including leucovorin (folinic acid), levamisole, methotrexate, PALA, cisplatin, and interferon. 5-FU is administered intravenously, either by bolus or continuous infusion. A variety of regimens and doses are used. A number of other chemotherapeutic agents commonly used in the treatment of GI cancers and their toxicities are listed in Table 11–4.

Cancer of the Esophagus

Epidemiology

Although cancer of the esophagus is the third most frequent GI cancer in the world, it is rare in the United States, with an overall survival rate of only about 10 percent.

The incidence of esophageal cancer varies widely around the world. High-risk and low-risk areas have greater than 100-fold differences in incidence. These differences strongly implicate a variety of risk factors. In Western nations, consumption of alcohol and tobacco significantly increases risk. In undeveloped countries, nutritional deficiencies of particular vitamins and trace elements seem to be important. In the esophageal "cancer belt," extending from northeastern China to the Middle East, ingestion of carcinogens in foodstuffs (e.g., nitrosamine preservatives or fungal toxin contamination) has been identified as a risk factor. Physical irritation of the esophageal

Table 11-4 • GI Cancers: Commonly Used Chemotherapeutic Agents and Toxicity

Chemotherapeutic Agent	Toxicity
5-Fluorouracil	Dermatologic: alopecia, hyperpigmentation, nail changes, radiation recall Ocular: conjunctivitis, lacrimal duct fibrosis Neurologic: cerebellar ataxia, acute encephalopathy GI: mucositis, nausea and vomiting, diarrhea Hematologic: marrow depression, megaloblastosis
Cisplatin	Hypersensitivity: anaphylaxis, rash Dermatologic: alopecia Ocular: retrobulbar neuritis Neurologic: peripheral neuropathy, acute encephalopathy GI: nausea and vomiting Renal: toxic nephropathy, hypomagnesemia, hypocalcemia Hematologic: marrow depression, hemolytic anemia Miscellaneous: hypotension
Mitomycin-C	Dermatologic: vesicant Pulmonary: chronic fibrosis GI: mucositis, nausea and vomiting, hepatic function changes Renal: toxic nephropathy Hematologic: marrow depression, hemolytic anemia
Methotrexate	Hypersensitivity: rash Ocular: conjunctivitis Neurologic: acute encephalopathy Dermatologic: alopecia Pulmonary: acute infiltrate GI: mucositis, nausea and vomiting, diarrhea, hepatic function changes, hepatic necrosis, fibrosis, and cirrhosis Renal: toxic nephropathy, hyperglycemia Hematologic: marrow depression, megaloblastosis
Doxorubicin	Hypersensitivity: rash, fever, chills Dermatologic: vesicant, alopecia, hyperpigmentation, nail changes, radiation recall Ocular: conjunctivitis Cardiac: cardiac necrosis GI: mucositis, nausea and vomiting, diarrhea Hematologic: marrow depression Miscellaneous: hemorrhagic cystitis
Bleomycin	Hypersensitivity: fever, chills Dermatologic: alopecia, hyperpigmentation, nail changes, radiation recall Pulmonary: chronic fibrosis GI: mucositis Hematologic: DIC Miscellaneous: hypotension, Raynaud's syndrome
Etoposide	GI: nausea and vomiting Hematologic: marrow depression, DIC
Nitrosureas	Neurologic: acute encephalopathy Pulmonary: chronic fibrosis GI: hepatic function changes Renal: toxic nephropathy Hematologic: marrow depression

Adapted with permission from Perry MC (1992). *The Chemotherapy Source Book*. Baltimore: Williams & Wilkins.

epithelium has also been associated with increased risk. Causes include: (1) accidental ingestion of lye, (2) severe achalasia (failure of the esophageal sphincter to relax during swallowing, which prevents emptying and causes stasis and ulceration of the mucosa), and (3) reflux of gastric acids from inadequate treatment of hiatal hernia. In fact, Barrett's esophagus, in which columnar epithelium replaces squamous epithelium in the distal esophagus as a result of chronic esophageal reflux, is considered a premalignant condition. Finally, certain rare hereditary conditions (e.g., tylosis) are also associated with increased risk of disease (Moses, 1991; Schein, 1992).

Pathophysiology

In the past, more than 90 percent of all cancers of the esophagus were squamous cell carcinomas.

In recent years, however, adenocarcinomas represent 40 percent of esophageal cancers (Blot et al., 1991). These occur primarily in the lower esophagus.

Cancers of the esophagus arise in the mucosa and tend to grow longitudinally through the esophageal wall. Tumors greater than 5 cm in length are more commonly associated with locally advanced and metastatic disease (Roth et al., 1993). The tumor spreads locally by direct extension through the layers of the wall; because the esophagus has no serosal layer, local spread can occur early in the disease, with invasion of any of the adjacent structures in the neck or chest (Harter, 1992a). Regional spread occurs through the lymphatic system, as high as the cervical and supraclavicular lymph nodes and as low as the celiac and gastric lymph nodes. The disease metastasizes most commonly to the liver, lung, pleura, adrenals, bone, and kidney.

Clinical Presentation

The primary symptom of cancer of the esophagus is dysphagia (difficulty swallowing), occurring in 90 percent of patients, with odynophagia (pain with swallowing) in 50 percent (Roth et al., 1993). Because of the distensibility of the esophagus, dysphagia indicates a significant degree of obstruction. As the obstruction worsens, patients may not even be able to swallow saliva. Significant weight loss frequently accompanies dysphagia. Patients may also complain of heartburn-like substernal or epigastric pain, possibly radiating into the back. Signs of local invasion include cough with swallowing (suggesting esophago-tracheal fistula), hoarseness (suggesting recurrent laryngeal nerve involvement), superior vena cava syndrome, and pleural effusion (Coia, 1994; Harter, 1992a; Medvec, 1988).

Diagnostic Work-Up and Staging

The diagnostic techniques used in the staging of cancer of the esophagus are listed in Table 11–2. Minimally invasive surgical techniques (e.g., thoracoscopy and laparoscopy) may be used increasingly in the future to improve the accuracy of staging (Jaklitsch et al., 1994). The AJCC TNM staging system is described in Table 11–5.

Five percent of patients with esophageal cancer also have a synchronous cancer of the head and neck, or lung at the time of diagnosis (Harter, 1992a). Thorough evaluation of these sites is important in the patient's work-up.

Table 11-5 • Cancer of the Esophagus: TNM Classification System

PRIMARY TUMOR (T)	
TX	Primary tumor cannot be assessed
T0	No evidence of primary tumor
Tis	Carcinoma in situ
T1	Tumor invades lamina propria or submucosa
T2	Tumor invades muscularis propria
T3	Tumor invades adventitia
T4	Tumor invades adjacent structures

REGIONAL LYMPH NODES (N)	
NX	Regional lymph nodes cannot be assessed
N0	No regional lymph node metastasis
N1	Regional lymph node metastasis

DISTANT METASTASIS (M)	
MX	Presence of distant metastasis cannot be assessed
M0	No distant metastasis
M1	Distant metastasis

STAGE GROUPING			
0	Tis	N0	M0
I	T1	N0	M0
IIA	T2	N0	M0
	T3	N0	M0
IIB	T1	N1	M0
	T2	N1	M0
III	T3	N1	M0
	T4	Any N	M0
IV	Any T	Any N	M1

Reprinted with permission from American Joint Committee on Cancer (1992). *Manual for Staging of Cancer* (4th ed.). Philadelphia: JB Lippincott.

Treatment with Curative Intent

Patients with cancer confined to the esophagus are treated with curative intent; however, there is no clear evidence as to the optimal treatment approach. Definitive surgical treatment includes: (1) subtotal or total esophagectomy to resect the tumor and (2) reconstruction to restore GI continuity, most commonly through mobilization of the stomach. The location of the tumor dictates the specific surgical technique employed. Because of the poor 5-year survival after resection and the significant postoperative morbidity, alternative treatment approaches have been explored.

Radiation therapy used as an alternative to surgery produces equivalent results in similarly staged patients. Preoperative or postoperative radiation has not demonstrated significant improvement in local control or survival when compared to surgery alone (Fisher & Brady, 1992).

Efforts to improve survival have led to the investigation of combined modality therapy, most commonly with a 5-FU based regimen. This has resulted in an improved 5-year survival, as high as

32 percent (Coia et al., 1991; Herskovic et al., 1992). Current studies are exploring the use of neoadjuvant chemotherapy, dose-intensive concurrent chemotherapy, and increased doses of radiation therapy. The most effective curative treatment for cancer of the esophagus has not yet been established. Combined modality therapy is probably equivalent to surgery, but the optimal combination, dose, and sequence of therapies to maximize local control and survival have not yet been determined.

Patients with lesions in the cervical esophagus pose a challenge in regard to treatment. These tumors are difficult to surgically resect because of their proximity to vital structures in the neck, often requiring laryngectomy. Treatment with radiation therapy is most often recommended for these patients, and their management is best understood when reviewing care of patients receiving radiation therapy to the head and neck.

Treatment for Palliation

In patients with locally advanced or metastatic cancer of the esophagus, an aggressive approach to palliation of symptoms can significantly improve their quality of life. Dysphagia from tumor obstruction is the most common problem, significantly limiting intake of food and fluids. Surgical methods to restore or maintain esophageal patency include: esophageal dilatation, insertion of a prosthetic endoesophageal tube or stent, endoscopic laser therapy, photodynamic therapy, and surgical resection or bypass (not a viable option for most patients). External beam radiation therapy or intraluminal brachytherapy, with or without chemotherapy, relieves dysphagia in 40 to 70 percent of patients and provides long-lasting effectiveness with minimal toxicity (Ahmad et al., 1994).

Radiation Therapy Techniques

The treatment field for esophageal cancer includes all gross and microscopic disease, with a margin of 5 cm above and below, as well as the locoregional lymph nodes at highest risk (Fisher & Brady, 1992). Patients may be placed in the prone position, to move the esophagus anteriorly, away from the spinal cord.

For definitive radiation therapy, a dose of 5000 cGy is generally given with chemotherapy. If administration of chemotherapy is not possible, higher radiation doses are needed, generally 6000 to 6500 cGy. Treatment is delivered using multiple fields. To minimize dose to the surrounding normal tissue, a boost of 1000 to 2000 cGy can be administered to the primary tumor with intraluminal brachytherapy, generally given in two to three fractions following external beam radiation. The radioactive source is placed through afterloading catheters positioned in a nasogastric tube or endoscope and administered via low or high dose-rate afterloading. (Fisher & Brady, 1992; Gaspar, 1994; Harter, 1992a; Minsky, 1994).

Cancer of the Stomach

Epidemiology

Before 1980, gastric cancer was the single most common cancer in the world; it was the leading cause of cancer death among men in the United States before 1945. The incidence, though, has decreased significantly worldwide (Parker et al., 1997). Despite its decreasing incidence, only 10 to 20 percent of gastric cancers are diagnosed at an early stage in the United States, and the disease continues to have poor survival rates.

Differences in the worldwide incidence of cancer of the stomach have led to the identification of dietary factors that increase the risk of developing this disease, in particular, high intake of nitrosamines used in salting, smoking, and pickling of meats, fish, and vegetables. It is believed that metabolites of nitrosamines are carcinogenic to the gastric lining. Improved refrigeration has resulted in a decrease in these dietary practices, and subsequently a decrease in gastric cancer incidence. In addition, improved refrigeration has led to an increased intake of raw fruits and vegetables (rich in vitamins A, C, and E) and dairy products, which may be protective against the development of gastric cancer. Other factors identified as increasing risk are chronic atrophic gastritis, helicobactor pylori infection, prior gastric surgery, smoking, low socioeconomic status, and family history (Alexander et al., 1993; Wang, 1988).

Pathophysiology

Approximately 95 percent of all cancers of the stomach are adenocarcinomas. Most arise in the antrum of the stomach. In recent years there has been an increased incidence of proximal tumors, located in or near the esophagogastric junction (Blot et al., 1991). These have a worse prognosis than distal tumors.

Gastric cancers arise in the mucosa of the stomach. They are classified based on their appearance as: (1) polypoid or fungating, (2) ulcerating with elevated borders, (3) ulcerating with infiltration, or (4) diffusely infiltrating (Alexander et al., 1993). Infiltrating lesions have a worse prognosis. As the tumor grows it can cause obstruction or hemorrhage. Gastric cancers spread locally by infiltration along the mucosal surface and by direct extension through the layers of the gastric wall, invading adjacent structures, including the esophagus, pancreas, liver, spleen, kidney, and colon. Gastric cancers spread regionally through the lymphatic system and metastasize by peritoneal seeding, throughout the abdominal and pelvic cavities, and/or by hematogenous dissemination, most commonly to the liver, lung, and bones.

Clinical Presentation

The primary symptom of cancer of the stomach is pain. Initial symptoms are vague and similar to those seen in benign gastric disorders, such as gastritis or ulcer disease. Complaints include epigastric distress, dyspepsia, abdominal fullness, bloating, distention after meals, and abdominal gas pains. With progression of disease, patients may complain of anorexia, nausea, and vomiting (secondary to obstruction of the gastric outlet), significant weight loss, and anemia (from chronic occult blood loss). Patients with lesions of the esophagogastric junction present with symptoms similar to those seen with cancer of the esophagus: dysphagia and substernal pain (Alexander et al., 1993; Frogge, 1993; Wang, 1988).

Diagnostic Work-Up and Staging

The diagnostic techniques used in the staging of cancer of the stomach are listed in Table 11–2. In some patients, surgical laparotomy is required to confirm the diagnosis and evaluate stage of disease. The AJCC TNM staging system is described in Table 11–6.

Treatment with Curative Intent

Surgery is the primary treatment for cancer of the stomach. Approximately 50 percent of patients are candidates for surgical resection at the time of diagnosis. The specific procedure depends on the location of the tumor within the stomach and the extent of disease. Controversy exists regarding the type of resection needed: subtotal versus total gastrectomy, limited versus extended lymphadenectomy, and the need for prophylactic splenectomy (Alexander et al., 1993). After resection, the remaining part of the stomach is anastomosed to the

Table 11-6 • Cancer of the Stomach: TNM Classification System

PRIMARY TUMOR (T)

TX	Primary tumor cannot be assessed
T0	No evidence of primary tumor
Tis	Carcinoma in situ: intraepithelial tumor without invasion of lamina propria
T1	Tumor invades lamina propria or submucosa
T2	Tumor invades muscularis propria or subserosa
T3	Tumor penetrates serosa (visceral peritoneum) without invasion of adjacent structures
T4	Tumor invades adjacent structures

REGIONAL LYMPH NODES (N)

NX	Regional lymph nodes cannot be assessed
N0	No regional lymph node metastasis
N1	Metastasis in perigastric lymph nodes within 3 cm of edge of primary tumor
N2	Metastasis in perigastric lymph nodes more than 3 cm from edge of primary tumor, or in lymph nodes along left gastric, common hepatic, splenic, or celiac arteries

DISTANT METASTASIS (M)

MX	Presence of distant metastasis cannot be assessed
M0	No distant metastasis
M1	Distant metastasis

STAGE GROUPING

0	Tis	N0	M0
IA	T1	N0	M0
IB	T1	N1	M0
	T2	N0	M0
II	T1	N2	M0
	T2	N1	M0
	T3	N0	M0
IIIA	T2	N2	M0
	T3	N1	M0
	T4	N0	M0
IIIB	T3	N2	M0
	T4	N1	M0
IV	T4	N2	M0
	Any T	Any N	M1

Reprinted with permission from American Joint Committee on Cancer (AJCC) (1992). *Manual for Staging of Cancer* (4th ed.). Philadelphia: JB Lippincott.

duodenum (Bilroth I) or jejunum (Bilroth II) to restore continuity of the GI tract.

Patients with T3 or N1 disease have a 38 to 67 percent risk of local recurrence after complete surgical resection (Minsky, 1996). Adjuvant treatment with chemotherapy alone has not significantly improved patient survival (Hermans et al., 1993). Adjuvant treatment with radiation therapy alone has also not demonstrated any clinical benefit. This has led to the development of new adjuvant trials using combined modality therapy with a 5-FU based regimen. Currently, the standard treatment following complete resection is observation alone.

For patients with unresectable tumors or with residual disease following surgery, combined modality therapy using a 5-FU based regimen may result in improved survival, but the data are conflicting and the optimal treatment approach has not yet been established.

Intraoperative radiation therapy has demonstrated improved survival in some studies, but more investigation of this approach is needed (DuBois, 1992). Because local failure continues to be a major problem for patients with gastric cancer, a variety of other approaches are also being investigated, including various combinations of chemotherapy, altered fractionation schedules, and treatment with particle therapy, including neutrons and helium ions (Smalley & Gunderson, 1992).

Treatment for Palliation

In patients with advanced gastric cancer, chemotherapy is commonly used with a variety of drugs, doses, and treatment schedules. The most commonly used agents include 5-FU, mitomycin-C, doxorubicin, cisplatin, methotrexate, etoposide, and methyl CCNU. Combination regimens are used more commonly than single agents. Chemotherapy administration has included both the systemic and intraperitoneal routes. Although some regimens have high response rates, none have significantly improved patient survival (Alexander et al., 1993).

The focus of care in most patients is palliation of symptoms. A variety of surgical procedures can be effective in relieving obstruction or bleeding. These include insertion of a stent if the lesion is at the esophagogastric junction, endoscopic laser therapy, or even a partial resection of the stomach (Alexander et al., 1993). Radiation therapy is effective in relieving symptoms of bleeding, obstruction, and pain in 50 to 75 percent of patients, particularly if used in combination with 5-FU (Smalley & Gunderson, 1992).

Radiation Therapy Techniques

The treatment field for gastric cancer includes all areas of gross and microscopic disease, as well as the local and regional lymph nodes. Because of the anatomical position of the stomach, the treatment field is quite large and includes significant amounts of normal tissue. Depending on the location of the tumor within the stomach (proximal or distal), the spleen, adrenal gland, kidney, duode-

num, pancreas, transverse colon, liver, spinal cord, heart, and remaining stomach may be included.

Doses of 4500 to 5000 cGy are used for adjuvant treatment, but doses as high as 6000 cGy to a limited field are needed for patients with unresectable or residual disease. Treatment can be delivered using a two-field or four-field technique, with a cone down after 4500 cGy. Patients are simulated and treated in the supine position. (Caudry, 1992; Minsky, 1996).

Cancer of the Pancreas

Epidemiology

Cancer of the pancreas is the fourth leading cause of cancer death among males and the fifth among females in the United States. It is one of the least curable of all malignancies; the overall 5-year survival is less than 5 percent, and most patients survive less than one year (Parker et al., 1997).

There are no clearly identified risk factors for pancreatic cancer. An association with cigarette smoking, diets high in fat and meat, previous partial gastrectomy, and occupational exposure to solvents and petroleum compounds has been observed (Warshaw & Castillo, 1992).

Pathophysiology

Cancers of the pancreas are most commonly of exocrine tissue. Ninety percent are adenocarcinomas arising from ductal cells. Anatomically, the disease occurs two times as frequently in the head of the pancreas as in the body or tail. The tumor grows rapidly, invading the pancreas and obstructing the pancreatic and common bile ducts. The tumor spreads locally into the duodenum, stomach, transverse colon, spleen, kidney, and diaphragm, and can invade the celiac nerve plexus and the surrounding major blood vessels. Pancreatic cancer spreads to local and regional lymph nodes and metastasizes by peritoneal seeding throughout the abdominal and pelvic cavities and by hematogenous dissemination, most commonly to the liver, lung, and bones (Brennan et al., 1993).

Pancreatic cancers of endocrine origin account for only 5 percent of all tumors and include islet cell tumors such as insulinomas. Treatment of these will not be addressed here.

Clinical Presentation

The initial symptoms of pancreatic cancer are nonspecific. Upper abdominal or epigastric pain is common. Initially the pain is dull and intermittent, often described as gnawing, possibly radiating to the back. With nerve invasion, the pain becomes continuous and more severe. In addition, significant weight loss is seen in most patients. The specific presentation of pancreatic cancer depends on the site of origin within the pancreas. Cancers in the head of the pancreas are more likely to cause obstruction of the common bile duct, leading to progressive jaundice. Cancers in the body and tail of the pancreas rarely present with jaundice and are more likely to present with pain (Brennan et al., 1993; Frogge, 1993).

Diagnostic Work-Up and Staging

The diagnostic techniques used in the staging of pancreatic cancer are listed in Table 11–2. Percutaneous transhepatic cholangiography (PCT) can detect common bile duct obstruction. Angiography can detect vascular invasion. The endoscopic retrograde cholangiopancreatography (ERCP) utilizes a fiberoptic endoscope passed into the duodenum. The ampulla of Vater is visualized and a catheter is passed into the opening. Biopsies can be obtained and a radiopaque contrast is infused to visualize the pancreatic and common bile ducts. A serum tumor marker specific for pancreatic cancer is POA (pancreatic oncofetal antigen). Although use of the AJCC TNM staging system is recommended (Table 11–7), patients are generally classified as "resectable" or "unresectable."

Treatment with Curative Intent

Curative treatment with surgical resection is an option for only 20 percent of patients and is recommended only for those who are in optimal physiologic health. The most common procedure is the pancreaticoduodenectomy (Whipple procedure), which involves resection of the head of the pancreas, as well as the duodenum, gastric antrum, bile duct, and gall bladder. More extensive resections may also be performed. The benefit of resecting the entire pancreas is the reduced likelihood of leaving behind microscopic residual disease. The disadvantage is that patients will have pancreatic dysfunction, developing malabsorption syndrome and brittle diabetes (Brennan et al., 1993).

For patients receiving radical surgery, the 5-year survival is quite low, less than 15 percent. Adjuvant therapy following surgical resection, with external beam radiation therapy in combination with 5-FU, improves the 2-year survival from 18 to 46 percent (Gastrointestinal Tumor Study

Table 11-7 • Cancer of the Pancreas: TNM Classification System

PRIMARY TUMOR (T)			
TX	Primary tumor cannot be assessed		
T0	No evidence of primary tumor		
T1	Tumor limited to the pancreas		
T1a	Tumor 2 cm or less in greatest diameter		
T1b	Tumor more than 2 cm in greatest diameter		
T2	Tumor extends directly to duodenum, bile duct, or perpancreatic tissues		
T3	Tumor extends directly to stomach, spleen, colon, or adjacent large vessels		

REGIONAL LYMPH NODES (N)			
NX	Regional lymph nodes cannot be assessed		
N0	Regional lymph nodes not involved		
N1	Regional lymph nodes involved		

DISTANT METASTASIS (M)			
MX	Presence of distant metastasis cannot be assessed		
M0	No distant metastasis		
M1	Distant metastasis		

STAGE GROUPING			
I	T1	N0	M0
	T2	N0	M0
II	T3	N0	M0
III	Any T	N1	M0
IV	Any T	Any N	M1

Reprinted with permission from American Joint Committee on Cancer (AJCC) (1992). *Manual for Staging of Cancer* (4th ed.). Philadelphia: JB Lippincott.

Group, 1985a). The use of combined modality therapy has also become a common approach for patients with unresectable disease, as it increases median survival from six months to up to one year (Gunderson & Willet, 1992). A neoadjuvant approach utilizing preoperative radiation therapy improves resectability in a significant number of patients with unresectable disease (Pilepich & Miller, 1980).

Treatment for Palliation

Patients with metastatic disease are often too debilitated to undergo aggressive treatment and may not be eligible for entry into a clinical trial. Chemotherapeutic agents, alone or in combination, including 5-FU, mitomycin-C, streptozocin, and doxorubicin, have demonstrated partial short-term response in some patients but have not demonstrated a significant long-term survival benefit. Because the median survival of patients with metastatic disease is only three months, the focus of care is on management of symptoms. Biliary tract obstruction can be relieved with surgical bypass, endoscopic stent placement, or radiologic placement of a percutaneous transhepatic biliary catheter. Duodenal obstruction may require a surgical bypass procedure. Radiation therapy can play an important role in palliation, providing pain relief in a significant percentage of patients (Brennan et al., 1993). Nerve blocks may also be effective in relieving the pain of patients with pancreatic cancer.

Radiation Therapy Techniques

The treatment field for pancreatic cancer includes all areas of gross and microscopic disease, as well as the local and regional lymph nodes. Because of the anatomic position of the pancreas, the treatment field is quite large and includes significant amounts of normal tissue. Depending on the location of the tumor within the pancreas (head, body, or tail), the stomach, small intestine, large bowel, spleen, liver, kidney, and spinal cord may be irradiated.

Doses of 5000 to 6000 cGy are used in the treatment of pancreatic cancer. Treatment is delivered using a two-field or four-field technique, with cone down after 5000 cGy. Patients are simulated and treated in a supine position(Gunderson & Willet, 1992).

Interstitial implantation with iodine-125 and intraoperative radiation therapy have been used, alone or with external beam radiation therapy, to deliver a boost to the target while minimizing dose to the surrounding normal structures. Neither of these has demonstrated a significant clinical benefit over the use of external beam radiation therapy alone (Brennan et al., 1993; Harter, 1992b). It is hoped that as the technology advances, intraoperative radiation therapy may play a greater role in the future treatment of pancreatic tumors (Merrick & Dobelbower, 1990).

Cancers of the Colon and Rectum

Epidemiology

Cancers of the colon and rectum represent the most common GI cancers and the third most common cause of death from cancer in the United States (Parker et al., 1997). Of all the GI cancers, colon and rectal cancers have the best survival rates. Patients with early disease (stages I and II) have a 5-year survival rate of 50 to 100 percent (NCI, 1995). Increased efforts at early detection should have a significant impact on improving survival from these cancers.

A number of factors contribute to the development of cancers of the colon and rectum (Cohen et al., 1993a, 1993b; Hampton, 1993). The higher incidence in Western developed nations, associated with diets high in fat and low in fiber, has supported theories of risk related to diet. High intake of animal fat causes increased release of bile acids into the intestine, which is thought to induce proliferation of mucosal cells. In addition, it has been suggested that carcinogens formed from the breakdown of particular food substances (particularly animal fats and cholesterol) coming into contact with intestinal mucosa may initiate malignant transformation. If stool transit time is prolonged, as with diets low in fiber, there is increased time of contact. Some dietary substances seem to play a protective role, decreasing risk. These include fiber, vegetables, vitamins C and E, calcium (which may modify mucosal proliferation), and selenium (which may deactivate carcinogens).

Genetic factors also play a role in increasing the risk of developing cancers of the colon and rectum. These factors are: (1) genetic syndromes associated with adenomatous polyps (e.g., familial adenomatous polyposis; and Gardner's, Oldfield's, Turcot's, and Peutz-Jeghers syndromes), (2) familial syndromes associated with increased risk of adenocarcinomas (e.g., hereditary nonpolyposis colorectal cancer), and (3) families with a history of colorectal cancer.

Other risk factors include inflammatory bowel disease and adenomatous intestinal polyps, especially villous adenomas larger than 2 cm.

Pathophysiology

As with most other GI malignancies, cancers of the colon and rectum arise in the mucosa. Almost 95 percent are adenocarcinomas. Most colorectal cancers occur in the distal portion of the large bowel, but in recent years there has been an increasing incidence of proximal tumors. In the proximal colon, tumors are more often exophytic and fungating, growing into the lumen. In the distal colon, tumors are more likely to be ulcerating and to grow into the wall circumferentially, leading to narrowing and constriction of the lumen. The tumor spreads to local and regional lymph nodes and metastasizes through the venous circulation, most commonly to the liver, lung, bones, and brain. Cancers of the colon may also metastasize through peritoneal seeding throughout the abdominal and pelvic cavities (Cohen et al., 1993a, 1993b; Hampton, 1993).

Clinical Presentation

The presenting signs and symptoms of colorectal cancer depend on the location of the tumor. Lesions in the proximal colon may become quite large before developing symptoms, most commonly anemia and abdominal cramping or pain. Many patients will have a palpable abdominal mass. Lesions in the distal colon most commonly present with bright red bleeding and constipation secondary to obstruction from the constricting lesion. Lesions in the rectum also present with bright red bleeding, alone or covering stool, and with a change in bowel habits (e.g., constipation or increased frequency of bowel movements). Stools may become mixed with mucus and decreased in caliber. Patients may also complain of urgency, a sense of incomplete evacuation, and rectal pressure or pain. Regardless of tumor location, patients may present initially with bowel obstruction or perforation. These presentations are generally associated with a poor prognosis (Cohen et al., 1993a, 1993b; Hampton, 1993).

Diagnostic Work-Up and Staging

The diagnostic techniques used in the staging of cancers of the colon and rectum are listed in Table 11–2. The AJCC TNM staging system is described in Table 11–8.

Treatment with Curative Intent

As with most other GI cancers, surgery is the treatment of choice for patients with cancers of the colon and rectum. Surgery encompasses resection of the tumor, with adequate proximal and distal margins, as well as resection of the vascular supply and the draining lymphatic system. Adequate lateral margins are also essential if the tumor is adherent to adjacent structures. For colon cancer, the procedure is most commonly a hemicolectomy with reanastomosis. For the relatively few patients with rectal cancer who present with small, well-differentiated, exophytic, mobile lesions, a variety of local procedures can effectively be used for cure, including local excision, electrocoagulation, fulguration, and endocavitary radiation. For most patients with rectal cancer, however, the surgeon must balance the need to assure adequate margins in the resection with the attempt to spare the anal sphincter and preserve continence. The specific surgical procedure depends on the location of the lesion. For tumors in the upper third of the rectum, a low anterior resection with reanastomosis is generally performed. For tumors in the middle and lower third of the rectum, an abdominal perineal resection with creation of a permanent colostomy was historically the recommended procedure. With the

Table 11-8 • Cancers of the Colon and Rectum: TNM Classification System

PRIMARY TUMOR (T)

TX	Primary tumor cannot be assessed
T0	No evidence of primary tumor
Tis	Carcinoma in situ
T1	Tumor invades submucosa
T2	Tumor invades muscularis propria
T3	Tumor invades through muscularis propria into subserosa, or into nonperitonealized pericolic or perirectal tissues
T4	Tumor directly invades other organs or structures, and/or perforates visceral peritoneum

REGIONAL LYMPH NODES (N)

NX	Regional lymph nodes cannot be assessed
N0	No regional lymph node metastasis
N1	Metastasis in 1 to 3 pericolic or perirectal lymph nodes
N2	Metastasis in 4 or more pericolic or perirectal lymph nodes
N3	Metastasis in any lymph node along course of a named vascular trunk, and/or metastasis to apical node(s) (when marked by the surgeon)

DISTANT METASTASIS (M)

MX	Presence of distant metastasis cannot be assessed
M0	No distant metastasis
M1	Distant metastasis

STAGE GROUPING

I	T1	N0	M0
	T2	N0	M0
II	T3	N0	M0
	T4	N0	M0
III	Any T	N1	M0
	Any T	N2	M0
	Any T	N3	M0
IV	Any T	Any N	M1

Reprinted with permission from American Joint Committee on Cancer (AJCC) (1992). *Manual for Staging of Cancer* (4th ed.). Philadelphia: JB Lippincott.

advent of new intraluminal stapling devices, many of these patients can now be treated with a low anterior resection with reanastomosis or a coloanal anastomosis (Cohen et al., 1993a, 1993b).

At the time of tumor resection, a temporary colostomy to divert the fecal stream may be created to relieve symptoms of obstruction or to facilitate healing of a distal anastomosis. Right-sided colostomies will drain liquid stool, and left-sided colostomies will drain more formed stool. If the patient is found to have up to three metastatic lesions within a single lobe of the liver, these may be resected. If postoperative radiation therapy is anticipated for rectal cancer, the surgeon may take measures to prevent the small intestine from descending into the pelvis. Techniques include filling of the pelvic dead space with omentum and forming a sling with absorbable mesh to hold the small intestine out of the pelvis (Hoover, 1993).

Cancers of the colon and rectum have different natural histories. The initial site of failure is based on tumor location in relation to the peritoneal reflection. Colon cancers, above the peritoneal reflection, tend to have a higher incidence of distant failure, whereas rectal cancers, below the peritoneal reflection, are more likely to have local recurrence. These differences in pattern of disease failure have led to the development of different treatment approaches.

The standard therapy for node positive colon cancer is adjuvant therapy with 5-FU based chemotherapy. Drugs most commonly used with 5-FU include leucovorin and levamisole. Because the development of distant disease is more common than local recurrence, and it is not currently possible to predict who is at high risk for local recurrence, the role of radiation therapy as adjuvant treatment in colon cancer is unclear. Whole-abdominal radiation therapy, from the dome of the diaphragm to the pelvic floor, is of limited use because of the need to keep the dose below 3000 cGy to avoid excessive toxicity. When 5-FU based chemotherapy is added to whole-abdominal radiation, local control is improved. A significant number of these patients, though, develop metastatic disease in the liver (Giri et al., 1993). Current studies are examining the use of adjuvant radiation therapy and chemotherapy in high risk patients with stage III disease.

The role of radiation therapy in the adjuvant treatment of rectal cancer is more clearly defined because local recurrence is more common than distant disease as the first site of failure. Pre- or postoperative adjuvant radiation therapy has demonstrated significant reduction in local recurrence (Twomey et al., 1989). The addition of a 5-FU based chemotherapy regimen further decreases local recurrence and also decreases systemic metastasis.

The standard approach has been to use radiation therapy postoperatively, after patients have been surgically staged with T3 disease or N1–2 disease. Postoperative combined modality therapy when compared to radiation alone decreases local recurrence by half and decreases systemic failure by about one third (GITSG, 1985b; Krook et al., 1991).

Preoperative radiation therapy has several potential advantages over postoperative treatment. These advantages include: (1) no postoperative tumor hypoxia, (2) decreased toxicity, and (3) downstaging of tumors with increased use of sphincter-sparing surgery (Mendenhall et al., 1993; Minsky, 1994). The randomized trials reported suggest improved local control but not improved survival. However, none used a standard dose of radiation (≥4500 cGy) or an optimal interval of time between completion of radiation therapy and surgery (4 to 6 weeks) (Martenson & Gunderson, 1993; Minsky, 1994). Randomized trials comparing preoperative and postoperative combined modality therapy are needed to determine the optimal approach. Additional questions to be answered include: (1) Is 5-FU better used alone or in combination with other chemotherapeutic agents? (2) What are the optimal chemotherapy doses? and (3) Is continuous infusion of 5-FU superior to bolus administration? These issues are being addressed in two current intergroup clinical trials.

Patients with locally advanced or unresectable rectal cancer, on initial presentation or at recurrence, have also benefited from preoperative radiation therapy. Patients presenting with recurrent disease tend to have a worse prognosis. Although 50 to 75 percent of unresectable lesions become resectable, long-term local control is achieved in only 36 to 45 percent of patients (Martenson, Jr. & Gunderson, 1992). The benefits of combined modality therapy over radiation alone include: (1) improved resectability, (2) sphincter preservation, (3) administration of systemic therapy early in treatment, and (4) the ability to tolerate higher doses of radiation therapy with less toxicity (Minsky, 1992). The current standard approach for patients with locally advanced or unresectable rectal cancer is preoperative radiation therapy, with or without chemotherapy.

Additional efforts to improve local control in patients with locally advanced and unresectable disease include the use of brachytherapy or intraoperative radiation therapy at the time of surgery to provide a boost to the primary site.

Treatment for Palliation

There is no standard therapy for patients with advanced colon or rectal cancer. A variety of 5-FU based chemotherapy regimens have been associated with a clinical response, but none have resulted in significant improvements in survival. Chemotherapeutic agents used with 5-FU include mitomycin-C, methotrexate, methyl-CCNU, and leucovorin. Irinotecan is a new drug showing promise for patients with metastatic disease. Patients with cancers of the colon and rectum who develop obstruction benefit from surgery to resect the tumor or divert the fecal stream by creation of a colostomy. For patients with rectal cancer, laser therapy can be effective in controlling rectal bleeding, and radiation therapy is very effective in reducing pain and controlling bleeding (Coia, 1994).

For patients with liver metastasis, whole-liver irradiation may be effective in relieving symptoms (Minsky & Leibel, 1989). Three-dimensional conformal radiation for the treatment of liver metastasis is under investigation.

Radiation Therapy Techniques

In treating rectal cancer, the primary tumor and local and regional lymph nodes are included in the treatment field. To enhance visualization of the rectum during simulation, contrast is instilled through a rectal catheter. Minimizing the dose to the small intestine is the major challenge in planning treatment. Techniques that can be used during simulation and treatment to displace the small intestine and minimize its dose include: (1) placing the patient in the prone position, (2) placing a pillow on the treatment table to compress the abdominal wall, (3) treating the patient with a full bladder, and (4) using computerized treatment planning (Minsky, 1993). The standard dose of radiation therapy for rectal cancer is 5000 to 5400 cGy, using a three- or four-field technique and cone down after 4500 to 5000 cGy. Patients with locally advanced or unresectable disease may require more than 6000 cGy to achieve an optimal response (Cohen et al., 1993b).

Cancer of the Anus

Epidemiology

Cancer of the anus is a very rare disease, representing only about 1 percent of all GI cancers diagnosed each year in the United States (Parker et al., 1997). Anal cancer has a significantly better survival than most other GI cancers. Even patients with stage III A disease have a 60 percent 5-year survival rate.

Cancer of the anus generally occurs more commonly in women than in men. In recent years, there has been an increased incidence in younger homosexual men, which has led to the belief that receptive anal intercourse increases risk of developing this disease in men. Other risk factors implicated include human papilloma virus or condylomata acuminata infections, HIV positive status, immunosuppression, prior radiation therapy, and cigarette smoking (Harter & Ahlgren, 1992; Shank et al., 1993).

Pathophysiology

Anal cancers arise from the mucosa (anal canal cancers) or from the skin (anal margin cancers). Squamous cell carcinomas account for about 65 percent and transitional cell carcinomas for about 25 percent of these cancers. Anal cancers grow locally by direct extension into the sphincter muscles and to the surrounding soft tissues. In addition, these cancers invade pelvic structures and spread to regional lymph nodes as high as the inferior mesenterics and as low as the inguinals. Distant metastasis is rare but occurs most commonly to the liver and lung (Shank et al., 1993).

Clinical Presentation

The initial symptoms of anal cancer are similar to those seen with benign anal problems such as hemorrhoids or fissures. Presenting symptoms include anal pressure or pain, bleeding, sensation of a mass, or pruritis. Lesions in the anal margin may present as small nodules with ulceration (Cantril & Schoeppel, 1988).

Diagnostic Work-Up and Staging

The diagnostic techniques used in the staging of anal cancers are listed in Table 11–2. The AJCC TNM staging system is described in Table 11–9.

Treatment with Curative Intent

Small superficial lesions of the lower anal canal or anal margin can be treated with local excision. For all other anal cancers, an abdominal perineal resection was historically the standard approach. Primary treatment with radiation therapy alone has been used as an alternative to surgery. Radiation therapy preserves anal function, but requires high doses of radiation with significant toxicity. Combined modality therapy uses lower doses of radiation with less toxicity and has demonstrated better results than surgery alone. The chemotherapeutic agents most commonly used are 5-FU and mitomycin-C. These are most commonly used concurrently with radiation therapy, but the optimal regimen has not yet been determined. Patients with anal cancer demonstrate excellent responses to combined modality therapy, with local control of 90 percent and 5-year survival of 80 percent. In addition, 43 to 80 percent have preservation of anal function (Harter & Ahlgren, 1992).

Table 11-9 • Cancer of the Anus:
TNM Classification System

PRIMARY TUMOR (T)

TX	Primary tumor cannot be assessed
T0	No evidence of primary tumor
Tis	Carcinoma in situ
T1	Tumor 2 cm or less in greatest dimension
T2	Tumor more than 2 cm but not more than 5 cm in greatest dimension
T3	Tumor more than 5 cm in greatest dimension
T4	Tumor of any size invades adjacent organs (e.g., vagina, urethra, bladder)

REGIONAL LYMPH NODES (N)

NX	Regional lymph nodes cannot be assessed
N0	No regional lymph node metastasis
N1	Metastasis in perirectal lymph nodes
N2	Metastasis in unilateral internal iliac and/or inguinal lymph node(s)
N3	Metastasis in perirectal and inguinal lymph nodes and/or bilateral internal iliac and/or inguinal lymph nodes

DISTANT METASTASIS (M)

MX	Presence of distant metastasis cannot be assessed
M0	No distant metastasis
M1	Distant metastasis

STAGE GROUPING

I	T1	N0	M0
II	T2	N0	M0
	T3	N0	M0
IIIA	T1	N1	M0
	T2	N1	M0
	T3	N1	M0
	T4	N0	M0
IIIB	T4	N1	M0
	Any T	N2	M0
	Any T	N3	M0
IV	Any T	Any N	M1

Reprinted with permission from American Joint Committee on Cancer (AJCC) (1992). *Manual for Staging of Cancer* (4th ed.). Philadelphia: JB Lippincott.

If the patient has persistent disease or recurrence after primary treatment, salvage therapy with abdominal perineal resection can be provided. An important consideration in evaluating response to treatment is the need to wait for up to 12 months after radiation is completed, as tumors may regress quite slowly (Shank et al., 1993).

Treatment for Palliation

A variety of chemotherapy regimens, alone or in combination, are used for patients with advanced disease. Agents commonly used include 5-FU, mitomycin-C, methotrexate, bleomycin, and cisplatin.

Radiation Therapy Techniques

In the treatment of anal cancer, the radiation treatment field encompasses the primary tumor as well as the local and regional lymph nodes. The patient is simulated and treated in the prone position. To enhance visualization of the rectum and anal canal during simulation, contrast is instilled through a rectal catheter. Minimizing the dose to the small intestine is the major challenge in planning treatment. Doses of 4500 to 5500 cGy are generally given, using a three- or four-field technique. If there is disease in the inguinal lymph nodes, they are boosted with electrons. There is controversy over the benefit of prophylactic irradiation for negative lymph nodes (Cummings, 1992).

Side Effects of Radiation Therapy

Side effects of radiation therapy for the treatment of GI cancers are based on the site of treatment and the tissues and organs included in the treatment field. Tissues with rapidly renewing cell populations are particularly sensitive and express the effects of radiation early. Throughout the GI tract, early effects generally include thinning of the exposed mucous membranes, with denuded areas and superficial ulcerations, and inflammation of the submucosa. Tissues with slower turnover rates, such as liver, kidney, and pancreas, are less sensitive and express the effects of radiation relatively late (Hall, 1994).

The minimal tolerance dose for a specific organ (TD 5/5) is that dose which produces a 5 percent probability of treatment complications in 5 years. There is no standardized method for determining normal tissue tolerance. In addition, if treated only partially, some organs can tolerate higher doses than if the entire volume is treated, as demonstrated in Table 11–10 (Emami et al., 1991).

Organ-Specific Effects of Radiation

The effects of radiation for the individual patient depend on the structures encompassed in the treatment field. The specific early and late effects on organs most commonly affected in the treatment of GI cancers are described in this section. The clinical signs and symptoms associated with the early effects of radiation are listed in Table 11–11.

Esophagus

The early effect of radiation therapy to the esophagus is esophagitis, with thinning of the mucosa

Table 11-10 • Normal Tissue Tolerance (5% Risk of Complications in 5 Years)

Organ	Tolerance Dose (cGy)		
	1/3 Volume	2/3 Volume	3/3 Volume
Esophagus	6000	5800	5500
Stomach	6000	5500	5000
Small Intestine	5000		4000
Colon	5500		4500
Rectum			6000
Liver	5000	3500	3000
Kidney	5000	3000	2300
Bladder		8000	6500
Femoral heads			5200

Adapted with permission from Emami B, Lyman J, Brown A (1991). Tolerance of normal tissue to therapeutic irradiation. *International Journal of Radiation Oncology, Biology, Physics, 21,* 109–122. Copyright 1991 by Elsevier Science Inc.

and inflammation of the submucosa. The most significant late effect of radiation is related to fibrosis of the submucosa and periesophageal connective tissue with subsequent narrowing of the lumen and stricture formation. Other late effects include atrophy of the mucosa with surface erosions, ulceration or perforation, decreased mucus secretion, and decreased esophageal motility from damage to the muscularis (Berthrong, 1986; Coia, Myerson, & Tepper, 1995; Cox et al., 1986).

Stomach

The early effect of radiation therapy to the stomach is gastritis, with thinning of the mucosa and development of superficial erosions. Ulceration and bleeding may also occur. The etiology of nausea and vomiting associated with gastric irradiation is complex and not fully understood. Theories suggest that nausea and vomiting result from stimulation of the vomiting center (VC) and the chemoreceptor trigger zone (CTZ) in the brain, which is mediated by neurotransmitters within the GI tract and in the central nervous system (e.g., dopamine, serotonin, histamines, and prostaglandins). With gastric irradiation, stimulation is most likely a result of local inflammation. Gastric irradiation also causes a reduction in secretion of hydrochloric acid and pepsinogen, resulting in a decrease in gastric acidity (Rubin et al., 1992). This is a late effect and may take years to resolve or may be permanent. Additional late effects include: (1) atrophy of the gastric mucosa, possibly leading to ulceration, hemorrhage, or perforation, and (2) fibrosis of the muscularis, which may result in contracture of the stomach or gastric outlet obstruction (Berthrong, 1986; Coia et al., 1995).

Pancreas

No early effects of pancreatic irradiation have been described. The symptoms patients experience during treatment are a result of the effects on the surrounding structures. Fibrosis of the exocrine glands, leading to decreased secretion of pancreatic enzymes, has been observed as a late effect. With the few long-term pancreatic cancer survivors, the clinical impact of this is unclear. The endocrine function of the pancreas is not affected by radiation. Posttreatment diabetes is not seen (Berthrong, 1986).

Liver

The radiation treatment fields for GI cancers generally include a relatively small percentage of the full volume of the liver. Therefore, it is very uncommon to see early effects. The primary late effect is a veno-occlusive lesion, which may lead to secondary degeneration of the liver with progressive fibrosis, cirrhosis, and liver failure (Rubin et al., 1992).

Small Intestine

Because of its anatomic structure and the rapid cell turnover of the mucosa, the small intestine is one of the most radiosensitive organs in the body. There are numerous mucosal folds throughout the small intestine, and the mucosa is covered by projections called villi which greatly increase its surface area and absorptive capacity. The crypts of Lieberkuhn at the base of each villus contain rapidly dividing undifferentiated cells. While undergoing maturation, these cells move toward the tip of the villus and function for only a few days before being sloughed off into the intestinal lumen. The entire epithelial population is replaced every 4 to 7 days (McCance & Huether, 1994). The early effect of radiation therapy to the small intestine is enteritis, involving cell depletion, with thinning of the mucosa and flattening of the villi. Hypermotility also occurs. These changes lead to (1) decreased absorption of nutrients and bile salts, (2) decreased or absent lactase with subsequent lactose intolerance, and (3) increased chyme transit time (Coia et al., 1995; Kaanders & Ang, 1994). The volume of small intestine included in the treatment field depends on the site of disease being treated, and the severity of radiation side effects will vary accordingly.

Late side effects result from injury throughout the small intestine wall. Submucosal fibrosis causes stricture formation and serosal fibrosis leads to formation of small bowel adhesions.

Table 11-11 • Acute Effects of Radiation Therapy: Signs and Symptoms

Acute Effect	Signs and Symptoms

Esophagus: Esophagitis	Dysphagia (difficulty swallowing, "lump in throat," "food sticking")
	Odynophagia (pain with swallowing)
	Substernal burning pain ("heartburn")
	    May be intermittent or continuous
	        May be associated with swallowing or with recumbent position

Stomach: Gastritis	Anorexia
	Dyspepsia ("heartburn")
	Epigastric burning pain ("heartburn")
	Nausea and vomiting
	    May begin 1–2 hours after first treatment and resolve after several hours or may
	        be continuous
	Hematemesis
	Melena

Small Intestine: Enteritis	Abdominal cramps and diarrhea (frequent watery stools)
Colon: Colitis	Abdominal cramps and diarrhea (frequent watery stools)
Rectum: Proctitis	Frequent stools Urgency, incontinence Tenesmus (persistent sensation of need to evacuate) Rectal pain (especially with passage of stools) Perianal pruritis Mucoid or bloody discharge
Bladder: Cystitis	Frequency Urgency, incontinence Dysuria Suprapubic pain Hematuria
Vagina: Vaginitis	Vaginal irritation, dryness, pruritis Mucoid discharge Dyspareunia (painful intercourse)
Ovary: Decreased hormone production	Hot flashes Vaginal dryness with dyspareunia
Bone marrow: Bone marrow suppression	Leukopenia Thrombocytopenia Anemia
Skin: Skin reaction	Erythema (erythema) Dry desquamation (pruritis, flaking, hyperpigmentation) Moist desquamation (vesicles, peeling of skin, oozing of serous fluid)

From Coia LR et al. (1991). Long-term results of infusional 5-FU, mitomycin-C, and radiation as primary management of esophageal cancer. *International Journal of Radiation Oncology, Biology, Physics, 20,* 29–36; Cox JD et al. (1986). Complications of radiation therapy and factors in their prevention. *World Journal of Surgery, 10,* 171–188; Kaanders JHAJ and Ang KK (1994). Early reactions as dose-limiting factors in radiotherapy. *Seminars in Radiation Oncology 4,* 55–67; Rostock RA et al. (1992). Radiation therapy in the treatment of colorectal cancer. In J Ahlgren and J Macdonald (Eds.), *Gastrointestinal Oncology* (pp. 359–381). Philadelphia: JB Lippincott.

Either of these can lead to small bowel obstruction (Rostock et al., 1992). Ischemic changes of the mucosa result in atrophy, with permanent alterations in absorption, and ulceration, with possible progression to perforation or fistula. There may also be changes in intestinal motility (Berthrong, 1986; Coia et al., 1995). Factors that increase the likelihood of radiation effects of the small intestine include: (1) prior abdominal surgery; (2) history of pelvic inflammatory disease or colitis; (3) history of cardiovascular disease, hypertension, or diabetes; and (4) thin body build (Scully et al., 1994).

Colon

The early effect of radiation to the colon is colitis, which involves mucosal thinning, superficial erosions or ulcerations, and submucosal inflammation. This may lead to decreased absorption of water. The late effects include fibrosis, but this rarely leads to obstruction.

Rectum

The early effect of radiation to the rectum is proctitis. This involves mucosal thinning, with superficial erosions or ulcerations, and submucosal inflammation, with increased mucus secretion.

Fibrosis develops as a late effect, which may result in decreased rectal compliance and volume. Vascular changes cause mucosal telangiectasias, which bleed easily, and ischemia with subsequent atrophy and ulceration (Coia et al., 1995; Rostock et al., 1992).

Bladder

The early effect of radiation therapy to the bladder is cystitis, with thinning and inflammation of the epithelial lining of the bladder. Because the cell turnover is relatively slow, the effects may not manifest until the end of treatment. There are also changes in the cell junctions and loss of the protective polysaccharide layer, which make the underlying tissues more vulnerable to hypertonic urine, urinary metabolites, and bacteria. In addition, edematous changes in the smooth muscle of the bladder wall result in decreased bladder compliance (Marks et al., 1995). Late effects include mucosal atrophy with ulceration and bleeding and fibrosis of the bladder wall with subsequent loss of compliance (Berthrong, 1986). These effects are rare at the doses used for GI cancers.

Sexual Organs

The effects of radiation on the sexual organs are manifested with changes in: (1) gonadal function (i.e., ovarian and testicular hormone production), (2) reproductive ability (i.e., fertility), and (3) sexual function (i.e., desire, arousal, orgasm). The radiation literature generally describes effects on the sexual organs after high dose treatment for a primary malignancy rather than at doses they receive when treated for GI cancers.

In females, early effects include: (1) vaginitis, with thinning and inflammation of the mucosa; (2) superficial ulceration of the cervix; and (3) decreased ovarian hormone production, with onset of menopausal symptoms. Late effects of the vagina include: (1) atrophy of the mucosa, with thinning, ulceration, and decreased lubrication, and (2) fibrosis of the vaginal wall, with narrowing, shortening, and loss of elasticity. The cervix and uterus may also become atrophied, and stenosis of the cervical os may develop. Within the ovary there may be permanent cessation of hormone production resulting in menopause. Estrogen deficiency also contributes to atrophy of the vaginal mucosa. Oocytes do not repopulate and are generally not sensitive to the effects of radiation. However, older women may become sterile earlier or at lower doses than younger women because they have fewer oocytes (Grigsby et al., 1995; Rubin et al., 1992).

In males, there are no early effects of radiation to the sexual organs in the treatment of GI cancers described in the literature. However, some men report burning with ejaculation, perhaps a result of urethritis from radiation. In addition, radiation will cause swelling of the prostate gland, resulting in increased frequency of urination. Testicular irradiation results from scatter, and generally involves a low dose of radiation. However, the germ cells are very radiosensitive, and patients may develop azoospermia early after exposure. Recovery to normal sperm counts may take many months and depends on the dose of exposure (Rubin et al., 1992).

Skin

Skin reactions from radiation include erythema, dry desquamation, and moist desquamation, as described in Chapter 8 in the text. Patients treated with radiation for GI cancers generally have only a mild skin reaction, except for those with the supraclavicular lymph nodes (i.e., some esophageal lesions), inguinal lymph nodes (i.e., anal lesions), or perineum in the treatment field.

Bone Marrow

With pelvic radiation, the pelvis, lower vertebrae, and proximal femur are included in the treatment field. Early effects of radiation on the bone marrow result in progressive depopulation of white blood cell, thrombocyte, and erythrocyte precursors, with subsequent decrease in the number of circulating peripheral blood cells (Fajardo, 1993; Kaanders & Ang, 1994). The timing and sequence of these effects are based on the life span of the mature peripheral cells: 1 to 2 days for granulocytes, 10 to 12 days for thrombocytes, and 120 days for erythrocytes. If large volumes of bone marrow are irradiated, chronic hypoplasia of the marrow can persist as a late effect. These changes rarely have clinical significance when less than 25 percent of the total body bone marrow is irradiated unless patients are also given chemotherapy that causes bone marrow suppression (Mauch et al., 1995; Rubin et al., 1992).

Nursing Care of Patients

Patient Assessment

The radiation oncology nurse's initial contact with the patient may be at the time of consultation, simulation, or first on-treatment visit. A baseline assessment addressing physiologic, psychologic, social, cultural, spiritual, and educational issues should be conducted at this time to identify actual or potential patient problems. The assessment described here is not intended to be comprehensive, but rather focuses on issues specific to patients with GI cancers about to undergo treatment with radiation therapy.

Although the patient's medical history can be obtained from a review of the chart, it is important to have patients tell their story in their own words to learn about their understanding of the disease and treatment and how they are coping. In eliciting the history, it is important to consider factors that place the patient at an increased risk of side effects if undergoing radiation therapy. Table 11–12 outlines the structure of the medical history of an initial patient assessment for patients with GI cancer.

Assessment before treatment should also focus on the patient's current symptoms, how they are managing these, and the effectiveness of these strategies. Table 11–13 outlines the structure of the symptom assessment, which should be obtained as part of an initial patient assessment for patients with GI cancer.

Patients receiving radiation therapy are seen at least weekly to evaluate their response to treatment. Nursing participation in these on-treatment or status check visits is essential to assure early detection of side effects and prompt initiation of interventions. Nursing interventions aim to assure optimal patient comfort and reduce the likelihood of requiring a break in treatment that may minimize treatment effectiveness. Specific symptoms to assess are discussed next and listed in Table 11–14.

Patient Education

One of the primary responsibilities of the radiation oncology nurse is the education of patients and families regarding treatment, possible side effects, and the management of symptoms.

It is important to consider the patient's and family's readiness to learn and to focus first on their specific areas of concern. It is difficult for patients to hear what is being explained to them if they are preoccupied by other thoughts and feelings. Addressing these first will clarify misconceptions, allay fears and anxieties, and communicate concern for them as individuals. Education should be a dialogue, not just a citing of information. Written patient education material can reinforce teaching, because patients may not remember much of what is verbally explained at the time of consultation.

Table 11-12 • Initial Patient Assessment: Medical History

HISTORY OF PRESENT ILLNESS
Presenting symptoms
Diagnostic work-up: tests completed, stage of disease
Prior treatments used in this disease or prior cancers

PAST MEDICAL HISTORY
Cardiac, pulmonary, hepatic, or renal disease
Gastric reflux, significant if the patient will be undergoing esophageal irradiation
Inflammatory bowel disease or pelvic inflammatory disease, significant if the patient will be undergoing pelvic irradiation

PAST SURGICAL HISTORY
Many patients will present for radiation after surgical treatment for their cancer. Specific GI surgeries may result in particular problems as described below (Hoebler & Irwin, 1992).
Esophagectomy with gastric pull-up: reduced stomach volume with early satiety and esophageal reflux with secondary esophagitis
Esophageal bypass with jejunal or colon interposition: dysphagia from stricture or nerve damage
Partial gastrectomy: anemia from vitamin B12 deficiency and dumping syndrome from rapid movement of food into small intestine
Whipple procedure: malabsorption from pancreatic enzyme deficiency (e.g., fat intolerance) and hyperglycemia from surgically-induced diabetes
Low anterior resection or coloanal anastomosis: loss of rectal reservoir, frequent urgent stools, inability to differentiate sensation of passing stool from gas, and fecal incontinence
Colostomy: if right-sided, decreased water absorption and liquid stools
Any abdominal or pelvic surgery: formation of adhesions and possible small bowel obstruction

MEDICATIONS
Over-the-counter and prescription medications
Allergies

Table 11-13 • Initial Patient Assessment: Symptom Assessment

NUTRITION

The nutritional assessment should screen for actual or potential problems requiring a more in-depth assessment by a dietitian.

Weight
  Usual and current weight
  Percent weight loss: (current weight ÷ usual weight) × 100 = % weight loss
    5% weight loss over 1 month or 10% weight loss over 3 months is considered significant

Food and fluid intake pattern
  Types of food generally eaten and amount: usual and current
  Usual intake of alcohol and caffeine
  Changes in appetite, anorexia

Serum albumin

Medical dietary problems (e.g., lactose intolerance, diabetic, pancreatic enzyme deficiency)

Personal, cultural, or religious dietary preferences (e.g., use of megadose vitamins; macrobiotic diet; ethnic diets high in spices, beans, or cheese; vegetarian diets, kosher diet)

Use of supplements
  Type, amount, frequency

Symptoms associated with eating (e.g., dysphagia, odynophagia, reflux, nausea or vomiting, cramping)

Symptoms that can affect appetite (e.g., pain, fatigue, nausea or vomiting, diarrhea, constipation, altered taste)

Social supports
  Presence of someone at home to help with buying and preparing food and to share meals with patient
  Ability to afford and obtain supplements

ELIMINATION

Usual bowel pattern
  Frequency, consistency, urgency, incontinence
  Changes since surgery
  Presence of an ostomy, usual pattern and consistency of stools, use of irrigation, patient's ability to manage pouch changes, frequency of pouch change
  Current use of laxatives, stool softeners, or antidiarrheal medications

Usual bladder pattern
  Frequency, dysuria, incontinence
  Changes since surgery
  History of frequent urinary tract infections

SEXUALITY

Sexual function (i.e., desire for sex, ability to become aroused, ability to experience orgasm)

Sexual activity (e.g., sexual partner, sexual preferences, frequency of sexual activities)

Use of birth control

Body image, self concept, and self esteem

Importance of future parenting

Changes since diagnosis and treatment (e.g., impact of rectal surgery or stoma, pain, fatigue, depression)

For females: menopausal status and associated symptoms

SKIN

Inspect the skin in the planned treatment field observing for the following:
  Unhealed incision line
  Stoma: evaluate fit of appliance and condition of peristomal skin
  External stents
  Area of skin breakdown

BONE MARROW

History of leukopenia, thrombocytopenia, anemia

Prior chemotherapy and bone marrow response

PAIN

Presence, location, quality, and severity of pain

Timing (e.g., continuous or intermittent)

Exacerbating and alleviating factors
Current analgesic regimen and its effectiveness

Table continued on following page

Table 11-13 • Initial Patient Assessment: Symptom Assessment (*Continued*)

FATIGUE
Severity (0–10 scale)
Timing during the day (e.g., often becomes worse as the day progresses)
Factors that may worsen fatigue (e.g., sleep disorder, pain, nutritional deficit, anemia, depression)
Effect on daily activity

PSYCHOSOCIAL
Ability to communicate thoughts and feelings
Coping with disease and previous treatment
Previous participation in decision-making and problem-solving related to illness
Symptoms of anxiety or depression
Family response to disease and previous treatment
Responsibilities at home for children or elderly dependents
Ability to manage care at home
Ability to arrange transportation for daily treatment
Support at home to help with household responsibilities and care of dependents

Provide specific instructions about measures to take to manage the symptoms. List specific foods to avoid and suggest foods to eat in their place; providing sample menus may be helpful. Review the precise dose and timing of medications on an ongoing basis; a written medication schedule may be helpful.

Assessment and Management of Specific Side Effects of Radiation

There are a number of measures patients should initiate at the onset of treatment to prevent or minimize the severity of potential side effects. These are described next. When assessing patients on treatment, it is essential to consider the specific structures in the treatment field. Knowledge of the potential acute effects of treatment and their associated signs and symptoms, as described in Table 11–11, should guide the assessment.

Esophagitis and Gastritis
PREVENTIVE MEASURES

To minimize discomfort from mucosal changes of the esophagus and stomach, instruct patients on dietary changes to make at the start of treatment to prevent irritation of the mucosa. Patients should avoid dry coarse foods (e.g., crackers, chips, pretzels, toast, raw vegetables), extremely hot foods and fluids, acidic and citrus foods and juices (e.g., tomatoes, oranges, grapefruit), strongly seasoned and spiced foods, and alcohol. If patients are taking medications that may exacerbate mucosal irritation (e.g., aspirin products, nonsteroidal anti-inflammatory medications, steroids), evaluate the reason for their use, and explore if alternate medications can be prescribed.

ASSESSMENT

Assess patients for the presence of discomfort or pain. A sudden marked increase in the severity of pain may indicate a secondary candida infection. If the esophagus is in the treatment field, difficulty swallowing without pain should be questioned. If the stomach is in the treatment field, assess for nausea or vomiting. If the patient reports blood in vomitus or black stools, further evaluation for upper GI bleeding should be initiated. Other specific items to include in the assessment are listed in Table 11–14. Assessment of patients with a significantly decreased oral intake and persistent nausea and vomiting should include evaluation for nutritional deficits, dehydration, and electrolyte imbalance.

TREATMENT

Topical anesthetics and systemic analgesics are commonly needed to treat pain from esophagitis. Xylocaine 2% jelly or viscous solution is commonly used alone or in combination with an antacid (e.g., Maalox) and an antihistamine (e.g., Benadryl), mixed in equal proportions. This is best used immediately before meals to decrease pain with swallowing. It is important to keep in mind that topical anesthetics will suppress the gag reflex, so they should be used selectively and patients should be instructed to eat slowly and sit upright for 30 minutes after meals to avoid pulmonary aspiration. Systemic narcotic analgesics in liquid form may be necessary to adequately control the pain of esophagitis and gastritis. If the patient develops a secondary candida infection, treatment with ketoconazole (Nizoral) or fluconazole (Diflucan) is indicated. Other medications that have been investigated for their effectiveness

Table 11-14 • Weekly On-Treatment Patient Assessment

NUTRITION
Ability to swallow different foods: solids, soft foods, liquids
 	
Pain with swallowing
 	
Nausea and/or vomiting
   Severity (ability to keep food and fluids down)
   Pattern during the day
   Frequency, duration
   Blood in vomitus
 	
Associated symptoms: queasiness, heartburn, indigestion, belching
 	
Impact of changes in oral intake and bowel elimination on *nutrition*
   Weight
 	
Impact of changes in oral intake and bowel elimination on *hydration and electrolyte status*
   Weakness, light-headedness, dizziness
   Orthostatic blood pressure and pulse changes
   BUN, Creatinine, electrolytes
 	
BOWEL ELIMINATION
Number of bowel movements per day
 	
Volume
 	
Consistency
 	
Timing during the day
 	
Incontinence
 	
Associated symptoms: abdominal cramps, urgency, tenesmus, mucus discharge, rectal bleeding, rectal pain, perianal pruritis
 	
Impact of diarrhea, mucus discharge, or incontinence on perianal skin
 	
URINARY ELIMINATION
Frequency
 	
Urgency
 	
Dysuria
 	
Incontinence
 	
Associated symptoms: suprapubic pain, hematuria, mucus shreds
	SEXUALITY
	Women: vaginal irritation, dryness, pruritis, discharge; dyspareunia
	
	Premenopausal women: changes in menses, hot flashes
	
	Impact of treatment side effects on sexual function and activity (e.g., fatigue, rectal pressure, vaginal discomfort)
	
	SKIN
	Inspect skin of treatment field
	   Erythema: redness, edema
	   Dry desquamation: pruritis; dry, flaky
	   Moist desquamation: red, moist, weeping
	
	High risk areas: supraclavicular and inguinal lymph nodes, perineum, peristomal area
	
	BONE MARROW SUPPRESSION
	Regular CBC (weekly if concurrent chemotherapy)
	
	PAIN
	Location
	
	Quality
	
	Severity
	
	Timing
	
	FATIGUE
	Change in energy level, tiredness, weakness
	
	Severity (0–10 scale)
	
	Timing during the day (e.g., often becomes worse as the day progresses)
	
	Need for rest periods during the day
	
	Ability to obtain a restful sleep at night
	
	Impact on daily activities
	
	Ability to manage care at home
	
	PSYCHOSOCIAL
	Coping with treatment
	
	Symptoms of anxiety or depression
	
	Family response to treatment

in treating esophagitis include sucralfate suspension, which may coat denuded mucosal regions, and antiprostaglandins, which may reduce inflammation (Coia et al., 1995).

Instruct patients to modify their diet further as symptoms of esophagitis develop. They should take small bites of food and chew thoroughly. Mixing food with sauces and gravies may initially make swallowing easier, but patients may have to liquify their food or switch to liquid nutritional supplements to ensure adequate intake. A variety of nutritional supplements are available that usually provide 30 calories per ounce (1 calorie per ml). Most products are also available in a high-calorie formula providing about 45 calories per ounce (1.5 calories per ml). Supplements that are easily available to patients include Carnation Instant Breakfast, Ensure, Sustacal, Boost, Nutren, Resource, Meritene, and Enrich. If taking supplements, patients should be encouraged to achieve a total intake of about 2000 calories. For patients with significant nutritional deficits, referral to a dietitian can be helpful in determining the precise calorie and protein needs and individualizing the nutritional interventions. For patients with financial difficulties, referral to a social worker can be helpful in identifying reimbursement alternatives.

For patients with symptoms related to gastroesophageal reflux, reducing meal size, sitting upright for 1 hour after meals, and elevating the upper body with pillows at bedtime may be helpful. Antacids may also be effective in reducing symptoms because of their ability to neutralize gastric hydrochloric acid. Antacids generally contain magnesium (e.g., Milk of Magnesia), which may induce diarrhea; aluminum (e.g., Amphojel or Basaljel), which may induce constipation; or a mixture of these two minerals. Combination products, as listed in Table 11–15, are recommended to minimize alterations in bowel elimination.

Because antacids affect patients differently, they should be supplemented with products containing only aluminum or magnesium as needed to control changes in bowel elimination. Liquid preparations are more effective than chewable tablets in reducing symptoms.

Other medications that may be helpful for gastroesophageal reflux and gastritis include: (1) metoclopramide, which increases pressure of the esophageal sphincter and promotes gastric emptying, (2) sucralfate, which coats denuded areas of mucosa, and (3) H2 receptor antagonists, which inhibit gastric acid secretion. Commonly used drugs and doses are listed in Table 11–15.

For nausea and vomiting, a variety of medications are available. The phenothiazines are dopamine antagonists and inhibit the chemoreceptor trigger zone (CTZ). Metoclopramide acts similarly in the brain and also acts within the GI tract, increasing gastric emptying. The 5-HT3 antagonists block serotonin receptors centrally in the brain and peripherally in the GI tract, which decreases transmission of signals to the CTZ and the vomiting center (VC). Antiemetics most com-

Table 11-15 • Commonly Used Medications for the Treatment of Esophageal Reflux and Gastritis

Medication	Administration
ANTACIDS: MAGNESIUM AND ALUMINUM	
Maalox	Dosages vary
Mylanta	1 and 3 hours after meals, at
Gaviscon	bedtime and as needed
METOCLOPRAMIDE	
Reglan	10 mg QID
Tablet (5 and 10 mg)	30 minutes before meals and
Solution (5 mg/5 ml)	at bedtime
SUCRALFATE	
Carafate	1 gm QID
Tablet (1 gm)	1 hour before meals and at bedtime
	Antacids should not be taken 30 minutes before or after sucralfate
H2 RECEPTOR ANTAGONISTS	
Cimetidine (Tagamet)	300 mg QID
Tablet (300 mg)	
Solution (300 mg/5 ml)	
Ranitidine (Zantac)	150 mg BID
Tablet (150 and 300 mg)	
Solution (75 mg/5 ml)	
Famotidine (Pepcid)	20–40 mg BID
Tablet (20 and 40 mg)	
Suspension (40 mg/5 ml)	

From McEvoy GK (1995). *Drug Information*. Bethesda, MD: American Society of Health-System Pharmacists.

Table 11-16 • Commonly Used Medications for the Treatment of Nausea and Vomiting

Medication	Administration
PHENOTHIAZINES	
Prochlorperazine (Compazine)	
Tablet (5 and 10 mg)	5–10 mg q 4–6 hours
Solution (5 mg/5 ml)	5–10 mg q 4–6 hours
Capsule (10, 15, and 30 mg)	15–30 mg in the AM, or 10 mg q 12 hours
Suppository (25 mg)	1 suppository q 12 hours
Thiethylperazine (Torecan, Norzine)	
Tablet (10 mg)	10 mg QD to TID
Suppository (10 mg)	10 mg QD to TID
METOCLOPRAMIDE	
Reglan	10 mg QID
Tablet (5 and 10 mg)	30 minutes before meals and
Solution (5 mg/5 ml)	at bedtime
5-HT3 SEROTONIN ANTAGONISTS	
Ondansetron HCl (Zofran)	
Tablet (4 and 8 mg)	8 mg TID
Granisetron (Kytril)	
Tablet (1 mg)	1 mg q 12 hours

From Cleri LG (1995). Serotonin antagonists: State of the art management of chemotherapy-induced emesis. *Oncology Nursing: Patient Treatment and Support, 2,* 1–19; and McEvoy GK (1995). *Drug Information.* Bethesda, MD: American Society of Health-System Pharmacists.

monly used for the treatment of nausea and vomiting related to abdominal irradiation are listed in Table 11–16. For patients with symptoms 1 to 2 hours after treatment, taking the antiemetic 1 hour before treatment is recommended. There are inconsistent recommendations regarding the benefit of eating a light meal just before receiving treatment or being treated on an empty stomach. Encourage patients to take the antiemetic as needed to assure comfort and adequate nutritional intake; taking the medication one hour before meals may be helpful, as well as resting after meals. Encourage a trial and error approach with food. Foods that are dry, cool, not too sweet, spicy, or fatty, and those with minimal odor, may be better tolerated. If vomiting is a problem, instruct the patients to increase their fluid intake to maintain adequate hydration. For patients with dehydration or electrolyte imbalance, intravenous hydration and electrolyte replacement may be needed during daily treatment visits.

Enteritis and Colitis

PREVENTIVE MEASURES

To minimize diarrhea and abdominal cramping, patients should initiate dietary changes at the start of treatment that include: (1) low fiber, to decrease irritation of the mucosa and GI motility, (2) low fat, to prolong transit time, and (3) low lactose, to handle lactase deficiency. Table 11–17 lists specific dietary recommendations. Some patients may develop constipation early in treatment with these dietary changes, so modifications may be required. Most patients should be instructed to continue this diet throughout treatment and until

Table 11-17 • Diet Recommendations to Prevent Diarrhea

FOODS LOW IN FIBER	
Protein foods	Tender meats baked or broiled, eaten with fat trimmed
	Poultry with skin removed
	Fish
	Eggs
Vegetables	Cooked squash, eggplant, carrots
	Potatoes without the skin
	Tomato paste and puree
	Vegetable juices
Fruits and juices	Bananas
	Cooked apples, peaches, apricots, plums
	Canned pineapple
	Strained cranberry sauce
	Fruit juices and nectars without pulp (e.g., apple, grape, cranberry)
Bread, cereal, and grains	White bread, rolls, bagels, English muffins
	Saltines, Graham crackers
	Cornflakes, Corn Chex
	Puffed rice, Cream of Rice, Rice Krispies
	White rice
	Spaghetti, noodles
FOODS LOW IN LACTOSE	
Milk	Milk treated with lactase enzyme (e.g., Lactaid, Dairy Ease)
Cheeses	Hard, aged, or processed cheeses
Miscellaneous	Yogurt
	Sherbet
	Low-lactose ice cream
	Lactose-free supplements
FOODS LOW IN FAT	
Fats	Use fats, oils, margarine, salad dressings sparingly
	Unsaturated oils only
Meat	Lean meats
	Fish (water-packed if canned)
	Poultry without the skin
RESTRICTIONS	
Avoid caffeine, alcohol, and spicy food	

From Nelson JK, Moxness KE, Jensen MD, and Gastineaus CF (1994). *Mayo Clinic Diet Manual: A Handbook of Nutrition Practices* (7th ed.). St. Louis: Mosby.

bowel patterns return to normal, generally 2 to 4 weeks after treatment is completed. These dietary modifications may be very difficult for some patients to accept. With increased general awareness of the value of high-fiber foods and with cultural or ethnic dietary norms (e.g., Indian and Asian diets high in vegetables, Spanish diets high in beans and spices), patients need thorough explanations of the reasons for the changes. A referral to a dietitian to assist in making appropriate food choices and planning meals can be beneficial.

Patients who have a left-sided colostomy and irrigate daily should maintain their usual irrigation routine until they begin to have spontaneous bowel movements in between irrigations or stools become liquid. At that time they should discontinue irrigation until bowels return to usual consistency after treatment is completed.

If the patient is being treated for pancreatic cancer following surgical resection, it is important to initiate pancreatic enzyme replacement if needed before beginning treatment, because enzyme deficiencies may cause diarrhea from malabsorption of fat.

ASSESSMENT

Specific items to include in ongoing assessment during treatment are listed in Table 11–14. This includes asking the patient about abdominal cramping and diarrhea. Patients receiving concurrent 5-FU may develop particularly severe diarrhea. If they also develop leukopenia from chemotherapy, they are at risk for infection since the damaged intestinal mucosa may provide a site of entry for microorganisms leading to systemic infection. As bowel movements become more frequent and fluid, evaluate the patient for weight loss, dehydration, and electrolyte imbalance. In addition, assess perianal skin for irritation or intensified radiation skin reaction.

TREATMENT

When the patient develops more than 3 watery bowel movements a day, medication should be initiated. Mild antidiarrheal medications such as Kaopectate and Pepto Bismol are generally not effective for radiation enteritis. Initial treatment is usually with anticholinergic medications, and if these are not effective at full dose, opium derivatives can be used. Bulk laxatives have also been recommended because of their ability to absorb fluid and increase stool bulk, but they should be taken with less liquid than when used for constipation. Table 11–18 lists commonly used antidiarrheal medications and their doses. These should be titrated to effect, which may require daily contact with the patient to ensure that they are taking the medication correctly and that diet modifications are appropriate. If the patient continues to have severe diarrhea, diet should be restricted further, eliminating all fruits and vegetables except for bananas and applesauce. If the diarrhea does not resolve with these dietary restrictions and the full dose of medication, a treatment break may be required.

A number of other medications have been investigated for their effectiveness in treating diarrhea from radiation enteritis. These include: (1) cholestyramine, to bind bile salts that may not be adequately absorbed if the terminal ileum is in the treatment field, (2) somatostatin analogues, which inhibit secretion of various gut peptides and reduce GI motility, (3) sucralfate, which forms a protective barrier over denuded intestinal mucosa, and (4) various salicylates, which reduce inflammation (Coia et al., 1995, Rostock et al., 1992).

Additional considerations in caring for patients with diarrhea include the need to ensure that patients are taking adequate amounts of fluids and nutrients to prevent dehydration, electrolyte imbalance, and weight loss. The nurse should encourage clear juices, broth, noncaffeinated tea, juices high in electrolytes (e.g., Gatorade), and lactose-free liquid supplements. Intravenous hydration and electrolyte replacement may be needed during daily treatment visits. In addition, the nurse should instruct patients on skin care to the perianal region to minimize the severity of radiation skin reaction.

Proctitis

PREVENTIVE MEASURES

Patients with rectal cancer often present with complaints of constipation and may use stool softeners and laxatives regularly before beginning treatment. Patients are generally advised not to use these medications once treatment begins. Some patients, however, may be reluctant to give them up in fear of developing constipation, but all stool softeners and laxatives should be stopped with the first development of loose or watery bowel movements.

ASSESSMENT

Specific items to include in ongoing assessment during treatment are listed in Table 11–14. This includes assessing patients for changes in bowel pattern, accompanying mucoid or bloody discharge, and rectal pain.

TREATMENT

For symptoms related to proctitis, warm water sitz baths several times a day, for 15 to 20 minutes at a time, may be helpful. Insertion of medication into the rectum during treatment is not recommended, because the integrity of the rectal mucosa can be compromised. Narcotic analgesics are often necessary to alleviate rectal pain. If patients are having significant amounts of mucus discharge or fecal incontinence, wide pantiliners or adult diapers will promote physical and psychological comfort. In addition, meticulous skin care to the perianal region is needed to minimize the severity of radiation skin reaction. Treatment of perianal pruritus with moisturizers is particularly important to assure comfort and minimize excoriation from scratching.

Cystitis

PREVENTIVE MEASURES

To minimize irritation of the bladder mucosa, encourage patients to avoid irritants such as caffeine,

Table 11-18 • Commonly Used Medications for the Treatment of Diarrhea

Medication	Administration
ANTICHOLINERGICS	
Loperamide HCl (Imodium) Tablet (2 mg) Capsule (2 mg) Solution (1 mg/5 ml)	The equivalent of 2 tablets initially, and then 1 tablet after each watery BM, up to 8 tablets a day
Diphenoxylate HCl with atropine sulfate (Lomotil) Tablet (2.5 mg) Solution (2.5 mg/5 ml)	Alternatively, the equivalent of 1–2 tablets 30 minutes before each meal and at bedtime
OPIATES	
Opium tincture Tincture (10% opium in 19% alcohol base) (.5 ml equivalent to 5 mg morphine)	.3–1 ml QID as needed Dilute with water or juice
Paregoric Tincture (.4% opium in 45% alcohol base) (5 ml equivalent to 2 mg morphine)	5–10 ml QID as needed *Note: opium tincture contains 25 times more morphine than paregoric*
BULK LAXATIVES	
Psyllium (Metamucil, Fiberall)	1–2 packages daily
Methylcellulose (Citrucel)	Take with only small amount of liquid

From McEvoy GK (1995). *Drug Information.* Bethesda, MD: American Society of Health-System Pharmacists.

alcohol, tobacco, and spices. In addition, instruct them to keep the urine dilute by drinking 1 to 2 liters of fluid a day, unless medically contraindicated.

ASSESSMENT

Although urinary changes are less likely to occur than bowel changes from pelvic radiation for a GI cancer, assess patients for specific symptoms at each visit as described in Table 11–14. Symptoms will be exacerbated by the presence of a urinary tract infection. Urine samples should be obtained for analysis and culture as needed.

TREATMENT

Symptoms of dysuria may be relieved with urinary anesthetics, which provide topical anesthesia to the bladder mucosa. Symptoms of frequency may arise from bladder spasms or from swelling of the prostate gland. Antispasmodics relax the smooth muscle of the bladder and alpha blockers may relieve bladder outlet obstruction. Table 11–19 lists medications and doses commonly used in treating urinary symptoms from pelvic radiation.

Sexual Effects

PREVENTIVE MEASURES

Patients receiving pelvic radiation should be told that they may continue sexual activity as desired

during treatment. Birth control measures should be used during treatment and for some months after treatment if the female patient or partner is premenopausal. Address the issue of fertility with patients interested in future parenting. Men should not develop permanent infertility, so sperm banking is not necessary. Women may become infertile, and in addition, because of postradiation changes in hormonal function and uterine anatomy, they will not be able to carry a fetus. Discuss the possibility of egg harvesting with in vitro fertilization and future surrogacy with female patients concerned about loss of fertility. However, this may not be an option for many patients because it requires the use of hormonal stimulation for at least 1 month, which may delay the onset of treatment. To minimize damage to the vaginal mucosa from the early effects of radiation, female patients should not use tampons during treatment.

ASSESSMENT

In asking patients about sexual issues, it is often helpful to begin with general questions about less sensitive issues, for example: "Other patients often have concerns about the effects of treatment on their sexuality. Do you have any concerns about this?" During the course of treatment, as a trusting relationship is established with the patient, nurses can move to more sensitive and specific sexual issues (e.g., ability to become aroused, ability to experience orgasm, satisfaction with sexual activity). Specific items to include in ongoing assessment during treatment are listed in Table 11–14. Patients' sexual concerns often become more pressing after treatment is completed. Assessing sexuality during follow-up visits is particularly important. Knowledge of the specific symptoms that may develop following treatment should be used to guide the assessment.

TREATMENT

If women develop vaginal irritation during the course of pelvic radiation, intercourse or manual stimulation of the vagina should be discontinued until these side effects have resolved after treatment is completed. Encourage women to use pantiliners as needed for discharge and to take warm water sitz baths for 15 to 20 minutes at a time as needed for cleanliness and comfort. The benefit of vaginal douching to relieve symptoms during treatment is debated. Since vaginal symptoms will be exacerbated by the presence of a vaginal infection, early diagnosis and prompt treatment of infection is essential.

Table 11-19 • Commonly Used Medications for the Treatment of Urinary Symptoms

Medication	Administration
URINARY ANESTHETIC	
Phenazopyridine HCl (Pyridium, Urodine) Tablet (100 and 200 mg)	200 mg TID
ANTISPASMODICS	
Oxybutynin Cl (Ditropan) Tablet (5 mg) Solution (5 mg/5 ml)	5 mg BID to TID
Flavoxate HCl (Urispas) Tablet (100 mg)	100–200 mg TID to QID
ALPHA BLOCKERS	
Terazosin (Hytrin) Tablet (1, 2, 5, and 10 mg)	Start with 1 mg q hs and increase gradually to achieve desired effect
Doxazosin (Cardura) Tablet (1,2,4, and 8mg)	

From Marks LB, Carroll PR, Dugan TC, and Anscher MS (1995). The response of the urinary bladder, urethra, and ureter to radiation and chemotherapy. *International Journal of Radiation Oncology, Biology, Physics,* 31, 1257–1280; McEvoy GK (1995). *Drug Information.* Bethesda, MD: American Society of Health-System Pharmacists.

Vaginal dryness is a common late effect of radiation to the vagina. After the early effects of radiation have resolved, instruct patients to insert a water-soluble moisturizer (e.g., Replens) into the vagina 3 times a week or more to minimize vaginal dryness. It is also important for patients to take measures to maintain vaginal patency. This requires regular (e.g., 2 to 3 times a week) sexual intercourse or the use of a vaginal dilator for 10 to 15 minutes at a time. To enhance comfort and ease at these times, water-soluble lubricants (e.g., Astroglide, K-Y Jelly) should be used during intercourse and when using the vaginal dilator. Estrogen replacement should be considered to maintain vaginal lubrication and elasticity unless medically contraindicated. Estrogen can be given systemically or through intravaginal topical application. For persistent dyspareunia, trying different positions during intercourse may minimize discomfort, and alternative methods of expressing sexual intimacy should be explored.

Men who have had pelvic surgery are at risk of developing erectile dysfunction as a result of their treatment. If patients report changes in erectile function, refer them to a urologist with expertise in this area. The etiology can be determined, and treatment options can be discussed.

For all patients reporting difficulties with sexual function during and following treatment, it is important to discuss alternative ways of expressing intimacy. The American Cancer Society (ACS) publishes an excellent book for patients on sexuality and cancer (ACS, 1988). See Chapter 13 for additional information on managing sexuality issues.

Skin Reaction

PREVENTIVE MEASURES

For patients with a colostomy, the appliance should fit correctly to prevent irritation of the skin as the stool becomes more fluid. Patients who are having difficulty with pouch changes and needing to change the pouch more often than every 4 to 5 days, can be referred to an enterostomal therapist for assessment and teaching. If the stoma is in the treatment field, the barrier used to affix the colostomy pouch may act as a bolus on the skin surface or may contain ingredients that increase the local skin reaction. Determine if there is a need to have the patient remove the pouch during treatment or use a different type of appliance for the duration of treatment (Hassey, 1987).

ASSESSMENT

Inspect the skin weekly during the course of treatment, paying particular attention to high risk

areas: supraclavicular lymph nodes (i.e., with some esophageal lesions), inguinal lymph nodes (i.e., with anal lesions), perineum, and peristomal skin. Specific items to include in ongoing assessment during treatment are listed in Table 11–14. For patients with a colostomy, the development of diarrhea may lead to leakage of stool under the barrier and will result in excoriation of the peristomal skin and a possible candida infection. Ask the patient how frequently the pouch needs to be changed to assure an adequate seal.

TREATMENT

Refer patients with a colostomy to an enterostomal therapist as needed during the course of treatment.

Bone Marrow Suppression

PREVENTIVE MEASURES

There are no specific measures known at present that patients can take to prevent developing bone marrow suppression from radiation; however, granulocyte-colony stimulating factor may be used for patients receiving combined modality therapy.

ASSESSMENT

Monitor complete blood counts (CBC) regularly during treatment, observing particularly for decreases in the number of granulocytes and platelets because of their short life span. Patients receiving concurrent chemotherapy or pelvic radiation are especially at risk; obtain a CBC at least weekly for these patients, and increase the frequency if the blood counts begin to drop. Also assess for associated signs and symptoms of bone marrow suppression. Patients with granulocyte counts below 500/mm^3 are at significantly increased risk of developing infection and with counts from 500 to 1000/mm^3 are at moderate risk. Assess these patients for signs and symptoms of infection (e.g., fever, chills, cough). Patients with platelet counts below 20,000/mm^3 are at significantly increased risk of bleeding and with counts from 20,000 to 50,000/mm^3 are at moderate risk. Assess these patients for signs and symptoms of bleeding (e.g., mucosal bleeding, bruising, petechiae). Patients with hemoglobin less than 8 g/dl have significant anemia. Assess these patients for fatigue, dizziness, tachycardia, and shortness of breath.

TREATMENT

If blood counts drop, patients should be instructed on infection and bleeding precautions. Patients may need to temporarily discontinue treatment to allow for recovery of blood counts.

There are varying opinions about appropriate cut-off levels.

Fatigue

PREVENTIVE MEASURES

Fatigue is a common side effect of radiation therapy; however, the etiology is unclear. Patients with a large treatment field, as in the treatment of many GI cancers, are particularly at risk. See Chapter 8 for further discussion on fatigue.

Conclusion

The radiation oncology nurse is responsible for educating patients and families regarding treatment with radiation therapy, the possible side effects of treatment, and the management of these side effects. This chapter has provided the medical framework for understanding the experience of the patient receiving treatment for a GI cancer and has discussed the specific nursing care required to support patients through this experience.

Unfortunately there is little research-based information to guide nurses in these activities. Much of what nurses do is based on anecdotal experience and is passed on as tradition. The challenge for radiation oncology nurses caring for patients with GI cancers is to now undertake research to evaluate the efficacy of specific interventions in achieving selected patient outcomes. Only then can nurses be sure of providing patients with optimal care during their treatment.

References

Ahlgren JD (1992). Principles of chemotherapy in gastrointestinal cancer. In J Ahlgren & J Macdonald (Eds.), *Gastrointestinal Oncology* (pp. 29–49). Philadelphia: JB Lippincott.

Ahmad NR, Goosenberg EB, Frucht H, & Coia LR (1994). Palliative treatment of esophageal cancer. *Seminars in Radiation Oncology, 4*, 202–214.

Alexander HR, Kelsen DP, & Tepper J (1993). Cancer of the stomach. In VT DeVita, Jr., S Hellman, & SA Rosenberg (Eds.), *Cancer: Principles and Practice of Oncology* (pp. 818–848). Philadelphia: JB Lippincott.

American Cancer Society (1988). *Sexuality and Cancer for the Man Who Has Cancer and His Partner.* Atlanta: ACS.

American Cancer Society (1988). *Sexuality and Cancer for the Woman Who Has Cancer and Her Partner.* Atlanta: ACS.

American Joint Committee on Cancer (AJCC) (1992). *Manual for Staging of Cancer* (4th Ed.). Philadelphia: JB Lippincott.

Annon JS (1976). *Behavioral Treatment of Sexual Problems: Brief Therapy.* New York: Harper and Row.

Auchincloss SS (1989). Sexual dysfunction in cancer patients: Issues in evaluation and treatment. In JC Holland & JH Rowland (Eds.), *Handbook of Psychooncology* (pp. 383–413). Oxford: Oxford University Press.

Berthrong M (1986). Pathologic changes secondary to radiation. *World Journal of Surgery, 10*, 155–170.

Blot WJ, Devesa SS, Kneller RW, & Fraumeni JF (1991). Rising incidence of adenocarcinoma of the esophagus and gastric cardia. *Journal of the American Medical Association, 265*, 1287–1289.

Brennan MF, Kinsella TJ, & Casper ES (1993). Cancer of the pancreas. In VT DeVita, Jr., S Hellman, & SA Rosenberg (Eds.), *Cancer: Principles and Practice of Oncology* (pp. 849–882). Philadelphia: JB Lippincott.

Cantril ST & Schoepel P (1988). Carcinoma of the anus: A review. *Seminars in Oncology Nursing, 4*, 293–299.

Caudry M (1992). Gastric cancer: Radiotherapy and approaches to locally unresectable or recurrent disease. In J Ahlgren & J Macdonald (Eds.), *Gastrointestinal Oncology* (pp. 181–187). Philadelphia: JB Lippincott.

Cleri LG (1995). Serotonin antagonists: State of the art management of chemotherapy-induced emesis. *Oncology Nursing: Patient Treatment and Support, 2*, 1–19.

Cohen AM, Minsky BD, & Schilsky RL (1993a). Colon cancer. In VT DeVita, Jr., S Hellman, & SA Rosenberg (Eds.), *Cancer: Principles and Practice of Oncology* (pp. 929–977). Philadelphia: JB Lippincott.

Cohen AM, Minsky BD, & Schilsky RL (1993b). Rectal cancer. In VT DeVita, Jr., S Hellman, & SA Rosenberg (Eds.), *Cancer: Principles and Practice of Oncology* (pp. 978–1005). Philadelphia: JB Lippincott.

Coia LR (1994). Gastrointestinal cancer. In LR Coia & DJ Moylan (Eds.), *Introduction to Clinical Radiation Oncology* (pp. 247–292). Madison, W: Medical Physics.

Coia LR, Engstron PF, Paul AR, Stafford PM, Hanks GE et al. (1991). Long-term results of infusional 5-FU, mitomycin-C, and radiation as primary management of esophageal cancer. *International Journal of Radiation Oncology, Biology, Physics, 20*, 29–36.

Coia LR, Myerson RJ, & Tepper JE (1995). Late effects of radiation therapy on the gastrointestinal tract. *International Journal of Radiation Oncology, Biology, Physics, 31*, 1213–1236.

Cox JD, Byhardt RW, Wilson F et al. (1986). Complications of radiation therapy and factors in their prevention. *World Journal of Surgery, 10*, 171–188.

Cummings BJ (1992). Anal canal. In CA Perez & LW Brady (Eds.), *Principles and Practice of Radiation Oncology* (pp. 1015–1024). Philadelphia: JB Lippincott.

DuBois JB (1992). Intraoperative radiation therapy in the treatment of gastrointestinal cancer. In J Ahlgren & J Macdonald (Eds.), *Gastrointestinal Oncology* (pp. 607–614). Philadelphia: JB Lippincott.

Dudas S (1993). Altered body image and sexuality. In SL Groenwald, M Goodman, MH Frogge & CH Yarbro (Eds.), *Cancer Nursing: Principles and Practice* (pp. 719–733). Boston: Jones and Bartlett.

Emami B, Lyman J, & Brown A (1991). Tolerance of normal tissue to therapeutic irradiation. *International Journal of Radiation Oncology, Biology, Physics, 21*, 109–122.

Fajardo LF (1993). Morphology of radiation effects on normal tissues. In CA Perez & LW Brady (Eds.), *Principles and Practice of Radiation Oncology* (pp. 114–123). Philadelphia: JB Lippincott.

Fisher SA & Brady LW (1992). Esophagus. In CA Perez & LW Brady (Eds.), *Principles and Practice of Radiation Oncology* (pp. 853–876). Philadelphia: JB Lippincott.

Frogge MH (1993). Gastrointestinal cancer: Esophagus, stomach, liver, and pancreas. In SL Groenwald, M Goodman, MH Frogge & CH Yarbro (Eds.), *Cancer Nursing: Principles and Practice* (pp. 1004–1043). Boston: Jones and Bartlett.

Gaspar LE (1994). Radiation therapy for esophageal cancer: Improving the therapeutic ratio. *Seminars in Radiation Oncology, 4,* 192–201.

Gastrointestinal Tumor Study Group (GITSG) (1985a). Pancreatic cancer: Adjuvant combined radiation and chemotherapy following curative resection. *Archives of Surgery, 120,* 899.

Gastrointestinal Tumor Study Group (GITSG) (1985b). Prolongation of the disease-free interval in surgically resected rectal cancer. *New England Journal of Medicine, 315,* 1294–1295.

Giri PGS, Fabian C, Estes N, Smalley SR, Reddy EK (1993). The role of whole abdominal irradiation in advanced stage colon cancer. *Seminars in Radiation Oncology, 3,* 68–73.

Goodman MG, Ladd LA, & Purl S (1993). Integumentary and mucous membrane alterations. In SL Groenwald, M Goodman, MH Frogge & CH Yarbro (Eds.), *Cancer Nursing: Principles and Practice* (pp. 734–800). Boston: Jones and Bartlett.

Grigsby PW, Russell A, Bruner D et al. (1995). Late injury of cancer therapy on the female reproductive tract. *International Journal of Radiation Oncology, Biology, Physics, 31,* 1281–1299.

Gunderson LL & Martenson JA (1993). Postoperative adjuvant irradiation with or without chemotherapy for rectal carcinomas. *Seminars in Radiation Oncology, 3,* 55–63.

Gunderson LL & Willet CG (1992). Pancreas and hepatobiliary tract. In CA Perez & LW Brady (Eds.), *Principles and Practice of Radiation Oncology* (pp. 985–999). Philadelphia: JB Lippincott.

Guyton AC (1991). *Textbook of Medical Physiology* (8th ed.). Philadelphia: W B Saunders.

Hall EJ (1994). *Radiobiology for the Radiologist* Philadelphia: JB Lippincott.

Hampton B (1993). Gastrointestinal cancer: Colon, rectum, and anus. In SL Groenwald, M Goodman, MH Frogge & CH Yarbro (Eds.), *Cancer Nursing: Principles and Practice* (pp. 1044–1064). Boston: Jones and Bartlett.

Harter KW & Ahlgren JD (1992). Cancer of the anal canal and anal margin. In J Ahlgren & J Macdonald (Eds.), *Gastrointestinal Oncology* (pp. 437–447). Philadelphia: JB Lippincott.

Harter KW (1992a). Esophageal cancer: Management with radiation. In J Ahlgren & J Macdonald (Eds.), *Gastrointestinal Oncology* (pp. 123–134). Philadelphia: JB Lippincott.

Harter KW (1992b). Pancreatic cancer: Radiotherapeutic approaches. In J Ahlgren and J Macdonald (Eds.), *Gastrointestinal Oncology* (pp. 215–225). Philadelphia: JB Lippincott.

Harter K W (1992c). Principles of radiotherapy. In J Ahlgren & J Macdonald (Eds.), *Gastrointestinal Oncology* (pp. 51–59). Philadelphia: JB Lippincott.

Hassey K (1987). Radiation therapy for rectal cancer and the implications for nursing. *Cancer Nursing, 10,* 311–318.

Hermans J, Bonenkamp JJ, Boon MC et al. (1993). Adjuvant therapy after curative resection for gastric cancer: Meta-analysis of randomized trials. *Journal of Clinical Oncology, 11,* 1441–1447.

Herskovic A et al. (1992). Combined chemotherapy and radiotherapy compared with radiotherapy alone in patients with cancer of the esophagus. *New England Journal of Medicine, 326,* 1593–1598.

Hill MC, Roberts IM, & Schwab F (1992). Imaging techniques in the diagnosis and staging of gastrointestinal cancer. In

J Ahlgren & J Macdonald (Eds.), *Gastrointestinal Oncology* (pp. 13–18). Philadelphia: JB Lippincott.

Hoebler L & Irwin MM (1992). Gastrointestinal tract cancer: Current knowledge, medical treatment, and nursing management. *Oncology Nursing Forum, 19,* 1403–1415.

Hoover Jr. HC (1993). Recent developments in the surgical management of rectal carcinoma. *Seminars in Radiation Oncology, 3,* 8–12.

Jaklitsch MT, Harpole DH, Healey EA, & Sugarbaker DJ (1994). Current issues in the staging of esophageal cancer. *Seminars in Radiation Oncology, 4,* 135–145.

Kaanders JHAM, & Ang KK (1994). Early reactions as dose-limiting factors in radiotherapy. *Seminars in Radiation Oncology, 4,* 55–67.

Kelsen D (1993). Neoadjuvant therapy for gastric cancers. *Oncology, 7,* 25–32.

Krook JE et al. (1991). Effective surgical adjuvant therapy for high-risk rectal carcinoma. *New England Journal of Medicine, 324,* 709–715.

Lawrence TS & Maybaum J (1993). Fluoropyrimidines as radiation sensitizers. *Seminars in Radiation Oncology, 3,* 20–28.

Marks LB, Carroll PR, Dugan TC, & Anscher MS (1995). The response of the urinary bladder, urethra, and ureter to radiation and chemotherapy. *International Journal of Radiation Oncology, Biology, Physics, 31,* 1257–1280.

Martenson Jr. JA & Gunderson LL (1992). Colon and rectum. In CA Perez & LW Brady (Eds.), *Principles and Practice of Radiation Oncology* (pp. 1000–1014). Philadelphia: JB Lippincott.

Mauch P, Constine L, & Greenberger J (1995). Hematopoietic stem cell compartment: Acute and late effects of radiation therapy and chemotherapy. *International Journal of Radiation Oncology, Biology, Physics, 31,* 1319–1339.

McCance KL & Huether SE (1994). *Pathophysiology: The Biologic Basis for Disease in Adults and Children* (2nd ed.). St. Louis: Mosby.

McEvoy GK (1995). *Drug Information.* Bethesda: American Society of Health-System Pharmacists.

Medvec BR (1988). Esophageal cancer: Treatment and nursing interventions. *Seminars in Oncology Nursing, 4,* 246–256.

Mendenhall WM et al. (1993). Preoperative irradiation for clinically resectable rectal adenocarcinoma. *Seminars in Radiation Oncology, 3,* 48–54.

Merrick HW & Dobelbower RR (1990). Aggressive therapy for cancer of the pancreas: Does it help? *Gastroenterology Clinics of North America, 19,* 935–962.

Minsky BD (1993). Pelvic radiation therapy in rectal cancer: Technical considerations. *Seminars in Radiation Oncology, 3,* 42–47.

Minsky BD (1994). The adjuvant treatment of esophageal cancer. *Seminars in Radiation Oncology, 4,* 165–169.

Minsky BD (1996). The role of radiotherapy in gastric cancer. *Seminars in Oncology , 23,* 390–396.

Minsky BD, Cohen AM, Kemeny N, et al. (1992). Enhancement of radiation-induced downstaging of rectal cancer by fluorouracil and high-dose leucovorin chemotherapy. *Journal of Clinical Oncology, 10,* 79–84.

Minsky BD & Leibel SA (1989). The treatment of hepatic metastases from colorectal cancer with radiation therapy alone or combined with chemotherapy or misonidazole. *Cancer Treatment Reviews, 16,* 213–219.

Moses FM (1991). Squamous cell carcinoma of the esophagus: Natural history, incidence, etiology, and complications. *Gastroenterology Clinics of North America, 20,* 703–716.

National Cancer Institute (NCI) (1995). *PDO Cancer Information Database*. Washington, DC: Author.

Nelson JK, Moxness KE, Jensen MD, & Gastineaus CF (1994). *Mayo Clinic Diet Manual: A Handbook of Nutrition Pracitices* (7th ed.). St. Louis: Mosby.

Parker SL, Tong T, Bolden S, & Wingo PA. (1997). Cancer statistics: 1997. *Ca-A Cancer Journal for Clinicians, 47*, 5-27.

Perry MC (1992). *The Chemotherapy Source Book*. Baltimore: Williams and Wilkins.

Pilepich MV & Miller HH (1980). Preoperative irradiation in carcinoma of the pancreas. *Cancer, 46*, 1945.

Raefsky EL & Wasserman TH (1992). Combined Modality Therapy. In M C Perry (Ed.). *The Chemotherapy Source Book* (pp. 110–129). Baltimore: Williams and Wilkins.

Rostock RA et al. (1992). Radiation therapy in the treatment of colorectal cancer. In J Ahlgren & J Macdonald (Eds.), *Gastrointestinal Oncology* (pp. 359–381). Philadelphia: JB Lippincott.

Roth JA, Lichter AS, Putnam JB, & Forastiere AA (1993). Cancer of the esophagus. In VT DeVita Jr., S Hellman, & SA Rosenberg (Eds.), *Cancer: Principles and Practice of Oncology* (pp. 776–817). Philadelphia: JB Lippincott.

Rotman M, & Torpie RJ (1992). Supportive care in radiation oncology. In CA Perez & LW Brady (Eds.), *Principles and Practice of Radiation Oncology* (pp. 1508–1516). Philadelphia: JB Lippincott.

Rubin P, Constine LS, & Nelson DF (1992). Late effects of cancer treatment: Radiation and drug toxicity. In CA Perez & LW Brady (Eds.), *Principles and Practice of Radiation Oncology* (pp. 124–161). Philadelphia: JB Lippincott.

Schein PS (1992). Gastrointestinal cancer: A global perspective. In J Ahlgren & J Macdonald (Eds.), *Gastrointestinal Oncology* (pp. 3–11). Philadelphia: JB Lippincott.

Scully R E, Mark EJ, McNeely WF, & McNeely BU (1994). Case records of the Massachusetts General Hospital. *New England Journal of Medicine, 330*, 627–632.

Shank B, Cohen AM, & Kelsen D (1993). Cancer of the anal region. In VT DeVita, Jr., S Hellman, & SA Rosenberg (Eds.), *Cancer: Principles and Practice of Oncology* (pp. 1006–1022). Philadelphia: JB Lippincott.

Smalley SR & Gunderson LL (1992). Stomach. In CA Perez & LW Brady (Eds.), *Principles and Practice of Radiation Oncology* (pp. 970–984). Philadelphia: JB Lippincott.

Twomey P, Burchell M, Strawn D, & Guernsey J. (1989). Local control in rectal cancer: A clinical review and metaanalysis. *Archives of Surgery, 124*, 1174–1179.

Wanebo HJ & Turk PS (1992). General surgical principles in gastrointestinal cancer. In J Ahlgren and J Macdonald (Eds.), *Gastrointestinal Oncology* (pp. 19–28). Philadelphia: JB Lippincott.

Wang JF (1988). Stomach cancer. *Seminars in Oncology Nursing, 4*, 257–264.

Warshaw AL & Castillo CF (1992). Pancreatic carcinoma. *New England Journal of Medicine, 326*, 455–465.

Wingo PA, Tong T, & Bolden S (1995). Cancer statistics: 1995. *Ca: A Cancer Journal for Clinicians, 45*, 8–30.

Male Genitourinary Cancers

KAREN E. MAHER

Male genitourinary (GU) cancers encompass the spectrum of cancer treatment and nursing care. Patients may receive surgery, chemotherapy, and radiation therapy concomitantly or as a single modality. This chapter focuses on the role of radiation therapy in the treatment of prostate, urinary bladder, testis, and penile cancers. These malignancies can profoundly affect multiple body systems, thus each site will be discussed individually, including specific radiation-related toxicities and nursing assessment and interventions. Sexuality is an integral aspect of male GU cancers with treatment sequelae affecting sexual functioning. A section is included to address nursing issues regarding this sensitive and important topic. Finally, future directions in therapy for male GU malignancies are discussed.

Anatomy

Prostate

The prostate gland is a small, walnut sized (4 to 6 cm long) organ shaped like an inverted pyramid. It lies posterior to the symphysis pubis, just inferior to the bladder, and in front of the rectum. (See Figure 12–1.) The superior portion of the gland is referred to as the base, and lies at the neck of the bladder. The seminal vesicles are superiorly positioned at the base and lie behind the bladder. The inferior region of the prostate is the apex. The posterior portion and median sulcus of the gland are easily palpated by digital rectal examination. The portion of the urethra that passes through the prostate is the prostatic urethra. The prostate provides a viscous alkaline secretion to semen.

Bladder

The bladder is located directly behind the symphysis pubis and in front of the rectum in males.

The lower portion, continuous with the urethra, is called the neck, and the upper segment is the apex. The region between the ureteral openings is the trigone. The bladder wall consists of an inner mucous layer of transitional epithelium (also called urothelium), a muscular coat of smooth muscle, and an outer layer of fibrous muscle (detrusor). The bladder has a storage capacity in health of approximately 500 ml. Sphincter muscles control urinary retention.

Testis

The testes are located in the scrotum. Their function is to produce spermatozoa and the male hormone testosterone. They are enclosed within the inelastic fibrous tunica albuginea. The testis is divided into numerous lobules that contain seminiferous tubules within which the spermatozoa originate. The lobules join a plexus that leads to the epididymis. The epididymis leads to the ductus deferens, through which sperm are conveyed to the urethra. The interstitial Leydig cells are located between the seminiferous tubules and are the source of testosterone.

Penis

The penis is a cylindrical organ suspended from the front and sides of the pubic arch. It is composed mainly of erectile tissue arranged in three columns and covered with skin. The two lateral columns are the corpora cavernosa penis. The median column is the corpus spongiosum and contains the urethra. Hyperemia of the genitals fills the corpora cavernosa with blood as the result of sexual excitement or stimulation, causing an erection. The cone-shaped head of the penis, glans penis, contains the urethral orifice. It is covered with the foreskin or prepuce.

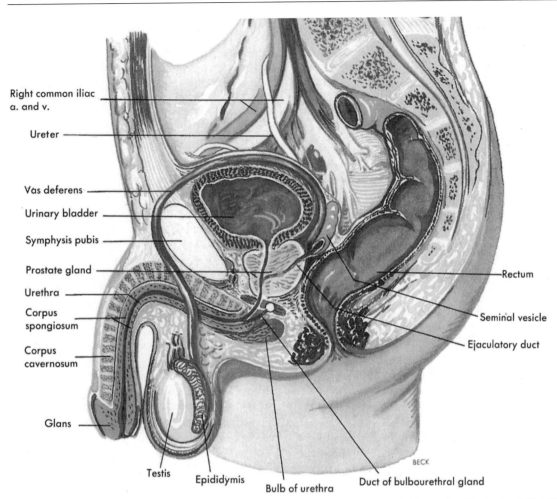

Figure 12-1 • Male pelvic organs. From Davis M (1994). Genitourinary cancers. In SE Otto (Ed.). *Oncology Nursing* (pp. 168–189). St. Louis: Mosby.

Prostate

Epidemiology and Risk Factors

Adenocarcinoma of the prostate is the most common cancer in men. Estimates for 1997 include 334,500 new cases and 41,800 deaths in the United States (Parker et al., 1997). This translates to an estimated 43 percent of all new male cancers and approximately 14 percent of all male cancer deaths that will be attributed to prostate cancer in 1997. The probability of developing an invasive prostate cancer in the 40 to 59 year age group is 1 in 103 and rises in the 60 to 79 year age group to a ratio of 1 in 8. The overall probability of developing an invasive prostate cancer in a lifetime is 1 in 6 (Parker et al., 1997). African-American men have the highest incidence of prostate cancer and are twice as likely as white American men to die

from the disease (Garnick, 1994). Many explanations have been proposed but none proved. Some possible explanations include: higher levels of circulating androgens in college-age African-American men; less access to health care, which may lead to later medical diagnosis and intervention; and fewer opportunities to try investigational therapies (Garnick, 1994). Due to the increasing number of men in the 60 to 79 age group, prostate cancer is a major health problem facing aging men and the health care system.

Genetic risk factors include age, race, and a positive family history of prostate cancer. Research in genetic predisposition to prostate cancer is in its infancy and has yet to describe the genetic alterations that cause prostatic tumors (Greco & Kulawiak, 1994). Hereditary prostate cancer accounts for a substantial proportion of early-onset prostate cancer. Overall about 9 percent of prostate cancer is estimated to be due to the effects of the hereditary prostate cancer gene in the population (Carter et al., 1993). Epidemiological studies have found no consistent correlation between prostate cancer with life style, dietary, or environmental factors such as: increased body fat, venereal disease, infections, sexual habits, number of sexual partners, vasectomy, tobacco use, or occupational exposure (Greco & Kulawiak, 1994; Maxwell, 1993). Exposure to cadmium has been shown to be associated with an increased risk of carcinoma of the prostate, and patients with carcinoma of the prostate often have elevated cadmium levels. A comparison of cadmium levels in serum and prostate tissue of high-risk and low-risk populations showed similar levels among controls and patients with benign prostatic hypertrophy and carcinoma. This suggests that elevated serum cadmium levels may well be a marker of, rather than a risk factor for, carcinoma of the prostate (Hanks et al., 1993).

Clinical Presentation

Patients presenting with early stage prostate cancer are usually asymptomatic. Symptoms become evident as the cancer increases in size or progresses systemically. The most common presenting features result from urinary tract obstruction due to the enlarged prostate gland. Urgency, nocturia, and hesitancy are the most common signs of an enlarged prostate gland with bladder neck obstruction. Frequently there is little to differentiate these symptoms from those due to benign prostatic enlargement, which may also be present. Less common signs include impotence or less firm penile erections; this information is often not elicited in history-taking and can be mistakenly ascribed as a normal response in an aging man (Garnick, 1993).

Prostate cancer growth frequently follows a predictable pattern. As the tumor increases in size, it progresses to the capsule margin, through the capsule, and into the seminal vesicles and bladder neck (Maxwell, 1993). Lymphatic spread is orderly with the pelvic lymphatics affected first. Hematogenous dissemination most frequently affects the bones, commonly the vertebrae, pelvis, femur, and ribs (Lind et al., 1993). Bone metastases most frequently present as osteoblastic lesions, however lytic lesions also occur. Spread of disease can involve the lungs and liver, with brain involvement an uncommon and late occurrence. Metastatic spread may herald the diagnosis with symptoms such as back pain secondary to vertebral metastases as the most common initial finding. In a small percentage of patients, the initial presenting symptoms may include acute urinary retention caused by bladder neck obstruction, bilateral hydronephrosis caused by tumor extension to the bladder wall and trigone, or spinal cord compression caused by epidural extension. Rarely, patients may have supraclavicular lymphadenopathy or abnormalities of hepatic function (Garnick, 1993).

Screening, Diagnosis, and Staging

Screening

The recent widespread availability of prostate-specific antigen testing and transrectal ultrasonography has increased awareness of prostate cancer in the community and among health care providers, and fueled the epidemic of prostate cancer detection efforts. The value of prostate cancer screening for early detection in asymptomatic men is controversial because of high cost and the inability to distinguish between indolent and aggressive tumors. The natural history of many localized prostate cancers is characterized by slow, asymptomatic local progression, and competing comorbidities may be greater than the risk of death from cancer (Fowler et al., 1995). Despite concern over the increasing incidence of prostate cancer, the effectiveness of screening remains questionable (Waldman & Osborne, 1994). Screening should demonstrate that cancer deaths are decreased as a result of detecting more cancers earlier. The empiric risk associated with familial and hereditary prostate cancer suggests the need for focused screening efforts on these groups of men (Carter et al., 1993). Prospective trials are under way to determine if screening does reduce prostate cancer deaths.

Prostate-Specific Antigen (PSA)

PSA is a highly immunogenic glycoprotein produced only by prostatic tissue. It is detected in prostate tissue, seminal fluid, and blood. Although PSA is prostate-specific, it is not prostate cancer-specific (Maxwell, 1993). It is generally agreed that digital rectal exam does not elevate PSA levels as an artifact when the two tests are conducted at the same time. Normal PSA values range from 0.4 to 4.0 ng/ml. Levels over 4 ng/ml indicate either benign prostatic hypertrophy or cancer. Levels over 10 ng/ml more clearly point to malignancy (Maxwell, 1993). In patients with prostate cancer, serum PSA levels are generally proportional to the clinical stage of the disease and volume of cancer in the gland. An increase in PSA of more than 80 ng/ml generally correlates with more advanced tumor stage, including metastatic disease (Garnick, 1993).

The half-life of PSA has been determined to be 2.2 to 3.2 days. Following radical prostatectomy, the interpretation of serum PSA values is straightforward. Any detectable level is an all but certain indicator of the presence of cancer. The interpretation of PSA after definitive irradiation is less clear. The fall of PSA following radiation therapy is gradual with a half-life of approximately 2 months. Data from Kavadi, Zagars, and Pollack (1994) reveal that serum PSA nadirs are reached by 12 months after completion of radiation therapy and little decline can be expected beyond that time. While these findings are still controversial, most investigators suggest that only patients whose PSA nadir falls <1 ng/ml can be said to have achieved a biochemical complete response. However, even such a low nadir value does not ensure durable disease control for patients with high pretreatment serum PSA levels (>30 ng/ml).

Failure of the PSA to return to normal or a secondary rise in PSA values after definitive irradiation or radical prostatectomy can predict residual localized cancer or the development of metastasis (Hanks, 1994). Following the initiation of hormonal therapy in disseminated disease, PSA values, if elevated, can decline to normal values. The persistence of such a decrease may help predict a favorable prolonged response to therapy (Garnick, 1993).

Diagnosis

The most common diagnostic procedures are digital rectal examination (DRE), PSA testing, and transrectal ultrasonography (TRUS). Prostate biopsy is most often accomplished via a TRUS guided transperineal or transrectal technique. Multiple planes of prostate anatomy can be visualized resulting in a more accurate sample procurement (Garnick, 1993). Tissue may also be obtained with fine-needle aspiration; and with specimens obtained at the time of transurethral resection.

Pathologic Classification

Some 95 percent of prostatic carcinomas arise in the acinar structures or distal ducts of the prostate gland and are adenocarcinomas (Hanks, 1994). Sarcomas, transitional cell, small cell and squamous cell carcinomas of the prostate are rare (Maxwell, 1993). The Gleason scoring system for pathologic grading of adenocarcinoma of the prostate has gained the widest acceptance (Gar-

nick, 1993). This system divides prostate cancer into five histologic patterns, ranging from 1 to 5. To determine the Gleason score, a histologic grade (1 to 5) is given to the primary and secondary patterns of tumor as seen microscopically. The grade numbers of the two patterns are added to obtain the Gleason score that will range from 2 through 10. The pathologist will report the score as 3+4 or 3+2; others may use 7/10 or 5/10 (Garnick, 1993). Accurate understanding of the differentiation of a given prostatic carcinoma is necessary to predict behavior and make the most accurate treatment decision (Hanks, 1994). Gleason score may be the strongest prognostic indicator for outcome. Overall survival correlates inversely with grade, thus the poorly differentiated tumors (Gleason 7, 8, 9) have the worst prognosis. (See Table 12–1.) Other technologies used to grade prostate tumors include DNA analysis, proliferative rate determination, nuclear-organizing regions, morphology, and chromosomal investigation (Maxwell, 1993).

Staging

When a prostate cancer has been confirmed, the patient undergoes a staging evaluation. Present standard staging may include blood chemistry studies, serum PSA, urine cytology, bone scan, computerized tomography, and magnetic resonance imaging. Although radionuclide bone scan is extremely sensitive in evaluating the skeleton for metastatic disease, it is costly and time consuming for the patient. In general, a bone scan is approximately 10 times more expensive than PSA (Chybowski et al., 1991). Chybowski et al. studied the correlation of positive bone scan with several

Table 12-1 • Gleason Scoring System

SCORE = DOMINANT PATTERN + SECONDARY PATTERN

Pattern 1	Uniform glands, well-defined tumor margin
Pattern 2	Less uniform glands, tumor margin less well defined
Pattern 3	Irregular glands of variable size, poorly defined tumor margin
Pattern 4	Fused glands with infiltrating cords, of variable size and patterns
Pattern 5	Few or no glands, cords or sheets of tumor cells infiltrating stroma

SCORE	GRADE
2, 3, 4	Well differentiated
5, 6, 7	Moderately differentiated
8, 9, 10	Poorly differentiated

Data from Hanks GE, Myers CE, & Scardino PT (1993). Cancer of the prostate. In VT De Vita Jr., S Hellman, and SA Rosenberg (Eds.), *Cancer Principles and Practice of Oncology* (p. 1079). Philadelphia: JB Lippincott; Hanks G (1994). The prostate. In JD Cox (Ed.), *Moss' Radiation Oncology, Rationale, Technique, Results* (p. 588). St. Louis: Mosby.

other parameters including PSA levels, in patients with newly diagnosed, untreated adenocarcinoma of the prostate. The most significant finding of the study was the negative predictive value of a low serum PSA concentration for bone scan findings. In 306 men with a serum PSA level of $\leq$20 ng/ml, only 1 (PSA 18.2 ng/ml) had a positive bone scan (negative predictive value 99.7 percent). This finding suggests that a staging radionuclide bone scan in a previously untreated patient with prostate cancer and a low serum PSA concentration may not be necessary.

Traditionally prostate cancer has been staged by the American Urological Association (AUA) system based on the Whitmore-Jewett system (Held et al., 1994). The tumor, node, metastasis (TNM) classification system (Table 12–2) is the newer and most commonly used staging system.

Treatment Modalities

The management of prostate cancer in all stages is controversial and may include watchful waiting, hormonal therapy, and curative treatment with surgery and/or radiation therapy. Treatment recommendations for individual patients are evolving and at times controversial, primarily due to recent advances in detection and treatment, rendering much of the existing literature outdated. In making treatment decisions, clinicians will consider the established value of various treatments in association with the patient's age and general health, comorbid conditions, factors concerning the quality of life and available resources (Catalona, 1994). Major considerations taken into account are serum PSA because of its relationship to the primary tumor and likely outcome, and Gleason grade and T-stage because they remain the major determinant of metastatic relapse (Zagars et al., 1995). See Table 12–3 for an overview of treatment options according to stage of disease.

Observation ("Watchful Waiting")

There is considerable controversy regarding aggressive treatment for low-stage prostate cancer.

Table 12-2 • TNM Staging System for Prostate Carcinoma

PRIMARY TUMOR (T)

TX	Primary tumor cannot be assessed		N1	Metastasis in single lymph node, $\leq$2 cm in greatest dimension	
T0	No evidence of primary tumor				
T1	Clinically inapparent tumor not palpable or visible by imaging		N2	Metastasis in single lymph node, >2 cm but >5 cm in greatest dimension; or multiple lymph node metastasis, none $\geq$5 cm in greatest dimension	
T1a	Tumor incidental histologic finding in $\leq$5% of tissue resected		N3		
T1b	Tumor incidental histologic finding in $\geq$5% of tissue resected			Metastasis in a lymph node >5 cm in greatest dimension	
T1c	Tumor identified by needle biopsy (e.g., because of elevated PSA)		DISTANT METASTASIS*** (M)		
			MX		
T2	Tumor confined within prostate*		M0	Presence of distant metastasis cannot be assessed	
T2a	Tumor involves half of lobe or less		M1	No distant metastasis	
T2b	Tumor involves more than half of lobe, but not both lobes		M1a	Distant metastasis	
			M1b	Nonregional lymph node(s)	
T2c	Tumor involves both lobes		M1c	Bone(s)	
T3	Tumor extends through the prostatic capsule**			Other site(s)	
T3a	Unilateral extracapsular extension		STAGE GROUPING		
T3b	Bilateral extracapsular extension				
T3c	Tumor invades the seminal vesicle(s)				
T4	Tumor is fixed or invades adjacent structures other than seminal vesicles				
T4a	Tumor invades any of: bladder neck, external sphincter, or rectum				
T4b	Tumor invades levator muscles and/or is fixed to pelvic wall				

REGIONAL LYMPH NODES (N)

NX	Regional lymph nodes cannot be assessed
N0	No regional lymph node metastasis

STAGE GROUPING

Stage 0	T1a	N0	M0	G1
Stage I	T1a	N0	M0	G2, 3–4
	T1b	N0	M0	Any G
	T1c	N0	M0	Any G
	T1	N0	M0	Any G
Stage II	T2	N0	M0	Any G
Stage III	T3	N0	M0	Any G
Stage IV	T4	N0	M0	Any G
	Any T	N1	M0	Any G
	Any T	N2	M0	Any G
	Any T	N3	M0	Any G
	Any T	Any N	M1	Any G

From American Joint Committee on Cancer (1992). *Manual for staging of cancer* (4th ed.). Philadelphia: JB Lippincott. Reprinted with permission.
* Tumor found in one or both lobes by needle biopsy, but not palpable or visible by imaging, is classified T1c
** Invasion into the prostatic apex or into, but not beyond, the prostatic capsule is not classified as T3, but as T2
*** When $\geq$1 site of metastasis is present, the most advanced category (pM1c) is used

Table 12-3 • Treatment Options in Prostate Cancer According to Stage of Disease

Stage	Treatment Options
T1a	
Projected life expectancy <10 yrs	Watchful waiting
Projected life expectancy >10 yrs	Radical prostatectomy, radiation, therapy, watchful waiting
T1b, T1c, T2a, T2b, T2c	
Projected life expectancy <10 yrs	Radiation therapy, hormonal therapy
Projected life expectancy >10 yrs	Radical prostatectomy, radiation therapy
T3 (clinically staged)	Radiation therapy, radical prostatectomy, ±hormonal therapy
T3 (surgically staged)	
Positive margin(s)	Radiation therapy
Extracapsular extension	Radiation therapy, watchful waiting
Seminal vesicle invasion	Radiation therapy, hormonal therapy, watchful waiting
Lymph node metastases (±prostatectomy)	Early or delayed hormonal therapy
Recurrence after surgery	
Without metastases	Radiation therapy
With metastases	Hormonal therapy
Recurrence after radiation	Hormonal therapy, radiation therapy
Persistently elevated PSA	
PSA ≥20 ng/ml	Hormonal therapy
PSA <20 ng/ml	Lymphadenectomy and radical prostatectomy, radiation therapy ± lymphadenectomy, hormonal therapy
Disseminated disease	Hormonal therapy
Hormone refractory disease	Radiation therapy, corticosteroid therapy, chemotherapy, supportive therapy, investigational trials

Modified from Catalona WJ (1994). Management of cancer of the prostate. *The New England Journal of Medicine, 331,* 999. Copyright 1994 Massachusetts Medical Society.

Because of the variable history and biologic behavior of prostate cancer, treatment of persons with low-grade and low-stage (clinically organ confined T_1 and T_2) tumors may be assigned to watchful waiting. Observation has resulted in low rates of death from prostate cancer (9 to 15 percent) among men with localized disease, raising a question about the need to treat all men with low-grade localized disease. These figures do not necessarily apply to younger men at higher risk, who are unrepresented in the studies of watchful waiting (Catalona, 1994).

A retrospective study by Albertson et al. (1995) examined conservatively treated patients age 65 to 75 years with low-stage prostate cancer. The authors concluded that men with conservatively treated low-grade (Gleason score 2 to 4) prostate cancer incur no loss of life expectancy. However, maximum estimated lost life expectancy for men with Gleason score 5 to 7 tumors was 4 to 5 years and for men with Gleason score 8 to 10 tumors was 6 to 8 years.

Hormonal Manipulation

Hormone dependent tumors occur in 80 to 90 percent of men with prostate cancer and hormonal intervention is most often used to manage metastatic disease (Held et al., 1994; Maxwell, 1993). The purpose of endocrine therapy is to decrease the circulating plasma testosterone to castration levels. Hormonal therapies act primarily on the hypothalamic-pituitary-testicular axis by inhibiting secretion of luteinizing hormone (LH) at the cellular level, or they act at the adrenal glands where approximately 5 percent of male testosterone is produced (Maxwell, 1993). Figure 12–2 depicts the hormonal effects on the prostate. The timing of hormonal therapy is controversial, because patients with metastatic disease who are not treated may have long intervals without symptoms, and the side effects of androgen deprivation (hot flashes, diminished muscle mass, decreased libido and sexual potency) are not trivial in asymptomatic, sexually active men. About 85 percent of patients have an objective response, however unequivocal evidence of a survival benefit is lacking. A decrease in the serum PSA is a good indicator of response (Catalona, 1994).

Pollack, Zagars, and Kopplin (1995) defined a particularly poor prognostic group comprised of patients with pretreatment serum PSA levels >30 ng/ml with any tumor grade, or serum PSA levels >10 ng/ml and ≤30 ng/ml with tumors grade 3 or 4 (MD Anderson Cancer Center grading). Within 3 years, 80 percent of high-risk patients treated

HORMONAL EFFECTS ON PROSTATE

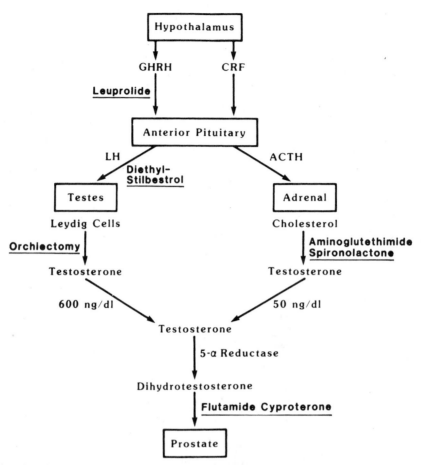

Figure 12-2 • Flow chart illustrating anatomic sites of action of hormonal therapy agents. From Perez CA (1992). Prostate. In CA Perez & LW Brady (Eds.), *Principles and Practice of Radiation Oncology* (pp. 1067–1116). Philadelphia: JB Lippincott.

with radiotherapy alone will be deemed failures based on biochemical criteria. Clearly, radiotherapy was insufficient treatment. In this setting, many patients would opt for combined treatment after weighing the side effects of early androgen ablation against the risk of early disease progression. The investigators retrospectively compared groups, as described above, that were treated with radiotherapy alone versus radiotherapy plus hormonal ablation using leuprolide with or without flutamide, or orchiectomy. It was reported that the incidence of rising PSA at 3 years for the radiotherapy group was 81 percent versus 15 percent for the radiotherapy plus hormonal ablation group. In addition, local relapse at 3 years was 34 percent and 15 percent, respectively. There was no difference between groups in terms of survival. The authors conclude the immediate benefit of the combined use of radiotherapy and early androgen ablation ("debulking") is a lengthening of the time to biochemical and/or disease failure. The benefit of long-term survival remains to be documented. The appropriateness of early end points is questioned, and longer follow-up is needed to determine if survival is affected by immediate combined treatment (Pollack et al., 1995).

Androgen ablation is achieved by bilateral orchiectomy and/or systemic hormonal therapy. Estrogen therapy is as effective as orchiectomy. Diethylstilbesterol in a daily dose of 1 to 3 mg may be effective. However, it has limited use due to excessive cardiovascular toxicity in doses over 1 mg daily. Luteinizing hormone-releasing hormone (LHRH) agonists, when administered over a long period, stimulate pituitary gonadotropin secretion for 4 to 5 days, after which gonadotropin, especially luteinizing hormone (LH), secretion is suppressed. The initial rise in serum testosterone concentrations may stimulate tumor growth, therefore should not be used in patients with spinal cord compression, pathological fracture, or urinary obstruction from tumor growth (Catalona, 1994; Maxwell, 1993). Non-steroidal antiandrogens, such as flutamide, act by blocking the binding of testosterone and dihydrotestosterone to its intracellular receptors. When flutamide is used in combination with LHRH agonists, a maximal androgen blockade is accomplished. Other hormonal agents such as progestins (megestrol acetate) act by primarily inhibiting the release of LH and also block androgen receptors. With all progestins, the serum testosterone concentrations gradually rise after 6 to 12 months of therapy. Adding a low dose of estrogen assists in maintaining testosterone suppression (Catalona, 1994).

Surgical Intervention

Radical prostatectomy is one option for patients with clinically localized (T1, T2a) tumors, whose life expectancy is 10 years or more, with the goal of treatment to eradicate the disease (Catalona, 1994). The operation involves the retropubic or perineal removal of the entire prostate including the capsule, seminal vesicles, and a portion of the bladder neck (Held et al., 1994). The retropubic approach is favored by most surgeons because it allows bilateral pelvic lymph node removal at the time of operation and may be "nerve sparing." Lymph node dissection is performed first and if metastatic disease is discovered, radical prostatectomy is usually aborted. Nerve sparing radical retropubic prostatectomy may preserve erectile function in many men by avoiding injury to the cavernosal neurovascular bundle. The decision to use the nerve-sparing technique depends on preoperative and intraoperative findings regarding the extent of the tumor and is most often performed in men with tumors detected at an early stage. Larger tumors that approach the prostate capsule margin require more tissue excision with wider surgical margins and thus eliminate the nerve-sparing technique of dissecting close to the prostate gland (Maxwell, 1993; Catalona, 1994).

The advisability of radical prostatectomy in men with bulky, high-grade tumors (T2b and c) has been questioned. These patients have a higher risk of cancer at the margins of the excised tissue especially if they undergo nerve sparing prostatectomy (Catalona, 1994). It is questionable if men with cancer that has spread beyond the prostate (T3) can be cured with a wide excision of the tumor because they may also have occult distant metastasis (Catalona, 1994).

Less than 15 percent of patients with lymph node metastases (stages N1 to N3) are cured with any treatment. Most clinicians recommend a pelvic lymphadenectomy to determine the nodal stage of the disease before proceeding to radical prostatectomy and sometimes before radiation therapy. In high surgical risk patients, the nodes may be sampled by laparoscope. In patients with nodal metastases, treatment options include hormonal therapy, radical prostatectomy, and radiation therapy. Because lymphadenectomy is not therapeutic, most surgeons do not perform a radical prostatectomy if nodal metastases are present. In a retrospective study comparing radical prostatectomy, radiation therapy, and watchful waiting in patients with positive lymph nodes, those treated with prostatectomy fared best, but they also had less advanced disease than the other patients. There is no evidence that radiation therapy benefits men with nodal metastases (Catalona, 1994).

Transurethral resection of the prostate (TURP) may be required to relieve symptoms of bladder outlet obstruction due to enlarged size of the prostate gland. TURP is a palliative procedure and not a definitive cancer operation.

Chemotherapy

Cytotoxic chemotherapy is largely ineffective in treating prostate cancer. The role of chemotherapy is most commonly reserved for use in hormone refractory disease. Objective responses are uncommon, complete responses are rare, and overall survival is not increased (Catalona, 1994; Maxwell, 1993). The most effective drugs include estramustine, vinblastine, and trimetrexate (Catalona, 1994; Held et al., 1994). Suramin is an investigational agent with an antitumor effect that may be related to its ability to bind to growth-promoting factors, such as interleukin-2, and inhibit their activity (Catalona, 1994; Held et al., 1994). There have been no reports of a complete response to suramin therapy and about a third of patients have had objective responses. The median interval between treatment and the progression of disease was about 6 months, and the median survival was about 1 year (Catalona, 1994).

Radiation Therapy

EXTERNAL BEAM THERAPY

Radiation therapy has been widely used for clinically localized (T1 or T2) disease with 15-year rates of disease-free survival ranging from 45 to 85 percent. Direct comparisons between surgical intervention and definitive irradiation are frequently impossible because of differences between the two populations treated: patients treated with radical prostatectomy are generally younger and healthier and have more well-differentiated tumors than patients treated with radiotherapy. Also, a staging lymphadenectomy is usually performed before prostatectomy to assess nodal status, perhaps the most important prognostic factor in clinically localized prostate cancer (Lee & Hanks, 1995). Because of the lack of randomized trials, comparing reported series is the only way to examine the relative efficacies of each treatment. Lee and Hanks (1995) describe 104 patients treated with radiotherapy in RTOG 7706 protocol who were similar to patients considered to be candidates for radical prostatectomy. Patients had clinical stage T1 or T2 tumors at the time of diagnosis and negative lymphadenectomies before definitive radiotherapy. Ten-year cause-specific survival for these men was 86 percent, and the absolute survival exceeded that of an age-matched population. When comparing this cohort with recent surgical series of similarly staged patients with negative lymphadenectomies, the results are equivalent. Similar to radical prostatectomy, radiation therapy does not cure men with occult metastasis, nor does it consistently eradicate all cancer cells within the treatment field (Catalona, 1994).

External beam irradiation has been the most common management of early prostate cancer (Hanks, 1994). For patients with stage T1 disease, the overall rate of survival with radiation therapy is equivalent to that of the general population. For patients with stage T2 tumors, survival ranges from a rate equivalent to that of the general population to a rate about 20 percent below that of the general population (Catalona, 1994). Patients with clinical T3 lesions are usually treated with radiation therapy because surgical removal of the prostate gland is difficult and gross and microscopic nodal cancer cells are often left behind (Garnick, 1993). Strict comparisons between therapeutic modalities are difficult to make because many patients in all series have not been surgically staged, and due to comorbid conditions were thought to be inappropriate candidates for radical surgery. The overall 10- to 15-year survival, disease-free survival, and cause-specific survival rates are comparable between radical prostatectomy and definitive irradiation (Garnick, 1993).

Zietman and Shipley (1993) analyzed therapeutic approaches for locoregionally confined prostate cancer over the last 30 years. The authors summarize that thus far, randomized trials have raised many questions and answered few. In many cases treatments previously used are now outmoded, and local symptom control and quality of life issues were largely ignored. A sufficient number of large, nonrandomized, prospective studies have been reported to suggest that men over 70 years of age with T1 and T2a well- or moderately differentiated tumors who are initially managed by observation and deferred treatment are unlikely to die from metastatic prostate cancer. However, many physicians and their patients will continue to opt for radical therapy until such a trial defines exactly the subgroups who have little to lose by a conservative policy (Zietman & Shipley, 1993).

RADIOTHERAPY TECHNIQUES

Although several techniques of radiation therapy have been used, the most common is external beam radiation to the prostate gland and periprostatic tissues. Optimal external beam treatment requires accurate knowledge of the target volume and maximal technical efforts to exclude from the high-dose treatment volume as much as possible of the low rectum and proximal anus (Shipley, 1988). Several basic technical principles have been described as important in planning and executing daily treatment. Day-to-day reproducibility of treatment is crucial to the delivery of a homogenous dose to the intended target volume. This may be achieved by using rigid immobilization devices. A planning computer tomographic (CT) scan is a major aid in determining the correct location of the prostate and seminal vesicles as well as other structures that lie within the treatment field. The planning CT should be obtained in the treatment position and include the immobilization device if used. In some centers this planning is achieved by three-dimensional (conformal) computer reconstructions of the prostate and seminal vesicles to more precisely define tumor/target volumes. Dose escalation may be achieved more safely with conformal treatment, with reduced frequency, and grade of toxicities (Hanks, 1994). A retrograde urethrogram, performed at simulation, is an accurate means of identifying the margin of the genitourinary diaphragm which lies approximately 1 cm below the inferior edge of the prostate. Simulation techniques include a cystogram and rectogram for localization of these important structures.

Using the linear accelerator, 62 to 74 Gy is given to the prostatic bed over a period of 7 to 8 weeks in 180 to 200 cGy fractions. Ideally, higher energy (>10 MV) photons are used. A whole or modified pelvic four-field approach is most common with all fields treated daily. Modified pelvic fields include treating the prostate, seminal vesicles, and selected regional lymph nodes such as the iliac nodal chains (Figure 12–3). The boost fields are shaped, as determined by the simulation or planning CT. The goal is to decrease dose to the posterior rectum, proximal anus, bladder, and urethra while treating the primary tumor mass.

BRACHYTHERAPY

Conceptually, brachytherapy offers the advantage of a highly confined radiation dose with a sharp gradient beyond the target volume, thus reducing morbidity. For prostate carcinoma, brachytherapy has been used for definitive treatment, or as a boost following external beam irradiation. Patients preferred for brachytherapy are those presenting with low-volume tumors where extracapsular spread is unlikely. This includes low-grade T1 and early T2a or T2b lesions. Combined treatment of external beam irradiation followed by an iodine-125 or palladium-103 boost may be offered to patients with a larger tumor volume and a higher risk of extraprostatic spread. These are patients with more elevated PSA and higher grade lesions. However, the ability of brachytherapy to improve local tumor control, survival, or morbidity for patients with prostate cancer remains controversial (Blasko et al., 1993).

Early techniques of permanent implants involved the use of iodine-125 seeds and gold-198, and required a surgical procedure for insertion. The doses of radiation were unevenly distributed, with poor results (Catalona, 1994). In the last 10 years, advances have occurred in noninvasive imaging, radioisotope development, and computer-based dosimetry. Permanent implants can now be planned, executed, and evaluated in a more accurate and reproducible manner (Blasko et al., 1993). Newer radioisotopes used in prostate brachytherapy include iridium-192 (temporary) and palladium-103 (permanent). The choice of isotope is primarily based on the grade of the lesion. Gleason scores of 2 to 6/10 are treated with iodine-125 whereas Gleason scores of 7 to 10/10 receive palladium-103. These implants are inserted with the guidance of transrectal ultrasound coupled with rigid template guidance systems, which allow direct visualization without the need for open surgery. Temporary implants generally are removed after 24 to 72 hours. The length of time is determined by the prescribed dose. The long-term outcome of these newer isotope

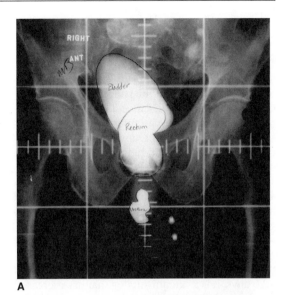

A

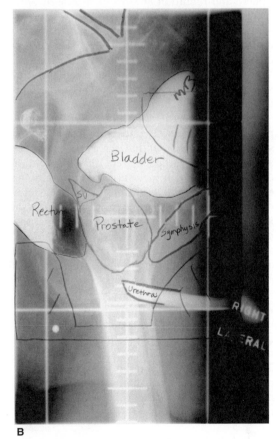

B

Figure 12-3 • Modified pelvic (periprostatic) irradiation treatment fields using a four-field box technique in prostate cancer as shown on simulation films. (A) Anterior and posterior fields (11 × 11 cm). (B) Opposed lateral fields (11 × 10 cm).

implants as compared to conventional external beam treatment is not yet known.

RADIOPHARMACEUTICAL THERAPY

"Bone seeking" systemically administered isotopes are being used in the palliative management of metastatic bone disease. These agents have proven effective for patients who have not responded to hormonal therapy, or whose disease is too widespread for local radiation to achieve pain control (Held et al., 1994). Bone pain in single sites frequently responds to external beam irradiation. For patients with multiple sites of painful bony metastases, hemibody irradiation achieved good palliation but with significant toxicity. An alternative method is the systemic administration of radiopharmaceuticals, such as strontium-89 (Sr-89). Sr-89 is a pure beta emitter with a half-life of 50.6 days. It is a calcium analog that has increased uptake and retention at sites of increased bone metabolism, such as osteoblastic metastatic lesions. Retention of Sr-89 at metastatic sites may be indefinite and substantially longer than the radioactive half-life of the agent (Porter et al., 1993). Thus Sr-89 can deliver therapeutic radiation for several months and can be repeated at 3-month intervals (Kan, 1995).

The mechanism by which Sr-89 produces pain relief is not well understood, but several studies have shown that the decrease in pain is not a placebo effect (Altman & Lee, 1996). One study of 126 patients with metastatic adenocarcinoma of the prostate with multiple bone metastases demonstrated a significant reduction of analgesic intake and sites of new pain, an improvement in physical mobility, and a delay in progression of symptoms in the group receiving local irradiation and strontium-89 versus the group receiving local radiotherapy alone (Porter et al., 1993).

Sr-89 is administered as a single intravenous injection usually as an outpatient procedure. Toxicities include myelosuppression, primarily leukocytes and platelets. An initial flare of bone pain may occur 2 to 3 days after injection and lasts 3 to 4 days. Precautions should be taken by care provider(s) against Sr-89 contamination from the patient's blood or excretions, especially if the patient is incontinent (Kan, 1995).

Bladder

Epidemiology and Risk Factors

Carcinoma of the bladder accounts for approximately 4 percent of cancers in the United States. An estimated 54,500 new cases are predicted for 1997 affecting 39,500 males and 15,000 females. Deaths from bladder cancer are estimated to be 11,700, or 2 percent of all cancer deaths in 1996 (Parker et al., 1996). Bladder cancer is almost two times more common in white men than in African-American men and is seen less commonly in Asian men and rarely in native Americans. The ratio of incidence in whites favors men to women 3 to 1. Most cases occur in men over 50 years of age, with the mean age at diagnosis being 65 years (Pearse, 1994).

Bladder cancers are largely carcinogen-induced (Pearse, 1994). The major risk factors are cigarette smoking, exposure to occupational and environmental toxins including aromatic amines, dyestuffs, organic chemicals and petroleum, rubber, paint, and aluminum. Cigarette smoking is the most important known preventable cause of bladder cancer. The risk correlates with the number of cigarettes per day, inhalation, and the duration of abuse. It is estimated that cigarette smoking alone accounts for 50 percent of bladder tumors in men and 30 percent in women (Pearse, 1994). There is a high incidence of squamous cell carcinoma of the bladder in Egypt that is linked to exposure to the parasite *Schistosoma haematobium*. Ingestion of other physical agents, such as coffee, alcohol, saccharin, and phenacetin, has been weakly linked to bladder cancer. None of these agents has consistently been related to bladder cancer incidence in humans (Lind et al., 1993).

Clinical Presentation

It is estimated that 70 to 80 percent of patients present with symptoms of gross, painless hematuria. Symptoms of vesical irritability such as pain, frequency, and urgency occur in 25 percent of patients. Up to 20 percent of patients are asymptomatic with the diagnosis made during evaluation of microscopic hematuria or pyuria (Pearse, 1994). Patients may present with manifestations of advanced local disease such as bladder neck obstruction or flank pain due to hydronephrosis as a result of ureteral obstruction.

Diagnosis and Staging

Cystoscopy is usually the first diagnostic procedure for patients presenting with unexplained hematuria and severe irritative voiding symptoms. A cystoscopic examination allows tumor visualization, an opportunity for tumor biopsy and selected mucosal biopsies, and resection of the lesion. The goal of biopsy is to obtain a histologic diagnosis and determine the presence or absence of muscular invasion. A bimanual examination, usually done under anesthesia, may detect tumor extension.

The purpose of staging in bladder cancer is to identify evidence of extravesical involvement. A staging evaluation is based upon the common sites of tumor spread, which include perivesical infiltration, regional lymph nodes, and dissemination to bone, lung, and liver. Appropriate tests include cystoscopy (as previously described), liver function studies, intravenous pyelography (IVP), chest radiograph, and computerized axial tomography (CT) of the abdomen and pelvis. The role of other imaging modalities such as transurethral ultrasound and magnetic resonance imaging (MRI) have yet to be defined.

Clinical staging systems for bladder cancer are seen in Table 12–4. The TNM classification is correlated with the Jewett-Strong findings and Marshall's modifications. The most important determinant for treatment is the presence or absence of muscle invasion. The depth of muscular

Table 12-4 • A Comparison of the Marshall-Jewett and TNM System in the Classification of Bladder Cancer

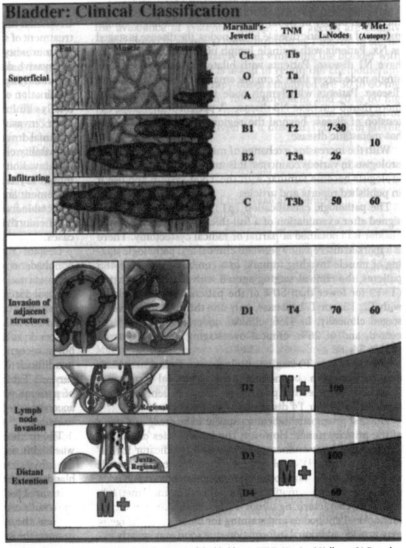

From Fair WR, Fuks ZY, Scher HI (1993). Cancer of the bladder. In VT DeVita Jr., S Hellman, SA Rosenberg (Eds.), *Cancer: Principles & Practice of Oncology* (pp. 1052–1072). Philadelphia: JB Lippincott. Used with permission.

invasion is the best indicator for risk of pelvic node involvement and systemic disease, and ultimately for survival.

Pathologic Classification

The bladder and upper urinary tract are lined with transitional epithelium, and 90 percent of all primary bladder neoplasms are transitional cell carcinomas. Dysplastic changes in the transitional epithelium are associated with the tendency to develop multiple and recurrent tumors. Due to the tendency toward multicentricity of transitional cell tumors, bladder biopsies are performed on suspicious areas as well as on normal appearing epithelium (Pearse, 1994).

Squamous cell carcinoma accounts for 7 percent of bladder tumors. These tumors tend to be large, solitary, and sessile and are associated with urinary tract infections, stones, and obstruction. Squamous cell carcinomas are the most prevalent form of bladder cancers in patients with schistosomiasis and are slightly more common in women.

Adenocarcinomas of the bladder account for only 2 percent of all primary bladder epithelial tumors. They may develop in any location of the bladder, but usually occur in the dome in association with remnants of the urachus (Pearse, 1994).

Tumor grade, or degree of cell differentiation, is not considered in staging but is a factor considered in treatment selection. The grades of bladder cancer are described as I to IV, with IV being the least well differentiated and with the poorest prognosis. Survival described as a function of grade and level of invasion is seen in Table 12–5.

Other pathologic diagnostic studies include urinary cytology and flow cytometry. Cytology is obtained by voided specimen or through saline bladder irrigation. Flow cytometry is a technique used to examine the DNA content of urine cells. It has been useful in providing prognostic information beyond grading and staging. Aneuploidy, or an abnormal amount of DNA per cell, is an indication of high-grade, high-stage transitional cell tumors (Lind et al., 1993).

Treatment Options

The selection of treatment options for patients with bladder cancer is dictated primarily by the presence or absence of muscle invasion and grade of the tumor.

Noninvasive Bladder Cancer

Superficial tumors of the bladder (clinical stage Ta, T1, Tis) remain in the epithelium and lamina propria. Approximately 70 to 80 percent of patients with newly diagnosed bladder cancer have superficial tumors. They are most often initially treated by transurethral resection of the bladder (TURB) and fulguration.

If multiple superficial tumors are found, or if they recur after TURB, intravesical chemotherapy is often administered. Chemotherapy is therapeutic in ablating superficial tumors and in delaying or preventing tumor recurrences. Due to the diffuse pattern of carcinoma in situ (Tis) intravesical therapy is frequently used in these patients. The effective intravesical agents include thiotepa, mitomycin-C, doxorubicin, VM-26, and bacillus Calmette-Guerin (BCG). BCG has been shown to be the most effective intravesical agent for Tis.

Intravesical drugs are instilled into the bladder through a urethral catheter and retained for up to 2 hours. Treatment is most often given weekly for 6 doses. Complete responses of up to 79 percent, reduction in rate of relapse, and prolonged disease-free survival have been reported (Lind et al., 1993). At the completion of therapy, patients are followed at regular intervals with urine cytology and cystoscopy.

Noninvasive tumors may be treated by other conservative (bladder-sparing) techniques including external beam irradiation, interstitial and intraoperative irradiation, and laser therapy. The high recurrence rate after initial therapy (40 to 80 percent) for superficial tumors warrants investigation of new methods to improve disease control (Pearse, 1994).

Invasive (Muscle Invading) Bladder Cancer

For patients with invasive bladder carcinoma (clinical stage T2, T3, T4a) no treatment is consistently successful or without morbidity and complications. The treatment of patients with invasive bladder cancer is undergoing dramatic change, incorporating many potentially effective and complementary therapies from several disciplines, including transurethral resection (TUR),

Table 12-5 • Survival as a Function of Grade and Depth of Invasion in Patients with Bladder Cancer

Grade	Survival (%)	Depth of Invasion	Survival (%)
1 and 2 (low-grade)	70–85	Ta, T1 (noninvasive)	60–85
3 and 4 (high-grade)	35–40	T2, T3 (invasive)	30–60

From Pearse HD (1994). The urinary bladder. In JD Cox (Ed.), *Moss' Radiation Oncology, Rationale, Technique, Results* (p. 529). St. Louis: Mosby. Used with permission.

cystectomy with continent urinary diversion, systemic chemotherapy, and irradiation.

SURGICAL INTERVENTION

Radical cystectomy has been the conventional treatment of muscle-invasive bladder cancer in the United States for the past two decades. Radical cystectomy includes removal of the bladder, prostate, and seminal vesicles in men, and the uterus, ovaries, fallopian tubes, urethra, and proximal vagina in women. Urinary diversion has traditionally been accomplished by ileal conduit. The disadvantages of reflux, having to wear a urostomy appliance, and impotence have been addressed with the more recent use of several continent, antirefluxing procedures and in selected patients preservation of the neurovascular bundles to maintain potency (Pearse, 1994).

Nodal metastasis found at pelvic lymphadenectomy is associated with poor survival. Five-year actuarial survival rates of 25 to 36 percent are reported in selected patients undergoing *meticulous* lymph node resection (Pearse, 1994).

Radical cystectomy is associated with excellent local control of the primary tumor, but has a high probability of subsequent distant metastases approaching 50 percent, generally occurring within 2 years of diagnosis. Thus, the question has been raised whether incorporating chemotherapy into treatment plans can reduce the rate of distant metastases and improve survival.

CHEMOTHERAPEUTIC INTERVENTION

Combination chemotherapy, given in the adjuvant and neoadjuvant settings, has been used to treat both advanced local tumors in the bladder and metastatic disease, with encouraging results reported for several series of patients (Kaufman et al., 1993). The chemotherapeutic agents most active against bladder carcinoma are cisplatin and methotrexate, with doxorubicin and vinblastine also demonstrating activity. Based on single-agent responses, combination therapy was developed that incorporated these four drugs and is now the most frequently used regimen (M-VAC).

Multiagent chemotherapy produces complete responses of 28 to 50 percent and partial responses of 21 to 28 percent (Held & Volpe, 1991). The pathologic complete response rate to neoadjuvant multiagent chemotherapy is in the range of 22 to 43 percent. This span of response demonstrates the need for definitive local therapy. In selected patients, treatment has been accomplished with cystectomy or irradiation. Cystectomy, usually recommended for deeply invasive tumors,

eliminates understaging error and the possibility of new bladder tumor formation (Pearse, 1994). Although systemic chemotherapy used as an adjuvant to radical cystectomy delays the appearance of recurrent disease, it has no established effect on overall survival (Kaufman et al., 1993).

DEFINITIVE RADIOTHERAPY

The goal of definitive radiotherapy is to preserve bladder function and optimize local and systemic control of disease. Despite the use of modern megavoltage equipment coupled with precise simulation and treatment techniques, local tumor control is achieved in only 50 percent of patients with muscle-invading tumors, and 5-year survival rates of 20 to 40 percent are less than optimal (Pearse, 1994). It should be noted that although radiation therapy is curative only in a minority of patients, many have limited survival due to multiple comorbid conditions that render them unsuitable for combined therapy or cystectomy alone.

To improve local and systemic disease, investigators began to look at combined modality regimens. In the 1980s, several studies indicated that selected patients with invasive bladder cancer could be successfully treated by TURB alone or in combination with radiotherapy with or without cisplatin. Two large randomized trials showed no significant advantage to immediate cystectomy as compared with cystectomy deferred until a recurrence after external-beam irradiation (Kaufman et al., 1993). Bladder-sparing definitive treatment for selected patients with invasive disease using combination radiotherapy and chemotherapy can be based on the following:

- Radical cystectomy is not curative in more than 50 percent of patients, mainly because of the appearance of distant metastases
- A thorough TURB of the primary tumor is important in any approach to sparing the bladder
- Maintaining bladder function after combined treatment with cisplatin and radiation is feasible
- Radiation combined with cisplatin is more effective against the primary tumor than radiation alone
- Multiagent chemotherapy combining cisplatin, methotrexate, and vinblastine with doxorubicin is significantly more effective than single-agent chemotherapy in terms of both the response rate and survival of patients with advanced bladder cancer (Kaufman et al., 1993).

Favorable prognostic factors in patients selected for definitive radiotherapy include stage T2 or T3a, solitary tumor without associated carcinoma in situ, papillary surface histology, absence of ureteral obstruction, grossly complete TURB, younger age, and good Karnofsky status (Pearse, 1994).

RADIOTHERAPEUTIC TECHNIQUES

Treatment planning is accomplished at simulation. This requires contrast inserted into the rectum and bladder to delineate these structures. Patients are treated with opposed anterior/posterior fields and opposed lateral fields. Each field is treated daily. The patient is instructed to void prior to daily therapy.

A four-field pelvic field with shaped corner blocks is the most frequent technique. The fields ensure coverage of iliac chains and obturator nodes and prostatic urethra. The anterior and posterior fields are shaped with symmetric inferior corner blocks that shield the medial border of the femoral heads. Corner blocks are used to block the abdominal wall superiorly and anal canal posteriorly (Pearse, 1994). See Figure 12–4. The cone-down boost is accomplished with a four-field approach or paired lateral fields.

Selection of total radiation dose may vary due to multiple factors that include the clinical stage, tumor volume, and the patient's medical condition. Most commonly, the radiation prescription will deliver 50.4 Gy in 5 to 6 weeks at 180 cGy fractions to the whole pelvis. Following this, a cone-down boost to the tumor volume (excluding normal bladder if possible) is given to a final dose of 64.8 to 68.4 Gy in 180 cGy fractions in a total of 7 to 8 weeks (Pearse, 1994).

In patients that receive concomitant chemotherapy, most often cisplatin, the treatment schema may be altered. A smaller four-field box technique is used to a dose of 45 Gy in 180 cGy fractions. At this point, evaluation of the tumor status is performed and depending upon findings, the patient will receive consolidation irradiation with a boost of 1980 cGy, to a total dose of 64.8 Gy to a modified pelvic field.

PERIOPERATIVE RADIOTHERAPY

There has been considerable debate about preoperative irradiation as an adjunct to cystectomy for invasive bladder cancer. One benefit is the downstaging of tumor to facilitate cystectomy. Parsons and Million (1988) reported a 15 to 20 percent survival advantage with preoperative irradiation when all comparable clinical series were reviewed.

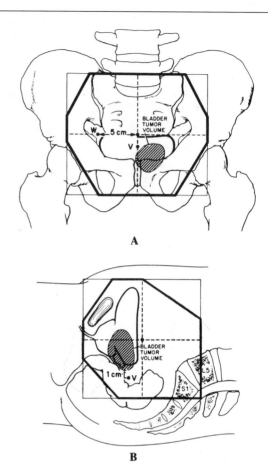

Figure 12-4 • Radiation treatment fields to the bladder tumor volume and pelvic lymph nodes for 4–25 MV x rays with an isocentric contoured four-field box technique. Fields are treated to 40–45 Gy and followed by a boost to the bladder tumor volume to approximately 65Gy. (A) Anterior and posterior fields. (B) Paired lateral fields. From Shipley WU (1988). Genitourinary cancer. In CC Wang (Ed.), *Clinical Radiation Oncology Indications, Techniques, and Results* (pp. 262–290). Littleton, MA: PSG Publishing.

However, overall comparable results of radical cystectomy versus radiotherapy plus cystectomy, fail to demonstrate a statistically significant survival benefit from such combined treatment.

Postoperative irradiation has not been adequately tested in patients with invasive bladder cancer, in part because of concern that radiation-induced complications following radical surgery would be excessive (Pearse, 1994).

INTERSTITIAL IRRADIATION

Brachytherapy in bladder cancer provides a means of administering a high dose of radiation to the tumor while sparing normal tissue. This method of irradiation should not be used alone with a curative intent except in superficial lesions involving limited areas. It is impractical to implant a tumor larger than 5 cm in diameter, and multiple-plane and volume implants are difficult in the bladder. Implants are most often performed on Stage T1 and T2 tumors, and T3 tumors (<5 cm) in conjunction with external beam irradiation. Poor prognostic indicators are T3 tumors, multiple TURBs, abnormal IVP, and a sessile or undifferentiated tumor. Despite good local control after implantation, there is an increase in distant failure associated with increasing stage (Pearse, 1994).

Treatment for Disseminated Bladder Cancer

Systemic chemotherapy has been used with limited success in metastatic bladder cancer. One of the most active regimens is methotrexate, vinblastine, doxorubicin, and cisplatin (M-VAC). This regimen has shown an improved response rate compared with single-agent cisplatin, but at the expense of increased toxicity. The overall response rate can be as high as 72 percent, however, the median survival is approximately 12 months, even in patients having resection of a residual mass after chemotherapy (Pearse, 1994).

Local radiation is useful in palliation of pain for patients with bony metastases. Osseous metastases are rarely solitary and respond slowly to irradiation. Approximately 50 percent of patients will obtain significant palliation of pain. Palliative radiation may use 50 Gy with conventional fractionation, 40 Gy in 3 to 4 weeks, 30 Gy in 2 weeks, and 15 to 25 Gy in 1 week (Pearse, 1994). The patient's overall condition and performance status will determine the most appropriate dose schedule.

Radiotherapy can also be effective in controlling pain and hematuria in patients with ulcerated and unresectable primary tumor lesions. Other local measures used to control bleeding are endoscopic resection and fulguration, arterial embolization, hyperthermia, intravesical instillations, and hydrostatic tamponade (Pearse, 1994). Local irritative symptoms can be made worse by radiotherapy.

Testis

Testicular cancer is a germ cell malignancy and one of the most successfully treated solid tumors. This is largely because of the development of effective chemotherapy for nonseminomatous cancers, utilization of tumor markers to monitor disease status, and new imaging techniques for staging and cancer detection. The majority of men diagnosed with testis cancer can look forward to long-term survival and cure.

Epidemiology and Risk Factors

The American Cancer Society estimates 7,200 new cases of testicular cancer in the 1997 and 350 deaths (Parker et al., 1997). Testis cancer is the most common solid tumor found in men between the ages of 15 and 35 years in the United States. It is much more common in whites (4.4 per 100,000 population per year) than in African-Americans (0.5 per 100,000 population per year). It is also slightly more common in an identical twin or a family member of a patient with a testis tumor than in men without a family history of the disease (Hussey, 1994).

Testis cancer is potentially curable even when diagnosed in advanced stage. Five-year survival rates for all stages combined are approximately 90 percent. More than 50 percent of patients are diagnosed with stage I disease confined to the testis, and approximately 15 percent are diagnosed with advanced disease in the abdomen or above the diaphragm. Germ cell tumors are usually rapidly progressive diseases necessitating early diagnosis and prompt treatment (Brock et al., 1993).

Cryptorchidism remains the best documented risk factor for the development of germ-cell tumors. A 10- to 40-fold increased risk of developing testicular cancer in the undescended testis has been reported, with an estimated 7 to 10 percent of all cases having a history of cryptorchidism (Hussey, 1994). It has been suggested that elevated temperature or atrophy contribute to risk of the disease. However, 25 percent of the cancers found in association with cryptorchidism occur in the contralateral normally descended testis, which suggests that a developmental defect is responsible for both the maldescent and the tumor. The risk of a man with cryptorchidism developing testicular cancer is directly related to the degree of maldescent: 1 in 20 if the testis is intraabdominal and 1 in 80 if it is within the inguinal canal (Hussey, 1994).

An increased incidence of testicular cancer has been linked to exogenous estrogens given to women as birth control pills or as diethylstilbestrol (DES) given to prevent spontaneous abortion. This increased risk ranges from 2.8 to 5.3 over the expected incidence in the male children of women exposed to DES, estrogen, or estrogen-progestin combinations (Lind et al., 1993).

Few (1 to 3 percent) testicular cancers occur bilaterally and may also occur synchronously or metachronously. Second testicular primaries have been noted up to 15 years later (Hussey, 1994).

Clinical Presentation

The most common presenting symptom of testicular cancer is a painless, firm scrotal enlargement. Often the mass or swelling is discovered accidentally. Low back pain associated with enlarged retroperitoneal nodes may occur. The patient may present with supraclavicular masses, cough, shortness of breath, and chest pain due to disseminated disease. Gynecomastia may also be evident.

Diagnosis and Staging

Diagnosis is made by radical inguinal orchiectomy. The rationale for this approach is that the lymphatic drainage of the testis is along its vascular supply to nodes in the retroperitoneum. Thus spillage of tumor is kept to a minimum because the primary tumor is distant from the incision site (Brock et al., 1993). Once the diagnosis is confirmed the patient will undergo staging work-up. Patients may be staged clinically on the basis of laboratory and radiographic findings, and/or pathologically on the basis of surgical results.

Initial physical examination includes palpation of the testes, abdomen, breasts, and supraclavicular regions for masses or enlargement. A nontransilluminating, firm, diffuse intratesticular mass should be considered cancer until proven otherwise. Diagnostic procedures include CT scans of chest, abdomen, and pelvis, chest radiograph, testicular ultrasound, and intravenous pyelogram. Pedal lymphangiography is useful in detecting lymph node metastases as small as 5 to 7 mm. However, because lymphangiography is not readily available in many institutions, investigators are relying on CT to evaluate patients for retroperitoneal nodal metastases. CT will detect nodes 1.5 to 2.0 cm or larger. Controversy remains regarding the use of lymphangiography for initial staging for testicular cancer patients. See Table 12–6 for AJCC staging systems for testicular cancer.

Initial laboratory studies should include CBC, chemistry profile with liver function studies, urinalysis, and biologic tumor markers, such as human chorionic gonadotropin and alphafetoprotein.

Biologic Markers

Serum marker proteins for testis tumors are an important part of the clinical assessment of disease status, and are used to monitor disease status and

Table 12-6 • TNM Staging for Cancer of the Testicle

PRIMARY TUMOR (T)
The extent of primary tumor is classified after radical orchiectomy

pTx	Primary tumor cannot be assessed (if no radical orchiectomy has been performed, Tx is used)
pT0	No evidence of primary tumor (e.g., histologic scar in testis)
pTis	Intratubular tumor: preinvasive cancer
pT1	Tumor limited to testis, including rete testis
pT2	Tumor invades beyond the tunica albuginea or into the epididymis
pT3	Involvement of the spermatic cord
pT4	Tumor invades the scrotum

REGIONAL LYMPH NODES (N)
NX	Regional lymph nodes cannot be assessed
N0	No regional lymph node metastasis
N1	Metastasis in a single lymph node, ≤ 2 cm in greatest dimension
N2	Metastasis in a single lymph node, >2 cm but ≤ 5 cm in greatest dimension; or multiple lymph nodes, none >5 cm in greatest dimension
N3	Metastasis in a lymph node >5 cm in greatest dimension

DISTANT METASTASIS (M)
MX	Presence of distant metastasis cannot be assessed
M0	No distant metastasis
M1	Distant metastasis

STAGE GROUPING
Stage 0	pTis	N0	M0
Stage I	Any pT	N0	M0
Stage II	Any pT	N1	M0
	Any pT	N2	M0
	Any pT	N3	M0
Stage III	Any pT	Any N	M1

From American Joint Committee on Cancer (1992). *Manual for staging of cancer* (4th ed.). Philadelphia: JB Lippincott. Used with permission.

response to therapy. The most sensitive and specific markers are alphafetoprotein (AFP) and the beta subunit of human chorionic gonadotropin (HCG). AFP and HCG are not normally detectable in adults, therefore any elevation should raise suspicion of a germ cell malignancy. (See Table 12–7.) Serum marker proteins should be obtained

Table 12-7 • Tumor Markers in Testicular Cancer

Histology	HCG	AFP
Seminoma	+/–	–
Embryonal carcinoma	+	+
Choriocarcinoma	+	–
Teratoma	–	–
Yolk sac	–	+

both prior to and after orchiectomy for assessment of the efficacy of removal of the primary tumor. The metabolic half-life of AFP is approximately 5 days and the half-life of HCG is estimated at 16 to 24 hours. The rate of disappearance of elevated tumor markers is useful in determining response to therapy. A postorchiectomy specimen should be obtained after sufficient time has elapsed to allow for metabolism of markers present at the time of orchiectomy.

HCG levels can also be elevated in patients who use marijuana and in a variety of nontesticular malignancies, such as stomach, pancreas, liver, and breast cancer. False positive elevation of AFP is rare. Abnormal HCG titers are found in 42 to 60 percent of patients with nonseminomatous testicular tumors and in 7 to 10 percent of those with pure seminomas (Hussey, 1994). Elevated AFP levels are not found in patients with pure seminomas or choriocarcinomas, and therefore any patient with a pathologic diagnosis of pure seminoma and an elevated AFP titer should be considered to have a mixed tumor.

Initial elevated markers are useful for determining the response to therapy and for following patients for disease progression. The rate of disappearance of elevated tumor markers is useful in monitoring response to treatment with HCG the most clinically helpful. A commonly used guideline is that a 10-fold decrease in the HCG level over a 3-week period is consistent with successful chemotherapy treatment. Less steep declines of HCG levels correlate with the emergence of drug-resistant disease. Reappearance of marker elevation often precedes the radiographic documentation of recurrent disease and is invaluable in detecting early relapse (Brock et al., 1993). Elevated HCG and/or AFP titers after orchiectomy usually indicate metastatic disease. Normal levels do not ensure that metastatic disease is not present because false negative results occur in 15 to 30 percent of patients (Hussey, 1994).

Other clinical markers are alkaline phosphatase that is elevated in 85 to 90 percent of patients with active seminoma, but can be falsely elevated in smokers, and serum lactic acid dehydrogenase (LDH) elevation that correlates with bulk of disease.

Pathologic Classification

Approximately 95 percent of testicular tumors arise in the primordial germ cell which is a multipotent stem cell. The multipotent cell can produce a variety of cell lines, which explains why a primary testicular cancer can have multiple histologic patterns. The remaining 5 percent of testicular cancers are stromal tumors (e.g., melanomas, rhabdomyosarcomas) or metastatic foci of other tumors such as lymphomas and leukemias (Davis, 1994; Hussey, 1994).

When a primordial germ cell is fertilized, it almost immediately divides into two groups of cells: (1) the extraembryonic or trophoblastic cells, and (2) the embryonic or somatic cells. The primordial germ cell has the capacity to differentiate either into an aggressive and invasive cell, the trophoblast, or into somatic cells, which develop into mature tissues and organs. Germ cell tumors can develop anywhere along this pathway (Hussey, 1994). (See Figure 12–5.)

Testicular cancer cell types are classified in terms of embryonal tissue (seminoma versus nonseminoma). This distinction is important because it influences treatment selection. Seminomas originate from the germinal epithelium of the seminiferous tubules. However, the origin of nonseminomatous tumors is more controversial. Most investigators believe that nonseminomatous cancer originates from the totipotential primordial germ cells (Hussey, 1994).

Histopathologically seminomas tend to have a uniform appearance. They comprise 35 to 40 percent of testicular malignancies. There are three types of seminoma: classic, anaplastic, and spermatocytic. Nonseminomatous malignancies, 55 to 60 percent of diagnoses, are of primarily 6 types: embryonal, choriocarcinoma, teratoma, teratocarcinoma, yolk sac, and non-germ cell tumors. (See Table 12–8.)

Treatment Options

Significant advances in the treatment of testicular cancer over the past 15 years have made this one of the most curable malignancies. Overall relative 5-year survival rates are in excess of 90 percent. Although the incidence of testicular cancer has risen 50 percent since 1970, the mortality rate for this disease has declined by more than 60 percent during the same period (Hussey, 1994).

Treatment of Seminoma Tumors

Pure seminomas are exquisitely radiosensitive and are characterized by an orderly pattern of metastasis. Even massive seminomas can be effectively treated by relatively low doses of irradiation. Relapse-free survival rates with orchiectomy and regional lymphatic irradiation are estimated to be 95 percent for stage I and 80 percent for stage II (Hussey, 1994). Prognostic factors in seminoma

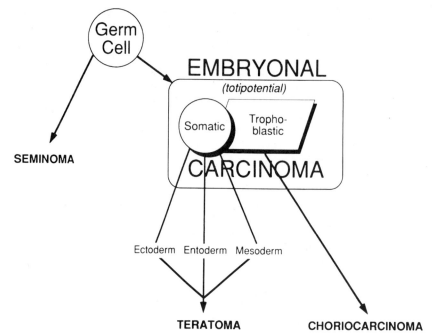

Figure 12-5 • Diagram illustrating the histogenesis of germ cell tumors of the testis. From Hussey DH (1994). The testicle. In JD Cox (Ed.), *Moss' Radiation Oncology Rationale, Technique, Results* (7th ed). (pp. 559–586). St. Louis: Mosby.

include stage of disease at presentation, bulk of disease, postoperative elevation of HCG, and spermatic cord involvement (Dosmann & Zagars, 1993).

Patients with stage I disease are most commonly treated with radical orchiectomy followed by regional lymphatic irradiation. Radical or-

Table 12-8 • Distribution and Characteristics of Testicular Cancers

Histology (%)	Characteristics
SEMINOMA (35–40)	
Classic (85)	Very radiosensitive
Anaplastic (10)	Does not appear to have worse prognosis
Spermatocytic (<10)	Rare, seen in patients >60 yrs
NONSEMINOMA (55–60)	
Embryonal (20)	Highly malignant, anaplastic
Teratocarcinoma (40)	Combination embryonal/ teratoma
Yolk sac (25)	Most common in children, poor prognosis in adults
Teratoma (5–10)	More aggressive in adults
Choriocarcinoma (1)	Associated with widespread dissemination
NON-GERM CELL TUMORS (10) Leydig cell, Sertoli cell, gonadoblastoma	Rare, ~10% malignant

chiectomy is considered a diagnostic procedure as well as the first phase of treatment. The procedure includes removal of the involved testis, epididymis, a portion of the vas deferens, and portions of the gonadal lymphatics and blood supply. The remaining testis undergoes hyperplasia and produces enough testosterone to maintain sexual capacity, sexual characteristics, and libido (Lind et al., 1993).

The characteristic paired anterior and posterior irradiation fields used in treating seminoma are seen in Figure 12–6. The lateral boundaries include the ipsilateral external iliac nodes, bilateral common iliacs, and paracaval and paraaortic nodes with a margin of at least 2 cm. The ipsilateral renal hilum is included with a more generous margin with left-sided than with right-sided tumors. If there has been scrotal violation, orchiopexy or other inguinal surgery extension of the radiation field should be considered to include these areas. Also included is gonadal shielding to prevent the majority of externally scattered photons from hitting the remaining testicle (Shipley, 1988; Hussey, 1994). The most common fractionation is 25 Gy in 150 cGy fractions for 5 days each week.

There is controversy regarding radiotherapy versus surveillance after radical orchiectomy for patients with stage I seminoma. Proponents of

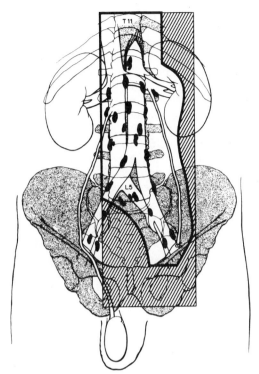

Figure 12-6 • Contoured anterior and posterior radiation treatment fields for clinical stage I or IIA left testicular cancer. The diagonally shaded area is an individually made 8 cm thick cerrobend block. From Shipley WU (1988). Genitourinary cancer. In CC Wang, (Ed.), *Clinical Radiation Oncology Indications, Techniques, and Results* (pp. 262–290). Littleton: PSG Publishing.

surveillance cite that only 15 to 20 percent of patients with stage I seminoma will relapse due to occult retroperitoneal metastasis, and therefore 80 to 85 percent of patients are needlessly irradiated (Stein et al., 1993). Relapses in patients with stage I testicular seminoma tend to occur later, sometimes more than 3 years after orchiectomy, in contrast to nonseminomatous germ cell tumors in which approximately 80 percent of relapses occur during the first year (Stein et al., 1993). It is also argued that relapsed patients can be successfully salvaged with radiotherapy and chemotherapy. The risk and concerns about impaired fertility are reasons for postorchidectomy surveillance in stage I seminoma, and is a therapeutic option for those patients not wishing to receive radiation. Surveillance is costly since repeated abdomino-pelvic CT scans at six-month intervals are required for several years (Thomas, 1994). A carefully conducted surveillance program requires an adherent patient. While mortality does not seem to be increased by using surveillance, long-term data are

required to decide whether the morbidity of increased relapse and salvage chemotherapy will be offset by the reduced application of radiotherapy (Abdeen et al., 1992; Hussey, 1994).

Stage IIA seminoma is treated with subdiaphragmatic radiation portals as in stage I. The dose is increased to 30 Gy and often followed by a boost to 35 Gy to involved nodes. There is considerable debate regarding the extension of radiation fields to include the uninvolved mediastinal/supraclavicular regions due to the usually orderly pattern of lymphatic spread. One argument against prophylactic mediastinal or supraclavicular radiation therapy in these patients is based on data that they have poor tolerance to chemotherapy and inferior outcome should they relapse after irradiation. Some investigators conclude mediastinal irradiation does not seem to influence overall outcome in stage IIA seminoma and is probably not necessary (Abdeen et al., 1992). However, there are data to suggest a relationship between the size of the largest abdominal metastasis and the risk of mediastinal or supraclavicular failure (Speer et al., 1995).

There is controversy regarding the optimal management of patients presenting with stage IIB disease. In patients with masses >10 cm, relapse rates are higher and it is argued that they should receive chemotherapy as the prime modality. In patients with abdominal disease measuring 5 to 10 cm in size, radiation may be used alone with chemotherapy reserved for relapse (Hussey, 1994).

Patients presenting with stage III nodally confined disease usually receive cisplatin based chemotherapy as the primary therapeutic regimen, with reported cure rates in excess of 90 percent (Brock et al., 1993). Radiotherapy can also be used initially for treatment of massive retroperitoneal disease (stage IIIB). Irradiation consists of abdominal portals followed by a boost to the clinically involved areas within the abdomen. The mediastinum and supraclavicular fossa may be treated adjuvantly.

Patients presenting with disseminated disease in sites such as lung and bone fare less well, but can have a 60 to 80 percent cure rate with cisplatin-based chemotherapeutic regimens (Brock et al., 1993). It is recommended that patients with bulky disease and any seminoma with an elevated AFP should receive primary chemotherapy.

Treatment of Nonseminoma Tumors

Patients with nonseminomatous tumors are treated initially with a radical orchiectomy. Treatment after orchiectomy depends on clinical and patho-logical staging of disease and biologic tumor marker levels. Radical retroperitoneal lymph node dissection (RPLND) has been the classic therapy for pathologic staging of nonseminomatous disease, and for removal of all nodes involving lymphatic drainage to the testis. This procedure is usually a modified bilateral resection. Many autonomic nerves necessary for erectile potency and for ejaculation are located in the area, therefore ejaculatory ability may be altered, even if erectile potency is maintained. Due to very positive results with cisplatin-based chemotherapy, surveillance programs are more commonly used in patients with negative RPLND (Davis, 1994).

Patients with nodal metastasis at surgery or who have persistently elevated biologic tumor markers postoperatively receive chemotherapy with cisplatin-based regimens. Although radiation therapy does not play a major role in the initial treatment of patients with nonseminomatous cancers, it may be used for patients who have persistent disease after chemotherapy or who require palliation for metastatic disease (Hussey, 1994).

Salvage Therapy

Patients with germ cell tumors that relapse from complete remission are candidates for salvage therapy. The therapeutic results with salvage chemotherapeutic regimens have not been as dramatic as those with initial therapy, primarily because of the lack of active agents for patients refractory to cisplatin. Salvage regimens include ifosfamide and high-dose cisplatin plus either VP-16 or vinblastine as third-line or fourth-line therapy. Durable remissions up to 34 months have been reported. High-dose chemotherapy with autologous bone marrow transplantation has been investigated in patients with refractory germ cell tumors (Brock et al., 1993).

Penis

Epidemiology and Risk Factors

Carcinoma of the penis is a rare disease in the United States accounting for 2 to 5 percent of all urogenital malignancies and less than 1 percent of all cancer deaths in male patients (Pedrick et al., 1993; Fair et al., 1993b). Tumors of the penis are a significant clinical problem in populations in which circumcision is not a common practice and personal hygiene is lacking. Most patients are over 50 years of age.

The risk of penile carcinoma correlates strongly with the existence of a foreskin and the irritative effects of smegma combined with the products of poor hygiene within the preputial sac. The annual age adjusted incidence of carcinoma of the penis in the United States is only 1 per 100,000, while the lifetime risk of penile cancer developing in uncircumcised males may be as high as 1 in 600 (Fair et al., 1993b).

There are no firm data to support the association of penile carcinoma with cervical carcinoma in sexual partners, number of sexual partners, herpetic infection, or sexually transmitted disease (Fair et al., 1993b).

Premalignant lesions of the penis have been identified that include leukoplakia, erythroplasia of Queyrat, carcinoma in situ (Bowen's disease), balanitis xerotica obliterans, and condyloma acuminatum giganticum (Buschke-Lowenstein tumor). Controversy exists as to the treatment of these lesions (Persky & deKernion, 1986).

Clinical Presentation

The most common presenting symptom of penile cancer is a mass or a persistent sore or ulcer on the glans or foreskin. Most lesions are painless, and there may be significant ulceration and bleeding (Fair et al., 1993b). Patients may present with locally advanced lesions, groin adenopathy, and significant anemia secondary to bleeding from the lesion. Urethral obstruction is uncommon.

Pathology

Most penile cancers are squamous cell carcinoma. Basal cell carcinomas and melanoma of the penis are both extremely rare.

Diagnosis and Staging

Diagnosis is made by incisional or preferably excisional biopsy. Work-up includes physical examination to determine extent of local invasion and inguinal lymph node status. Imaging studies to evaluate pelvic and abdominal lymph nodes is done by CT or MRI.

The clinical staging systems for penile cancer are shown in Figure 12–7, which correlates the TNM system with the Jackson staging system.

Treatment Options

Treatment options range from local excision to radical penectomy; or radiation therapy using external beam treatment or brachytherapy with surgery reserved for salvage. The best management of the primary lesion is controversial due

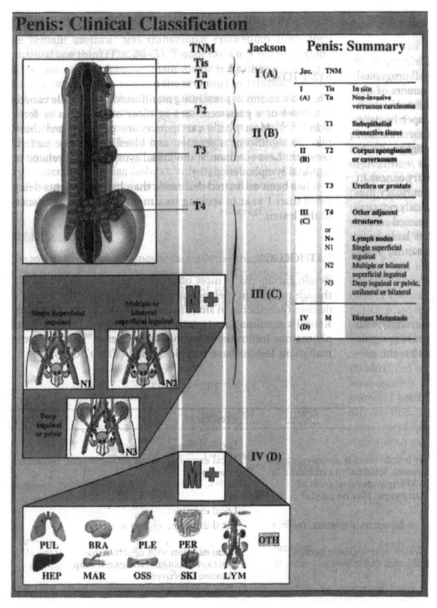

Figure 12-7 • Clinical classification of penile cancer. (From Fair WR, Fuks ZY & Scher HE (1993). Cancer of the urethra and penis. In VT DeVita Jr., S Hellman & SA Rosenberg (Eds.), *Cancer: Principles & Practice of Oncology* (4th ed.), (pp. 1114–1125). Philadelphia: JB Lippincott.)

to the lack of controlled clinical trials in this rare disease.

Surgery

Surgery involves removal of the lesion with adequate margins to minimize the risk of local recurrence. Partial or total penectomy is indicated depending upon the size of the lesion, level of invasion, and location on the shaft. Total penectomy with excision of both corpora and creation

of a perineal urethrostomy is performed for extensive lesions approaching the base of the shaft.

The incidence of false positive lymph nodes on clinical examination averages 40 percent because of the association of inflammatory inguinal lymphadenopathy associated with ulcerated or infected penile lesions. Clinical assessment of the lymph nodes should be delayed until after a 4 to 6 week course of antibiotics. Overall, 40 to 50 percent of patients with positive inguinal nodes can be rendered disease free by surgical resection. The significant morbidity that may accompany groin dissection and the lack of controlled prospective studies to document the benefit of early "prophylactic" versus late "therapeutic" groin dissection has led many surgeons to delay lymphadenectomy until clinical evidence of lymph node involvement occurs (Fair et al., 1993b). The most common surgical complications include lymphedema (19 to 45 percent) and wound infection. Persistent lymphedema can be problematic, but may be managed with compression stockings, elevation, and immobilization.

Controversy also exists regarding the benefit obtained by pelvic node dissection if there are pelvic nodal metastases. Although positive pelvic nodes indicate a very poor prognosis, there are reports of 20 to 29 percent cure rates with surgical resection in these patients (Fair et al., 1993b).

External Beam Radiation Therapy

Radiotherapy is an effective treatment for smaller penile cancers such as T1, T2, and small T3 tumors. The main advantage of radiation therapy is preservation of the penis and an associated decrease in functional and psychosexual morbidity. When external beam irradiation is used, the method of delivery is with a custom-made plastic or wax mold to ensure a uniform dose distribution and to provide bolus. Circumcision may be recommended prior to treatment to minimize radiation morbidity. The whole shaft of the penis is treated to 40 Gy in 200 cGy fractions and the primary lesion is then boosted to a total dose of 60 to 65 Gy. Superficial lesions can be treated with orthovoltage or electron beams carried to a similar dose.

External beam irradiation of stage I to III tumors usually produces 70 to 80 percent local control rates, and most local failures that appear in the remainder of patients can be salvaged with surgery without affecting the ultimate disease-free survival (Fair, Fuks, & Scher, 1993b; Ravi et al., 1994). If prophylactic or therapeutic lymph node dissection cannot be performed, external beam radiotherapy to the inguinal and pelvic lymph nodes to a dose of 45 to 50 Gy can provide permanent control in a substantial percentage of patients (Fair et al., 1993b). Radiotherapy is also used for symptomatic relief in patients with painful bony metastases.

Acute radiation effects include edema of the penis and mucocutaneous reactions. The most common late effect of treatment is meatal-urethral stricture. The incidence of stricture following radiotherapy compares favorably with the incidence of stricture following penectomy. These strictures can be managed by dilation or simple plastic surgery (McLean et al., 1993). Mucosal changes and telangiectasias are the most frequent long-term sequelae. There is little information in the literature on long-term penile function in patients who have been successfully treated with radiation therapy.

Brachytherapy

Interstitial brachytherapy has been used for many years in the treatment of localized carcinoma of the penis. Techniques using radium needles and iridium-192 ribbons are reported (McLean et al., 1993). Results for patients with T1, T2, and small T3 lesions include a local control rate of 80 percent with excellent cosmetic results, minimal late sequelae, and no significant impairment of penile function. The total treatment takes approximately 5 to 7 days to deliver a homogenous dose to the target volume (McLean et al., 1993).

Chemotherapy

Chemotherapy is used for invasive or metastatic penile cancers. Cisplatin-based regimens have shown activity in squamous cell tumors.

External beam irradiation has been delivered concomitantly with chemotherapeutic drugs such as single-agent bleomycin, and regimens using mitomycin-c and 5-fluorouracil to enhance response in patients with early- and late-stage invasive tumors. Equivalent outcome has been reported with combined modality therapy compared with surgery in low-stage tumors, with the advantage of preserved sexual function (Modig et al., 1993).

Nursing Care During Radiotherapy for a Genitourinary Malignancy

Site-specific toxicities can be expected during a course of radiotherapy for a genitourinary (GU) malignancy. The gastrointestinal and genitourinary systems are most affected by radiotherapy for GU cancers because these organs are located within the treatment fields. However, patients may also experience alterations in the integumentary system and sexuality in addition to the more general effects of a course of radiotherapy such as fatigue, anorexia, and myelosuppression. It is often difficult to separate symptoms as they may occur in multiple systems simultaneously. Assessment and teaching regarding expected toxicities and self-care strategies are important nursing care activities.

Bowel

Pathophysiology of Radiation Effects

The small intestinal mucosa is one of the most radiosensitive tissues in the body. The radiation tolerance of the small bowel is generally regarded as approximately 45 Gy, 1.8 Gy daily fractions, 5 days per week. Acute radiation enteritis is often increased and appears earlier in patients receiving chemotherapy. Drugs commonly used in patients treated for a GU malignancy include cisplatin and 5-fluorouracil. Adding chemotherapy does not significantly enhance late effects (Coia et al., 1995). The rectum and rectosigmoid tolerate higher doses of radiation than does the small bowel. They are nevertheless relatively easily damaged by radiation, and their presence in the radiation field often limits the dose or justifies technical modifications in pelvic irradiation (Stevens, 1994).

Clinical Symptoms

ACUTE EFFECTS

Diarrhea is the most common acute manifestation of radiotherapy to the abdomen and pelvis. Alteration in bowel elimination patterns may vary from mild to moderate (2 to 4 stools per day) to severe (which may be defined as 8 or more stools in a 24-hour period). Severe watery diarrhea is uncommon. The patient may also experience abdominal cramping, tenesmus, proctalgia, and occasionally hematochezia. One or more of these side effects occur to varying degrees in a third to half of the patients treated (Shipley et al., 1994). Acute radiation enteritis is directly related to the dose rate and the volume of bowel irradiated. Onset of symptoms is variable but generally begins when the patient has received a total dose in the range of 1500 to 3000 cGy. Without intervention symptoms usually increase in severity as treatment continues.

LATE EFFECTS

Late sequelae of radiation therapy to the bowel are a complex problem, with the major determinants being the total radiation dose, daily dose fractionation, and volume of bowel irradiated. Late bowel damage occurs much less frequently than acute damage. Slow healing mucosal ulcers can result in cicatricial luminal narrowing, perforation, fistula formation, and chronic blood loss. The injury to the intestinal wall results in edema with loss of fibrillar appearance of collagen and obliterative vascular injury. This results in progressive fibrosis, shortening, constriction, and stenosis of the irradiated portion of the bowel. Adhesions between loops of bowel cause further functional and obstructive symptoms (Stevens, 1994).

Functional changes include malabsorption secondary to enteritis and narrowing of the intestine, causing stricture and possible obstruction. Vascular changes within the mesentery contribute to fibrosis and ischemia of the intestine. Typically symptoms manifest within 6 to 18 months following completion of irradiation and include diarrhea, abdominal cramping, nausea, vomiting, malabsorption, and obstruction. Jonler et al. (1994) reported that 31 percent of patients who received definitive irradiation for prostate carcinoma still had some intestinal symptoms at the time of follow-up (median 31 months). The authors state that the frequency of bowel dysfunction following radiation therapy is higher than previously reported, and 18 percent of all patients found they were still significantly bothered by these symptoms. The major problems that may require major medical or surgical intervention are intestinal obstruction (because of the luminal size, this occurrence is rare in the large bowel), severe bleeding, fistula formation, and intractable diarrhea (Coia et al., 1995).

Treatment Modifications

A variety of treatment modification techniques may be used to minimize radiation dose to the small bowel and lessen sequelae. See Chapter 11 for detailed information on radiation modification techniques.

Management of Intestinal Treatment Effects

Refer to Chapter 11 for a discussion on the management of gastrointestinal radiation effects.

Bladder

The urinary bladder is unavoidably irradiated during conventional treatment for many pelvic malignancies. Since a large proportion of patients receiving such treatment survive many years, much information has been accumulated about early and late reactions to radiation and the radiation tolerance of the bladder (Pearse, 1994).

Pathophysiology of Radiation Effects

The pathophysiology of acute and chronic radiation-induced bladder injury is not fully understood. The limited understanding derives mainly from animal models. Early and late effects of radiation are readily observed clinically and can be demonstrated pathologically. The tolerance of the bladder to fractionated irradiation is 65 to 70 Gy. Severe late effects may occur in 5 percent of patients receiving 60 to 65 Gy to the entire bladder and in 50 percent of patients receiving 70 to 75 Gy (Pearse, 1994).

Overall patients at higher risk for acute and postirradiation bladder sequelae are those in whom treatment is preceded by ulceration, infection, intravesical chemotherapy, and fibrotic changes from multiple open or transurethral resections. Bladder cancer patients at higher risk of acute and late effects include those previously listed and patients who have undergone surgical procedures to the bladder within 3 weeks of onset of radiation therapy, obstructive uropathies, bladder infections, and large necrotic tumor. In patients who have undergone pelvic surgery for a GU malignancy, irradiation is usually withheld until 4 to 6 weeks postoperatively to allow for healing and help prevent severe radiation reactions.

Systemic chemotherapeutic agents may affect bladder function through excretion of active metabolites in the urine or by increasing the severity of radiation effects when used concurrently. The systemic chemotherapeutic agents most commonly observed to cause considerable toxicity are cyclophosphamide and its analog ifosfamide. The uroprotectant mesna is useful in preventing urotoxicity resulting from ifosfamide administration. Multiple studies have incorporated chemotherapy and radiotherapy in the treatment of invasive bladder cancer. The clinical symptoms of combined modality therapy such as frequency and urgency, dysuria, hemorrhagic cystitis, and shrunken bladder are identical to those seen with radiation alone. In addition, the incidence of severe complications after combined modality therapy is fairly low, ranging from 0 to 15 percent (Marks et al., 1995).

Transient mucosal erythema may appear during the first 24 hours after irradiation. Mild, early mucosal reaction with acute cystitis symptoms may begin as early as 1500 cGy and is likely to occur by 3000 to 4000 cGy (in 3 to 4 weeks). There may be a slight reduction in bladder capacity caused by increased bladder irritability secondary to edema. Curative radiation therapy for treatment of a primary bladder cancer will likely deliver 60 to 65 Gy to the bladder and is likely to cause acute effects. Cystoscopically, the bladder mucosa appears as it would in acute cystitis. Desquamation is rare. Microscopic findings include acute inflammation of the bladder mucosa and submucosa, engorged capillaries, round cell infiltration, and edema. As the radiation dose increases, the mucosa continues to inflame and becomes an intense red (Pearse, 1994).

Multiple series confirm that mild transient side effects are common and that severe late urinary complications are noted in 2 to 5 percent of patients. In patients undergoing irradiation for cancer of the prostate, the risk of serious late bladder injury is fairly low (0 to 10 percent) when standard irradiation techniques are used (Pearse, 1994). The majority of the bladder can be irradiated to approximately 30 to 50 Gy, with small volumes of the bladder receiving 60 to 65 Gy, with a fairly low rate of serious complication. The risk of serious bladder injury increases dramatically when the daily fraction size is increased and in patients treated with one to two fields per day compared to those treated with multiple fields daily (Marks et al., 1995).

Bladder complications are more frequent in bladder cancer patients and are likely due to several factors. The volume of bladder irradiated is greater and the presence of the tumor itself may make the bladder more sensitive to radiation damage. The diseased bladder is also likely to be somewhat dysfunctional because of the tumor. In a review of 10-year survivors of bladder cancer treated with definitive radiotherapy ($\geq$50 Gy in ~15 fractions), 68 percent had well-functioning bladders. Only 10 percent of patients developed contracted bladders; 6 percent were functional and 4 percent required cystectomy. The remainder had either active bladder tumor or had a cystectomy for tumor control (Marks et al., 1995). Perez and associates noted that 80 percent of observed urinary tract complications occurred within 48 months. Although the bladder is a highly innervated organ, the acute changes in reservoir function do not seem to be caused by changes in nerve function (Marks et al., 1995).

Clinical Symptoms

ACUTE SYMPTOMS

Acute cystitis symptoms include dysuria, hesitancy, urgency, and an increase in urinary frequency including nocturia. As the dose escalates, bladder capacity may be further reduced. Patients may experience both tenesmus and bladder spasms that potentiate all symptoms. Rarely patients have hematuria. Acute irritative symptoms frequently occur 3 to 5 weeks after the initiation of therapy, and usually subside gradually 2 to 8 weeks after completion of treatment. An inflamed bladder mucosa may lead to an infection that will require intervention. These mild, short-term reactions are reversible and usually subside with mucosal healing, pharmacological interventions, and a treatment break as needed.

LATE SYMPTOMS

Most late complications are related to bladder contracture, bleeding, and symptomatic cystitis. Incontinence is not common. The development of incontinence is likely related to surgical manipulations of the bladder neck and urethra. In a study designed specifically to address this issue, incontinence was seen in 5.4 percent (7 out of 130) of patients who had prior transurethral prostate resection (TURP), compared to 1 percent (1 out of 105) of patients who had not (Marks et al., 1995).

Nursing Management of Bladder Effects

ACUTE EFFECTS

Management of early reactions are focused on symptomatic relief. Nursing management is comprised of pretreatment assessment, weekly evaluation while treatment is being delivered, and follow-up monitoring. Initial pretreatment assessment of bladder function includes documentation of patterns of urinary elimination. Assessments will incorporate the frequency of voids, amount of urine output per void, and any sensations that may have changed with prior treatment. Past history of urinary tract infections and medications used for treatment should be noted. Urinary diversions created by surgery need to be evaluated as well as changes produced by chemotherapy. Once a baseline assessment of urinary elimination is obtained, the nurse may begin teaching the patient anticipated radiation effects (McCarthy, 1992).

Instructing patients to maintain an adequate intake of fluids will promote frequent voiding and decrease the potential for infection by diluting the bacterial population. Recommended fluid intake is 1 to 2 L per day. If voided urine is clear to light yellow in color, hydration is probably adequate. In addition, teaching patients to avoid foods that irritate the bladder mucosa may help to delay the onset of cystitis and decrease symptoms. These foods include coffee, tea, alcohol, spices, and tobacco products.

Encourage patients to report any signs of bladder irritation, such as dysuria, frequency, urgency with decreased urine volume, and any signs of hematuria or excessive mucous shreds in the urine. The nurse should also be aware of the baseline hemoglobin and hematocrit values as well as any coagulation studies. If hematuria occurs, these values will be monitored over the course of treatment. Hematuria usually causes minimal blood loss and rarely an anemia, but early documentation will assist in assessment of future problems.

The irritative voiding symptoms are due to mucosal ulceration of the bladder, which increases the potential for infection. Initial treatment consists of ruling out infection, and if present, antibiotic therapy is indicated. Infection often escalates bladder spasm and complicates radiation treatment delivery. Antispasmodics help relieve dysuria and provide relief from bladder spasms. Treatment of either infection or spasm is sometimes inseparable, and optimal comfort is obtained if they are treated simultaneously.

Phenazopyridine hydrochloride (Pyridium) is frequently used for dysuria symptoms. When taken orally the majority of drug enters the urine unchanged, where it acts as a topical analgesic within the bladder. The patient's urine will be colored orange/red when taking the drug.

Reduction in irritative voiding symptoms and improvement in urine flow rates is related to the relaxation of smooth muscle. Symptoms such as mild urinary frequency are frequently due to a modest reduction in bladder capacity. To increase storage capacity antispasmodic medications such as oxybutynin chloride (Ditropan) and flavoxate hydrochloride (Urispas) relax the bladder smooth muscle by inhibiting the muscarinic effects of acetylcholine. Side effects of such therapy include hypertension, palpitations, arrhythmia, and additional stimulation of the central nervous system. Such drugs should be used cautiously in those with cardiovascular diseases and hyperthyroidism. Relaxation of bladder smooth muscle can also be produced by a blockade of the alpha-1 adenoreceptors in the bladder. An alpha-1 adrenergic blocker such as terazosin (Hytrin) can decrease bladder outlet obstruction without affecting contractility. Terazosin 1 mg at bedtime, with escalating doses based on response, can markedly decrease obstructive symptoms and nocturia. Use with caution in patients with hypertension who may be on antihypertensive medication.

LATE EFFECTS

Late dysfunction may be manifested by diminished bladder capacity, irritative voiding symptoms and infrequently, incontinence. As most effects of radiation and chemotherapy are minor or moderate in severity and transitory, an evaluation consisting of a history, physical examination, and urinalysis is usually adequate to assess the degree of bladder dysfunction and begin a plan of management. The pretreatment assessment will be helpful when evaluating the changes in function over time.

Patients should be evaluated for the presence of irritative (urinary frequency, urgency, dysuria) or obstructive (decrease in the force or caliber of the urinary stream) symptoms. If the patient is experiencing incontinence, it should be differentiated as urge incontinence (occurring at the time of a sensation of bladder fullness and associated with an imminent desire to urinate) or stress incontinence (occurring during activity and not associated with urgency). Women with bladder cancer who experience large volume or continuous incontinence should be evaluated for the presence of a urinary tract fistula (Marks et al., 1995).

The abdomen and suprapubic region should be palpated to assess for the presence of bladder distention or tenderness. Inspect the external genitalia to exclude inflammatory conditions. On occasion, a gynecological examination in women with bladder cancer may be performed to assess for a urinary tract fistula or the presence of gynecological inflammatory disease.

Urinalysis will reveal the presence of red and white cells as well as bacteria. Urinary infection can greatly exacerbate the late effects of irradiation and should be treated promptly. A urinary cytology is necessary in uninfected patients who present with irritative symptoms occurring late after radiation or cyclophosphamide administration (Marks et al., 1995).

A urodynamic evaluation should be performed in patients with symptoms of incontinence, inability to empty not due to anatomic obstruction, or severe irritative voiding symptoms not associated with infection or secondary malignancy. Management of bladder incontinence should be accomplished by referral to either a urologist or urodynamic multidisciplinary team for complete assessment and treatment. Evaluation of late effects include radiographic evaluation, especially for patients with excessive hematuria or an increasing serum creatinine. Cystography and cystoscopy are indicated in those patients who suffer severe late effects of irradiation associated with severe bladder dysfunction. As bladder dysfunction increases secondary to advances in cancer treatment, Continence Nurse Specialists may be utilized as resources for patients (Jeter et al., 1990; McCarthy, 1992).

Severe reductions in bladder capacity not responding to pharmacotherapy may be managed with bladder augmentation using a segment of intestine (Marks et al., 1995). Defects in urethral resistance are less common. Mild sphincteric insufficiency may respond to pharmacotherapy. Severe sphincteric insufficiency may be managed with periurethral injection of polytetrafluoroethylene or collagen. Patient controlled, low-pressure sphincters may be placed surgically. However, placement of such devices after radiation may be associated with a higher rate of complications compared to implantation in patients who have not received pelvic irradiation.

Urethral strictures are most often managed with simple endoscopic incision. Open surgical repair may be necessary in those with recurrent or complex strictures. Intermittent self-catheterization may be an option in selected patients with fixed strictures of the urethra and compliant, adequate capacity bladders (Marks et al., 1995). Generally self-catheterization is performed with clean technique.

Severe hemorrhage caused by radiation should be evaluated by cystoscopy and treated with selective cauterization of bleeding points followed by irrigation with various agents such as alum, silver nitrate, or dilute formalin. Patients with persistent, recurrent, or severe hemorrhage may require bladder diversion or substitution (Marks et al., 1995). Vesicovaginal fistulas may be corrected using a variety of surgical approaches.

Additional Irradiation-Related Toxicities

Patients undergoing radiation therapy for a GU malignancy are at risk for alterations in skin integrity, fatigue, and myelosuppression. When lower energy (electron beam or orthovoltage therapy) treatments are used for penile cancers, skin reactions are commonly experienced. Assessment and nursing management of each is discussed at length in Chapter 8. GU cancer patients are at no greater risk for these toxicities, however these effects may be enhanced if chemotherapy is administered concomitantly.

Fatigue and malaise are very common among patients undergoing irradiation for a GU malignancy. Greenberg et al. (1993) studied 15 men who were receiving irradiation for localized prostate cancer. Each patient rated fatigue daily on a visual analog scale, recorded hours slept, and completed the Beck Depression Inventory weekly. Serum IL-1 was measured at baseline and each Friday. Mean fatigue scores for each subject increased at week 4 then plateaued and rose again in weeks 6 and 7. In week 6, the last week of full volume radiation, subjects slept most compared to all other weeks, including week 7 when treatment was coned down. Ranked serum IL-1 tended to rise between weeks 1 and 4, as fatigue scores rose.

These data suggest that localized radiation treatment is associated with increased fatigue and sleep requirements independent of depressive symptoms. Relative serum IL-1 changes may be one signal for the systemic reaction and subjective fatigue associated with the acute effects of irradiation.

When large volumes of active bone marrow are irradiated the effect on the marrow can cause myelosuppression. Approximately 40 percent of active marrow is located in the pelvis. Thus, GU cancer patients (especially prostate and bladder) are at relatively high risk for bone marrow depression. The patient population frequently includes the elderly who may have compromised marrow as a result of aging. However, overall these patients infrequently have myelosuppression that necessitates intervention such as a treatment break. The exceptions include those patients who are receiving concomitant chemotherapy.

Rare Long-Term Complications

Other infrequent long-term sequelae of megavoltage conventional external beam radiotherapy include leg edema and genital edema, which have almost always been reported in association with a preirradiation staging pelvic lymphadenectomy. With the use of megavoltage and multiple treatment beams, reports of fibrosis of the subcutaneous tissues and radionecrosis of the femoral head or pubic bone are rare (Shipley et al., 1994).

The possible increase in the incidence of secondary malignancy is a major concern for all patients undergoing radiation therapy for a GU malignancy. Bagshaw and colleagues (1988) at Stanford University evaluated 914 patients who underwent radiation therapy for prostate cancer and found no significant difference between the observed and expected second malignancy incidence rates (Bagshaw et al., 1988).

Effects on Sexuality

Treatment for a GU cancer often affects sexual functioning (Shipes & Lehr, 1982). Surgery, chemotherapy, and irradiation will each have an impact on sexuality and the combined effects can enhance sexual dysfunction. Altered sexual function associated with nerve and vascular damage or hormonal ablation may be temporary or permanent. In certain patients, impotence can be devastating, assuming a focus of such importance that other aspects related to recovery and survival seem trivial in comparison. Patients may choose, or refuse, some forms of treatment because of the potential for impotence. Patients with GU cancers span the age continuum with men treated for testicular cancer generally younger than those receiving treatment for bladder, prostate, or penile malignancies. The physio-psychosocial issues of fertility and potency are the predominant domains of human sexuality.

Fertility

Spermatogenesis in men appears to be more sensitive to fractionated irradiation than to single doses. The sensitizing effect of fractionation is thought to be mainly due to the long cell cycle of the primitive stem cell which results in a significant population of cells in a relatively radioresistant phase of the cell cycle.

The severity of the impairment in spermatogenesis, and length of recovery, depends on the radiation dose to the testis. In the typical patient receiving irradiation for pure seminoma, the remaining testis receives a dose in the range of 30 to 180 cGy. An even greater dose is delivered to the contralateral testis if the hemiscrotum is irradiated. Doses of this magnitude usually produce temporary oligospermia or azospermia followed by recovery 18 to 24 months later (Hussey, 1994). A marked but transient suppression of sperm production is evident with dosages as low as 15 cGy with more prolonged periods of aspermia reported with higher doses. At 200 to 300 cGy, full recovery of sperm production requires 3 years; at 400 to 600 cGy, the interval is about 5 years; and above 600 cGy, sterility appears to be permanent (Sherins, 1993). Issues of fertility associated with sexual dysfunction, such as treatment-induced impotence, are less common. Generally men undergoing surgical procedures and/or irradiation for bladder, prostate, or penile carcinoma are older and their concerns are more centered on potency than fertility.

Patients may become fertile during the recovery phase, and they should be informed of this possibility. Mutations induced in stem cells may produce abnormal spermatozoa. Fortunately, the spermatozoa arising from these stem cells tend to have poor fertilization potential. The frequency of the mutations depends on the radiation dose delivered. No genetic abnormalities from ionizing radiations have been demonstrated in men, which perhaps reflects the ability to repair such damage (Hussey, 1994). Patients are advised to practice birth control during and after paraaortic irradiation. The length of time is not entirely clear but generally 24 months are recommended, to allow for recovery of spermatogenesis.

Whenever possible, a testicular shield should be used to minimize the dose delivered to the testicles of male patients undergoing pelvic irradiation. See Figure 12–8. This apparatus works principally by shielding the testicles from radiation scattered from within the patient. Such shielding devices can reduce testicular exposure to about 1 percent of the dose delivered to the midpelvis (Hussey, 1994).

Impotence

The etiology of radiation-associated impotence is not fully understood. Based on a series of imaging and functional studies, impotence has been judged to be secondary to radiation-induced endarteritis of the branches of the internal pudendal and penile arteries, which course laterally to the prostate and are frequently in the region of high-dose radiation. Other possible causes of radiation-associated impotence, such as significant functional changes in the pudendal nerve or endocrine secretions, are possible but less likely. Reduced testosterone levels may be noted within a few weeks after irradiation to the testis, but they usually return to normal within 6 to 12 months, presumably because of compensatory hypersecretion of LH by the pituitary. Uncompensated Leydig cell damage could be responsible for the impotence seen in some men who have been treated with pelvic irradiation (Hussey, 1994). Sexual dysfunction at any age is often the combined result of various psychological, neurological, hormonal, and vascular factors (Shipley et al., 1994).

Shipley et al. (1994) reviewed several series that reported on the maintenance of full potency after radiation therapy for early prostate cancer. Potency was reported to be 30 to 61 percent at 5 years. See Figure 12–9. Litwin and colleagues (1995) assessed health-related quality of life in 214 men treated for clinically localized prostate cancer and 273 men without prostate cancer. The patients with cancer were in three groups: radical prostatectomy, primary pelvic irradiation, and observation alone. Findings from this study include that men who underwent radical surgery or radiation reported poorer sexual function (decreased frequency and quality of erections, decreased morning erections, decreased frequency of intercourse, and decreased ability to achieve sexual climax) than those without prostate cancer (control group). In sexual function and other health-related domains (physical and social function, general health perceptions, energy/fatigue), all prostate cancer groups scored significantly worse than the control group. Specifically, patients undergoing surgery were statistically indistinguishable from those receiving radiation. This study demonstrated that in prostate cancer patients, sexual function is a domain that is directly affected by treatment and is distinct from general health-related quality of life. The authors conclude that providers interacting with prostate cancer patients should advise them that treatment is unlikely to affect general health-related quality of life, but may be associated with clinically significant changes in sexual functioning. Any survival gains from surgery or radiation must be balanced with expected decrements in some areas of sexual function and other health-related domains (Litwin et al., 1995).

Jonler and associates (1994) measured quality of life in patients with prostate cancer 14 to 60 months (median 31 months) after definitive prostate irradiation. Potency and other treatment-related sequelae were assessed retrospectively. The authors judged that the 77 percent of patients who recalled establishing full or partial erections before radiation therapy may have been high compared to previous reports. Of patients able to have erections prior to radiation therapy, only 16 percent were able to have erections firm enough for

Figure 12-8 • Testicular shield (clamshell). (A) Open; (B) closed.

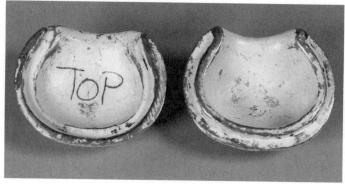
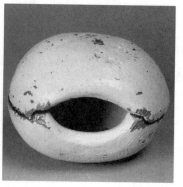

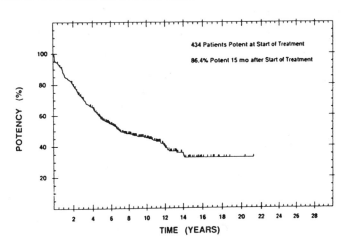

Figure 12-9 • Actuarial incidence of maintenance of potency in 914 patients treated with external beam radiation therapy at Stanford University as a function of time after treatment. From Shipley WU, et al. (1994). Treatment related sequelae following external beam radiation for prostate cancer: a review with an update in patients with stages T1 and T2 tumor. *The Journal of Urology, 152,* 1799–1805.

intercourse at time of follow-up, 37 percent had not had any erections after radiation therapy, and 29 percent reported they perceived sexual dysfunction as a substantial problem. Despite this, 81 percent of the patients were satisfied with the choice of radiation therapy as a treatment modality for prostate cancer (Jonler et al., 1994).

Sexual desire diminished among 77 percent of men ranging in age from 53 to 80 years (mean 70 years) after definitive irradiation for localized prostate cancer, as reported by Helgason and colleagues (1995). Of all men, 50 percent reported that quality of life had decreased much or very much due to a decline in the erectile capacity following external radiation therapy. Also reported was a reduction in sexual desire and orgasmic function. The authors conclude that quality of life decreases in most patients experiencing reduced sexual functioning. The findings suggest that health care providers may have underestimated the importance of intact sexual functioning for the well-being among older men with prostate cancer (Helgason, 1995).

In a study by Opjordsmoen and Fossa (1994) 30 patients were followed for a median of 80 months after treatment for penile cancer. Treatment included local/laser excision(n = 5), radiation therapy(n = 12), partial penectomy(n = 9), and total penectomy(n = 4). The patients who underwent partial or total penectomy tended to have the poorest outcome with regard to sexual function and enjoyment. Although the four patients without a penis functioned the worst on these two variables, their global well-being and social activity tended to be better than the average observed for the whole group. This suggests radically treated patients adapt relatively well to the new

situation in terms of subjective well-being and overall social function. The majority reported preferring higher long-term survival to saving penile organ function, but some claimed that, if asked again, they would choose a treatment with lower long-term survival to increase their chance of remaining sexually potent.

The importance of sexuality as a consideration in treatment outcomes is demonstrated in these studies. These data underscore the importance of establishing a therapeutic relationship to allow patients and their partners to explore how alterations in sexuality will affect their lives.

Alterations in Sexuality

Malignancies of the bladder, prostate, testis, and penis, and their treatment outcomes, may affect libido, erection, orgasm, and ejaculation in the male patient. (See Table 12–9.) Patients are often reluctant to ask questions or discuss concerns related to sexual topics. Loss of sexual potency may be viewed as a major threat to the maintenance of a satisfactory sexual relationship. Although many patients with a GU malignancy are older men, it is important to not assume that sexuality is no longer an important element in their lives.

Nurses in concert with colleagues in medical oncology, urology, and other related specialties will be involved in the sexual rehabilitation of the patient with a GU malignancy. The nurse is often the most accessible member of the health team, and consequently is the professional most frequently asked to assist in formulating a comprehensive plan of care related to alterations in sexuality. There are several areas of importance related to sexuality, some specific to radiation therapy and others more generic, for radiation oncology nurses to consider.

Table 12-9 • Treatment Related Sexual Dysfunctions

Treatment	Decreased Libido	Erectile Problems	Retrograde Ejaculation
PROSTATE			
Transurethral resection prostate	Rarely	Rarely	Almost always
Radical prostatectomy	Rarely	Frequently	Always
Radiation therapy	Rarely	Frequently	Rarely
Bilateral orchiectomy	Frequently	Almost always	Occasionally
Hormonal therapy	Almost always	Almost always	Occasionally
BLADDER			
Radical cystoprostatectomy	Rarely	Almost always	Always
TESTIS			
Orchiectomy (unilateral)	Rarely	Rarely	Rarely

Adapted from Held JS, Osborne DM, Volpe H et al. (1994). Cancer of the prostate: treatment and nursing implications. *Oncology Nursing Forum, 21*, 1517–1529, and Shipes E & Lehr S (1982). Sexuality and the male cancer patient. *Cancer Nursing, 5,* 375. Used with permission.

Site-Specific Interventions

Usually patients with testicular cancer are younger men (15 to 34 years old) and in a crucial stage of life. Cancer treatment can produce organic problems and sexual anxieties that can lead to dysfunction (Shell, 1994). Unilateral orchiectomy rarely causes organic sexual dysfunction. Extensive surgery (retroperitoneal lymph node dissection), radiation, and chemotherapy may cause erectile and orgasmic dysfunction. Educating the patient and his partner includes information that normal sexual desire and pleasurable sensations, erection, and orgasm will probably continue. If sexual desire is lost, serum testosterone should be checked; replacement therapy may be needed. Alpha-adrenergic stimulating drugs can increase ejaculation and occasionally the intensity of orgasm for some patients who have had retroperitoneal lymph node dissection. Testicular prosthesis can remedy patient embarrassment from loss of the testicle. It is important to reinforce the fact that cancer is not contagious through sexual activity and that radiation therapy will not contaminate the partner (Shell, 1994).

Sperm banking may be an option if the number and motility of sperm are adequate. In men with testicular cancer, human chorionic gonadotropin is often secreted from the tumor. This hormone stimulates increased estrogen production and can adversely affect the contralateral testis (Sherins, 1993). Sperm banking is costly and there is no guarantee that future artificial insemination will be successful. If the patient wishes sperm banking, it should be completed before chemotherapy or radiation is initiated.

Penile implants are an option for selected patients with impotence. The patient and partner may choose from several different types of prosthesis. A comparison of two types is seen in Figure 12–10 and Table 12–10. Noninvasive devices such as the vacuum erection device are being used more commonly. Injection of vasoactive agents into the penile corpora cavernosa is effective and becoming more widely utilized.

Penile cancer results in the greatest risk of sexual dysfunction (Shell, 1994). If partial penectomy is done, the penile stump usually becomes erect with stimulation and is long enough for penetration with antegrade ejaculation. If the entire glans penis is removed, a perineal urethrostomy is created behind the scrotum. When it is stimulated to orgasm, ejaculation takes place through the perineal urethrostomy. Counseling for the patient and his partner includes methods of sexual stimulation and satisfaction that can include use of a phallic shaped vibrator as a substitute penis for partner satisfaction (Shell, 1994). If total penectomy has occurred, stimulation of the mons pubis, perineum, and scrotum can produce orgasms with pleasurable contractions in the remaining cavernous musculature. If partial penectomy has occurred, men report erections and orgasms of normal or near normal intensity with the phallic stump. Female partners should be advised to have a yearly Pap smear since they may be at increased risk for cervical cancer from exposure to the human papilloma virus (Schover, 1988).

Sexual dysfunction after cystectomy is similar to that after radical prostatectomy, except that the patient may also have undergone urethrectomy and will have a urinary diversion. More patients are choosing continent internal urinary reservoir or ileocolonic neobladder and report remaining more sexually active than men with appliances (Schover, 1988).

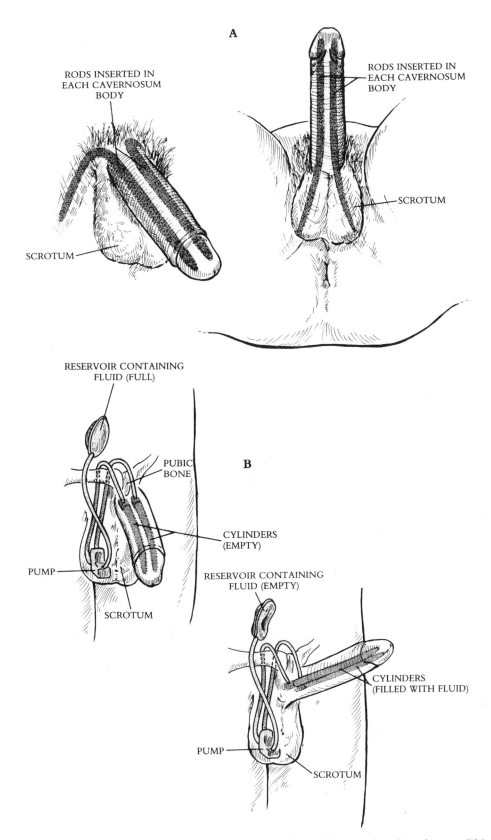

A

RODS INSERTED IN
EACH CAVERNOSUM
BODY

RODS INSERTED IN
EACH CAVERNOSUM
BODY

SCROTUM

SCROTUM

RESERVOIR CONTAINING
FLUID (FULL)

PUBIC
BONE

B

CYLINDERS
(EMPTY)

RESERVOIR CONTAINING
FLUID (EMPTY)

PUMP

SCROTUM

CYLINDERS
(FILLED WITH FLUID)

PUMP

SCROTUM

Figure 12-10 • Penile prostheses can be of two types. (A) Two semirigid silicone rods are implanted into the penis. (B) In the second type two expandable cylinders are inserted into the penis and are connected by a tubing system to a fluid filled bulb. From Denney N & Quadagno D (1992). *Human sexuality*. St. Louis: Mosby.

215

Table 12-10 • Comparison of Inflatable and Semirigid Penile Prostheses

Factor	Type of Prosthesis	
	Semirigid	Inflatable
Ease of concealment	May need special briefs; noticeable in locker room or public urinal	No problem, self-contained version may not lie down completely
Size of erection	Some loss of length and thickness	Normal thickness, some loss of length (self-contained version cannot add thickness)
Function during sexual intercourse	80–90% patients satisfied	80–90% patients satisfied
Infection during healing	Occurs in 1–2% of patients	Occurs in 1–2% of patients
Prosthesis erodes through spongy tissue inside penis	Less than 5% of patients	No problems
Prolonged pain after healing	Rare	Rare
Need to repair prosthesis	Rare	5–15% reoperation rates
Usual hospital stay*	2–4 days	2–5 days
Total costs*	$6000–10,000	$10,000–12,000

From Schover L. (1988). *Sexuality and cancer: for the man who has cancer; and his partner.* American Cancer Society. New York and *Shell JA (1994). Impact of cancer on sexuality. In SE Otto (Ed.), *Oncology Nursing,* (pp. 737–760). St. Louis: Mosby. Reprinted with permission.

Research

A greater understanding of the molecular biology and genetics surrounding prostate cancer development and the development of both hormonal repressiveness and refractory mechanisms should be a major focus of basic research efforts. It is unlikely that any new, effective treatment modalities will emerge until these mechanisms of hormonal resistance are better understood (Garnick, 1993). Basic research in prostate cancer is focused on the role of hormones, growth factors, oncogenes, tumor-suppressor genes, and apoptosis (programmed cell death) in the development and progression of prostate cancer (Catalona, 1994). Clinical drug studies that are in process or planned include the evaluation of high-dose lovastatin (to block cholesterol synthesis in cancer cells), taxol, retinoids, and interferon. In addition, clinical trials will evaluate radical prostatectomy as compared with watchful waiting, hormonal therapy before either prostatectomy or radiation therapy, and adjuvant radiation therapy or hormonal therapy after radical prostatectomy. This research will provide important insights to help resolve the current controversies concerning the treatment of patients with prostate cancer and may lead to reduced morbidity and mortality rates (Catalona, 1994).

Quality of Life Outcomes

The consequences of therapy for GU cancers continue to wield an impact on patients for years after therapy is completed. Although many aspects of day-to-day life return to normal for these men, some functions may be profoundly altered (Litwin et al., 1995). With the emergence of the "outcomes movement" as a major aspect of health care delivery and evaluation, consumers and providers want to know more about the outcome of cancer care than survival rates alone (Ganz, 1995).

Cost

In the age of managed care, health care costs are increasingly becoming major factors in determining whether new or expensive therapies come into use in clinical practice. A course of radiation therapy is costly. It is estimated that a definitive course of treatment for a patient with prostate cancer is approximately $8000 to $11,000. Treatment for patients with locally extensive and metastatic disease is also expensive. The annual cost for an antiandrogen agent such as flutamide and the LHRH analog, leuprolide, is approximately $9300 ($3600 for flutamide, $5700 for leuprolide). In contrast, a 1-year supply of diethylstilbestrol (DES) costs less than $100. However, avoiding cardiovascular complications associated with DES and eliminating the need for prophylactic radiation therapy to the breasts to avoid gynecomastia may offset the cost associated with LHRH analog therapy and antiandrogen agents. Bilateral orchiectomy costs approximately $2000 to $3000, including surgeon's fees and associated hospital costs (Garnick, 1993). Also to be considered are the substantial costs during terminal phases of illness and supportive care required. Managing complications can become expensive. Surgical procedures for impotence and incontinence can result in additional physician and hospitalization costs (Garnick, 1993). The point of these data is to emphasize that cost is often a consideration, by both patient and insurer, when selecting a therapeutic modality. How much a treatment costs and the data related to outcome continue to have a major impact in today's health care environment.

Summary

Contemplating the future of radiation therapy and nursing care of male patients experiencing a GU malignancy brings to the forefront several issues. A major focus is how to balance therapies and their associated cost and morbidity with disease outcome and quality of life. As patients and their families demand more information on all aspects of treatment and care, they will look to nurses for education and guidance in making therapeutic decisions. Nursing's role is evolving to one of policy maker. Now and in the future nursing will be responsible for analyzing information to help colleagues and patients/families to make treatment decisions. Nurses are encouraged to study the issues surrounding national and local policies regarding health care allotment, availability, and regulation. Nurses in radiation oncology have the ability and responsibility to influence and create public and nursing policy that allows patients and families to attain the optimum level of health within the cancer treatment continuum.

Acknowledgments

The author wishes to acknowledge the invaluable assistance of Harper D. Pearse, MD, Professor of Urology and Radiation Oncology, Oregon Health Sciences University, Portland, Oregon; and Mark F. Schray, MD, Department of Radiation Oncology, Legacy Portland Hospitals, Portland, Oregon, in the preparation of this manuscript.

References

Abdeen N, Souhami L, Freeman C, Yassa M, & Roman T (1992). Radiation therapy of testicular seminoma: A 15-year survey. *American Journal of Clinical Oncology, 15,* 87–90.

Albertson PC, Fryback DG, Storer BE, Kolon TF, & Fine J (1995). Long-term survival among men with conservatively treated localized prostate cancer. *Journal of the American Medical Association, 274,* 626–631.

Altman GB, & Lee CA (1996). Strontium-89 for treatment of painful bone metastasis from prostate cancer. *Oncology Nursing Forum, 23,* 523–527.

American Joint Committee on Cancer. (1992). *Manual for staging of cancer* (4th ed.). Philadelphia: JB Lippincott.

Bagshaw MA, Cox RS, & Ray GR (1988). Status of radiation therapy of prostate cancer at Stanford University. *National Cancer Institute Monograph, 7,* 47.

Blasko JC, Grimm PD, and Ragde H (1993). Brachytherapy and organ preservation in the management of carcinoma of the prostate. *Seminars in Radiation Oncology, 3,* 240–249.

Brock D, Fox S, Gosling G, Haney L, Kneebone P, Nagy C, et al. (1993). Testicular cancer. *Seminars in Oncology Nursing, 9,* 224–236.

Carter BS, Bova GS, Beatty TH, Steinberg GD, Childs B, Isaacs WB, et al. (1993). Hereditary prostate cancer: Epidemiological and clinical features. *The Journal of Urology, 150,* 797–802.

Catalona WJ (1994). Management of cancer of the prostate. *The New England Journal of Medicine, 331,* 996–1004.

Chybowski FM, Keller JJL, Bergstralh EJ, & Oesterling JE (1991). Predicting radionuclide bone scan findings in patients with newly diagnosed, untreated prostate cancer: Prostate specific antigen is superior to all other clinical parameters. *The Journal of Urology, 145,* 313–318.

Coia LR, Myerson RJ, & Tepper JE (1995). Late effects of radiation therapy on the gastrointestinal tract. *International Journal of Radiation Oncology, Biology, Physics, 31,* 1213–1236.

Davis M (1994). Genitourinary cancers. In SE Otto (Ed.), *Oncology Nursing,* (pp. 168–189). St. Louis: Mosby.

Dossman MA, & Zagars GK (1993). Postorchiectomy radiotherapy for stages I and II testicular seminoma. *International Journal of Radiation Oncology, Biology, Physics, 26,* 381–390.

Fair WR, Fuks ZY, & Scher HE (1993a). Cancer of the bladder. In VT DeVita Jr., S Hellman, & SA Rosenberg (Eds.), *Cancer: Principles & Practice of Oncology* (pp. 1052–1072). Philadelphia: JB Lippincott.

Fair WR, Fuks ZY, & Scher HE (1993b). Cancer of the urethra and penis. In VT DeVita Jr., S Hellman, & SA Rosenberg (Eds.), *Cancer: Principles & Practice of Oncology,* (4th ed), (pp. 1114–1125). Philadelphia: JB Lippincott.

Fowler JE, Braswell NT, Pandey P, & Seaver L (1995). Experience with radical prostatectomy and radiation therapy for localized prostate cancer at a veterans affairs medical center. *The Journal of Urology, 153,* 1026–1031.

Ganz PA (1995). Impact of quality of life outcomes on clinical practice. *Oncology, 9*(11 supplement). pp. 61–65.

Garnick MB (1993). Prostate cancer: Screening, diagnosis, and management. *Annals of Internal Medicine, 118,* 804–818.

Garnick MB (1994). The dilemmas of prostate cancer. *Scientific American,* April 1994, 72–81.

Greco KE, & Kulawiak L (1994). Prostate cancer prevention: Risk reduction through life-style, diet, and chemoprevention. *Oncology Nursing Forum, 21,* 1504–1510.

Greenberg DB, Gray JL, Mannix CM, Eisenthal S, & Carey M (1993). Treatment-related fatigue and serum interleukin-1 levels in patients during external beam irradiation for prostate cancer. *Journal of Pain and Symptom Management, 8,* 196–200.

Hanks G (1994). The prostate. In JD Cox (Ed.), *Moss' Radiation Oncology Rationale Technique, Results,* (pp. 559–586). St. Louis: Mosby.

Hanks GE, Myers CE, and Scardino PT (1993). Cancer of the prostate. In VT DeVita Jr., S Hellman, & SA Rosenberg (Eds.), *Cancer Principles & Practice of Oncology* (pp. 1073–1113). Philadelphia: JB Lippincott.

Held JS, Osborne DM, Volpe H & Waldman AR (1994). Cancer of the prostate: treatment and nursing implications. *Oncology Nursing Forum, 21,* 1517–1529.

Held J, & Volpe H (1991). Bladder preserving combined modality therapy for invasive bladder cancer. *Oncology Nursing Forum, 18*, 49–57.

Helgason AR, Fredrikson M, Adolfsson J, & Steineck G (1995). Decreased sexual capacity after external radiation therapy for prostate cancer impairs quality of life. *International Journal of Radiation Oncology, Biology, Physics, 32*, 33–39.

Hussey DH (1994). The testicle. In JD Cox (Ed.), *Moss' radiation oncology rationale, technique, results* (pp. 559–586). St. Louis: Mosby.

Jeter K, Faller N, & Norton C (1990). *Nursing for continence.* Philadelphia: WB Saunders.

Jonler M, Ritter MA, Brinkmann R, Messing EM, Rhodes PR, & Bruskewitz RC (1994). Sequelae of definitive radiation therapy for prostate cancer localized to the pelvis. *Urology, 44*, 876–883.

Kan MD (1995). Palliation of bone pain in patients with metastatic cancer using strontium-89 (Metastron). *Cancer Nursing, 18*, 286–291.

Kaufman DS, Shipley WU, Griffin PP, Heney NM, Althausen AF, & Efird JT (1993). Selective bladder preservation by combination treatment of invasive bladder cancer. *The New England Journal of Medicine, 329*, 1377–1382.

Kavadi VS, Zagars GS & Pollack A (1994). Serum prostate-specific antigen after radiation therapy for clinically localized prostate cancer: prognostic implications. *International Journal of Radiation Oncology, Biology, Physics 30*, 279–287.

Lee RW & Hanks GE (1995). External-beam radiotherapy for early-stage prostate cancer. *Advances in Oncology, 11*, 13–19.

Lind J, Kravitz K, & Greig B (1993). Urologic and male genital malignancies. In SL Groenwald, MH Frogge, M Goodman, & CH Yarbro (Eds.), *Cancer Nursing Principles and Practice*, (pp. 1258-). Boston: Jones and Bartlett.

Litwin MS, Hays RD, Fink A, Ganz PA, Leake B, & Leach GE et al. (1995). Quality-of-life outcomes in men treated for localized prostate cancer. *Journal of the American Medical Association, 273*, 129–135.

Marks LB, Carroll PR, Dugan TC & Anscher MS (1995). The response of the urinary bladder, urethra, and ureter to radiation and chemotherapy. *International Journal of Radiation Oncology, Biology, Physics, 31*, 1257–1280.

Maxwell MB (1993). Cancer of the prostate. *Seminars in Oncology Nursing, 9*, 237–251.

McCarthy CP (1992). Altered patterns of elimination. In KH Dow & LH Hilderley (Eds.), *Nursing Care in Radiation Oncology.* Philadelphia: WB Saunders.

McLean M, Akl AM, Warde P, Bissett R, Panzarella T, & Gospodarowicz M (1993). The results of primary radiation therapy in the management of squamous cell carcinoma of the penis. *International Journal of Radiation Oncology, Biology, Physics, 25*, 623–628.

Modig H, Duchek M, & Sjodin J (1993). Carcinoma of the penis. *Acta Oncologica, 32*, 653–655.

Opjordsmoen S, & Fossa SD (1994). Quality of life in patients treated for penile cancer. A follow-up study. *British Journal of Urology, 74*, 652–657.

Parker SL, Tong T, Bolden S, & Wingo PA (1997). Cancer statistics, 1997. *CA: A Cancer Journal for Clinicians, 47*, 5–27.

Parsons JT, & Million RR (1988). Planned preoperative irradiation in the management of clinical stage B2-C (T3) bladder carcinoma. *International Journal of Radiation Oncology, Biology, Physics, 14*, 797–810.

Pearse HD (1994). The urinary bladder. In JD Cox (Ed.), *Moss' Radiation Oncology, Rationale, Technique, Results* (pp. 518–554.). St. Louis: Mosby.

Pedrick TJ, Wheeler W, & Riemenschneider H (1993). Combined modality therapy for locally advanced penile squamous cell carcinoma. *American Journal of Clinical Oncology, 16*, 501–505.

Perez CA (1992). Prostate. In CA Perez & LW Brady (Eds.), *Principles and Practice of Radiation Oncology*, (pp. 1067–1116). New York: JB Lippincott.

Persky L, & deKernion J (1986). Carcinoma of the penis. *CA: A Cancer Journal for Clinicians, 36*, 258–272.

Pollack A, Zagars GK, & Kopplin S (1995). Radiotherapy and androgen ablation for clinically localized high-risk prostate cancer. *International Journal of Radiation Oncology, Biology, Physics, 32*, 13–20.

Porter AT, McEwan AJB, Powe JE, Reid R, McGowan DG Lukka H, et al. (1993). Results of a randomized phase-III trial to evaluate the efficacy of strontium-89 adjuvant to local field external beam irradiation in the management of endocrine resistant metastatic prostate cancer. *International Journal of Radiation Oncology, Biology, Physics, 25*, 805–813.

Purdy JA (1995). Current techniques in three-dimensional CT simulation and radiation treatment planning. (article review) *Oncology, 9*, 1238–1240.

Ravi R, Chaturvedi HK, & Sastry D (1994). Role of radiation therapy in the treatment of carcinoma of the penis. *British Journal of Urology, 74*, 646–651.

Schover L (1988). *Sexuality and cancer: for the man who has cancer and his partner.* New York: American Cancer Society.

Shell JA (1994). Impact of cancer on sexuality. In SE Otto (Ed.), *Oncology Nursing*, (pp. 737–760). St. Louis: Mosby.

Sherins RJ (1993). Gonadal dysfunction. In VT DeVita Jr., S Hellman, and SA Rosenberg (Eds.), *Cancer principles and practice of oncology* (pp. 2395–2406) Philadelphia: JB Lippincott.

Shipes E & Lehr S (1982). Sexuality and the male cancer patient. *Cancer Nursing, 5*, .375.

Shipley WU (1988). Genitourinary cancer. In CC Wang (Ed.), *Clinical Radiation Oncology Indications, Techniques, and Results* (pp. 262–290). Littleton: PSG Publishing.

Shipley WU, Zietman AL, Hanks GE, Coen JJ, Caplan RJ, Won M, et al. (1994). Treatment related sequelae following external beam radiation for prostate cancer: a review with an update in patients with stages T1 and T2 tumor. *The Journal of Urology, 152*, 1799–1805.

Speer TW, Sombeck MD, Parsons JT, & Million RR (1995). Testicular seminoma: a failure analysis and literature review. *International Journal of Radiation Oncology, Biology, Physics, 33*, 89–97.

Stein ME, Kessel I, Luberant N & Kuten A (1993). Testicular seminoma Stage I: Treatment results and long-term follow-up (1968–1988). *Journal of Surgical Oncology, 53*, 175–179.

Stevens KR (1994). The colon and rectum. In JD Cox (Ed.), *Moss' Radiation Oncology Rationale, Technique, Results* (pp. 462). St. Louis: Mosby.

Strohl RA (1992). The elderly patient receiving radiation therapy: treatment sequelae and nursing care. *Geriatric Nursing*, May/June, 153–159.

Thomas G (1994). Alternative management options to radiation therapy for stage I and IIA testicular seminoma. *In-*

ternational Journal of Radiation Oncology, Biology, Physics,
28, 547–548.

Waldman AR, & Osborne DM (1994). Screening for prostate
cancer. *Oncology Nursing Forum, 21*, 1512–1517.

Zagars GK, Pollack A, & von Eschenbach AC (1995). Prostate
cancer and radiation therapy—the message conveyed by
serum prostate-specific antigen. *International Journal of
Radiation Oncology, Biology, Physics, 33*, 23–35.

Zietman AL, & Shipley WU (1993). Randomized trials in
loco-regionally confined prostate cancer: past, present,
and future. *Seminars in Radiation Oncology, 3*, 210–
220.

Gynecologic Cancer

STEPHANIE MITCHELL

Endometrial, cervical, and ovarian are the three most common gynecological cancers, with vulvar and vaginal cancers being the fourth and fifth respectively. An estimated 76,200 new cases and 25,000 deaths from cervical, endometrial and ovarian cancers occur per year (American Cancer Society, 1997). Gynecological cancers occur in women of all ages, but during the last decade the incidence of cervical cancer has increased in women under 50 years. Endometrial, ovarian, vulvar, and vaginal cancers increase with age, with ovarian cancer causing more deaths than any other gynecologic cancer. A majority of women will be diagnosed with carcinoma in situ, a precancerous condition, which is now more frequent than invasive carcinoma of the cervix, vulva, and vagina. Most gynecologic cancers are discovered in early stages when they are highly curable, but many women with ovarian cancer are diagnosed in advanced stages of the disease.

Nursing care of the woman with a gynecologic cancer can be very challenging for the radiation oncology nurse. Many women experiencing gynecologic problems may have feelings such as fear, guilt, or embarrassment, which may prevent them from seeking appropriate medical attention. Often women with these feelings will delay seeking medical attention until the symptoms have progressed and the tumor is in an advanced stage (Sorensen & Rosenow, 1987). The patient who has undergone surgery, pelvic irradiation, and/or brachytherapy may have a number of issues, from very basic skin care to the more complex sexual concerns. Radiation therapy plays a major role in most gynecologic cancers. It is important that the nurse understand the stresses that a patient may experience during treatment thereby helping patients cope with the side effects of treatment as well as any lifestyle changes they may be facing.

The purpose of this chapter is to (1) familiarize the nurse with the five most common gyneco-logic cancers, cervical, endometrial, ovarian, vulvar, and vaginal, and (2) provide a detailed discussion of the nursing care and management of the side effects women receiving treatment for a gynecologic malignancy may experience.

Anatomy

The female reproductive system consists of internal organs and external organs. The internal organs include the ovaries, uterus and vagina, and the mons pubis, labia majora, labia minora, and the vestibule of the vagina comprise the external genitalia. The uterus is situated in the middle of the pelvis between the bladder and the rectum, and is divided into two parts, the body and the cervix. The body and the cervix are further divided by a narrowing of the uterus called the isthmus. Two pairs of ligaments play an important role in providing support for the uterus and cervix: the uterosacral ligaments and the cardinal ligaments. The uterosacral ligaments support the lower uterus and consist of fibrous tissue with smooth muscle. The cardinal ligaments arise from the upper margins of the cervix and insert into the fascial covering of the pelvic diaphragm.

The uterus consists of three layers: serosal, muscular, and mucosal. The serosal layer is formed by the peritoneum covering the uterus. The muscular layer, or myometrium, consists of smooth muscle and elastic fibers, and the mucosal layer, which is the innermost lining of the uterus, is known as the endometrium (Thompson, McFarland, Hirsch, Tucker & Bowers, 1989). The lower part of the uterus is known as the cervix. The opening to the uterus is called the cervical os or opening. The uterus has a rich network of lymphatics and blood vessels which drain to various areas in the pelvis.

The vagina is a tubular canal measuring on the average 10 to 15 cm in length and decreases in length with age. The vagina extends from the vestibule to the uterus and is located between the bladder and the rectum. The cervix produces two lateral fornices which project into the vagina, and are of clinical importance because palpation can easily be done through this thin wall. The vagina is made up of a thick mucous membrane that is constantly in contact with each other and kept moist by cervical secretions. The vagina is composed of three layers: the mucosa, the muscularis, and the adventitia. The mucosa is the outer layer and consists of folds called rugae, the muscularis is composed of smooth muscle fibers, and the adventitia is thin connective tissue.

The vulva includes the mons veneris, the labia majora and minora, the clitoris, and the vulvar vestibule. The mons veneris is the fatty prominence, which is covered by hair during puberty. The labia majora and minora are underneath and contain sebaceous glands. Anteriorly they are split to form the clitoris, which is an erectile structure consisting of a glans, a body, and two crura. The main arterial supply for the vulva is the pudendal artery which has different branches that supply different areas. The superficial artery supplies the labia, the artery of the bulb supplies the vestibule bulb and the erectile tissues of the vagina, the corpus cavernosum supplies the corresponding organ, and the dorsal artery of the clitoris supplies the dorsum of that organ. Lymphatics that drain the vulva are primarily situated along the line of the inguinal ligament and along the saphenous vein. The femoral lymph nodes lie below the cribriform fascia and consist of only two or three lymph nodes.

The ovaries are two oval structures in the upper part of the pelvic cavity, between the uterus medially and the lateral pelvic wall. They are suspended by the mesovarium, which extends from the surface of the broad ligaments. The glandular elements of the ovaries are described as the interstitial, thecal, and luteal cells.

Cervical Cancer

The American Cancer Society estimates 14,500 new cases of invasive carcinoma of the cervix and 65,000 new cases of carcinoma in situ in 1997 (Parker et al., 1997). The overall 5-year survival rate is 67 percent. The survival rate for women diagnosed with carcinoma in situ is 100 percent, compared to 90 percent for early and localized disease (American Cancer Society, 1997). Early detection is important in the prevention and treatment of cervical cancer. The American Cancer Society recommends that women 18 years and older and sexually active younger women undergo annual Pap smears until they have three consecutive negative tests. At this time, the Pap tests may be performed less frequently at the discretion of the clinician and woman (American Cancer Society, 1997).

There are several risk factors that increase a woman's chances for cervical cancer. These include:

1. venereal disease, especially those attributed to the (HPV) human papillomavirus and herpes simplex type 2 virus,
2. early age at first intercourse,
3. multiple sex partners,
4. cigarette smoking,
5. history of cervical intraepithelial neoplasia,
6. in utero exposure to diethylstilbestrol (DES),
7. large number of pregnancies,
8. and low socioeconomic status.

The development of cervical cancer seems to be related to multiple injuries and insults and is almost nonexistent in a celibate population (Thompson, 1990). There is increasing evidence that cervical cancer may be related to HPV infection. Early signs and symptoms of cervical cancer include serosanguineous or yellowish vaginal discharge, painless, intermittent, postcoital, intermenstrual, or postmenopausal vaginal bleeding, and an increase in the length and amount of menstrual flow. Late signs and symptoms may include dysuria, urinary retention, urinary frequency or hematuria, rectal bleeding, constipation, or bowel obstruction, which appears in advanced stages because of invasion of the bladder and/or rectum. Other late symptoms may include abdominal or pelvic pain, lower extremity edema, and painful intercourse.

If a positive Pap test shows atypia or mild dysplasia, the test should be repeated in a few weeks. If the results are persistent, the patient is usually followed closely at least every 6 months. If a Pap test shows dysplasia or malignant cells, a colposcopy is usually performed. This test allows the clinician to assess, with magnification, the proper sites for biopsy. If a colposcope is unavailable, another useful test is the Schiller test. Iodine is used to stain the normal tissue in the cervix, leaving the cancerous tissue unstained. When the entire lesion cannot be identified by colposcopy, or a colposcopic biopsy suggests microinvasion, a cone biopsy is usually performed (Perez et al., 1992a). This includes surgically removing both epithelial and endocervical tissue from the cervix in a cone-shaped segment. For more extensive disease, patients may be examined under anesthesia to enable the clinician to examine the entire cervix with the abdominal muscles relaxed. If a lesion of the cervix is noted, punch biopsies may be taken in all four quadrants of the cervix for diagnosis. It is also recommended that dilatation and curettage of the endocervical canal and endometrium be performed to determine if the tumor has extended upward (Perez et al., 1992a). This determination is important in the initial staging because it may modify the treatment plan. Staging of cervical cancer is outlined in Table 13–1. Further studies that may be performed in patients with more than microinvasive disease are CT scan, intravenous pyelography, ultrasound, or MRI to evaluate whether the disease is localized or has metastasized to regional lymph nodes or other sites outside of the pelvis. It is also recommended that cystoscopy, and in some cases proctoscopy, be performed in advanced disease to establish if the tumor has invaded the bladder or the rectum. A chest x ray may also be done to rule out lung metastasis.

When discussing treatment options, cervical cancer is divided into two types: premalignant (noninvasive) cancer and invasive cancer. Noninvasive cancer of the cervix includes mild dyplasia (cervical intraepithelial neoplasia) (CIN I), moderate dysplasia (CIN II), and severe dysplasia (carcinoma in situ) (CIN III). Treatment options depend on the patient's age, desire to maintain fertility, and size and location of the lesion. Specific treatment options for cervical neoplasms are outlined in Table 13–2.

The majority of invasive cancers are predominantly squamous cell carcinomas. Treatment of invasive carcinoma is dependent on the patient's age, physical condition, tumor volume, and the desire to maintain ovarian function. Surgery is limited to patients with early disease or stage I

Table 13-1 • International Federation of Gynecology and Obstetrics (FIGO) Staging for Cervical Cancer

TNM	FIGO	Definition
TX		Primary tumor cannot be assessed
T0		No evidence of primary tumor
Tis		Carcinoma in situ
T1	I	Cervical carcinoma confined to the uterus
T1a	IA	Preclinical invasive carcinoma, diagnosed by microscopy only
T1a1	IA1	Minimal microscopic stromal invasion
T1a2	IA2	Tumor with an invasive component 5 mm or less in depth taken from the base of the epithelium and 7mm or less in horizontal spread
T1b	IB	Tumor larger than T1a2
T2	II	Cervical carcinoma invades beyond the uterus but not to the pelvic wall or to the lower third of the vagina
T2a	IIA	Tumor without parametrial invasion
T2b	IIB	Tumor with parametrial invasion
T3	III	Cervical carcinoma extends to the pelvic wall and/or involves the lower third of the vagina and/or causes hydronephrosis or nonfunctioning kidney
T3a	IIIA	Tumor involves the lower third of the vagina, with no extension to the pelvic wall
T3b	IIIB	Tumor extends to the pelvic wall and/or causes hydronephrosis or a nonfunctioning kidney
T4	IVA	Tumor invades the mucosa of the bladder or rectum and/or extends beyond the true pelvis
M1	IVB	Distant metastasis
REGIONAL LYMPH NODES		
NX		Regional lymph nodes cannot be assessed
N0		No regional lymph node metastasis
N1		Regional lymph node metastasis
DISTANT METASTASIS		
MX		Presence of distant metastasis cannot be assessed
M0		No distant metastasis
M1		

Source: Beahrs OH et al. (Eds.) (1993). Handbook for staging of cancer. From *Manual for Staging of Cancer* (4th ed.). Philadelphia: JB Lippincott. Reprinted with permission.

Table 13-2 • Treatment Options for Cervical
Intraepithelial Neoplasia

Observation	If the lesion is small and the patient is compliant for return visits, pregnant, or immunosuppressed
Cryosurgery	A single- or double-freeze technique using CO_2 or nitrous oxide
Electrocautery	Less popular because of discomfort and the potential for more scar formation
Laser vaporization	No anesthesia, can treat the disease area leaving normal epithelium untouched
Hysterectomy	Usually done in women who are finished with childbearing

Adapted from Nolte S & Hanjani P (1990). Intraepithelial neoplasia of the lower genital tract. *Seminars in Oncology Nursing, 6,* pp. 183–185. Reprinted with permission.

(and in some institutions, stage IIa) and as an exenterative procedure for patients with recurrent disease. Surgery is frequently the choice for younger women because of their desire to maintain ovarian function and to avoid vaginal atrophy or stenosis (Fuller et al., 1990). Radiation is most often the overall treatment choice because it can be used in early or advanced stages of the disease, or in combination with surgery. Radiation therapy usually consists of external beam to treat the whole pelvis and the parametria, and intracavitary brachytherapy to treat local disease. Treatment for stage IA disease may consist of intracavitary radiation of doses between 6000 and 8000 cGy. For bulky stage IB a dose of approximately 4000 to 5000 cGy to the whole pelvis and an intracavitary dose to a total of 8500 cGy. In stages IIA, IIB, and III whole pelvic radiation may consist of 4000 to 5000 cGy, sometimes with an additional parametrial boost, and a total intracavitary dose of 7500 to 9000 cGy (Perez, 1993). Radiation therapy is sometimes used preoperatively to treat bulky IB disease, or in some women postoperatively after a hysterectomy.

The most common areas of metastasis are lymph nodes, lungs, liver, and bone. The disease can also locally extend to other pelvic organs. With metastasis, chemotherapy has been used with only short-term responses (Thombes, 1991). Patients with advanced or recurrent carcinoma of the cervix, who have bleeding and/or pelvic pain, can be treated with brachytherapy or external beam radiation for palliation in doses of 3000 to 5000 cGy (Perez, 1993). One of the more promising chemotherapy agents being used by the Gynecologic Oncology Group (GOG) is cisplatin, where a 50 percent response rate was observed (Thompson, 1990). Total pelvic exenteration may be an option for women who have no evidence of extra pelvic spread. This includes removal of the bladder, uterus, cervix, vagina, and urethra, along with the formation of ureteral and intestinal diversions. Because of the high morbidity of this procedure, it is recommended for very few women. Radiation therapy has been used for the treatment of cervical cancer for a long time and continuing clinical trials will be focusing on the use of brachytherapy (including number of fractions, dose per fraction, and total doses), and the use of radiation sensitizers (Perez, 1993).

Endometrial Cancer

The American Cancer Society has estimated that 34,900 new cases of cancer of the endometrium occurred in 1996 along with an estimated 6,000 deaths (Parker et al., 1997). It is now the most common gynecologic cancer in the United States. Ninety-five percent of endometrial cancers occur in women over 40 years old (Park et al., 1992). Because the majority of women diagnosed with endometrial cancer are postmenopausal, the symptoms of abnormal uterine spotting or bleeding are easily detected and often the cancer is diagnosed at an early stage. The overall 5-year survival rate is 83 percent, 94 percent if discovered at an early stage, and 67 percent if diagnosed at a regional stage (American Cancer Society, 1997). The American Cancer Society (1997) recommends that women over 40 years of age have annual pelvic exams, and women at a high risk for endometrial cancer should have an endometrial tissue sample evaluated at menopause.

A number of risk factors are associated with endometrial cancer. These include: failure of ovulation, nulliparity, obesity, the presence of estrogen-producing ovarian tumors, diabetes, hypertension (which may be linked to obesity), and prolonged use of unopposed estrogen therapy. Because estrogen therapy has been linked to an increased incidence of endometrial cancer, the benefits and risks of using estrogen to relieve such symptoms as "hot flashes" and painful intercourse, should be discussed by the woman and her physician (American Cancer Society, 1997). In contrast, combined estrogen and progesterone therapy have not been noted to increase the risk of endometrial cancer (NCI, 1995a).

Signs and symptoms of endometrial cancer may include abnormal uterine staining or bleeding, and abnormally heavy menses in premenopausal women. Other causes of vaginal bleeding may be attributed to any of the following: bacterial vaginitis, cancer of the vagina or cervix, urinary tract infections, or even metastatic disease from breast, gastric, colon, or other carcinomas (Hubbard & Holcombe, 1990). Since a majority of women with endometrial cancer are postmenopausal, the early sign of uterine bleeding prompts the woman to seek medical attention. Thus, endometrial cancer is likely to be diagnosed at an early stage.

The majority of endometrial cancers are adenocarcinomas. The detection and diagnosis of endometrial cancer is obtained by a thorough pelvic exam, cervical biopsies, endocervical curettage, endometrial biopsy, and/or fractional dilatation and curettage (D&C). Fractional D&C allows the clinician to measure the depth of the endometrial cavity as well as any cervical involvement (Berkowitz et al., 1990). This type of procedure is sometimes done if endometrial biopsies have been negative and bleeding persists. Other tests that may be done prior to surgery are urinary imaging studies, renal scans, cystoscopy and proctoscopy to determine if the tumor has spread to the bladder or rectum, routine blood and urine studies, and a chest x ray. Ultrasound and/or magnetic resonance imaging (MRI) may be done to help determine uterine invasion as well as nodal involvement.

Staging of endometrial cancer is completed surgically from exploratory laparotomy, total abdominal hysterectomy-bilateral salpingo-oophorectomy (TAH-BSO), lymph node sampling, and peritoneal washings. Table 13-3 lists FIGO staging for endometrial carcinoma. Staging is based on anatomical stage, histopathological grade, depth of the myometrial invasion, and metastatic spread. Patients that cannot undergo surgery for medical reasons can be clinically staged, but the preferred method of staging is by TAH-BSO (Park et al., 1992).

Treatment choices for endometrial cancer include surgery and/or external beam radiation therapy and brachytherapy; surgery is the first choice in all stages (Table 13–4). Radiation therapy may be used preoperatively for bulky disease, but is usually given after surgery to decrease the risk of pelvic and vaginal recurrence. Some institutions may still use preoperative radiation in patients

Table 13-3 • FIGO Staging for Endometrial Cancer

TNM	FIGO	Definition
TX		Primary tumor cannot be assessed
T0		No evidence of primary tumor
Tis		Carcinoma in situ
T1	I	Tumor confined to the corpus uteri
T1a	IA	Tumor limited to the endometrium
T1b	IB	Tumor invades up to or less than one-half of the myometrium
T1c	IC	Tumor invades more than one-half of the myometrium
T2	II	Tumor invades the cervix but not beyond the uterus
T2a	IIA	Endocervical glandular involvement only
T2b	IIB	Cervical stromal invasion
T3	III	Local and/or regional spread as specified in T3a, b, N1 and FIGO IIIA, B, and C below
N1		
T3a	IIIA	Tumor involves the serosa and/or adnexa and/or cancer cells in ascites or peritoneal washings
T3b	IIIB	Vaginal involvement (direct extension or metastasis)
N1	IIIC	Metastasis to the pelvic and/or para-aortic lymph nodes
T4	IVA	Tumor invades the bladder mucosa or the rectum and/or the bowel mucosa
M1	IVB	Distant metastasis (excluding metastasis to the vagina, pelvic serosa, or adnexa; including metastasis to intraabdominal lymph nodes other than paraaortic, and/or inguinal lymph nodes)

HISTOPATHOLOGIC GRADE

GX		Grade cannot be assessed
G1		Well differentiated
G2		Moderately differentiated
G3–4		Poorly differentiated or undifferentiated

Source: Beahrs OH et al. (Eds.) (1993). Handbook for staging of cancer. From *Manual for Staging of Cancer* (4th ed., pp. 174–175). Philadelphia: JB Lippincott. Reprinted with permission.

Table 13-4 • Usual Treatment Approaches
for Endometrial Cancer

Stage	Treatment		
IA G1	TAH-BSO		
IA G2, 3	TAH-BSO	+/−EBRT	+/−Brachytherapy
IB G1	TAH-BSO		
IB G2, 3	TAH-BSO	+/−EBRT	+/−Brachytherapy
II	TAH-BSO	+EBRT	+Brachytherapy
III	Treatment individualized		
IV	Hormone therapy sometimes offered		

with gross lesions involving the cervix or with lesions involving the upper vagina. Patients with a high grade lesion (grade III), deep myometrial invasion (at least half), and/or cervical involvement may require postoperative radiation. Patients with stage I or II disease who cannot undergo a hysterectomy can be treated with radiation alone using external beam radiation and brachytherapy (Berkowitz et al., 1990).

Postoperative treatment of stage I disease is not clear cut. It is recommended that the degree of tumor differentiation be assessed in patients with stage I disease, and the depth of myometrial invasion be considered in adjuvant radiation therapy recommendations. Poorly differentiated tumors have been associated with a higher incidence of vaginal vault recurrence, deep myometrial invasion, and spread to pelvic and aortic lymph nodes (Berkowitz et al., 1990). If the tumor is poorly differentiated or has other poor prognostic features, the treatment may include surgery along with external radiation to treat the nodal areas and upper vagina, as well as intracavitary vaginal radiation to reduce the risk of vaginal vault recurrence. Otherwise, surgery alone may be used in stage I disease (Berkowitz et al., 1990).

Patients with stage II endometrial cancer usually require surgery combined with radiation therapy because of cervical involvement, the increased risk for pelvic node metastasis and pelvic recurrence (Berkowitz et al., 1990). Radiation therapy as a sole modality of treatment for stage I or stage II disease is used when patients cannot undergo a hysterectomy for medical reasons. Stage III disease includes a variety of presentations and, for example, may include local and/or regional spread with possible ovarian metastasis. Because of the various areas of spread in stage III disease, it is important for the clinician to individualize the treatment plan. If possible, the treatment of choice is surgery followed by radiation therapy.

Vaginal recurrences after treatment of endometrial cancer are frequently small, nonulcerated, benign-appearing plaques (Komaki, 1994). The treatment of choice for these recurrences is usually external beam pelvic radiation therapy followed by brachytherapy (Komaki, 1994). Metastatic disease has been palliated with local irradiation or progestational therapy to try to control pain and bleeding (Berkowitz et al., 1990). Side effects of progestational therapy may include fluid retention, phlebitis, or thrombosis. Occasionally total body hair loss occurs at very high radiation doses.

Ovarian Cancer

The American Cancer Society has estimated that 26,800 new cases of ovarian cancer were diagnosed in 1996 and 14,200 deaths occurred (Parker et al., 1996). Ovarian cancer accounts for only 5 percent of all cancers in women, but causes more deaths than any other cancer of the female reproductive system (American Cancer Society, 1997). Ovarian cancer is a challenge for the health care professional since there is no known cause of the disease, and effective screening techniques are yet to be identified. Therefore, many women are diagnosed with ovarian cancer at later stages of the disease. Few risk factors have been identified with ovarian cancer, but some women are at a higher risk than others. These risk factors include nulliparity, advancing age, North American or Northern European descent, a personal history of breast, colon, or endometrial cancer, and a family history of ovarian cancer (NIH Consensus Statement, 1994). The NIH consensus statement concluded that women with two or more first-degree relatives with ovarian cancer have a 7 percent lifetime risk of ovarian cancer. In women with one affected relative, the lifetime risk is 5 percent and for women with no affected relatives the risk is 1 in 70.

The risk of developing ovarian cancer increases with age and peaks between the ages of 40 to 70 (Ball et al., 1990). Women may have vague complaints of gas, abdominal discomfort, urinary frequency, or other gastric symptoms that may delay the diagnosis. A careful pelvic exam occasionally may detect an ovarian mass. Late symptoms of ovarian cancer include abdominal distention, palpable tumor, pain, dyspnea, and weight loss. Screening tests that may be performed if ovarian cancer is suspected include serum CA-125, bimanual rectovaginal pelvic exam, and transvaginal ultrasound. An elevated CA-125 may also be found in women with other non-ovarian malignancies. It is estimated that a CA-125 is elevated in approximately 80 percent of women with epithelial ovarian cancers (NIH Consensus Statement, 1994). Studies to evaluate the liver, kidneys, bowel, bladder, lungs, and regional lymph nodes may be performed, since ovarian cancer tends to metastasize to these organs.

The FIGO staging system for ovarian cancer is listed in Table 13–5. The treatment of choice for all stages of ovarian cancer is a total abdominal hysterectomy and bilateral salpingo-oophorectomy. The surgical technique is quite specific for staging of ovarian carcinoma and includes, for example, multiple biopsy procedures including the diaphragm as well as an omentectomy. Stage IA-grade 1 and most stage IB-grade 1 ovarian cancers generally do not require postoperative adjuvant therapy. Chemotherapy is the preferred treatment of choice following surgery for stage I poorly differentiated tumors and stage II, III, and IV (NIH Consensus Statement, 1994). One American study concluded that intravenous or intraperitoneal cisplatin and paclitaxel are the optimal first-line

chemotherapy drugs following surgery for ovarian cancer, and are being used by most oncologists in the U.S. (NIH Consensus Statement, 1994). If a patient has a clinically complete response, then a "second look" surgery is sometimes performed to remove any remaining tumor and evaluate treatment response. Table 13–6 lists treatment options for ovarian cancer.

Currently, the usual role of radiation therapy in ovarian cancer is for treatment of localized symptoms and palliation. Occasionally, whole-abdominal radiation therapy is used postoperatively in patients with residual disease, but this treatment option has fallen out of favor in the United States. Phosphorous-32 (P-32), a beta emitter, is used in some institutions to treat microscopic disease in the peritoneum. P-32 is a colloidal substance that is instilled through a catheter that has been inserted into the peritoneal sac of a patient with ovarian cancer. The procedure for the insertion of the catheter is similar to that of a paracentesis. Ascitic fluid may be removed from the patient prior to the insertion of P-32. The procedure can be done on an outpatient basis using a procedure room in the Radiation Oncology Department. The patient lies on a stretcher in a position that is favorable for a paracentesis. Once the catheter is inserted, the patient is taken to the simulator for an x ray to verify the placement of the

Table 13-5 • FIGO Staging for Ovarian Cancer

TNM	FIGO	Definition
TX		Primary tumor cannot be assessed
T0		No evidence of primary tumor
T1	I	Tumor limited to ovaries (one or both)
T1a	IA	Tumor limited to one ovary; capsule intact, no tumor on ovarian surface, no malignant cells in ascites or peritoneal washings
T1b	IB	Tumor limited to both ovaries; capsules intact, no tumor on ovarian surface, no malignant cells in ascites or peritoneal washings
T1c	IC	Tumor limited to one or both ovaries with any of the following: capsule ruptured, tumor on ovarian surface, malignant cells in ascites or peritoneal washings
T2	II	Tumor involves one or both ovaries with pelvic extension
T2a	IIA	Extension and/or implants on the uterus and/or tube(s); no malignant cells in ascites or peritoneal washings
T2b	IIB	Extension to other pelvic tissues; no malignant cells in ascites or peritoneal washings
T2c	IIC	Pelvic extension (2a or 2b) with malignant cells in ascites or peritoneal washings
T3 and/or N1	III	Tumor involves one or both ovaries with microscopically confirmed peritoneal metastasis outside the pelvis and/or regional lymph nodes
T3a	IIIA	Microscopic peritoneal metastasis beyond the pelvis
T3b	IIIB	Macroscopic peritoneal metastasis beyond the pelvis 2 cm or less in the greatest dimension
T3c	IIIC	Peritoneal metastasis beyond the pelvis more than 2 cm in the greatest N1 dimension and/or
	IV	regional lymph metastasis
M1		Distant metastasis

Source: Beahrs OH et al. (Eds.) (1993). Handbook of staging of cancer. From *Manual for Staging of Cancer* (4th ed., pp. 178–179). Philadelphia: JB Lippincott. Reprinted with permission.

Table 13-6 • Treatment Options for Ovarian Cancer

Stage	Treatment
IA or IB, grade 1	No further treatment
IA, IB, grade 2, 3	Single-agent chemotherapy
IC	P-32 or combination chemotherapy
II, gross residual disease	Combination chemotherapy including cisplatin
II, III <2 cm residual disease	Combination chemotherapy including cisplatin (or whole abdominal pelvic radiation)
III >2 cm residual disease; IV	Combination chemotherapy including cisplatin
Refractory disease	Chemotherapy, immunotherapy, intraperitoneal therapy, hormonal therapy

Source: Eriksson JH & Walczak JR (1990). Ovarian Cancer. *Seminars in Oncology Nursing, 6*, 218. Reprinted with permission.

catheter. The patient returns to the procedure room and P-32 is brought to the procedure room by a member of the physics staff. The P-32 is instilled through the patient's catheter with either a syringe or a closed IV pressurized delivery method. Once all of the P-32 has been instilled, the catheter is removed and the patient is instructed to change positions on a specified plan to allow the isotope to be evenly distributed to the entire peritoneal sac. Once this is done the patient is allowed to return home. Chapter 3 provides a more in-depth discussion of the issues involved in radiation pro-tection.

If a woman with ovarian cancer relapses there is no realistic hope for cure. Patients who relapse within 6 months have a poor response rate to any kind of treatment. Those who relapse after 6 months have a greater chance of responding to platinum-containing regimens. A small percentage of patients may benefit from surgery. Some of these patients are disease free for 2 or more years (NIH Consensus Statement, 1994). Surgery may also be used for palliation as well as radiation therapy to treat localized symptoms. If the patient relapses a second time other chemotherapy regimens such as ifosfamide, hexamethylmelamine, tamoxifen, 5-FU, etoposide, and others have been used with a 15 percent response rate. Although there have been response rates suggested with these regimens, there has been no overall survival benefit demonstrated (NIH Consensus Statement, 1994). Therefore, quality of life is a very important consideration. The health care providers need to educate patients regarding the prognosis and treatment options so that patients can make informed decisions about selecting therapy.

Vaginal Cancer

Vaginal cancer represents 1 to 2 percent of all gynecologic malignancies (Perez et al., 1992b). There has been a decrease in the incidence of vaginal cancers, possibly due to increased screening for cervical cancers. There are two histologic types of vaginal cancer: squamous cell and adenocarcinoma. The two must be distinguished because each type has its own different pathogenesis and natural history (NCI, 1995b).

It is not clear what factors may increase the risk of vaginal cancer. It is thought that the human papillomavirus (HPV) is a promoting factor in cervical, vulvar, and vaginal cancers, but this theory has not yet been established. The human papillomavirus DNA have been identified in the female genital tract as well as in vaginal lesions, concluding that this virus may be a factor. It is also thought that vaginal intraepithelial neoplasia (VAIN) may be a predisposing factor to invasive carcinoma of the vagina, and that exposure to diethylstilbestrol (DES) in utero may be another predisposing factor for adenocarcinoma of the vagina in young women. Although this has not been determined, the history of VAIN and exposure to DES should concern the clinician (Chamorro, 1990).

Women presenting with a vaginal carcinoma may report intermittent or postcoital bleeding and vaginal discharge. Women with more advanced disease may present with complaints of dysuria and pelvic pain (Perez et al., 1992b).

During the pelvic examination the entire vagina as well as the cervix and vulva are examined. Bimanual palpation of the vagina and the rectum are performed. The distinction must be made between cervical cancer and vulvar cancer to make the diagnosis of vaginal cancer. If the lesion extends to the cervix and/or vulva, and biopsies are positive, then the diagnosis of primary vaginal cancer cannot be made (Perez et al., 1992b). If the lesion is confined to the vagina alone, cervical biopsies are still performed to rule out a primary cervical cancer. Biopsies of the vagina may be taken using the Schiller's test and colposcopy is performed to better visualize the vaginal lesions. Tests that may be performed to evaluate the extent of the disease are cytoscopy and proctosigmoidoscopy. Other tests are chest x ray, intravenous pyelogram, CT scan, and MRI, and sometimes barium enema or air contrast.

The examination for staging of vaginal cancer is performed jointly by the gynecologic and radiation oncologists with the patient under anesthesia. It is crucial to determine if the lesion is a primary vaginal cancer or metastatic spread, since the vagina is the most common site of spread from the ovary, endometrium, cervix, and bowel (Thombes, 1991). If the cervix contains the same histologic type of lesion as the vagina, the lesion is classified as cervical carcinoma and not vaginal carcinoma. If the lesion is primarily in the vagina, and biopsies are negative for the cervix, staging is done clinically using the International Federation of Gynecology and Obstetrics standards as listed in Table 13–7 (FIGO) (Perez et al., 1992b). There are several types of vaginal cancer: squamous cell carcinoma, verrucous cell carcinoma, small cell carcinoma, and benign epithelial and mixed tumors and melanomas. Squamous cell carcinoma is the most common histologic type of vaginal cancer, comprising 80 to 90 percent of primary vaginal carcinomas. These lesions are primarily found in older women and are most often located in the upper, posterior wall of the vagina (Perez et al., 1992b). Clear cell adenocarcinomas are rare and usually occur in women under thirty. Other rare malignancies include sarcomas.

Treatment differs between vaginal in situ and vaginal carcinoma. Vaginal in situ cancer is much less common than cervical cancer but is increasing in incidence in young women (Nolte & Hanjani, 1990). Treatment options include excision of the lesion, laser vaporization, intravaginal 5-FU, radiation therapy, and vaginectomy. Vaginectomy is usually performed when there are multiple lesions. However, due to the high morbidity of this procedure, radiation is usually the treatment of choice (Perez et al., 1992b). An intracavitary application delivering 6500 to 8000 cGy and sometimes higher may be used to the involved vaginal mucosa (Perez et al., 1992b).

Treatment of vaginal carcinoma primarily includes surgery, external beam radiation, and brachytherapy. The type of treatment is dependent on the stage, size, and location of the lesion, as well as the presence or absence of the uterus and whether there has been any previous pelvic radiation (NCI, 1995b). In lesions of the upper vagina that are 0.5 cm or less, surgery may be the treatment of choice, including a hysterectomy, pelvic lymphadenectomy, and partial vaginectomy. However, external beam radiation therapy and brachytherapy play the major role in the treatment of vaginal cancer. Very small lesions may require intracavitary radiation alone (Komaki, 1994). There are many treatment options for stage I disease and the treatment plan is individualized for the patient. External beam radiation therapy may be used along with brachytherapy (tandem and ovoids or vaginal cylinder). Perez et al. (1992b) suggest that for superficial lesions involving more than one vaginal wall, treatment may include only brachytherapy with an intracavitary cylinder covering the entire vagina that delivers a total dose of 6500 to 8000 cGy. If the lesion is deeper and involves only one wall, a single implant may be used to deliver a surface dose of 8000 to 10,000 cGy. Stage II tumors are usually treated with external beam radiation to the whole pelvis and a combination of interstitial and intracavitary implants are used to a total dose of 7000 to 7500 cGy. Stage III and IV tumors are often treated the same as stage II disease but to a higher total dose, usually around 8000 cGy. The radiation tolerance of the vagina is high and doses of 10,000 cGy to the top of the vagina (apex) are associated with few long-term complications (Perez et al., 1992b).

Currently there are ongoing studies investigating the effects of concurrent chemotherapy and radiation. The most promising drugs being used are mitomycin, 5-fluorouracil, cisplatin, and carboplatin. Chemotherapy by itself plays a minor role in the treatment of vaginal cancer (Chamorro, 1990).

Table 13-7 • FIGO Staging for Vaginal Cancer

TNM	FIGO	Definition
TX		Primary tumor cannot be assessed
T0		No evidence of primary tumor
Tis	0	Carcinoma in situ
T1	I	Tumor confined to the vagina
T2	II	Tumor invades paravaginal tissues but not to the pelvic wall
T3	III	Tumor extends to the pelvic wall
T4	IVA	Tumor invades the mucosa of the bladder or rectum and/or extends beyond the true pelvis
M1	IVB	Distant metastasis

Source: Beahrs OH et al. (Eds.) (1993). Handbook for staging of cancer. From *Manual for Staging of Cancer* (4th ed., p. 182). Philadelphia: JB Lippincott. Reprinted with permission.

Vulvar Cancer

Carcinoma of the vulva is the fourth most common gynecologic cancer among women. It occurs approximately three times more frequently than vaginal cancer (Komaki, 1994). Vulvar cancer is external and usually superficial and should be detected and diagnosed at an early stage. It is thought that vulvar cancer may arise from lesions known as vulvar intraepithelial neoplasia (VIN). Upon examination, any lesions or pruritus found are usually biopsied.

VIN in recent years has increased in younger women and poses a threat of progression to invasive cancer. There have been reported cases of VIN spontaneously regressing as well as progressing to invasive carcinoma (Nolte & Hanjani, 1990). The few identifiable risk factors associated with VIN are human papillomavirus (HPV) and herpes simplex type II virus. Other factors identified as possible risk factors include obesity, hypertension, diabetes, cervical cancer, early menopause, and chronic vulvar irritation (Clark, 1994). The appearance of VIN may vary, but may appear as fleshy, warty, white, red, or brown lesions of the vulva or perianus. The treatment of choice for VIN is based on the presence of unifocal disease, minimal disease, or multifocal/extensive disease (Nolte & Hanjani, 1990). See Table 13–8 for a listing of treatment options.

The most common symptom of vulvar cancer is a lump or mass on the vulva and a history of vulvar itching. Less common presenting symptoms include bleeding, discharge, or dysuria. Women in more affluent societies seek medical treatment at an earlier stage than women from less affluent societies. It is still common for women in poor areas to have much more advanced stages, usually presenting with large groin masses (Hacker et al., 1992). Biopsies are usually taken of any masses, warts, or vulvar abnormality to determine the underlying diagnosis. Before treatment begins biopsies of the cervix and vagina are appropriate to rule out any other genital tract malignancy (Hacker et al., 1992). See Table 13–9 for FIGO staging for vulvar cancers.

Vulvar carcinomas are predominantly squamous cell and arise on the labia minora, clitoris, fourchette, perineal body, or medial aspects of the labia majora (Hacker et al., 1992). The most common site for vulvar cancer is the labia majora, which comprises 50 percent of the cases. The labia minora, clitoris, and Bartholin's gland are less frequently involved. The Gynecologic Oncology Group (GOG) has proposed a grading system for vulvar squamous cell carcinoma. The GOG has also reported that the higher the tumor grade the higher the risk of lymph node spread. Other types of vulvar squamous cell carcinoma include adenoid squamous cell carcinoma, squamous cell carcinoma with tumor giant cells, sebaceous cell carcinoma, and spindle cell squamous cell carcinoma (Hacker et al., 1992). Other rare types of carcinomas arising in the vulva are verrucous carcinoma, basal cell carcinoma, Merkel cell carcinoma, and transitional cell carcinoma. Other types arise from the Bartholin's gland and include adenocarcinoma, which accounts for 5 percent of vulvar cancers, adenosquamous carcinoma, and adenoid cystic carcinoma, which arises within the gland and comprises 15 percent of Bartholin gland carcinomas. Carcinomas of the sweat glands are rare and comprise 10 percent of vulvar tumors. Vulvar malignant melanoma accounts for 10 percent of all primary lesions of the vulva. Sarcomas are another type of carcinoma arising in the vulva and surrounding tissues. Examples of these sarcomas are leiomyosarcoma, which is the most frequently seen sarcoma, malignant fibrous histiocytoma, epithelioid sarcoma, and malignant rhabdoid tumor (Hacker et al., 1992).

Although radical vulvectomy is the established treatment of choice for vulvar cancer, increasingly there is an effort to decrease the extent of the surgery to preserve function and achieve a high cure rate. Although many lesions are treated with radical vulvectomy and bilateral groin

Table 13-8 • Treatment Options for Vulvar Intraepithelial Neoplasia

Surgical excision	Treatment of choice, reserved for unifocal and minimal disease
Cryosurgery	Uncommon because of slow healing and severe pain
Laser surgery	Used with good cure rates reported at 90%
Laser vaporization	Usually done under anesthesia and complications include pain and discharge, which dissipate in 4–5 days
Skinning vulvectomy	Better postoperative and cosmetic results with a high cure rate, which involves the excision of vulvar skin and the substitution of a split-thickness skin graft
Investigational modalities	Currently interferon is being used to treat VIN. It is inexpensive, safe and effective therapy

Adapted from Nolte S & Hanjani P (1990). Intraepithelial neoplasia of the lower genital tract. *Seminars in Oncology Nursing, 6*, pp. 186–187. Reprinted with permission.

Table 13-9 • FIGO Staging for Vulvar Cancer

TX	Primary tumor cannot be assessed
T0	No evidence of primary tumor
Tis	Carcinoma in situ (preinvasive cancer)
T1	Tumor confined to the vulva or to the vulva and perineum, 2 cm or less in greatest dimension
T2	Tumor confined to the vulva or to the vulva and perineum, more than 2 cm in greatest dimension
T3	Tumor invades any of the following: lower urethra, vagina, or anus
T4	Tumor invades any of the following: bladder mucosa, upper urethral mucosa, or rectal mucosa, or is fixed to the bone

REGIONAL LYMPH NODES

NX	Regional lymph nodes cannot be assessed
N0	No regional lymph node metastasis
N1	Unilateral regional lymph node metastasis
N2	Bilateral regional lymph node metastasis

Source: Beahrs OH et al. (Eds.) (1993). Handbook for staging of cancer. From *Manual for Staging of Cancer* (4th ed., p. 186). Philadelphia: JB Lippincott. Reprinted with permission.

dissection, many smaller lesions are responsive to less radical procedures. For example, if the lesion is less than 2 cm in diameter and the depth of invasion is less than 5 mm, a simple vulvectomy is usually sufficient (Otte, 1992). Stage II and III lesions require more extensive surgery than stage I. Radical vulvectomy with inguinal and femoral node resection is the treatment of choice for stage III disease (NCI, 1995c).

Radical vulvectomy for vulvar cancer usually includes removal of the lesion and the surrounding skin from the mons pubis to the perianus, inguinal, and femoral lymph nodes. Simple vulvectomy or wide excision is usually done when patients have a lesion that is 2 cm or less (Komaki, 1994). Radiation therapy may also be used postoperatively if there are narrow surgical margins, large tumors, or positive nodes. Preoperative radiation may be used to improve the surgical outcome for patients with locally advanced disease. This approach using chemotherapy plus radiation therapy is being explored in clinical trials. A GOG study conducted by Homesley and associates (1986) showed a favorable response using radiation therapy as an alternative to pelvic node resection after radical vulvectomy and groin node lymphadenectomy. The study consisted of half the group receiving 4500 to 5000 cGy tumor dose to the groin and pelvis and the other half receiving pelvic node resection. The 2-year survival rates estimated 68 percent for radiation therapy and

54 percent for pelvic node resection (Homesley et al., 1986). Thus, for patients with positive groin nodes, postoperative radiation therapy to the pelvis is often indicated.

Current studies being conducted by the GOG are combined chemotherapy and radiation therapy as an adjuvant to surgery for advanced disease. Several studies being conducted by the GOG are looking at using 5-FU with or without cisplatin and radiation therapy as an alternative to extensive surgical resection (NCI, 1995c).

Recurrent disease should be detected as early as possible, so that appropriate treatment can be initiated before the disease advances. Standard treatment options for recurrent vulvar cancer include wide local excision with or without radiation, radical vulvectomy, and pelvic exenteration. Radiation therapy alone with or without 5-FU may be curative in some patients with local recurrence (NCI, 1995c).

Pelvic Radiation

During external beam radiation the patient may either lie on her stomach or on her back for treatment. The typical daily dose of radiation to the pelvis for gynecological cancer is 180 to 200 cGy. Many institutions use a four-field approach with portals of 15 × 15 to 15 × 18 cm. The doses of external beam radiation vary from institution to institution but range from 4000 to 5000 cGy for cervical cancer. Intracavitary radiation may consist of applicators called intrauterine tandem and colpostats. This technique is done in the operating room under anesthesia because the cervix must be dilated to introduce the tandem into the uterus. The colpostats are placed on either side of the cervix and packing is put in place to hold the applicators. The usual dose may range from 3000 to 5000 cGy in addition to external beam depending on the treatment plan and stage of the disease. (See Chapter 3 for a discussion of brachytherapy.)

Vaginal and endometrial cancers may require high- or low-dose rate intracavitary implants using a vaginal cylinder. High-dose rate implants can be done as an outpatient, whereas with low-dose rate implants the patient needs to stay in the hospital for a few days. In some instances the radiation treatment for vaginal cancer is similar to cervical cancer. If the patient has a lesion in the upper third of the vagina and her uterus and cervix are intact an intrauterine tandem and vaginal colpostats may be used.

Nursing Interventions and Teaching during Radiation Therapy

During radiation therapy the nurse must be aware of the potential side effects women will experience during pelvic radiation to initiate appropriate teaching and anticipate potential problems. Table 13–10 lists both the acute side effects and the long-term side effects of pelvic radiation. As with any treatment it is difficult to exactly predict who will experience what side effects and when these side effects will occur during the treatment.

Generally during the first few weeks of radiation the patient experiences very few side effects. Patients will experience one or more of the acute side effects listed in the table and it is important that the nurse be aware of them to initiate appropriate teaching.

Side Effects of Radiation Therapy

Effects on the Skin

Prevention of skin breakdown in the perineal area is a challenge for the radiation oncology nurse. Initial teaching of skin care is important because a majority of patients will have some type of skin irritation or breakdown due to the location and the

Table 13-10 • Side Effects of Pelvic Radiation

Acute Reactions	Long-Term Reactions
COMMON	COMMON
Fatigue	Early menopause/sterility
Skin reddening and irritation	Decreased vaginal secretions
Diarrhea	Mild vaginal stenosis
Decreased blood counts	
Bladder inflammation	
Vaginitis	
Hemorrrhoids	
UNCOMMON	UNCOMMON
Nausea and vomiting	Occasional small amount of bleeding from bladder or rectum
	Chronic diarrhea
	Urinary frequency
	Marked vaginal stenosis
	RARE
	Bowel complications requiring surgical procedure
	Urinary complications requiring surgical procedure
	Second malignancies

amount of skin folds in the perineum. As treatment progresses, the patient may experience dry, itchy, and flaky skin (dry desquamation), sometimes leading to moist desquamation, in which the skin becomes raw and painful and may drain serous exudate. This breakdown puts the patient at risk for infection. Obese women may have more of a problem because of the extra skin and skin folds in the groin and perineum. The perineum is at higher risk for skin breakdown because of the increased warmth and moisture and lack of ventilation. The patient should be taught to keep the perineal area dry, wash with warm water, and pat the area dry. The patient should wear cotton underwear or, if the patient is able to, wear no underwear while at home. Commercial lotions, creams, perfumes, powders, tape, or deodorants on the skin in the radiation field, as well as any restrictive clothing, should be avoided. In addition, the patient should avoid extreme heat and cold to the area being irradiated. These extreme temperatures are contraindicated because they may further compromise the acute vascular responses in the capillaries, making the skin very susceptible to injury.

It is important that the patient be aware of the potential for skin breakdown so that if any reddening or itching of the area occurs they will notify the radiation oncologist or nurse. If dry desquamation has started, sitz baths or frequent tub baths using lukewarm water will help soothe the area as well as increase blood flow. Sometimes an aloe vera based lotion can be applied to the perineum 2 to 3 times a day. The patient must remember to remove the lotion prior to treatment because the lotion may increase the skin reaction. If moist desquamation occurs, the patient needs to cleanse the area with one-quarter strength hydrogen peroxide and saline and apply A&D ointment, lanolin, or Aquaphor to the affected area 3 times a day. If the perineal area worsens, it may be necessary to stop the treatment and prescribe silver sulfadiazine to the affected area until the area improves enough to resume treatment. Patients allergic to sulfa drugs should not use silver sulfadiazine. To help keep the perineum dry, a blow-dryer set on cool or a fan may be used. These skin reactions are quite painful, and the nurse needs to assess the patient's level of pain and assure that appropriate analgesics are prescribed by the radiation oncologist.

Once radiation therapy is complete the skin will begin to heal within about 2 weeks. Frequently, patients are frustrated because they think their skin will suddenly improve after they have completed their radiation therapy. It is reassuring to the patients if they are aware of the fact that they will notice improvement of their skin week to week, not day to day. It is, however, important that the patients continue any skin treatment regimen that has been prescribed until they return for a follow-up visit in 2 to 4 weeks. See Chapter 8 for an in-depth discussion of skin care.

Diarrhea

Morphological changes in the small bowel can be detected as early as 12 hours after the first radiation treatment. Radiation therapy to the pelvis most frequently results in diarrhea and may begin anywhere from 1500 to 3000 cGy (McCarthy, 1992). It is difficult to determine which patients will have diarrhea and to what extent. Some patients may have an increase in the number and consistency of stools while others may have diarrhea that requires a radiation treatment break to allow the bowel to recover. The nurse needs to carefully assess changes in the patient's bowel patterns during radiation therapy. Frequent soft stools may not indicate diarrhea and may not require intervention, but loose or watery stools are an indication that the patient is experiencing diarrhea. The goal of the radiation oncology nurse should include prevention, treatment, teaching, and resuming normal bowel elimination. Prevention may include starting the patient on a low fiber diet during pelvic irradiation.

If diarrhea persists even when the patient is on a low fiber diet, appropriate antidiarrheal medications are prescribed. The nurse needs to instruct the patient to keep a record of when the diarrhea is occurring. Some patients may have a pattern of diarrhea, occurring directly after the radiation, after meals, or no identifiable pattern may occur. The first choice for antidiarrheal medication is usually loperamide (Imodium), 2 mg capsules. If Imodium doesn't control the diarrhea, diphenoxylate (Lomotil) may be prescribed by the radiation oncologist. The usual dosage for both of the above medications is usually 1 to 2 tablets after each loose stool, not to exceed 8 doses per day. If the patient is having severe diarrhea (more than 8 stools a day), which is not controlled by Imodium or Lomotil, opiates can be used to decrease peristalsis. These medications include opium tincture, 0.5 to 1.0 ml orally every 4 hours; paregoric elixir, 4 ml orally every 4 hours; or codeine, 15 to 30 mg orally every 4 hours (Lydon et al., 1992).

The nurse should evaluate the patient's and family's understanding of the medication. Teaching must be done to ensure that the patient will take the medication correctly to return to the usual pattern of elimination. It may be necessary for the patient to be on a clear liquid diet during severe bouts of diarrhea and be monitored for dehydration and electrolyte imbalances. If the diarrhea is severe, it may necessary to draw blood to check the patient's blood urea nitrogen and check orthostatic blood pressure to make sure the patient is not dehydrated. It may also be necessary to draw serum potassium and sodium as well. The patient may require fluid and electrolyte replacement as well as a treatment break to rest the bowel. Sitz baths with lukewarm water for 10 minutes can be used to cleanse the anus after episodes of diarrhea in place of frequent friction cleanses to wipe the anus.

Hemorrhoids may present another problem during pelvic radiation. Many women do not have problems with existing hemorrhoids or are unaware of their presence until treatment begins. Radiation may cause the hemorrhoids to become enlarged and inflamed. Sitz baths and any over-the-counter hemorrhoid cream with hydrocortisone will help ease the discomfort. The patient should avoid use of the cream before radiation treatment. In general the patient's hemorrhoids will return to their preirradiated status after the completion of radiation therapy.

Several long-term bowel complications related to radiation therapy exist. The possibility of a radiation-induced fistula, small bowel obstruction, and perforation are late complications and are relatively rare. Small bowel obstruction increases with continued pelvic radiation and abdominal surgeries and may occur up to several years after the completion of therapy. If a bowel obstruction occurs, the patient may only need to be on a clear liquid diet to rest the bowel, or it may be necessary to perform a colostomy or ileostomy to relieve the obstruction. Fistula formation can be caused by two factors: recurrent disease or radiation induced. Once recurrent disease is ruled out treatment must be aggressive to promote healing. Small bowel and rectovaginal fistulas are very painful and require a temporary colostomy to rest the affected bowel and allow healing. In most patients this is a temporary intervention, and once the fistula has healed the colostomy can be reversed. Good hygiene is very important to eliminate the odor associated with fistulas. Items that may assist with odor control are charcoal-impregnated dressings, skin cleansers, and air deodorizers (Thompson, 1990). See Chapter 11 for additional information on management of diarrhea.

Cystitis

Cystitis is the inflammation of the bladder and or ureter characterized by pain, urgency, hematuria, and urinary frequency. During radiation therapy the bladder may become irritated with cystitis starting mid to late in the treatment. Occasionally, it has been known to occur after the first week of treatment. Cystitis may be caused by a number of factors other than radiation, such as bacterial infection, viruses, fungi, and chemical agents.

The bladder is relatively tolerant to radiation. Therapeutic doses greater than 6000 to 7000 cGy over a 6 to 7 week period generally result in cystitis. A diagnosis of radiation-induced cystitis is usually made after a normal urine culture is obtained. The nurse should encourage the patient to increase fluids and take frequent sitz baths to relieve suprapubic pain. If antibiotics are warranted for infection, encourage the patient to take the entire regimen. Education is important for the nurse to reassure the patient that when the radiation therapy is complete the urinary symptoms will subside or if an infection is present, the antibiotics should relieve the discomfort. It is sometimes necessary for the radiation oncologist to prescribe an antispasmodic/analgesic medication such as Pyridium Plus. Patients should be warned that this medication will cause their urine to become orange and may stain undergarments. The medication may also be released as an orange color in the sweat glands.

One long-term urinary complication is a vesicovaginal fistula, which usually requires the patient to have a urinary diversion until the fistula heals. Another complication that is caused by radiation fibrosis is the formation of ureteral strictures that may require placement of ureteral stents. See Chapter 12 for additional discussion of genitourinary effects and their management.

Vulvovaginitis

Pelvic irradiation frequently results in erythema, inflammation, mucosal atrophy, inelasticity, and ulceration of the vaginal tissue (Lydon et al., 1992). Eventually adhesions will form in the vagina causing stenosis and closure of the vagina, resulting in painful intercourse and pelvic exams, and inability of the clinician to examine the entire vaginal canal. Some signs and symptoms of post-irradiation vaginitis include vaginal discharge, spontaneous and contact bleeding, pruritus, painful intercourse, and dysuria. Upon examination there may be erythema, inflammation, ulcerations, and possibly stenosis or necrosis of the vagina. The pain, inflammation, and erythema may last up to several weeks after therapy is complete (Lydon et al., 1992). Abitol and Davenport (1974) studied 97 patients treated for carcinoma of the cervix; 41 were treated with surgery alone, 37 with radiation alone, and 19 with combined therapies. Of patients who received radiation therapy alone or in combination with surgery, 41 had narrowing or obliteration of the vagina, 43 patients had pelvic fibrosis and 34 patients had pain and discomfort on pelvic examination. In the group that had surgery alone, only 7, 2, and 4 patients, respectively, had the same reactions (Abitol & Davenport, 1974). Adhesions may form weeks to months after radiation and must undergo lysis soon after they form to prevent stenosis. Patients who are treated for cervical cancer have a higher incidence of stenosis because higher doses of radiation are given to the cervix and vagina in an effort to eliminate the tumor. It is important that the nurse is aware of these symptoms and side effects to focus on the management and prevention of vaginal mucositis and stenosis.

Most often, treatment includes vaginal dilatation either by frequent sexual intercourse, a vaginal dilator, or a combination of the two. It is important that the nurse be comfortable with her or his own sexuality to develop a good relationship with the patient, and promote open discussions about sexual function concerns during and after radiation therapy. If the woman is sexually active or desires to resume sexual activity, the nurse should encourage this as long as the woman does not experience pain or bleeding during intercourse. If the woman is sexually active once a week or less, the nurse should encourage the use of a vaginal dilator as well. If the woman is not sexually active then a vaginal dilator is recommended. Vaginal dilators come in different sizes and it is important that the patient is fitted to the right size to prevent pain and discomfort. The nurse should give the patient written as well as verbal instructions on use of the dilator. It is best if the nurse provides the dilator for the patient, rather than have the patient buy one, as it may be difficult for a patient to obtain. The patient can use the dilator at any time during the day and should be encouraged to use it at least 2 to 3 times a week for up to 2 years. Some patients may have more scarring than others and instruction on dilatation sometimes needs to be individualized to the number of times per week and the number of years required to use one. Some patients may need to use the dilator indefinitely. A towel, lubricant, such as

K-Y jelly, and dilator are the necessary items needed for dilatation. The patient should apply the lubricant to the dilator and then lie supine on the bed with her knees bent. The dilator should be inserted slowly, turning it as it is being advanced. Turning the dilator as it is advanced sometimes promotes easier insertion and less discomfort. The dilator should be advanced as far as is comfortable and left in place for 10 to 15 minutes. After removal, the dilator should be washed with hot soapy water and dried.

Another treatment for vaginitis that may be used along with vaginal dilatation is the use of estrogen creams, which have been shown to promote epithelial regeneration and improve the appearance of the vagina. Patients have also been noted to have less bleeding, dyspareunia, and narrowing of the vaginal canal (Lydon et al., 1992). One drawback with using estrogen creams is that they are absorbed systemically and create high levels of estrogen in the circulation. Therefore it may be contraindicated with women who have estrogen-dependent tumors or endometrial cancer.

Infections

Another side effect that may be seen during radiation, although less frequently than mucositis, is vaginal infection. The normal noninfected vagina is maintained by four factors (Lydon et al., 1992):

1. Secretion of normal estrogen levels necessary to maintain the epithelial lining
2. Availability of glycogen in vaginal tissue
3. Presence of adequate numbers of lactobacilli to produce lactic acid
4. Adequate lactic acid to maintain acidity of the vagina (pH 4 to 4.5)

A change in any one of these factors can increase the woman's risk of infection. High-dose pelvic irradiation results in estrogen deprivation, which in turn causes mucosal atrophy and loss of the epithelial lining of the vagina (Lydon et al., 1992). Organisms most commonly associated with vaginitis are: Candida, Trichomonas, and Gardnerella vaginalis.

The nurse must be aware of these symptoms to initiate appropriate teaching with the patient, so that if any symptoms appear the patient will notify the radiation oncologist or the nurse. The treatment of choice is usually an antifungal medication for Candida and Gardnerella and a systemic antiprotozoan medication for Trichomonas. Patients should be instructed to not scratch the affected area, but to apply cool compresses and sitz baths to the perineum, which may help relieve the itching and burning. See Table 13–11 for additional discussion of treatment options.

Fatigue

Fatigue is the overwhelming sense of exhaustion and decreased capacity for physical and mental work, regardless of adequate sleep or rest (Thompson et al., 1989). During radiation therapy, a number of women may report feeling tired or drained of energy. Unfortunately it is not understood exactly why patients become fatigued during radiation therapy. Aistars (1987) suggests three sources of stressors: physiological, psychological, or situational. Physiological stressors may include such factors as the accumulation of waste products in the body as a result of radiation, chemotherapy or tumor necrosis, a hypermetabolic state related to active tumor growth, infection, fever, or surgery, the tumor competing with

Table 13-11 • Treatment Options for Vaginal Infections

Infection	Description	Treatment*
Trichomoniasis (a protozoan)	Inflammation of the vagina Painful intercourse Copious discharge or yellow/green discharge	Metronidazole (Flagyl), 2 g one time dose
Candida albicans (a yeast)	Erythematous labia with excoriations Severe perivaginal pruritus Thick curdlike discharge or thin discharge without odor	Nystatin vaginal suppository qd for 14 days Miconazole nitrate 2% vaginal cream, one at bedtime for 7 days Clotrimazole, 500 mg tab one time vaginally
Gardnerella (a bacterium)	Less erythema, mild or moderate Gray or white thin discharge Discharge has fishy odor	Metronidazole (Flagyl), 500 mg po bid for 7 days Ampicillin, 500 mg po qid for 7 days

* Sexual partners should be treated as well or the organism will be passed back and forth.
Adapted from Thompson JM et al. (Eds.) (1989). *Mosby's Manual of Clinical Nursing* (pp. 1285–1287). St. Louis: Mosby. Reprinted with permission.

the body for nutrients, an inadequate intake of nutrition, or pain. Psychological stressors may include anxiety, depression, or grief. Situational stressors may include sleep pattern disturbance, immobility, crisis, and fear of diagnostic tests (Aistars, 1987). Fatigue does not affect everyone during radiation therapy. Patients may already be fatigued from surgery or chemotherapy and the nurse needs to obtain information about the patient's pattern of fatigue.

Assessment of the patient's level of fatigue and reassurance that it is not uncommon for people to feel this way during radiation therapy are an important intervention for the radiation oncology nurse. The nurse may need to monitor the patient's blood counts periodically to evaluate presence of anemia. Encouraging the patient to decrease usual activities, and eliciting family members and friends to help with chores such as shopping and cleaning until after the therapy is completed, may be helpful in reducing the patient's fatigue. It is also helpful if patients plan rest periods or naps regularly. Some patients complain that they feel most tired right after receiving a radiation treatment. It is helpful for patients to take naps immediately after their treatment, which may help to conserve their energy for the rest of the day. If the patient is working it may be necessary to decrease work hours during the course of radiation therapy.

It is important that the nurse inform the patient that the fatigue may last for several months after radiation therapy is completed. This can be very debilitating for the patient and family and interfere with the patient's quality of life. It is important that ongoing assessment of the fatigue is pursued by both the radiation nurse and oncologist. See Chapter 8 for additional suggestions in the management of radiation-induced fatigue.

Altered Patterns of Sexuality

Sexuality is an important part of everyday life and is often overlooked by health care providers. Pleasurable sexual touching between a man and a woman is always possible, regardless of the physical problems or medical history (Schover, 1988). It is important that the nurse initiate questions with the patient and significant other concerning sexual and reproductive practices. Vincent and associates (1975) found that 70 percent of the patients received no information about the sexual implications of their disease before, during, or after treatment, 56 percent of the patients wanted more information about sex than they received,

and 79 percent said they would not ask the physician for more information than they received.

An individual's sexuality is influenced by many factors, including *developmental components* such as age, life stage, and knowledge of sexual and reproductive functioning; *psychological factors* such as body image, self-concept, self-esteem, and attitudes of significant others; *sociocultural factors* such as values, beliefs, ethnicity, religious preference, socioeconomic class, and family traditions; and *gender factors* that incorporate individual sexual experiences and personal sexual relationships (Dow, 1992).

The patient may be experiencing a number of treatment side effects that may decrease the individual's sexual desire. Because radiation treatment fields for gynecologic cancers usually include the vagina, a decrease in vaginal secretions and sensation may occur. Vaginal stenosis and/or vaginal shortening may be a late effect if the woman is not sexually active and chooses not to use a vaginal dilator. Other factors that may inhibit sexual desire are changes in body image such as loss of pubic hair and radical surgeries as for vulvar cancer. When a woman and her partner are resuming sexual activity, she may likely experience discomfort and pain. In a study of 27 women, Jenkins (1988) identified the reasons for problems with sexual adjustment were: painful intercourse (67 percent), vaginal dryness (60 percent), and feeling of a narrowed or shortened vagina (53 percent). The nurse should initiate questions and concerns of the patient to establish and anticipate any problems. The patient needs to be aware of the physical and hormonal changes that will occur from surgery and radiation and how this may affect her sexual functioning.

A conversation with the patient and her partner concerning misconceptions and/or fears they may have about resuming sexual activity should be initiated. Some patients believe that sex may make their cancer get worse or that their partner will contract cancer through intimate contact. The nurse is in a good position to bring up questions for the patient and dispel many of these myths. Many couples have different beliefs in sexual practices. Some couples believe that sexual intercourse is for procreation and that alternative sexual practices are not acceptable. The nurse must have an open mind and accept the couple's sexual practice (Cartwright-Alcarese, 1995).

Sexuality is an important health care issue and more education is needed in this area. Smith suggests that nurses can begin gathering information on the subject of sexuality by reading textbooks and journals that talk about human sexuality, both in wellness and illness. Workshops and conferences also offer a format for discussion on the issues and questions nurses may have (Smith, 1989).

The PLISSIT model developed by Annon (1974) discusses strategies for handling sexual dysfunction. Using this model with women who have been treated with radiation therapy for a gynecologic cancer may be helpful to those who are not comfortable approaching the subject of sexuality with the patient. This model gives the health care worker guidance in working with the patient.

The P in PLISSIT stands for *permission*, which is the first level in discussing the side effect of sexual dysfunction. This introduces the topic of sexuality and lets the patient know it is common to have sexual concerns and that sharing feelings with the health care team and partner is acceptable. The nurse may initiate a discussion with the patient about whether the patient is sexually active or had been sexually active prior to the illness. The nurse could ask, "Many women who have this type of treatment have many concerns about how this will affect their sexual activity. Do you have any concerns?" (Cartwright-Alcarese, 1995). If patients are hesitant about discussing their sexual dysfunction, providing the patient with matter-of-fact, general statements related to pelvic radiation for gynecological cancer can communicate that it is appropriate to ask questions and receive information regarding this topic (Cartwright-Alcarese, 1995). Printed information such as handouts and pamphlets that are helpful may be obtained from the American Cancer Society.

The LI in PLISSIT stands for *limited information*, which is the second level in discussing sexual dysfunction. This part of the model deals with telling the patient and her partner what they need to know as well as what they want to know. Each person may have different areas of concern such as the effect of radiation on the ability to have sexual intercourse, the effect on the ovaries, and the possibility of injury from sexual intercourse. The nurse may start by saying, "Radiation therapy to treat gynecologic cancer can cause changes in the vagina that may have an effect on sexual intercourse. There are measures to take to prevent and minimize these effects. Would you feel comfortable discussing these?" (Cartwright-Alcarese, 1995).

The SS in PLISSIT stands for *specific suggestions*, which is the third level in discussing sexual

dysfunction. This includes giving the patient and her partner specific interventions to prepare for sexual intercourse. For example, vaginal dryness is a common problem and instructing the patient to use a water-based lubricant such as K-Y jelly, Ortho Personal lubricant, Surgilube, Today Personal lubricant, or Astroglide may be helpful (Schover, 1988). Teaching the patient to relax the abdominal muscles will help decrease the discomfort during penetration and intercourse. Instruct the patient to do Kegel exercises once or twice a day. This includes tightening the vaginal muscles, counting to 3 and releasing pelvic tension. It is helpful to instruct the patient to do these exercises 10 times once or twice a day (Schover, 1988). Other problems women may experience that may decrease their sexual desire include a shortened vaginal canal, which can cause pain during sexual intercourse and can be remedied by the woman changing positions and exploring new positions that are more comfortable. Vaginal stenosis, as discussed earlier, can be alleviated by frequent sexual intercourse or vaginal dilatation using a dilator or both. Decreased vaginal sensation can be overcome by increasing the amount of foreplay, by having the woman's partner caress other areas of her body. Vaginal irritation can be a problem during sexual intercourse. It may be helpful to instruct the patient to have her partner withdraw before ejaculation or wear a condom, because semen has been noted to cause a burning sensation in the vagina (Cartwright-Alcarese, 1995).

The IT in PLISSIT stands for *intensive therapy*. If the problems a woman is experiencing are too complex or are beyond the scope of the nurse, a professional therapist consultation may be required. Table 13–12 provides a list of resources and organizations that may be helpful for some women experiencing deeper, underlying problems.

Summary

Many women with a gynecologic cancer may experience obstacles to overcome during the course of treatment, whether it is with surgery, radiation, or chemotherapy. The oncology nurse can provide initial teaching about the disease and the common side effects and their management. Gynecological cancers can be very challenging for the radiation oncology nurse because of the wide scope of care these women need, from physical to psychosocial to psychosexual.

Table 13-12 • Resources for Patients Experiencing Sexual Dysfunction

BOOKS

Baumanni CU (1990). Erotic partner massage. New York: Startling Publications.

Comfort A (1993). The new joy of sex: A gourmet guide to lovemaking (2nd ed.). New York: Crown Publications.

Hooper A (1992). The ultimate sex book. New York: Dorling Kinderley.

Inkeles G (1992). The new sensual massage (1st ed.). New York: Bantam Books.

Keesling B (1993). Sexual pleasure. Alameda, CA: Hunter House.

Russell S & Kolb J (1992). The tao of sexual massage. New York: Simon & Schuster.

Sandford W, Hawley N, & McGee E (1992). Sexuality. In J Pincus & W Sanford (Eds.). The new our bodies, ourselves (pp. 204–236). New York: Simon & Schuster.

Schover LR (1988). Sexuality and cancer: For the woman who has cancer, and her partner. Atlanta: American Cancer Society. (Free publication of the American Cancer Society.)

ORGANIZATIONS

American Association of Sex Educators, Counselors, and Therapists
Suite 1717
435 North Michigan Avenue
Chicago, IL 60611
312-644-0828
(Provides names of sex therapists around the country)

Cancer Care
1180 Avenue of the Americas
New York, NY 10036
212-302-2400
(Call for local facility)

Resolve
1310 Broadway
Somerville, MA 02144-1731
617-623-0744
(Helpline of the National Consumer Advocacy Organization for Infertile People)

The Wellness Community
2200 Colorado Avenue
Santa Monica, CA 90404-3506
310-453-2300
(Offers free psychosocial support to patients with cancer. Call for local facility.)

Source: Cartwright-Alcarese F (1995). Resources for patients experiencing sexual dysfunction. *Oncology Nursing Forum, 22,* p. 1231. Reprinted with permission.

References

Abitol MM & Davenport JH (1974). The irradiated vagina. *Obstetrics and Gynecology, 44,* 249–256.

Aistars J (1987). Fatigue in the cancer patient: A conceptual approach to a clinical problem. *Oncology Nursing Forum, 14,* 25–30.

American Cancer Society (1997). *Cancer Facts and Figures.*

Annon JS (1974). *The behavioral treatment of sexual problems.* New York: Harper and Row.

Ball HG, Bell DA & Griffin TW (1990). Cancer of the ovary. In RT Osteen (Ed.), *Cancer Manual* (8th ed., pp. 266–270). Massachusetts: American Cancer Society.

Beahrs OH, Henson DE, Hutter RVP & Kennedy BJ (Eds.) (1993). *Handbook for staging of cancer. From Manual for Staging of Cancer* (4th ed.). Philadelphia: JB Lippincott.

Berkowitz RS, Young RH, & Tak WK (1990). Cancer of the endometrium. In RT Osteen (Ed.), *Cancer Manual* (8th ed., pp. 265–266). Massachusetts: American Cancer Society.

Cartwright-Alcarese F (1995). Addressing sexual dysfunction following radiation therapy for gynecologic malignancy. *Oncology Nursing Forum, 22,* 1227–1232.

Chamarro T (1990). Cancer of the vulva and vagina. *Seminars in Oncology Nursing, 6,* 198–205.

Clark JC (1994). Gynecologic cancers. In SE Otto (Ed.), *Oncology Nursing* (2nd ed., pp. 190–220). St. Louis: Mosby-Year Book.

Dow KH (1992). Altered patterns of sexuality. In KH Dow & LJ Hilderley (Eds.), *Nursing Care in Radiation Oncology* (pp 149–159). Philadelphia: WB Saunders.

Fuller AF, Young RH, & Tak WK (1990). Cancer of the cervix, vulva, and vagina. In RT Osteen (Ed.), *Cancer Manual* (8th ed., pp. 257–265). Massachusetts: American Cancer Society.

Hacker NF, Berek JS, Julliard JF & Lagasse LD (1984). Preoperative radiation therapy for locally advanced vulvar cancer. *Cancer, 54,* 2056–2061.

Hacker NF, Eifel P, McGuire W & Wilkinson EJ (1992). Vulva. In WJ Hoskins, CA Perez & RC Young (Eds.), *Principles and Practice of Gynecologic Oncology* (pp. 537–566). Philadelphia: JB Lippincott.

Homesley HD, Bundy BN, Sedlis A & Adcock L (1986). Radiation therapy versus pelvic node resection for carcinoma of the vulva with positive lymph nodes. *Obstetrics and Gynecology, 68,* 733–740.

Hubbard JL & Holcombe JK (1990). Cancer of the endometrium. *Seminars in Oncology Nursing, 6,* 206–213.

Jenkins B (1988). Patients' reports of sexual changes after treatment for gynecological cancer. *Oncology Nursing Forum, 15*, 349–354.

Komaki R (1994). The endometrium, the vagina, the vulva, and the female urethra. In JD Cox (Ed.), *Moss' Radiation Oncology Rationale, Technique and Results.* (7th ed., pp. 617–712). St. Louis: Mosby-Year Book.

Lydon J, Purl S & Goodman M (1992). Integumentary and mucous membrane alterations. In SL Groenwald, MH Frogge, M Goodman & CH Yarbro (Eds.). *Manifestations of Cancer and Cancer Treatment.* (2nd ed., pp. 594–635). Boston: Jones and Bartlett.

McCarthy CP (1992). Altered patterns of elimination. In KH Dow & LJ Hilderley (Eds.). *Nursing Care in Radiation Oncology* (pp. 126–148). Philadelphia: WB Saunders.

National Cancer Institute. (1995a). PDQ-Endometrial cancer. Bethesda, MD: Author.

National Cancer Institute. (1995b). PDQ-Vaginal cancer. Bethesda, MD: Author.

National Cancer Institute. (1995c). PDQ-Vulvar cancer. Bethesda, MD: Author.

NIH Consensus Statement (1994). Ovarian Cancer: Screening, Treatment, and Followup. Apr 5–7; *12*, 1–30.

Nolte S & Hanjani P (1990). Intraepithelial neoplasia of the lower genital tract. *Seminars in Oncology Nursing, 6*, 181–189.

Otte DM (1992). Gynecologic cancers. In SL Groenwald, MH Frogge, M Goodman & CH Yarbro (Eds.). *The Care of the Individual with Cancer.* (2nd ed., pp. 845–885). Boston: Jones and Bartlett.

Park RC, Grigsby PW, Muss HB & Norris HJ (1992). Corpus: epithelial tumors. In WJ Hoskins, CA Perez & RC Young (Eds.). *Principles and Practice of Gynecologic Oncology* (pp. 663–686). Philadelphia: JB Lippincott Company.

Parker SL, Tong T, Bolden S & Wingo PA (1997). Cancer statistics, 1997. *CA-A Cancer Journal for Clinicians 47*, 5-27.

Perez CA (1993). Radiation therapy in the management of cancer of the cervix. *Oncology, 7*, part I 89–96, part II 61–69.

Perez CA, Kurman RJ, Stehman FB & Thigpen JT (1992a). Uterine cervix. In WJ Hoskins, CA Perez & RC Young (Eds.). *Principles and Practice of Gynecologic Oncology* (pp. 591–613). Philadelphia: JB Lippincott.

Perez CA, Gersell DJ, Hoskins WJ & McGuire WP (1992b). Vagina. In WJ Hoskins, CA Perez & RC Young (Eds.). *Principles and Practice of Gynecologic Oncology* (pp. 567–579). Philadelphia: JB Lippincott.

Schover LR (1988). Sexuality and cancer: For the woman who has cancer, and her partner. Atlanta: American Cancer Society.

Smith DB (1989). Sexual rehabilitation of the cancer patient. *Cancer Nursing, 12*, 10–15.

Sorensen KR & Rosenow A (1987). Assessing women experiencing gynecologic conditions. In J Luckman & KR Sorensen (Eds.). *Medical-surgical Nursing: A Psychophysiologic Approach* (3rd ed.) (pp. 1731–1804). Philadelphia: WB Saunders.

Thombes MB (1991). Gynecologic malignancies. In SB Baird (Ed.), *A Cancer Source Book for Nurses* (6th ed., pp. 228–242). Atlanta: American Cancer Society, Inc.

Thompson JM, McFarland GK, Hirsch JE, Tucker SM, & Bowers AC (Eds.). (1989). Chapter ten. *Mosby's Manual of Clinical Nursing* (2nd ed., pp. 968–975). St. Louis: Mosby.

Thompson LJ (1990). Cancer of the cervix. *Seminars in Oncology Nursing, 6*, 190–197.

Vincent CE, Greiss FC & Linton EB (1975). Some marital-sexual concomitants of carcinoma of the cervix. *Southern Medical Journal, 68*, 552–558.

Cancers of the Head and Neck

RYAN R. IWAMOTO

Head and neck cancer accounts for approximately 8.5 percent of all malignancies and includes malignant tumors of the upper aerodigestive tract, paranasal sinuses, and the major and minor salivary glands (Parker et al., 1997). In addition, tumors of the skin, soft tissue, bone, and neurovascular structures in the head and neck and tumors of the parapharyngeal space are also considered head and neck cancers.

Over 90 percent of all head and neck cancers are squamous cell carcinomas. Most of the remaining head and neck cancers are adenocarcinomas of salivary origin, melanomas, and tumors of somatic soft tissues. Head and neck cancers affect more men than women by a factor of 2 to 1. Approximately 57,000 new cases of head and neck cancers and approximately 14,000 deaths will occur each year (Parker et al., 1996). (See Table 14–1.)

Epidemiology and Etiology

The use of tobacco (cigarette, cigar, pipe, and smokeless tobacco), alcohol, and the combination of both are the best established and most significant carcinogens of mucosal malignancy in the oral cavity, oropharynx, hypopharynx, and larynx. The additive effect of using both tobacco and alcohol in the incidence of head and neck cancer has been well demonstrated.

These products are associated with over 95 percent of the cases of squamous cell carcinoma of the head and neck (Schleper, 1989; Spitz, 1994). Other etiologic factors include malnutrition, excessive mouthwash use, poor oral hygiene, viral exposure (Epstein-Barr virus, herpes simplex virus, and human papillomavirus), and occupational risk factors such as exposure to wood dust, organic compounds, and coal products.

The familial occurrence of head and neck cancer supports the role of heredity in this disease group (Trizna & Schantz, 1992). However, the roles of environmental and genetic factors are difficult to separate. Several well-characterized entities are associated with risk and prognosis of head and neck cancer. These include Lynch-II syndrome, Bloom syndrome, Fanconi's anemia, xeroderma pigmentosum, ataxia telangiectasia, and Li-Fraumeni syndrome.

Significant increases in the incidence of oral and pharyngeal cancers are seen in African-American men (Ries et al., 1994). For those younger than 65 years of age, the incidence rate among African-American men is nearly double that of white men. In men older than 65 years, white men have slightly higher incidence rates than African-American men.

Early detection is key to successful control of the disease. Five-year disease-free cure rates remain about 30 to 40 percent regardless of tumor size. Poor prognosis is due to size of tumor at diagnosis, presence of regional lymph node disease, and distant metastasis. Metastasis to regional lymph nodes has often already occurred when the patient first seeks medical care. Head and neck cancers are typically very aggressive locally and spread initially to anatomic sites within the head and neck region.

As evidenced by the risk factors for head and neck cancer, prevention of head and neck cancer may be accomplished by smoking cessation, moderation of alcohol consumption, and increased consumption of fruits and vegetables. It has been suggested that these actions could lead to the prevention of approximately 75 percent of the cases of head and neck cancers in Western countries (Boyle et al., 1992).

History and Physical Examination

Many head and neck squamous carcinomas are preceded by various precancerous lesions. These lesions may present in the form of leukoplakia or erythroplakia. A review of the patient's medical history includes an emphasis on exposure to carcinogens, a positive family history of cancer, lifestyle habits, and occupation. Symptoms may include unilateral nasal obstruction or discharge, persistent mucosal ulceration, persistent hoarseness, odynophagia, dysphagia, pharyngitis, and cervical adenopathy. Regional metastasis in the neck is the only presenting symptom in more than a third of patients with head and neck cancers.

Squamous cell head and neck cancers generally originate on the surface of the mucosal lining of the upper aerodigestive tract. The typical mucosal lesion can appear as an ulceration, a roughened or thickened area, a fungating cauliflower-like lesion, or a combination of all of these. The majority of head and neck tumors invade locally, deep into the underlying structures as well as along tissue planes or nerves. Lymphatic spread occurs both locally at the primary site and regionally through lymphatic channels. Prognosis is strongly influenced by the number of positive nodes. Infection, necrosis, or bleeding may evolve as the tumor grows. In addition, inflammation and pressure of the tumor can cause nerve impingement or muscle dysfunction at the primary site.

Diagnosis

In most patients, the primary head and neck tumor can be visualized by a thorough head and neck examination and a biopsy performed for diagnosis (Shah & Lydiatt, 1995). This examination includes a careful examination of the scalp, face, oral cavity, and oropharynx. A mirror or endoscopic examination of the nasal cavity, nasopharynx, hypopharynx, and larynx is also completed. A careful examination of the regional lymph nodes of the neck as well as the thyroid and salivary glands is an integral part of a complete head and neck examination. Finally the cranial nerves are evaluated.

The evaluation of supraglottic and hypopharyngeal tumors is usually made through indirect laryngoscopy. Direct laryngoscopy is used for obtaining a biopsy specimen. With salivary gland cancers, fine-needle aspiration cytology is performed. CT scanning is critical for the diagnosis of nasal cavity and paranasal sinus cancers. CT scans are also useful in determining the extent of disease, bony involvement, and metastasis. Chest x ray is used to diagnose any associated pulmonary disease. In addition, liver function is evaluated with blood chemistries.

Staging

Classification of head and neck cancers is listed in Table 14–2. Accurate staging provides the basis

for appropriate selection of therapy. The tumor-nodes-metastasis (TNM) staging system by the American Joint Committee on Cancer and the International Union Against Cancer is recommended for clinical staging.

Treatment

Surgery and radiation therapy alone or in combination are the cornerstones of curative treatment in head and neck cancer. Although the goal of treatment may be to cure, preservation of form and function in the head and neck region is also an important consideration in treatment decisions (Shah & Lydiatt, 1995). The choice of treatment depends on histology, location, and size of the primary tumor, and involvement of cervical lymph nodes. In general, either surgery alone or radiation therapy alone can be used effectively for early-stage disease (Sloan & Goepfert, 1991). If surgery can be done safely and without significant disruption of normal function or cosmesis, as in early oral cavity tumors, surgery is preferable (Shah & Lydiatt, 1995). Otherwise, in early oropharyngeal and laryngeal tumors, radiotherapy is favored. In most advanced stage cancers, single modality treatment is inferior to combined therapy. Combined surgery and radiotherapy for advanced disease offers improved locoregional control and enhanced survival (Sweeney et al., 1994). The status

Table 14-1 • Head and Neck Cancer: Estimated New Cancer Cases and Estimated Cancer Deaths in the United States, 1997

Site	Total	Male	Female
ESTIMATED NEW CANCER CASES FOR 1997			
Buccal cavity and pharynx	30,750	20,900	9,850
Lip	4,550	3,600	950
Tongue	6,400	4,200	2,200
Mouth	11,000	6,700	4,300
Pharynx	8,800	6,400	2,400
Endocrine			
Thyroid	16,100	4,700	11,400
ESTIMATED CANCER DEATHS FOR 1997			
Buccal cavity and pharynx	8,440	5,600	2,840
Lip	2,090	1,500	590
Tongue	1,820	1,200	620
Mouth	2,500	1,400	1,100
Pharynx	2,030	1,500	530
Endocrine			
Thyroid	1,230	450	780

From: Parker SL, Tong T, Bolden S, & Wingo PA (1996). Cancer statistics, 1997. *CA: A Cancer Journal for Clinicians, 47,* 5–27. Used with permission.

Table 14-2 • Classification of Head and Neck Cancers

PRIMARY TUMOR (T)

General: for all sites

TX	Primary tumor cannot be assessed
T0	No evidence of primary tumor
TIS	Carcinoma in situ

ORAL CAVITY, OROPHARYNX

T1	Greatest diameter of primary tumor < or = 2 cm
T2	>2 cm or = 4 cm
T3	>4 cm
T4	Massive tumor, with deep invasion into maxilla, mandible, pterygoid muscles, deep tongue muscle, skin, soft tissues of neck

HYPOPHARYNX

T1	Tumor confined to one subsite of hypopharynx
T2	Tumor invades more than one subsite of hypopharynx or an adjacent site, without fixation of hemilarynx
T3	Tumor invades more than one subsite of hypopharynx or an adjacent site, with fixation of hemilarynx
T4	Tumor involves adjacent structures (e.g., cartilage or soft tissues of neck)

NASOPHARYNX

T1	Tumor confined to one subsite
T2	Involvement of two subsites within nasopharynx
T3	Extension into nasal cavity or oropharynx
T4	Invasion into skull and/or cranial nerve(s)

LARYNX

Glottic

T1	Limited to true vocal cords; normal vocal cord mobility; may include anterior or posterior commissure
T2	Supra- or subglottic extension; normal or impaired mobility
T3	Confined to larynx proper; vocal cord fixation
T4	Cartilage destruction and/or extension out of larynx to other tissues

Supraglottic

T1	Limited to subsite of supraglottis; normal vocal cord mobility
T2	Extension to glottis or adjacent supraglottic subsite; normal vocal cord mobility
T3	Confined to larynx proper; cord fixation and/or extension into hypopharynx or preepiglottic space
T4	Massive tumor, cartilage destruction and/or extension out of larynx

Subglottic

T1	Limited to subglottic region
T2	Extension to vocal cord(s)
T3	Limited to larynx; vocal cord fixation
T4	Massive tumor; cartilage destruction and/or extension out of larynx

NODAL METASTASIS (N)

NX	Nodes cannot be assessed
N0	No regional lymph node metastasis
N1	Single, ipsilateral node: < or = 3 cm
N2A	Single, ipsilateral node: >3 cm or = 6 cm
N2B	Multiple, ipsilateral nodes: all < or = 6 cm
N3A	Ipsilateral node(s): one >6 cm
N3B	Bilateral nodes (each side subclassed)
N3C	Contralateral node(s), only

DISTANT METASTASIS (M)

MX	Presence of distant metastasis cannot be assessed
M0	No distant metastases
M1	Distant metastasis present

STAGE GROUPINGS

Stage I	T1, N0, M0
Stage II	T2, N0, M0
Stage III	T3, N0, M0; T1, T2, or T3 with N1, M0
Stage IV	T4, N0 or N1, M0
	Any T, N2 or N3, M0
	Any T, Any N, M1

From Beahrs OH, Henson DE, Hutter RVP, Kennedy BJ (1993). *Manual for Staging Cancer.* 4th Ed., Philadelphia: JB Lippincott. Used with permission.

of neck nodes is a critical prognostic factor because the neck remains the most common site of treatment failure.

Surgery

A variety of surgical techniques are employed in the treatment of head and neck cancer. Surgery may involve conventional resectional surgery, endoscopic surgery, laser surgery, cryotherapy, and electrocautery. Surgical approaches will be discussed more fully in the section on site-specific head and neck cancers.

Radiation Therapy

Radiation may be delivered by external beam, interstitial implantation, or surface-contact. Radiation therapy can be used as curative treatment of the primary tumor and as an adjuvant therapy to surgery, delivered either preoperatively or postoperatively. Preoperative irradiation can shrink the tumor before resection and make unresectable lesions resectable and increase the chance of negative surgical margins. However, preoperative irradiation can increase postoperative complications. Postoperative radiation therapy reduces operative morbidity and allows tailoring of radiotherapy to operative findings with respect to margins, nodal status, and tumor spread. Radiotherapy can also manage cervical lymph node metastases either electively or when there are clinically-proven positive lymph nodes.

Radiotherapy can be delivered externally or internally. External beam radiotherapy can encompass large volumes and give a uniform dose. Electron beam therapy can be used alone or combined with photon beam therapy for certain primary tumor sites. Intraoral cone therapy is used to treat small oral cancers. Brachytherapy is used alone or combined with external beam therapy in the treatment of head and neck cancers. Improved local control with brachytherapy has been demonstrated in floor of mouth and tongue cancers.

Conventional fractionation for curative treatment of head and neck cancer involves daily treatment of 1.8 to 2.0 Gy, Monday through Friday, by continuous course to a total dose in the range of 60 to 70 Gy (Sweeney et al., 1994). The exact total dose is dependent on the site and volume of cancer, its proclivity for spread, and the intent of treatment. Palliative doses to alleviate symptoms such as pain and bleeding are likely to be lower, such as 3000 cGy. Smaller field sizes are used in order to minimize side effects. Larger tumors tend to need higher doses while smaller tumors may be cured with 60 to 70 Gy. The patient without a clinically palpable neck node is traditionally treated with doses of 50 Gy to 55 Gy. Several different angles of the beam to treat the tumor are used to lessen the deleterious effects of radiation on the interposed normal tissues. The fields of delivery for external radiotherapy are usually planned by computer. Regions needing additional treatment use smaller field sizes. Higher doses can also be delivered through the insertion or implantation of radioactive material such as gold or iridium via seeds, needles, removable catheters, or surface contact (Mendenhall et al., 1991). The interstitial technique is particularly useful in the tongue base, tonsillar fossa, and oral cavity. Surface exposure is occasionally used to deliver additional radiation to the nasopharynx or to a maxillectomy cavity. New radiation fractionation schemes such as hyperfractionation and acceleration of the dose are being used to improve local tumor control of head and neck cancers and decrease late radiation injury (Dische, 1994).

The survival rate is 40 percent for patients with advanced squamous cell carcinoma of the head and neck whose tumors are completely resected and 20 percent for those with unresectable tumors treated with radiotherapy alone. A study was conducted to evaluate the influence of cigarette smoking on the efficacy of radiation therapy in head and neck cancer (Browman et al., 1993a). The patients who continued to smoke during radiation therapy had a lower rate of complete response (45 vs. 74 percent) and poorer 2-year survival (39 vs. 66 percent) than the patients who did not smoke or who had quit before treatment started.

TREATMENT SET-UP

Simulation and treatment planning for head and neck irradiation involve the use of imaging scans to precisely localize the tumor and surrounding structures. Immobilization devices such as masks and head holders are created to ensure accurate positioning for daily treatment. Figure 14–1 illustrates the Aquaplast Mask, which is used for immobilizing the head. Obturators for the mouth may be used to protect normal tissues and move structures such as the tongue out of the treatment field (Strohl, 1989).

Chemotherapy

Although chemotherapy is able to reduce or eradicate clinically detectable squamous cell cancers, by itself it is not curative. A number of chemother-

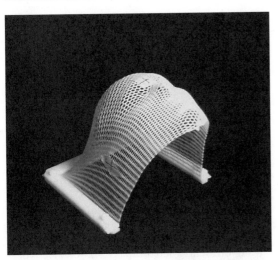

Figure 14-1 • Aquaplast mask for head immobilization (courtesy of WFR/Aquaplast Corporation, Wydoff, New Jersey).

apeutic agents are effective in significantly reducing head and neck tumor volume. Methotrexate, bleomycin, cisplatin, and 5-fluorouracil are the best established chemotherapeutic agents for head and neck cancers (Aisner et al., 1995; Hamasaki & Vokes, 1992; Tobias, 1992). The mainstay of treatment for recurrent head and neck cancer has been chemotherapy with cisplatin/5-fluorouracil or methotrexate. Paclitaxel has also shown activity in treatment of head and neck cancer (Forastiere, 1994). Principal toxicities include neutropenia, peripheral neuropathy, arthralgias, and myalgias.

Combined Modality

Combined modality approaches have been developed to enhance locoregional disease control, reduce distant metastases, and preserve anatomic function. These approaches include: neoadjuvant chemotherapy followed by standard therapy with surgery and/or radiation therapy; adjuvant chemotherapy after surgery or radiotherapy with or without neoadjuvant chemotherapy, and neoadjuvant chemotherapy concurrent with radiotherapy (Dimery & Hong, 1993). Although combined-modality approaches show promise in improving control of head and neck cancers, toxicities are increased. Concomitant chemotherapy and radiotherapy has resulted in statistically significant improved disease-free and overall survival for patients with head and neck cancer (al-Sarraf, 1994; Forastiere, 1992; Vokes, Awan, & Weichselbaum, 1991).

Infection has been found to be a significant factor in morbidity and mortality of patients with head and neck cancer undergoing multimodality therapy (Hussain et al., 1991). An analysis of 662 hospital admissions of 169 head and neck cancer patients revealed that infections contributed to 44 percent of deaths. Risk factors that predicted for or were associated with infection include: foreign bodies such as IV catheters and gastrostomy tubes, ethnicity, performance status, alcohol intake, and nutritional status.

Site-Specific Head and Neck Cancers

Oral Cavity and Oropharynx

Anatomy

The oral cavity includes the anatomical structures of the mouth including the lips, buccal mucosa, gingiva, tongue, floor of mouth, hard and soft palates, and teeth. A smooth mucous membrane covers the gingiva, hard and soft palates, buccal mucosa, and lips. The tongue is a muscular organ that is used for chewing, swallowing, and speech. The tongue also contains taste buds in the mucous membrane. The anatomy of the oropharynx includes the base of the tongue, palatine arches with tonsils, and posterior oropharyngeal wall. The mucosa of the pharynx is made up of a stratified squamous epithelium.

Epidemiology and Risk Factors

Cancers of the oral cavity and oropharynx account for 4 percent of all cancers in men and 2 percent of all cancers in women. Patients tend to be men, 50 to 65 years of age. There is a downward trend in the age group most affected. A history of smoking and tobacco use and alcohol abuse are significant risk factors. Poor oral hygiene, chronic mechanical irritation from ill-fitting dentures and plates, poor dentition with sharp, jagged teeth, and chronic oral infections are predisposing factors in the development of carcinoma of the tongue, gingiva, and other sites in the oral cavity. More than 90 percent of oral cancers are squamous cell carcinomas.

Clinical Presentation

The patient may present with a painless oral lesion. In some instances, pain may be present at the primary site and commonly is reported as referred pain to the ear or jaw. Lesions in the oral cavity and oropharynx tend to be poorly delineated, and not confined by the anatomic midline. Although squamous cell carcinomas generally grow along mucosal surfaces, in advanced lesions, these tumors spread submucosally and infiltrate into deeper structures. This deep invasion may occur along preformed pathways of muscle fascia or nerves, and regional lymph node metastases frequently occur. Distant metastases occur from cancer cells spreading through the lymphatic system and blood vessel embolization.

Treatment

Treatment is determined by the size of the lesion as well as the presence or absence of metastases. Surgery and radiation have comparable cure rates in early-stage lesions. The choice of treatment in early-stage lesions depends on functional and cosmetic results, the patient's general health, and patient preference. The role of adjuvant chemotherapy remains controversial. Platinum-based chemotherapeutic regimens have shown promise in providing complete and partial responses. Combined therapy is generally the rule for oral cavity lesions.

Surgical resection of the primary tumor with adequate margins (usually 2 cm) and reconstruction are performed. A neck dissection is completed to remove all the nodal groups in the accessible cervical region. Ipsilateral neck dissection is often completed because of the high frequency of metastasis to the ipsilateral nodes. Resection of early-stage oral cavity cancers may be completed with carbon dioxide (CO_2) laser. Laser use has resulted in reduced patient morbidity, decreased hospital stay, and improved recovery (McCaffrey, 1992).

Radiation therapy for primary tumors of the oral cavity can be delivered by external beam or combined external and interstitial implant methods. Radiation is used to treat clinically uninvolved nodal areas with 45 Gy to 55 Gy; areas of known disease receive a higher dose. For T1 and T2 tumors, external beam irradiation is delivered to the primary tumor and first echelon of lymph nodes with a boost via brachytherapy or intraoral cone. A minimum of 60 Gy to 70 Gy is delivered to achieve the 80 to 85 percent cure rate of T1–T2 disease. For floor of mouth cancers, local control of 88 to 98 percent for T1 lesions and 72 to 88 percent for T2 lesions is achieved with radiotherapy alone. Local control of oral tongue cancers with radiation therapy alone is 85 to 95 percent for T1 lesions and 65 to 85 percent for T2 lesions. Early

lesions of the tonsillar region are effectively managed with radiotherapy alone.

For advanced cancers of the oral cavity, surgery is combined with preoperative or postoperative irradiation. Overall 5-year survival of oral cavity tumors is approximately 50 percent, and oropharyngeal lesions is about 35 percent.

Larynx

Anatomy

The larynx is composed of three distinct areas: glottic, supraglottic, and subglottic. The glottic region encompasses the true vocal cords and includes the functions of phonation, airway protection during swallowing, and coughing. The supraglottic area encompasses the false vocal cords, arytenoid area, epiglottis, and aryepiglottic folds. This portion of the larynx interfaces superiorly with the hypopharynx. The supraglottic larynx functions as an air passage and mainly as a shield and sphincter to protect the airway. The subglottic portion of the larynx is the airway below the true vocal cords and above the first tracheal ring and represents the mucosa within the cricoid cartilage.

Epidemiology and Risk Factors

Squamous cell carcinoma of the larynx is the classic smoker's cancer of the head and neck and generally occurs after many decades of cigarette use. Its occurrence in nonsmokers is extremely unusual. Alcohol consumption increases the risk of cancer of the larynx. Hoarseness and other vocal complaints are common symptoms. The incidence of laryngeal carcinoma in the United States is 4.2 in 100,000. Approximately 80 percent of laryngeal carcinomas are found in persons over 50 years of age, with the highest incidence occurring in the sixth decade of life. Over 90 percent of laryngeal cancers are squamous cell in origin, ranging from well-differentiated to undifferentiated tumors, the majority being moderately well-differentiated. Tobacco and alcohol use and a history of exposure to ionizing radiation have been implicated as etiologic factors. Tumors in each region of the larynx involve distinct signs, symptoms, treatment regimens, and rehabilitation measures. Glottic carcinomas tend to be slow-growing, well-differentiated, and metastasize late. Supraglottic carcinomas account for 35 percent of laryngeal cancers and are aggressive with both direct extension and lymph node metastasis. Approximately one-half of patients with laryngeal cancer will present with lymph node involvement.

Clinical Presentation

The patient may complain of pain and poorly defined throat and neck discomfort that occurs during swallowing. Many patients complain of referred ear pain in combination with throat pain. Symptoms of cancers in the glottic area occur early and allow opportunity for early diagnosis. Cancers of the supraglottic region can be silent and generally present at a more advanced stage. Cancers of the subglottic larynx are rare. The symptoms of tumor involvement in the subglottic larynx include stridor.

Treatment

Treatment of early lesions is generally successful and equally effected by surgery or radiation therapy alone; at least 60 Gy of radiation is used. Choice of treatment is dictated by morbidity anticipated in the glottic area. Limited surgery may be performed, with radiation therapy reserved for recurrent disease or second primaries. Laser may be used to treat small glottic lesions. Endoscopic treatment of early laryngeal cancer using the CO_2 laser has been shown to be effective in several recent studies (McCaffrey, 1992). Induction chemotherapy followed by definitive radiation to the larynx and neck is another option. Early supraglottic lesions are amenable to conservative surgical techniques, but treatment needs to include both the primary site as well as the neck. This is often accomplished by external radiation to both areas, including at least 66 Gy to the primary site.

Some supraglottic tumors are initially treated with radiation therapy. If disease recurs following radiation therapy, salvage total laryngectomy with ipsilateral neck dissection is then performed.

Advanced lesions of either the glottic or supraglottic larynx generally require total laryngectomy and postoperative radiation therapy to both the larynx and neck fields. Positive neck nodes require surgical neck dissection. Radiation therapy is the treatment of choice for suspected, but unconfirmed, nodal metastases.

The outcome of glottic carcinoma treatment is dependent on the presence of vocal cord fixation, which almost reduces by one-half the 95 percent cure rate achievable in T1, and 80 to 85 percent cure rate achievable in T2 glottic lesions. Advanced (T3–T4) lesions with nodal metastases entail a less than 30 percent, 5-year survival rate. Supraglottic laryngeal cancer is generally more lethal. Survival rates are usually 10 to 25 percent worse than the corresponding glottic lesion. The prognosis for primary subglottic cancer is generally poor.

Hypopharynx and Cervical Esophagus

Anatomy

The hypopharynx surrounds the larynx and extends from the inferior border of the oropharynx to just above the cricopharyngeus muscle portion of the upper alimentary tract. Included are the pyriform sinuses, the lower posterior pharyngeal wall, and the posterior surface of the larynx. The cervical esophagus borders on and includes the cricopharyngeus muscle region, which includes the upper esophageal sphincter. This area represents a substantial narrowing of the hypopharyngeal lumen. The lower border of the cervical esophagus is generally considered to be the thoracic inlet.

Epidemiology and Risk Factors

The incidence of hypopharyngeal cancer is approximately 8 in 100,000. Specific sites within the hypopharynx that are commonly affected are the pyriform sinus (70 percent), the postcricoid area (15 percent), and the posterolateral wall (15 percent). Common etiologic factors include excessive smoking and alcohol consumption. Most lesions in the hypopharynx are squamous cell in origin. There is a tendency for submucosal spread, which often results in multiple separate primary tumors.

Clinical Presentation

Presenting symptoms include dysphagia, odynophagia, and referred ear pain. Advanced tumors of the pyriform sinuses and pharyngeal wall with extension into the larynx may have the associated symptoms of hoarseness or aspiration.

Treatment

Early tumors (T1 and T2) of the hypopharynx are rare and are treated with definitive radiation therapy with surgery reserved for salvage therapy. For early stage tumors, good local control (70 to 80 percent) is achieved with radiation therapy alone. Primary treatment involves large treatment portals to encompass the primary site as well as the cervical and mediastinal lymphatic regions. Opposed lateral fields are used to treat the upper neck and primary tumor and an anterior supraclavicular field is used to treat the lower neck. The total dose of radiation is at least 60 Gy. Interstitial radiation may be used with external beam therapy. Occasionally a small lesion confined to the lateral wall of the pyriform sinus or pharynx may lend itself to complete excision by pharyngectomy with reconstruction.

Combined modality approach with surgery, radiation, and chemotherapy is usually necessary to control the disease since the majority of patients with hypopharyngeal carcinomas present with advanced primary tumors. A partial or total pharyngectomy is required and may also include a partial or total laryngectomy or laryngo-esophagectomy. Approximately 75 percent of patients with hypopharyngeal cancers present with cervical metastases and require a radical or bilateral neck dissection. Postoperative external radiation to approximately 60 Gy usually begins 3 to 6 weeks following surgery. Overall survival is generally less than 30 percent.

Nasopharynx

Anatomy

The nasopharynx extends anteriorly to the plane of the choanae, which demarcates the nasal cavity. The lateral walls incorporate the eustachian tube orifices and a part of the pharyngeal wall, with inferior limits at the level of the palate. Superiorly, the nasopharynx includes the mucosa overlying the skull base and the sphenoid rostrum.

Epidemiology and Risk Factors

The incidence of nasopharyngeal carcinoma in the United States is only 0.6 in 100,000. Squamous cell carcinomas account for 98 percent of nasopharynx cancers. Nasopharyngeal carcinomas entail a different epidemiologic and etiologic spectrum, not associated with tobacco use, and are relatively uncommon in Caucasians. Factors postulated include genetic predisposition, increased size of the nasopharynx in southern Chinese, and environmental relationships to the ingestion of salted fish and foods. Nasopharyngeal cancer is endemic in parts of southern China where it is the most common malignancy of the head and neck. Environmental factors, particularly the Epstein-Barr virus, rather than genetic susceptibility are implicated.

Clinical Presentation

Patients tend to be younger and symptoms are varied and poorly localized. These symptoms include nasal obstruction, epistaxis, hearing impairment, tinnitus, and otitis media. More extensive disease may result in throat pain and neurologic or ocular symptoms. In many patients an enlarged node in the neck may be the first indication of nasopharyngeal carcinoma. Late symptoms include poorly localized headaches and facial pain, which can signify bone erosion and pressure on the fifth cranial nerve.

Treatment

Because of the complex anatomy of the nasopharynx and relative inaccessibility by surgery, radiation therapy is used as the principal treatment to the primary site and nodal areas. Radiation therapy employs a wide field encompassing the entire nasopharynx and extends from the skull base to the supraclavicular region, including all cervical nodal areas. Doses are generally 65 to 70 Gy. Induction platinum-based chemotherapy regimens are also used. Selected patients with recurrent or metastatic carcinoma of the nasopharynx receive aggressive combination chemotherapy.

Survival is related to the pretreatment volume of disease and histology. The rare T1 keratinizing lesion without palpable adenopathy may have an 80 percent, 5-year survival. Patients with advanced local (T3–T4) or regional disease will have only a 10 to 20 percent, 5-year survival. The delayed appearance of disseminated distant metastases is a significant problem and is responsible for more deaths than uncontrolled local or regional disease.

Nasal Cavity and Paranasal Sinuses

Anatomy

The nasal cavity begins at the limen nasi and ends at the posterior nares where it leads to the nasopharynx. The olfactory nerves enter the nasal cavity through the cribriform plate and distribute the nerves over the septum and superior nasal turbinates. The upper half of the nasal cavity is lined with a nonciliated columnar epithelium. The lower half of the nasal cavity is the respiratory portion and is lined with ciliated columnar epithelium. Numerous collections of lymphoid tissue and mucous glands lie beneath the epithelium. The paranasal sinuses include the maxillary sinuses, the frontal sinuses, the ethmoid sinuses, and the sphenoid sinus.

Epidemiology and Risk Factors

Primary nasal cavity carcinomas are rare. The maxillary sinus is the most commonly affected site. Squamous cell carcinoma is the predominant histology, although adenocarcinomas are seen. Adenocarcinomas are more commonly diagnosed in the ethmoid sinus. The incidence of nasal cavity carcinoma is increased in persons with occupations in nickel plating, furniture manufacturing, or leather working and in those exposed to chromate compounds, hydrocarbons, nitrosamines, dioxane, mustard gas, isopropyl alcohol, and petroleum.

Clinical Presentation

In early stages of the disease, the patient may be asymptomatic. Therefore most tumors are not discovered until they are advanced. Symptoms of cancers of the nasal cavity and paranasal sinuses include chronic sinusitis as well as a stuffy nose, sinus headache, dull facial pain, rhinorrhea, epistaxis, cheek hypoesthesia, trismus, and loose teeth. When the tumor extends in the area of the sphenoid sinus, compression of the third, fourth, and sixth cranial nerves can result in diplopia. In addition, pressure on the optic nerve can result in gradual loss of vision. General prognosis is more favorable if the tumor is located anterior and inferior to the plane connecting the medial canthus to the angle of the mandible.

Treatment

Although early carcinomas of the nasal cavity and paranasal sinuses are effectively treated with either surgery or radiation therapy alone, combined therapy with surgery and radiation is standard.

Maxillectomy is the treatment of choice for tumors in the maxillary sinus. More extensive disease with invasion into the floor of the orbit may necessitate combining radial maxillectomy with orbital exenteration. The craniofacial approach is used to resect tumors involving the skull base. Overall prognosis is poor with lesions recurring in the surgical cavity and invading the intracranial cavity.

Salivary Gland

Anatomy

There are three pairs of major salivary glands in the mouth: parotid, submandibular, and sublingual. The parotid glands lie below and anterior to the external ear. The parotid ducts open at the level of the second upper molar teeth. The submandibular glands lie below the mandible and their ducts (Wharton's) open on the underside of the tongue in the floor of the mouth. The sublingual glands lie in the sublingual folds in the floor of the mouth and have a number of small ducts that open in the floor of the mouth.

Epidemiology and Risk Factors

The parotid gland is the most common site for malignant lesions. The average age of patients is 55 years. A variety of histologies are seen, with mucoepidermoid lesions predominant within the parotid gland and adenoid cystic carcinomas predominant elsewhere.

Clinical Presentation

Patients frequently present with swelling of a salivary gland. Other symptoms include head and neck pain, rapid expansion of the mass, poor facial or mouth mobility, and facial nerve weakness.

Treatment

Surgical resection is the treatment of choice, with radiation therapy playing an adjuvant role and chemotherapy a palliative one. Surgical exploration of the gland and proximate nodal lymphatics is the approach of choice with removal of the entire gland and tumor. Neck dissection of enlarged lymph nodes is also performed. Elective ipsilateral neck dissection is warranted for high-grade mucoepidermoid and squamous cell lesions. Postoperative radiation therapy is used to eradicate residual disease.

The 5-year survival for high-grade mucoepidermoid malignancies is approximately 40 percent. Adenoid cystic carcinomas demonstrate a 5-year survival rate of 70 to 80 percent. Survival drops to 40 percent at 10 years, and 22 percent at 20 years. Neutron beam therapy for unresectable salivary gland tumors has been used with excellent local control as well as cosmetic outcome (Awan et al., 1991).

Thyroid

Anatomy

The thyroid gland lies anterior to and partially surrounds the thyroid cartilage and the upper rings of the trachea. The thyroid produces and secretes thyroxine.

Epidemiology and Risk Factors

Cancers of the thyroid usually occur between the ages of 25 to 65 years. Occasionally teenagers are affected. The estimated new cases per year are 16,100, with 11,400 cases occurring in women (Parker et al., 1997). The clinical behavior of the tumor varies widely from the aggressive anaplastic cancer to the relatively indolent well-differentiated papillary carcinomas. Differentiated thyroid cancers are either of papillary of follicular types. Anaplastic carcinomas usually display giant or spindle cells. Areas of anaplastic or undifferentiated cells may occur in differentiated thyroid cancer and are associated with poor outlook. Very poorly differentiated follicular carcinomas also carry a poor prognosis. Distant metastases are uncommon. The only specific epidemiological risk factor for thyroid cancer is childhood exposure to radiation.

Clinical Presentation

The usual presentation is a palpable nodule on the thyroid. Most cancers are less than 2 cm in diameter. Diffuse enlargement and rapid growth of the tumor may suggest an anaplastic spindle or giant cell carcinoma. Other physical findings for thyroid cancer include hardness and fixation of the gland, vocal cord paralysis, and displacement or narrowing of the trachea or esophagus. Thyroid function is evaluated using radioactive iodine scans to help define whether the thyroid nodules are functional or not. Diagnosis is completed with needle biopsy.

Treatment

Surgery is performed to remove all suspicious nodules. Total thyroid lobectomy is usually performed. Prognosis is related to the age of the patient and the extent of primary disease. Prognosis worsens with each decade of age over 50 years. Radioactive iodine ablation of residual thyroid tissue and its use for treatment of metastases is highly successful. Well-differentiated papillary and follicular thyroid cancers are highly curable.

Nursing Care of Patients with Head and Neck Cancer Receiving Radiation Therapy

The care of persons with head and neck cancer receiving radiation therapy involves management of the side effects of therapy as well as addressing the psychosocial issues that accompany the disease and treatment. Assessing the patient's and family's ability to participate in care is crucial. By involving the patient and family in the plan of care, the effectiveness of nursing care will be maximized (Madeya, 1996).

Skin Reactions and Fatigue

As in other areas, skin reactions occur within the treatment field. Areas such as the collar line along the neck are especially vulnerable to skin irritation and breakdown (Strohl, 1989). Monitoring the condition of the skin within the treatment field and recommending appropriate techniques for cleansing and moisturizing the skin will protect the skin and minimize further skin breakdown.

Fatigue commonly occurs during radiation therapy to the head and neck region. Malnutrition as a result of the disease or treatment exacerbates the fatigue. See Chapter 8 for more information on skin care and fatigue during radiation therapy.

Nutritional Effects

Approximately one-third of patients with advanced cancer of the head and neck are severely malnourished (Goodwin & Byers, 1993). Another one-third of patients suffer from mild malnutrition. Both physiological and psychological factors lead to decreases in food intake in head and neck cancer patients (Grant et al., 1989). Nutritional deficits are a result of disease, both local and systemic, premorbid nutritional habits, treatment (surgery, chemotherapy, and radiation therapy), poor dental health, and alcohol abuse (Zemel et al., 1991). Impaired nutritional status in the head and neck cancer patient predisposes the patient to increased morbidity, reduced immunocompetence, impaired would healing, and poor tolerance to therapy.

Patients receiving radiation therapy experience nutritional problems during and after therapy. These problems occur as a result of depleted energy stores, increased energy expenditure, as well as decreased oral intake of foods resulting from the side effects of radiation therapy. Studies have demonstrated the nutritional consequences of head and neck irradiation. Donaldson (1977) reported that of 122 patients who received radiation therapy to the oral cavity, oropharynx, and hypopharynx, 93 percent lost an average of 3.7 kg during the 6- to 8-week course of therapy. Close to 9 percent of these patients lost greater than 10 percent of their body weight during that time, and many of the subjects were malnourished before starting the therapy. In another study by Johnson and associates (1982), 68 percent of the patients who received radiation therapy to the head and neck region (N = 31) lost 5 percent of their pretreatment weight within 1 month after treatment. The average overall weight loss was 10 percent. The patients who lost weight tended to have greater severity and longer duration of side effects associated with the irradiation than those who did not lose weight.

The size of the treatment field also affects the nutritional status of patients. An evaluation of patients who received irradiation to the head and neck region revealed that patients who had a treatment field size greater than 7 cm suffered more nutritional consequences (weight loss) than those whose treatment field size was less than 7 cm (Pezner & Archambeau, 1985). Similar results were reported by Hearne and colleagues (1985), who found that radiation treatment field sizes of the head and neck region greater than 64 cm² were associated with weight loss and a greater duration of treatment-related morbidity. In addition, pretreatment nutritional status or dietary habits were not predictive of weight loss in these patients.

Nutritional assessment of the patient receiving head and neck irradiation includes evaluating dietary intake as well as anthropometric measurements, laboratory tests of albumin, glucose, and electrolytes, and physical examination (Grant et al., 1989). Oral intake of food and fluids can be supported by nutritional counseling and provision of nutritional supplements (Grant et al., 1989).

Wilson and associates (1991) evaluated the eating strategies of 11 patients with head and neck cancer during and after radiation therapy. Three general areas of eating strategies were identified by the patients. The first area involved strategies related to food choice and modification. Patients selected foods by trial and error based on particular symptoms experienced. The second area related to accepting assistance from others such as a spouse in meal preparation or health care provider in advice about nutrition or prescription of medications. The third area of eating strategies involved adopting a positive attitude about eating and nutrition.

Adequate nutritional support given before therapy will reduce therapy-related complications in severely malnourished patients. As a result, patients feel better, have a higher tolerance to therapy with fewer complications, and achieve a higher response rate to therapy.

Alterations in the Mouth

Stomatitis, moniliasis, dysphagia, taste alterations, xerostomia, dental caries, osteoradionecrosis, and trismus are side effects that occur with irradiation of the mouth. Nutritional problems frequently result from these side effects.

Early Side Effects

Stomatitis

The oral mucosa is composed of stratified squamous cells that form a nonkeratinized epithelium. These cells have a high turnover rate of approximately 10 to 14 days. The epithelial cells of the mouth are very radiosensitive. Stomatitis (also called mucositis) is inflammation that can occur along the mucous membranes lining the mouth. This reaction occurs approximately 2 to 3 weeks after the start of therapy. There is progressive involvement of the oral mucosa with vasocongestion and edema of the tissue (Donaldson, 1984; Sonis & Clark, 1991). A pseudomembrane can form and then slough off, leaving a friable epithelial layer. Superficial ulcerations and bleeding may occur. With prolonged irradiation to the head and neck area, chronic ulcers may form. In addition, irritants in the mouth such as chewing tobacco and alcohol, and trauma such as inadvertently biting the buccal mucosa or injuries from hard-bristled toothbrushes or irregularly shaped teeth, can cause a break in the epithelial layer of the mucosa and form an ulcer. If a patient has large metallic tooth fillings within the treatment field, the adjacent mucosa is at risk for developing an enhanced reaction from scatter radiation.

ASSESSMENT

Assessment for oral stomatitis involves the daily evaluation of the oral cavity (Beck, 1979). The patient may initially report hypersensitivity or pain in the mouth. Pain may also be noted when eating, or there may be difficulty with chewing foods and drinking fluids. An examination of the mouth is crucial (Eilers et al., 1988). Inspect the lips for dryness, cracks, and lesions. Note color of the tissues (pale to red) and the presence of edema. In order to inspect all mucosal surfaces have the patient remove dentures if present. The oral cavity is then inspected using a penlight. A moistened tongue blade or gloved finger is used to check the buccal mucosa, the palate, under the tongue, and along the inner aspects of the upper and lower lips. The gingiva and back of teeth are also carefully inspected.

On examination, mild to moderate patchy erythema may be noted. As stomatitis progresses, edema of the tissues is seen as well as an increase in erythema. Erythema may involve the entire mucosal surface. A confluent or patchy whitish-yellow membrane may form. Open lesions may occur along any of the mucosal surfaces. With this level of stomatitis, the patient usually experiences moderate to severe pain and has difficulty eating.

A variety of mouth assessment tools are available. Eilers and associates (1988) describe the Oral Assessment Guide. This tool consists of assessments in eight categories including voice, swallowing, lips, tongue, saliva, mucous membranes, gingiva, and teeth. The MacDibbs Mouth Assessment was developed to measure radiation-induced oral mucositis (Dibble et al., 1996). This tool assesses objective signs and subjective symptoms in patients. Items are grouped into four sections: patient information, examination, potassium hydroxide smear, and herpes simplex virus culture. The patient information section includes assessment of pain, dryness, eating, talking, swallowing, tasting, and saliva production.

NURSING INTERVENTIONS

Dental Consultation. A thorough oral examination by a dentist prior to the start of head and neck irradiation is important. Many patients have preexisting odontogenic disease and need dental prophylaxis prior to starting irradiation (Lockhart & Clark, 1994). Complications associated with head and neck irradiation can be prevented by treating diseased oral sites before initiation of cancer therapy (Peterson & D'Ambrosio, 1994). Radiation therapy can often cause changes in oral tissues that require long-term management by a dentist.

Mouth Care. The purpose of mouth care is to remove debris, lubricate the mucosa, and promote comfort. Patients who are at risk for developing stomatitis should perform mouth care at least 4 times a day—after meals and at bedtime. For patients who have active stomatitis, mouth care needs to be provided at least every 2 hours while awake. Brushing with a soft-bristled toothbrush and daily flossing between teeth is effective in removing debris from the teeth and periodontal areas. However, if severe stomatitis is present, a soft sponge-tipped applicator, although less effective, can help remove debris. For some patients, a gauze-covered finger is the most comfortable way to gently remove debris from the oral cavity. An irrigating syringe or gravity drip container (tube feeding bag or intravenous solution bag/bottle) with tubing can be used to gently irrigate the oral cavity. A red rubber-tipped catheter may be attached to the tubing or syringe to facilitate the irrigation (Mosco, 1986). Mouthwashes can help to further cleanse, lubricate, and comfort the oral cavity. Numerous agents have been suggested, including saline, sodium bicarbonate solutions, dilutions of hydrogen peroxide, and a combination of these solutions. In general, commercially prepared mouthwashes should be avoided if they contain alcohol or detergents; these ingredients can be painful on open lesions in the mouth and cause more dryness. Lemon-glycerine swabs can also further irritate the mouth because of the drying effects of glycerine and should be avoided (Daeffler, 1980; Van Drimmelen & Rollins, 1969; Wiley, 1969). Lanolin or petrolatum jelly may be applied to the lips to keep them moist and soft.

Ferraro and Mattern (1984) described the preparation and use of sucralfate suspension to promote healing of oral stomatitis. Sucralfate is a compound of sulfated sucrose and aluminum hydroxide that has been used for gastric and duodenal ulcers. Sucralfate acts by forming an adherent complex to the ulcer and creates a protective barrier against further injury. Wilkes (1986) described the healing effects of sucralfate suspension for chemotherapy-induced oral mucositis. She reported lesions that measured 1 to 2 cm healed within 2 to 3 days. There was also high patient satisfaction with the pain relief obtained from the medication. A study by Makkonen and associates (1994) evaluated the effectiveness of sucralfate to prevent radiation-induced mucositis. Forty patients with head and neck cancer were randomized to use either sucralfate mouthwashes 1 g 6 times a day (n = 20) during irradiation or placebo (n = 20). All patients developed varying degrees of mucositis after reaching a radiation dose of about 30 Gy. No difference in visually assessed degree of mucositis or oral pain was reported between groups. However, in the patients treated with sucralfate, less topical anesthetic was used and these patients' salivary lactoferrin and albumin levels were lower. These results suggest that sucralfate has a slight protective effect on the oral mucosa.

Minimizing Mouth Irritants. Poorly fitting dentures can be a source of irritation in the mouth. For the patient with moderate to severe stomatitis, dentures should be worn only during meals if tolerated to minimize further trauma to the mucosa. Chewing tobacco and smoking cigarettes, pipes, or cigars, as well as alcohol consumption, should also be avoided. For patients who have large metallic tooth fillings, the radiation oncologist should be consulted to determine whether a piece of gauze may be placed between the tooth and the mucosa to minimize an enhanced mucosal reaction from the radiations (Jones & Hafermann, 1986).

Dietary Modifications. When pain in the oral cavity occurs, the diet should consist of soft, bland, and moderate temperature foods. Soft foods are less likely to traumatize the tissues and are easier to chew and swallow. A bland, moderate temperature diet eliminates seasonings, alcohol, and hot or very cold foods that may further irritate the mucosa (see Table 14–3). Blended foods can help make the consistency of the foods less painful to chew and swallow. The patient should also appropriately increase oral fluid intake to maintain hydration (Grant, 1986).

Table 14-3 • Soft and Bland Diet to Minimize Pain and Discomfort Related to Stomatitis and Esophagitis

Type of Food	Foods to Include	Foods to Avoid
Eggs	Any except moderately or highly seasoned preparations	
Meat, fish, poultry	Beef, salmon, chicken, lamb, sole, duck, liver, halibut, turkey, veal, shellfish, pork, sweetbreads	Smoked, seasoned, or barbecued meat, fish, and poultry, any tough meats
Bread and cereal	Soft breads, cooked cereals, macaroni, pasta without spicy sauces	Toast, hard crackers, pretzels, uncooked cereals (unless soft), grainy cereals and breads
Vegetables	All cooked vegetables	Raw vegetables, potato chips
Fruits	Applesauce, baked apple, peeled ripe banana *Canned:* Apricots, peaches, pears *Fresh:* Ripe peeled peaches, pears, watermelon, honeydew melons	Raw fruits, berries, figs, citrus fruits, tomatoes, grapefruit, orange, pineapple, plums, prunes
Juices	Apple, apricot, peach, pear, prune	Berry, grape, tomato
Dairy products	Milk, buttermilk, plain yogurt, cream, cottage cheese, cream cheese, mild cheeses	Strong cheeses
Fats	Butter, margarine, salad oil, mayonnaise	Any other fats
Desserts	Puddings (cornstarch, rice, tapioca), breads, custard, gelatin, ice cream, plain sherbet, plain cake, plain cookies, cream pies, cheesecake	Highly seasoned pastries, berry pies, desserts containing nuts
Soups	Mild cream soups, mild broths or bouillons, cold blenderized soups: cucumber, potato	Highly seasoned soups, tomato soup
Beverages	Coffee if tolerated, tea if tolerated, cocoa, Postum, chocolate, malted milk, eggnog	Coffee if not tolerated, carbonated beverages, beer, wine, liquor
Miscellaneous	Salt in moderation, mild herbs, thyme, basil, oregano, sugar in moderation, jelly in moderation	Pepper, tabasco sauce, other spices, chili powder, paprika, nutmeg, cinnamon, large amounts of concentrated sweets, nuts

Pain Control. Stomatitis can cause moderate to severe pain. Topical or systemic analgesics used before meals can help promote comfort while eating. Topical anesthetics are useful for mild to moderate pain as a result of stomatitis. For moderate to severe pain from stomatitis, systemic analgesics are used in addition to topical anesthetics. Topical anesthetic agents such as lidocaine viscous help to numb the oral mucosa. Diphenhydramine, dyclonine hydrochloride, and topical analgesic mouthwashes that include acetaminophen are also used. These agents should be used approximately 15 minutes before meals. Nonsteroidal anti-inflammatory medications may also be used. For severe oral discomfort, systemic narcotic analgesics should be used 30 to 60 minutes before meals. Sustained-release and immediate-release narcotics are used for continuous severe mouth pain. Stool softeners must be provided to prevent constipation from the narcotic medications. For some patients, the narcotic medications cause nausea and antiemetics are given (Olsen & Creagan, 1991).

Moniliasis

Moniliasis is an infection by parasitic fungi such as the *Candida albicans* yeast. Moniliasis can increase the severity of stomatitis (Laskiewicz,

1982). This infection usually occurs in immunosuppressed individuals as a result of overgrowth of the fungi. Moniliasis is a common occurrence in patients treated with chemotherapy or steroid medications, regardless of the site of radiation treatment. Moniliasis can also occur when radiation-induced mucositis has altered the protective barrier of the oral cavity. Although the infection frequently occurs on the tongue, all mucous membranes of the oral cavity are susceptible to infection.

Moniliasis appears as soft, curd-like white patches or may be confluent and cover most of the tongue or mucosal surface. The white patches can be scraped off and areas of erythema will be seen on the mucosa. With severe infections, the yeast may also infect the esophagus.

ASSESSMENT

The daily oral examination includes inspecting for moniliasis. The patient may complain of painful areas or tenderness in the oral cavity. Some report an increased dryness in the mouth, unrelated to xerostomia. Frequently patients will report seeing the white patches in their mouth or on the tongue. A sample may be obtained to test for the presence of fungi.

NURSING INTERVENTIONS

The patient is instructed to continue mouth care. Antifungal medications are administered as prescribed and the patient's mouth is examined to determine the resolution of the infection. Reinfections may occur and should be monitored.

Dysphagia and Odynophagia

Dysphagia refers to difficulty swallowing and odynophagia refers to pain with eating. These symptoms often occur in combination with stomatitis and xerostomia, side effects also associated with head and neck irradiation. Dysphagia occurs approximately 2 to 3 weeks after starting irradiation, peaks toward the end of the course of radiation, and can continue for as long as 6 months following therapy (Lindsey, 1986). The patient first has difficulty eating solid foods and may progress to difficulties with swallowing fluids. Some patients who wear dentures may find that their dentures do not fit properly as a result of the soft tissue changes.

ASSESSMENT

The patient will report difficulty or pain with eating and swallowing. A decrease in amount of food eaten may be noted and weight loss is monitored. The mouth is inspected for signs of stomatitis and xerostomia.

NURSING INTERVENTIONS

Patients who experience dysphagia/odynophagia need to perform mouth care prior to and after meals. (See Mouth Care: Stomatitis.) Appropriate anesthetics and/or analgesics are used to control pain in the mouth.

A soft, bland, and moderate-temperature diet will be more comfortable to eat (see Table 14–3). Small, frequent meals (i.e., 6 to 8 small meals a day) can provide daily nutritional needs over a longer period of time. In that way, each meal is not overwhelming and early satiety is less of a problem (Grant, 1986). Dietary supplements (e.g., Carnation Instant Breakfast, Ensure, Resource, Sustacal) that are commercially available will add to the daily caloric and protein intake. The use of such nutrient-dense supplements will allow a decrease in the volume that must be consumed. Some patients find these supplements taste too sweet. This sweetness can be lessened by adding a few drops of bitters, which are used in cocktail drinks (Larpenteur, 1984) or ½ to 1 teaspoon of instant coffee.

Taste Alterations

Taste is influenced by many factors. These factors include color and smell of food, emotional state of the individual, and learned social responses. The taste buds (receptors) are located on the tongue, soft palate, glossopalatine arch, and posterior wall of the pharynx. There are four primary sensations: sour, sweet, salty, and bitter. Most taste buds respond to three or four of the primary sensations. The perception of taste occurs in the brain. Taste acuity tends to be highest before meals and rapidly decreases during meals. In addition, taste buds degenerate with age (Guyton, 1971). Taste changes have been reported in cancer patients (Chencharick & Mossman, 1983; Williams & Cohen, 1978). Patients may report a decrease in taste acuity (hypogeusia) for foods and fluids or an unpleasant taste (dysgeusia) in their mouths. An increase in the threshold for sweet recognition and a decrease in the threshold for bitter recognition as evidenced by meat aversions has also been noted.

Radiation therapy to the head and neck area affects the taste buds. At 1000 cGy there is a disruption of the architecture of the taste buds with atrophy and degeneration (Beumer et al., 1979). According to Donaldson (1977), the most susceptible sensations to irradiation are bitter and sour. Mossman and Henkin (1978) reported that peak impairment of taste acuity occurred after 3 weeks of radiation therapy. They also found that changes in bitter and salty tastes occurred earliest and lasted the longest. In addition, sweet sensations were the last to change and returned to normal in approximately 7 weeks after the completion of therapy. Many patients lose all sense of taste (ageusia), which is described as "mouth blindness" (MacCarthy-Leventhal, 1959). Although in some patients taste returns in 60 to 120 days after therapy is completed, for others it may take up to a year or longer (Conger, 1973; Mossman et al., 1982).

Microscopically, irradiation damages the microvilli of taste cells as well as their cell surfaces. Olfactory bulb changes are also noted at low doses of radiation (Cooper, 1968). Therefore an altered sense of smell may affect taste sensations in some patients.

ASSESSMENT

Taste alterations can be a persistent problem and should be assessed during the course of treatment and in follow-up visits to the clinic (Strohl, 1983). Some patients report a "bad" or "burnt" taste in their mouths. These patients usually find coffee and chocolates to be especially distasteful. Other patients report decreased or heightened taste sensations. A decreased appetite is usually noted and the patient's weight is monitored. The oral cavity is inspected for mucosal changes and foods not eaten are assessed. Strohl (1984) reported that before receiving information about taste changes, several patients had accused their families of trying to poison their food. With decreased sense of taste or smell, there is also a reduced awareness of hazards such as smoke, natural gas, and spoiled foods.

NURSING INTERVENTIONS

Enhancing Palatability of Foods. The palatability of foods can be enhanced by the use of seasonings, sugar, and so forth if tolerated. Patients can avoid or modify the foods that taste bad. For instance, patients who have meat aversions may find cold cooked chicken, mild cheeses, and fish to be more palatable sources of protein (Gallucci & Iwamoto, 1981). In addition, marinating and/or cooking meats in sweet sauces can help disguise the taste of certain meats (Strohl, 1984). Varying temperatures of food or having foods of different textures may also increase palatability. Presentation of the food in a pleasing manner and away from cooking or other unpleasant odors will enhance appetite. Some patients have found that their sense of smell is less affected than taste and will take a deep sniff of the food before placing the food in their mouths. These patients claim that this procedure offers some sense of "taste." Other patients have reported being able to taste sweet and sour foods (e.g., certain salad dressings and Chinese foods) when other foods lack taste. In this instance, salad dressings may be added to other foods to enhance taste (Strohl, 1984). Lemon drops and plain soft mints can help refresh the mouth and minimize unpleasant tastes (Pehanrich, 1983; Strohl, 1984). Instruct patients to chew food thoroughly to allow more particles to interact with sensory receptors and alternate between food substances to counteract sensory adaptation (Moore et al., 1991). Use of commercially available synthetic odors or odor amplifiers may help relieve blandness (Moore et al., 1991). Cigarette smoking has been associated with decreased olfaction and should be avoided (Moore et al., 1991).

Other Measures. Performing routine mouth care before and after meals can help clear residual tastes and refresh the mouth for meals. Modifying pain, fatigue, and depression can also benefit the patient. These factors can greatly influence a person's taste sensations as well as appetite (Gallucci & Iwamoto, 1981). Analgesics may be used as needed before meals to control pain. The patient should be encouraged to rest before and after meals. The nurse can provide support, counseling, and antidepressants, if prescribed, to help alleviate depression. Allow the patient and family to be involved in deciding which measures to use to increase the palatability of foods. If the patient continues to lose weight, consult a dietitian to plan a program for nutritional repletion.

Xerostomia

Xerostomia, or mouth dryness, occurs when the salivary glands are affected by irradiation. When xerostomia is present, there is an increased risk for dental caries, periodontal diseases, stomatitis, disturbed oral sensations, dysphagia, and altered taste (Navazesh & Ship, 1983). Saliva is important for lubrication of food during chewing and swallowing, chemical digestion, and taste. Saliva is also important for the cleaning of teeth, maintaining denture stability and retention, and speech.

Xerostomia has been reported after 1 week (or 1000 cGy) of radiation therapy (Kashima et al., 1965). The severity of xerostomia peaks at the end of a course of irradiation and continues to be a problem at 6 months or longer after completion of therapy (Donaldson, 1977; Mossman et al., 1982). Dreizen and associates (1976) reported that patients who received head and neck irradiation had an 83 percent reduction in saliva flow at 6 weeks (1000 cGy per week). They also noted that xerostomia continued to progress to a 93 percent reduction in salivary flow rates at 3 months after therapy. The quality and quantity of saliva is changed to a thick, ropy, acidic substance. With prolonged irradiation, postirradiation atrophy and fibrosis of the salivary glands is reported (Eneroth et al., 1972). Anaerobic microbes flourish when xerostomia occurs. The increased acidity of the saliva decreases the buffering properties of the saliva. Therefore microbial plaques form on the teeth, causing increased dental caries. An increase in candidiasis is also reported with xerostomia (Jones et al., 1980).

ASSESSMENT

Patients may report a dry mouth or "cotton mouth"—worse at night or upon arising in the morning. Abnormalities or decreases in taste sensations are also reported. Patients may also note tenderness or pain in the mouth, a burning sensation, difficulty with dentures, difficulty speaking, and increased sensitivity of teeth. On examination of the oral cavity, the mucosa appears dry and dull and there may be pallor or increased erythema. Salivary secretions appear thick and viscid and dentures (if present) may not fit correctly. Candidiasis may also be noted.

NURSING INTERVENTIONS
Enhancing Mouth Wetness. The patient is encouraged to increase fluid intake of juices and water. This provides comfort as well as calories and hydration. Sugarless lemon-flavored drinks can produce maximal salivary stimulation without the need for rinsing. For some patients, sucking on a hard, highly flavored sugarless candy or chewing sugarless gum stimulates some saliva production.

Saliva substitutes have been beneficial to some patients. Although the effect lasts only a few minutes, the saliva substitutes are helpful when other fluids are not available. The saliva substitutes are usually made out of mineral oil, inert glycols, and carboxymethyl cellulose. These substances coat the mucous membrane with a thin, slippery film and provide lubrication to the tissues. Fluoride is usually a part of the solution to help prevent dental caries. The saliva substitute may be applied before meals, at bedtime, and whenever needed. The patient is instructed to use as little solution as possible to produce comfort (approximately 2 ml).

Other substances may be used to provide lubrication of the oral cavity. Some patients have found using a small amount of a vegetable oil such as olive oil in the mouth provides long-lasting relief of mouth dryness. The vegetable oil may be placed in the mouth at bedtime to minimize the experience of waking up in the middle of the night with the tongue adhered to the roof of the mouth.

Other Measures. Mouth care should be performed before and after meals, at bedtime, and as needed during the day. This care regimen will refresh the mouth and wet the oral tissues. Commercial mouthwash with detergents and/or alcohol should be avoided because of its drying effect. Lemon-glycerine swabs should also be avoided because of the drying effect of glycerine.

Foods that are dry or "thick" (biscuits, crackers, peanut butter) and require large amounts of saliva to chew and swallow should be avoided unless they can be moistened or thinned. The patient should use sauces and gravies on foods and have fluids with all meals and snacks. Patients should increase their total fluid intake to 2500 to 3000 ml/day unless contraindicated (Grant, 1986).

Pilocarpine, a cholinergic alkaloid, has been shown to be effective in increasing salivary flow and producing symptomatic relief in head and neck cancer patients with radiation-induced xe-

rostomia (Greenspan & Daniels, 1987; Johnson et al., 1993; LeVeque et al., 1993). Five milligrams of pilocarpine are taken orally three times a day. Side effects include transient sweating, flushing, rhinitis, headache, nausea, and urinary frequency. Pilocarpine is contraindicated in patients with uncontrolled asthma, acute iritis, or narrow-angle glaucoma.

Late Side Effects

Dental Caries

Dental caries may occur as a late effect from radiation therapy to the head and neck region. When xerostomia occurs, there is a change in the character of saliva. The saliva becomes a thick, viscid, and acidic mixture that promotes plaque formation on teeth. This plaque is an excellent substrate for bacterial growth and attack. With the build-up of plaque, gingival inflammation and recession can occur and eventually lead to osteoradionecrosis. The symptoms of dental injury may initially be an increased sensitivity to sweets, heat, and cold.

The saliva of irradiated head and neck cancer patients has also been shown to contain fewer electrolytes, such as calcium, potassium, nitrogen, phosphorus, chloride, and carbonate. This leads to a lessened buffering capacity, which causes demineralization of tooth enamel (Dwyer, 1979). In addition, there is an alteration of the oral flora composition, which can lead to caries formation.

Dreizen and associates (1976) reported increased xerostomia at 3 months after radiation therapy and associated this with a higher incidence of dental caries. Dental caries may occur 3 to 12 months following a course of irradiation.

ASSESSMENT

Assessment for the onset of caries formation includes assessing tooth sensitivity to sweets as well as hot and cold temperatures. Toothaches also occur. Two to 3 weeks before the start of irradiation, the patient should be examined by a dentist for the following:

1. Diagnostic evaluation of teeth, including radiography,
2. Restorative dental therapy with extraction of nonrestorable teeth,
3. Review of oral care requirements during radiation therapy, including the use of topical fluoride applications, and
4. A thorough examination of the oral cavity for xerostomia, stomatitis, and gingival inflammation (National Institutes of Health, 1989).

NURSING INTERVENTIONS

Patients can be instucted in several measures to relieve xerostomia. Mouth care should be performed before and after meals and at bedtime. Topical fluoride applications need to be performed daily at bedtime until the xerostomia is relieved. The dentist will advise the patient on the use of an appropriate molded tray that fits the contour of the teeth. The fluoride gel is placed in the tray, and these trays are then placed in the mouth. The patient bites down on the trays for approximately 2 to 5 minutes, after which the trays are removed and cleansed. The patient may expectorate the excess fluoride gel but not rinse the mouth. The patient should perform this treatment after mouth care is done at bedtime and should try not to drink fluids after the treatment with fluoride.

Osteoradionecrosis

Osteoradionecrosis occurs as a result of radiation damage to the maxilla or mandible. This is a rare occurrence and appears as decreased marrow cellularity and vascularity, fibrosis, and fatty degeneration. As a result, the patient is more susceptible to infections and poor wound healing (Beumer et al., 1979). Up to 20 percent of patients may experience osteoradionecrosis (Bedwinek et al., 1976; Morrish et al., 1981; Larson et al., 1983). There is a greater incidence of osteoradionecrosis with higher doses of irradiation. Osteoradionecrosis has also been linked to denture wearing and to the continued use of alcohol and tobacco (Beumer et al., 1979; Parsons, 1984). It is thought that trauma and irritants cause the breakdown of the gingiva leading to a chronic, nonhealing wound.

Treatment for osteoradionecrosis includes surgically resecting the diseased tissue and bone, antibiotic therapy to treat underlying infections, and hyperbaric oxygen therapy to improve tissue healing (Davis, 1981; Hart & Mainous, 1976; Mansfield et al., 1981).

Patients may initially seek medical help for a persistent jaw or tooth ache. There may be exposed bone in the oral cavity or nonhealing gingival ulcers, especially over areas of tooth extraction. Occasionally, a patient may experience trauma or fracture to the bone structure and require emergency care.

ASSESSMENT

The patient complains of a persistent tooth or jaw ache. Patients who are at high risk are those who have received radiation therapy in the past year, wear dentures, and continue to consume alcohol and tobacco. The oral examination may reveal irregularity of teeth alignment or gums, a nonhealing wound on the gingiva or other mucosal surfaces covering bone, or exposed bone.

NURSING INTERVENTIONS

While a patient is undergoing radiation therapy to the head and neck region, thorough and systematic mouth care needs to be performed. Assess the use of dentures to be sure that they properly fit. Arrange for frequent follow-up visits with the dentist, radiation oncologist, and surgeon for monitoring and early identification of osteoradionecrosis. Maintain optimum caloric and protein intake to promote wound healing.

Trismus

Trismus is tonic contractions of the muscles of mastication and is seen as a chronic effect from head and neck irradiation. Trismus occurs as a result of scar formation on the muscles of mastication and appears to be more common in patients who have had head and neck surgery. Patients with trismus may experience a reduced capacity to open their mouths. Openings of as little as 10 to 15 mm are seen (Beumer et al., 1979). These patients are unable to place foods in their mouths and have difficulty chewing foods. Unless treated, trismus is progressive.

Medical management of trismus may involve surgery to release the muscles of mastication. Dynamic bite openers may be used to stretch the muscles and increase the size of the mouth opening.

ASSESSMENT

The patient reports difficulty opening mouth to normal width. Pain in the jaw and mouth may also be present. When measured, there is a decrease in the width of mouth opening.

NURSING INTERVENTIONS

Patients are encouraged to prevent trismus with frequent exercises of the muscles of mastication; i.e., chewing exercises. For patients with trismus, assist the patient in using the dynamic bite openers, exercise the muscles of mastication, and make modifications in the diet to soft and liquid consistency as needed. See Table 14–4 for instructions on exercises to minimize trismus.

Alterations in the Pharynx

The early side effects that occur with irradiation of the pharynx include pharyngitis. Prolonged pharyngitis without relief can lead to malnutrition and metabolic derangements.

Table 14-4 • Exercises for Trismus

1. Open mouth as wide as possible 20 times in succession 3 times a day.
2. Place heels of both hands under jaw, push up with hands while stretching mouth open. The pressure provides resistance to the mandible as it opens and thereby strengthens the muscles.
3. Place middle and index fingers on mandibular teeth and thumb on maxillary teeth. Use fingers in twisting motion to pry the mouth open. Hold open as wide as possible for 2 seconds, then relax. Repeat 10 times with the right hand and then repeat with the left hand. Repeat the entire sequence 4 times a day.

Data from Ritchie et al. (1985). Dental care for the irradiated cancer patient. *Quintessence International, 16*, 837–842; Sullivan & Fleming (1986). Oral care for the radiotherapy-treated head and neck cancer patient. *Dental Hygiene, 60*, 112–114.

Early Side Effects

Pharyngitis

The epithelial cells of the pharynx are highly radiosensitive. Donaldson (1984) reported that with prolonged radiation of the pharynx there is a local inflammatory reaction with a loss of superficial epithelium. Edema can then occur in the submucosa of the pharynx and lead to ulceration. Irritants such as smoking and alcohol consumption can further traumatize the mucosa. Patients who receive radiation therapy to the pharynx also tend to lose weight in spite of intensive nutritional counseling and support (Enig et al., 1985). Pharyngitis can occur approximately 2 to 3 weeks from the start of treatment. For some patients, the pharyngitis spontaneously resolves after a few weeks, but for others it persists until the end of treatment.

ASSESSMENT

Patients may report a "lump" or "fullness" in their throats and have difficulty swallowing foods. It is common to hear patients say that although their throat is not painful, the food "just doesn't go down." Other patients may complain of a mild to severe sore throat. The oropharynx is examined using a moistened tongue blade to gently depress the midpoint of the tongue while asking the patient to say "ah" or yawn. The palatine arches and the posterior oropharyngeal wall are also inspected. Indirect laryngoscopy may reveal erythema, edema, and ulceration of the laryngopharynx.

NURSING INTERVENTIONS

To minimize throat pain have patients gargle with warm saline before and after meals. Systemic narcotic analgesics are sometimes needed to control the pain from pharyngitis. Nonsteroidal anti-inflammatory agents can help decrease the local inflammation in the pharynx. Analgesics should be used 30 to 60 minutes before meals. Antacids in chewable tablet or liquid form can also provide temporary relief of pharyngitis if taken immediately before meals. Anesthetic lozenges can provide some comfort during the day. If aspirin is tolerated, a gargling solution made with two tablets of aspirin in a large glass of warm water may provide topical relief for pharyngitis. Topical anesthetics may also be applied but caution must be used with swallowing lidocaine viscous because it can hinder the gag reflex and cause aspiration. Hilderley (1986) describes a "radiotherapy mixture" that contains Mylanta, lidocaine viscous, and diphenhydramine elixir. This mixture is taken before meals and at bedtime to control pain.

Dietary Modifications. A soft, bland, and moderate temperature diet is best tolerated (see Table 14–3). Use of a blender or food processor can help make certain foods easier to swallow. Small frequent meals and snacks can help spread the nutritional intake over a longer period of time. Commercial nutritional supplements can help to increase the patient's caloric and protein intake. Avoid irritants such as tobacco and alcohol. Maintain hydration with juices and water.

If the patient continues to lose weight in spite of nutritional support and counseling, tube feedings should be considered. As a temporary measure, tube feedings can provide the daily nutritional requirements for the patient and help the patient maintain body weight until the pharyngitis resolves. Percutaneous endoscopic gastrostomy (PEG), jejunostomy, or small caliber nasogastric tube are commonly used. A dietitian should be consulted for expert advice and planning to meet the patient's individual nutritional needs.

Psychosocial Issues Associated with Head and Neck Cancer

Although head and neck cancers comprise a small portion of all cancers, they create a significant psychological and social threat to quality of life and lifestyle. The head and neck region is highly significant to body image. It is a visible, prominent area that provides expression of intellect and emotion, representation of self, and serves as the primary way for communication with others. In addition, the emphasis on physical attractiveness within this society imposes additional social consequences upon the individual (Dropkin, 1989). Many changes occur as a result of the disease and treatment. Often patients are unable to return to work, and avoid routine activities such as eating in restaurants and attending social gatherings. Many seek seclusion as a result of their changed appearance and regress to old habits of alcohol and tobacco consumption (Mathog, 1991; Mood et al., 1991).

Rehabilitation for the patient with head and neck cancer begins when treatment decisions are being made since the specific treatment selected will dictate the functional impairment following treatment (Logemann, 1994). Patient education is extremely important in this process. A study evaluating the informational needs of 32 patients who had head and neck surgery revealed that most patients experienced fear, anxiety, and pain and reported not receiving information about the postoperative changes in breathing, swallowing, speaking, and appearance (Glavassevich et al., 1995).

Giving patients an opportunity to speak with other patients and to learn about the procedures for rehabilitation will help the patient in coping with the disease and treatment. Pretreatment counseling with speech pathologists, social workers, and other rehabilitation specialists is important. A pretreatment psychosocial assessment may help identify preexisting psychosocial problems. This counseling will help reduce the patient's and family's fears and assure them of rehabilitation possibilities following treatment to improve functional status.

Psychosocial recovery is dependent on the impact of facial disfigurement and dysfunction, and the patient's ability to cope with these changes. The patient needs to learn self-care and begin the process of resocialization within the family and community. The patient's family also needs to be included in addressing psychosocial and rehabilitation issues because they share concerns about cancer and its meaning, disrupted social relations, and the experience with hospitalization, treatment, and future plans (Mah & Johnston, 1993).

Social support is key to successful rehabilitation. In a study by Baker (1992) of 51 head and neck cancer survivors, perceived social support and degree of dysfunction, rather than facial disfigurement or mode of treatment, was significantly correlated with rehabilitation. Likewise, Hanucharurnkul (1989) found that socioeco-

nomic status and social support were significant predictors of self-care during radiation therapy for head and neck cancer.

Head and neck cancer can be devastating to sexual functioning because of the high visibility of the disfigurement (Metcalfe & Fischman, 1985). Since head and neck cancer patients are usually between the ages of 45 and 65 years old, they are experiencing the physiological and emotional sexual changes associated with aging. In addition, if the patient has chronically abused alcohol, the patient has already begun experiencing the negative effects of alcohol on sexual functioning. Facial changes as a result of surgery can cause the patient to fear social rejection or abandonment, and decrease the time interacting with others. Nasogastric tubes, a laryngectomy, or other extensive surgery may prevent verbal communication.

Tools have been developed to measure quality of life in patients with head and neck cancer. The Head and Neck Radiotherapy Questionnaire is a valid measure of acute morbidity due to radiation therapy to the head and neck region (Browman et al., 1993a). This tool may be useful as an outcome measure for clinical trials of radiation treatment strategies. It is an interviewer-administered 22 question tool that covers symptoms related to the oral cavity, throat, skin, digestive function, energy, and psychosocial issues.

A pilot study was conducted by Rathmell and associates (1991) to determine which measures of quality of life would be of most use in following patients participating in clinical trials for head and neck cancer. Questions related to quality of speech, ability to eat, levels of energy and activity, and aspects of psychological well-being detected the largest effects on quality of life. This study found that quality of life impairment was consistently greater in those patients treated by surgery plus radiotherapy as compared to those treated by radiotherapy alone.

The relation of addressing psychosocial issues and compliance with therapy is significant. It is noted that there is a 30 to 50 percent noncompletion rate for national clinical trials for head and neck cancer (Mood et al., 1991). Noncompliance significantly hinders the success of treatment. The course of radiation therapy can be discouraging because it is long with multiple side effects. Patients and families must be adequately prepared to understand the intent of treatment in order to endure the long course of treatment (Strohl, 1989). Careful pretreatment and posttreatment assessment and intervention is crucial for successful rehabilitation.

Conclusion

The care of persons with head and neck cancer receiving radiation therapy is a challenge. The many physiological and psychosocial needs require creativity to successfully manage patient care. The nurse caring for these patients can meet these challenges during radiation therapy by skillful assessments and timely interventions.

References

Aisner J, Hiponia D, Conley B, Jacobs M, Gray W, & Belani CP (1995). Combined modalities in the treatment of head and neck cancers. *Seminars in Oncology, 22,* 28–34.

al-Sarraf M (1994). Cisplatin combinations in the treatment of head and neck cancer. *Seminars in Oncology, 21,* 28–34.

Awan AM, Vokes EE, & Weichselbaum RR (1991). Recent advances in radiation therapy for head and neck cancer. *Hematology/Oncology Clinics of North America, 5,* 635–655.

Baker CA (1992). Factors associated with rehabilitation in head and neck cancer. *Cancer Nursing, 15,* 395–400.

Beck S (1979). Impact of a systematic oral care protocol on stomatitis after chemotherapy. *Cancer Nursing, 2,* 185–199.

Bedwinek JM, Shukovsky LJ, Fletcher GH, & Daly TE (1976). Osteoradionecrosis in patients treated with definitive radiotherapy for squamous cell carcinoma of the oral cavity and naso- and oropharynx. *Radiology, 119,* 665–667.

Beumer J, Curtis T, & Harrison RE (1979). Radiation therapy of the oral cavity. Sequelae and management. Pt I. *Head and Neck Surgery, 1,* 301–312.

Boyle P, Macfarlane GJ, Zheng T, Maisonneuve P, Evstifeeva T, & Scully C (1992). Recent advances in epidemiology of head and neck cancer. *Current Opinion in Oncology, 4,* 471–477.

Browman GP, Levine MN, Hodson DI, Sathya J, Russell R, Skingley P, Cripps C, Eapen L, & Girard A (1993a). The head and neck radiotherapy questionnaire: a morbidity/quality-of-life instrument for clinical trials of radiation therapy in locally advanced head and neck cancer. *Journal of Clinical Oncology, 11,* 863–872.

Chencharick JD & Mossman KL (1983). Nutritional consequences of the radiotherapy of head and neck cancer. *Cancer, 51,* 811–815.

Conger A (1973). Loss and recovery of taste acuity in patients irradiated to the oral cavity. *Radiation Research, 53,* 338–347.

Cooper GP (1968). Receptor origin of the olfactory bulb response to ionizing radiation. *American Journal of Physiology, 215,* 803–806.

Daeffler R (1980). Oral hygiene measures for patients with cancer. II. *Cancer Nursing, 3,* 427–432.

Davis JC (1981). Soft tissue radiation necrosis: The role of hyperbaric oxygen. *HBO Review, 2,* 153–167.

Dibble SL, Shiba G, MacPhail L, & Dodd MJ (1996). MacDibbs Mouth Assessment: A new tool to evaluate mucositis in the radiation therapy patient. *Cancer Practice, 4,* 135–140.

Dimery IW & Hong WK (1993). Overview of combined modality therapies for head and neck cancer. *Journal of the National Cancer Institute, 85,* 95–111.

Dische S (1994). Radiotherapy-new fractionation schemes. *Seminars in Oncology, 21,* 304–310.

Donaldson S (1977). Nutritional consequences of radiotherapy. *Cancer Research, 37,* 2407–2413.

Donaldson, SS (1984). Nutritional support as an adjunct to radiation therapy. *Journal of Parenteral and Enteral Nutrition, 8,* 302–310.

Dreizen S, Brown LR, & Handler S (1976). Radiation-induced xerostomia in cancer patients. *Cancer, 38,* 273–278.

Dropkin MJ (1989). Coping with disfigurement and dysfunction after head and neck cancer surgery: a conceptual framework. *Seminars in Oncology Nursing, 5,* 213–219.

Dwyer J (1979). Dietetic assessment of ambulatory cancer patients with special attention to problems of patients suffering from head and neck cancers undergoing radiation therapy. *Cancer, 43,* 2077–2086.

Eilers J, Berger AM, & Petersen MC (1988). Development, testing, and application of the oral assessment guide. *Oncology Nursing Forum, 15,* 325–330.

Eneroth CM, Henrikson, CO, & Jacobson PA (1972). Effects of fractionated radiotherapy on salivary gland function. *Cancer, 30,* 1147–1153.

Enig B, Winther E, & Hesson I (1985). Changes in food intake and nutritional status in patients treated with radiation therapy for cancer of the larynx and pharynx. *Nutrition and Cancer, 7,* 229–237.

Ferraro JM & Mattern JQA (1984). Sucralfate suspension for stomatitis. (Letter). *Drug Intelligence and Clinical Pharmacy, 18,* 153.

Forastiere AA (1992). Chemotherapy of head and neck cancer. *Annals of Oncology, 3,* 11–14.

Forastiere AA (1994). Paclitaxel (Taxol) for the treatment of head and neck cancer. *Seminars in Oncology, 21,* 49–52.

Gallucci BB & Iwamoto RR (1981). Taste alterations in patients with cancer. Nursing care of the cancer patient with nutritional problems. *Report of the Ross Oncology Nursing Roundtable,* 40–46.

Glavassevich M, McKibbon A, & Thomas S (1995). Information needs of patients who undergo surgery for head and neck cancer. *Canadian Oncology Nursing Journal, 5,* 9–11.

Goodwin WJ & Byers PM (1993). Nutritional management of the head and neck cancer patient. *Medical Clinics of North America, 77,* 597–610.

Grant MM (1986). Nutritional interventions: Increasing oral intake. *Seminars in Oncology Nursing, 2,* 36–43.

Grant M, Rhiner M, & Padilla GV (1989). Nutritional management in the head and neck cancer patient. *Seminars in Oncology Nursing, 5,* 195–204.

Greenspan D & Daniels TE (1987). Effectiveness of pilocarpine in post-irradiation xerostomia. *Cancer, 59,* 1123–1125.

Guyton AC (1971). The chemical senses: Taste and smell. In AC Guyton. *Textbook of Medical Physiology.* Philadelphia: WB Saunders.

Hamasaki VK & Vokes EE (1992). Chemotherapy in head and neck cancer. *Current Opinion in Oncology, 4,* 504–511.

Hanucharurnkul S (1989). Predictors of self-care in cancer patients receiving radiotherapy. *Cancer Nursing, 12,* 21–27.

Hart GB & Mainous EG (1976). The treatment of radiation necrosis with hyperbaric oxygen. *Cancer, 37,* 2580–2585.

Hearne B, Dunaj J, Daly J, Strong E, Vikram B, LePorte BJ, & DeLosse JJ (1985). Enteral nutritional support in head and neck cancer: Tube versus oral feeding during radiation therapy. *Journal of the American Dietetic Association, 85,* 669–677.

Hilderley LJ (1986). Relieving radiation esophagitis. *Oncology Nursing Forum, 13,* 71.

Hussain M, Kish JA, Crane L, Uwayda A, Cummings G, Ensley JF, Tapazoglou E, & al-Saffaf M (1991). The role of infection in the morbidity and mortality of patients with head and neck cancer undergoing multimodality therapy. *Cancer, 67*, 716–721.

Johnson CA, Keane TJ, & Prudo SM (1982). Weight loss in patients receiving radical radiation therapy for head and neck cancer: A prospective study. *Journal of Parenteral and Enteral Nutrition, 6*, 399–402.

Johnson JT, Ferretti GA, Nethery WJ, Valdez IH, Fox PC, Ng D, Muscoplat CC, & Gallagher SC (1993). Oral pilocarpine for post-irradiation xerostomia in patients with head and neck cancer. *New England Journal of Medicine, 329*, 390–395.

Jones D & Hafermann MD (1986). A radiolucent bite-block apparatus. *International Journal of Radiation Oncology, Biology, Physics, 13*, 129.

Jones MT, Aldred M, & Walter DM (1980). Prevalence and intraoral distribution of *Candida albicans* in Sjögren's syndrome. *Journal of Clinical Pathology, 33*, 282–287.

Kashima HK, Kirkham WR, & Andrews RJ (1965). Post-irradiation sialadenitis. *American Journal of Roentgenology Radium Therapy and Nuclear Medicine, 94*, 271–291.

Larpenteur M (1984). Cutting the sweetness of supplements. *Oncology Nursing Forum, 11*, 69.

Larson DL, Lindberg RD, Lane E, & Goepfert H (1983). Major complications of radiotherapy in cancer of the oral cavity and oropharynx: A ten-year retrospective study. *American Journal of Surgery, 146*, 531–536.

Laskiewicz BM (1982). The management of patients undergoing synchronous combined chemotherapy and radiotherapy. *Journal of Laryngology and Otology, 96*, 265–275.

LeVeque FG, Montgomery M, Potter D, Zimmer MB, Rieke J W, Steiger BW, Gallagher SC, & Muscoplat CC (1993). A multicenter, randomized, double-blind, placebo-controlled, dose titration study of oral pilocarpine for treatment of radiation-induced xerostomia in head and neck cancer patients. *Journal of Clinical Oncology, 11*, 1124–1131.

Lindsey AM (1986). Cancer cachexia: Effects of the disease and its treatment. *Seminars in Oncology Nursing, 2*, 19–29.

Lockhart PB & Clark J (1994). Pretherapy dental status of patients with malignant conditions of the head and neck. *Oral Surgery, Oral Medicine, Oral Pathology, 77*, 236–241.

Logemann JA (1994). Rehabilitation of the head and neck cancer patient. *Seminars in Oncology, 21*, 359–365.

MacCarthy-Leventhal EM (1959). Post-radiation mouth blindness. *Lancet, 2*, 1138–1139.

Madeya ML (1996). Oral complications from cancer therapy: part 2-nursing implications for assessment and treatment. *Oncology Nursing Forum, 23*, 808–819.

Mah MA & Johnston C (1993). Concerns of families in which one member has head and neck cancer. *Cancer Nursing, 16*, 382–387.

Makkonen TA, Bostrom P, Vilja P, & Joensuu H (1994). Sucralfate mouth washing in the prevention of radiation-induced mucositis: a placebo-controlled double-blind randomized study. *International Journal of Radiation Oncology, Biology, Physics, 30*, 177–182.

Mansfield MJ, Sanders DW, Heimbach RD, & Marx RE (1981). Hyperbaric oxygen as an adjunct in the treatment of osteoradionecrosis of the mandible. *Journal of Oral Surgery, 39*, 585–589.

Mathog RH (1991). Rehabilitation of head and neck cancer patients: consensus of recommendations from the International Conference on Rehabilitation of the Head and Neck Cancer Patient. *Head and Neck, 13*, 1–2.

McCaffrey TV (1992). Head and neck cancer surgery. *Current Opinion in Oncology, 4*, 499–503.

Mendenhall WM, Parsons JT, Mendenhall NP, & Million RR (1991). Brachytherapy in head and neck cancer: selection criteria and results at the University of Florida. Part 1. *Oncology, 5*, 87–93.

Metcalfe MC & Fischman SH (1985). Factors affecting the sexuality of patients with head and neck cancer. *Oncology Nursing Forum, 12*, 21–25.

Mood DW, Parzuchowski J, Grant MM, & Ensley J (1991). Psychosocial care needs of patients with head and neck cancers. *Head and Neck, 13*, 3–4.

Moore GK, Getchell T, Mistretta C, Mozell M, & Kern R (1991). Taste/smell. *Head and Neck, 13*, 7–8.

Morrish RB, Chan E, Silverman S, Meyer J, Fu K & Greenspan D (1981). Osteoradionecrosis in patients irradiated for head and neck carcinoma. *Cancer, 47*, 1980–1983.

Mosco MF (1986). Oral irrigation tip. *Oncology Nursing Forum, 13*, 88.

Mossman KL & Henkin RT (1978). Radiation-induced changes in taste acuity in cancer patients. *International Journal of Radiation Oncology, Biology, Physics, 4*, 663–670.

Mossman K, Shatzman A, & Chencharick J (1982). Long term effects of radiotherapy on taste and salivary function in man. *International Journal of Radiation Oncology, Biology, Physics, 8*, 991–997.

National Institutes of Health (1989). Oral complications of cancer therapies: diagnosis, prevention, and treatment. Consensus Development Conference Statement, 7, 1–11.

Navazesh M & Ship II (1983). Xerostomia: Diagnosis and treatment. *American Journal of Otolaryngology, 4*, 283–292.

Olsen KD & Creagan ET (1991). Pain management in advanced carcinoma of the head and neck. *American Journal of Otolaryngology, 12*, 154–160.

Parker SL, Tong T, Bolden S, & Wingo PA (1996). Cancer statistics, 1996. *Ca:A Cancer Journal for Clinicians, 46*, 5–27.

Parsons JT (1984). The effect of radiation on normal tissue of the head and neck. In R Million & N Cassis (Eds.). *Management of Head and Neck Cancer: A Multidisciplinary Approach*. Philadelphia: JB Lippincott.

Pehanrich M (1983). A tip for the taste buds. *Oncology Nursing Forum, 10*, 60.

Peterson DE & D'Ambrosio JA (1994). Nonsurgical management of head and neck cancer patients. *Dental Clinics of North America, 38*, 425–445.

Pezner R & Archambeau JO (1985). Critical evaluation of the role of nutritional support for radiation therapy patients. *Cancer, 55*, 263–267.

Rathmell AJ, Ash DV, Howes M, & Nicholls J (1991). Assessing quality of life in patients treated for advanced head and neck cancer. *Clinical Oncology, 3*, 10–16.

Ries LAG, Miller BA, Hankey BF, Kosary CL, Harras A, & Edwards BK (1994). SEER Cancer Statistics Review, 1973–1991. National Institutes of Health, National Cancer Institute. NIH Publ., 94–2789.

Ritchie JR, Brown JR, Guerra LR, & Mason G (1985). Dental care for the irradiated cancer patient. *Quintessence International, 16*, 837–842.

Schleper JR (1989). Prevention, detection, and diagnosis of head and neck cancers. *Seminars in Oncology Nursing, 5*, 139–149.

Shah JP & Lydiatt W (1995). Treatment of cancer of the head and neck. *Ca:A Cancer Journal for Clinicians, 45*, 352–368. .

Sloan D & Goepfert H (1991). Conventional therapy of head and neck cancer. *Hematology-Oncology Clinics of North America, 5*, 601–625.

Sonis S & Clark J (1991). Prevention and management of oral mucositis induced by antineoplastic therapy. *Oncology, 5,* 11–18.

Spitz MR (1994). Epidemiology and risk factors for head and neck cancer. *Seminars in Oncology, 21,* 281–288.

Strohl R (1983). Taste sensations after radiation therapy. *Oncology Nursing Forum, 10,* 80.

Strohl R (1984). Understanding taste changes. *Oncology Nursing Forum, 11,* 81–84.

Strohl RA (1989). Radiation therapy for head and neck cancers. *Seminars in Oncology Nursing, 5,* 166–173.

Sullivan MD & Fleming TJ (1986). Oral care for the radiotherapy-treated head and neck cancer patient. *Dental Hygiene, 60,* 112–114.

Sweeney PJ, Haraf DJ, Vokes EE, Dougherty M, & Weichselbaum RR (1994). Radiation therapy in head and neck cancer: indications and limitations. *Seminars in Oncology, 21,* 296–303.

Tobias JS (1992). Current role of chemotherapy in head and neck cancer. *Drugs, 43,* 333–345.

Trizna Z & Schantz SP (1992). Hereditary and environmental factors associated with risk and progression of head and neck cancer. *Otolaryngologic Clinics of North America, 25,* 1089–1103.

Van Drimmelen J & Rollins HF (1969). Evaluation of a commonly used oral hygiene agent. *Nursing Research, 18,* 327–332.

Vokes EE, Awan AM, & Weichselbaum RR (1991). Radiotherapy with concomitant chemotherapy for head and neck cancer. *Hematology/Oncology Clinics of North America, 5,* 753–767.

Wiley SB (1969). Why glycerol and lemon juice? *American Journal of Nursing, 69,* 342–344.

Wilkes GM (1986). Sucralfate suspension for mucositis. *Oncology Nursing Forum, 13,* 71–72.

Williams LR & Cohen MH (1978). Altered taste thresholds in lung cancer. *American Journal of Clinical Nutrition, 31,* 122–125.

Wilson PR, Herman J, & Chubon SJ (1991). Eating strategies used by persons with head and neck cancer during and after radiotherapy. *Cancer Nursing, 14,* 98–104.

Zemel M, Maves M, Mickelson S, & Kaplan J (1991). Nutrition in head and neck cancer. *Head and Neck, 13,* 10–12.

Hodgkin's Disease and Non-Hodgkin's Lymphoma

ELLEN SITTON

Lymphomas are cancers arising from cellular components of the lymphoreticular system and are divided into two distinct clinical entities, Hodgkin's disease (HD) and non-Hodgkin's lymphoma (NHL). Hodgkin's disease rarely starts in areas other than the lymph nodes and generally spreads in an axial manner. Non-Hodgkin's lymphoma is a complex group of diseases that may present in the lymph nodes or in extranodal tissue and spreads in a variety of patterns. HD and NHL are among the most radiosensitive malignancies and radiation therapy plays a major role in treatment. The incidence of lymphomas in the United States is increasing attributed in part to the increased incidence of NHL, and to a lesser degree, HD, in patients with acquired immunodeficiency syndrome (AIDS). The increase incidence of NHL is most marked in the elderly.

This chapter focuses on the diagnosis and radiation-related treatment of HD and NHL. Epidemiology, presentation of disease, staging, and treatment of both HD and NHL are presented. Because both diseases may be treated in almost any location within the body, detailed radiation-related nursing care may be found in other chapters discussing site-specific management of radiation side effects.

Lymph Nodes and Lymphatic Vessels

The lymphocyte is the principal component of lymphoma. Lymphomas may arise in any lymphoid tissue. Hodgkin's disease almost always arises in the lymph nodes. About 20 to 40 percent of circulating white blood cells are lymphocytes.

Lymphocytes develop and mature in the primary lymphoid organs, which include the bone marrow and the thymus. Lymphocytes are stored and activated in the secondary lymphoid organs including the lymph nodes, lymph vessels, spleen, tonsils, adenoids, appendix, and unencapsulated lymphoid tissue lining the respiratory, alimentary, and genitourinary tracts.

Lymph nodes are structures ranging from 1 to 30 mm in size that are found throughout the body in a network that drains and filters tissue fluid. Most lymph nodes are located near the axis, or center, of the body. The spleen filters antigens in the blood, and the unencapsulated lymph tissue underlining mucous membranes interacts with antigens and prevents their entry into the systemic circulation. Most areas of the body, except for a few organs such as the central nervous system and bones, contain lymph vessels. These vessels transport immune cells (e.g., T and B lymphocytes) and foreign antigens to the circulatory system via the thoracic duct, which empties into the left subclavian vein. Lymphocytes recirculate throughout the body by exiting the blood vessels or lymphatic tissue and infiltrating tissues. They may then reenter the circulation via lymphatic vessels and reside in lymphatic tissue.

Lymphocytes recognize antigens and induce adaptive (specific) immune responses. Subpopulations of lymphocytes are currently identified by immunohistochemistry staining of cell surface molecules with highly specific monoclonal antibodies. The surface markers are known as cluster of differentiation (CD) antigens or CD markers. The monoclonal antibodies and the markers have been assigned CD numbers. The T and B lymphocytes are two major subpopulations of lymphocytes and are responsible for specific immune responses. CD5 is a marker for both T and B cell populations while CD1, CD3, and CD7 are markers only for T cells and CD21, CD22, CD37, and CD40 are markers only for B cells (Gallucci & McCarthy, 1995).

Afferent lymphatics drain into the lymph node where lymph travels through the lymph node and empties through the efferent lymphatic at the hilar area (see Figure 15–1). Blood vessels enter and exit through the hilar region. Lymphocytes from the blood may enter through venules in the paracortex.

Lymph nodes have an external capsule surrounding an interconnecting system of spaces called sinuses that facilitate maturation and differentiation of lymphocytes. Subcapsular sinuses are immediately below the capsule, and medullary sinuses are deeper within the node. Lymphoid tissue is made up of the cortex, paracortex, and medullary cords. Immediately inside the capsule is the cortex, which consists of primary follicles.

B lymphocytes, which proliferate upon antigen stimulation, are concentrated in the follicles. Some T lymphocytes are also found in the follicles. The germinal center of the follicles is surrounded by a tightly bound layer of lymphocytes known as the mantle, which also contains B lymphocytes. The paracortex is a dense cellular mass around the mantle. No sharp delineation exists between cortex and paracortex or between paracortex and medullary cords. Immunohistochemistry techniques demonstrate that T lymphocytes are the primary cells in the paracortex. The medulla with its medullary cords extending into the area of the paracortex is the area near the efferent lymphatic vessel of the lymph node. The medullary cords are composed of mature B lymphocytes (i.e., plasma cells) and some small lymphocytes. Histiocytes are found in the subcapsular and medullary sinuses of the lymph nodes. Phagocytosis occurs in the medullary sinus, the cortex, and paracortex.

Radiosensitivity of the lymph nodes is largely related to B and T lymphocytes, with B cells gen-

Figure 15-1 • Structure of a normal lymph node. From Fajardo LF (1994). Lymph nodes and cancer. *Frontiers of Radiation Therapy and Onocology, 28,* p. 2.

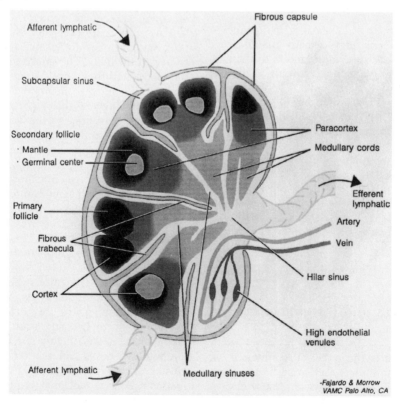

erally more radiosensitive than T cells (Fajardo, 1994a). Lymphocytes are relatively radiosensitive and radiation-induced lymphocyte death occurs in interphase rather than during mitosis, which is the phase instrumental in the death of most types of cells. Radiation change in the lymph node may be structural or functional and is dose-dependent. Alterations of immune function occur after total lymphatic irradiation. Effects of total lymphoid irradiation include rapid reduction of blood lymphocytes as well as reduction of cells in the spleen, lymph nodes, and thymus (Fajardo, 1994a). Blood counts show that B cells begin to reappear at the second week while T cells begin to reappear at the second month. Approximately 2 years are required for near normal values to return. Immune response in HD may be depressed for years and approximately 30 percent of patients are permanently anergic.

Hodgkin's Disease

Epidemiology

Cancer statistics from the American Cancer Society estimate 7500 new cases of Hodgkin's disease (HD) and 1480 deaths in 1997 (American Cancer Society, 1997). Incidence in males compared to females is approximately 1.4 to 1.0 HD is more common in developed countries than in underdeveloped countries. Incidence in developed countries has a bimodal peak at age 20 to 24 and again at age 75 to 80. HD is rare in children under 10. Histology and sites of involvement vary with age. There is an increase risk of HD in siblings.

The etiology of HD is unknown. No definitive evidence of infectious etiology has been found in spite of clinical signs and symptoms including fever, chills, and leukocytosis. Epstein-Barr virus (EBV) has been implicated in the etiology of HD with the EBV genome detected in 20 to 80 percent of tumor specimens (Mueller et al., 1989; Pallesen et al., 1991; Pallesen et al., 1993). HD may be a result of genetic factors and response to diverse pathologic processes including viral infections, occupational exposures (e.g., woodworking), and other environmental stimuli (DeVita et al., 1993; Urba & Longo, 1992).

A large study of 6700 homosexual men with HIV demonstrated that acquired immune deficiency disease (AIDS) appears to increase the risk of HD somewhat and increase the risk of NHL to a much greater extent (Hessol et al., 1992; Priest et al., 1993). HD in the HIV patient is likely to present with extranodal advanced disease that is very aggressive and associated with short survival (Kaufman & Longo, 1995). Two-thirds present with extranodal disease and bone marrow is involved in 50 percent.

In the last 30 years, survival of patients with HD has improved considerably with better imaging, improved radiation therapy techniques, more effective combination chemotherapy, and prospective clinical studies.

Presentation

Initial presentation of 90 percent of HD is superficial lymphadenopathy, which is usually painless. Involvement of axial lymph nodes with positive cervical (>80 percent), mediastinal (>50 percent) or paraaortic nodes is most common and spread of disease is almost always along contiguous lymph nodes. Contiguity of spread is a very important concept upon which treatment is based. The treatment of uninvolved lymph node areas rests on the assumption of predictable patterns of spread. Enlarged nodes may have a history of waxing and waning prior to diagnosis. The most frequent presenting site is cervical adenopathy. Asymptomatic mediastinal adenopathy found on routine chest x ray is not an uncommon presentation. A third of patients present with systemic, or B, symptoms: fever (≥38°C), drenching night sweats, or weight loss of greater than 10 percent of body weight. The presence of B symptoms has an adverse effect on prognosis. Some patients experience pruritus and pain in enlarged lymph nodes following ingestion of alcohol. Other symptoms are related to location and extent of disease.

Enlarged nodes may cause pressure symptoms. In the mediastinum, enlarged nodes may cause cough, dyspnea, dysphagia, pleural effusions, and on occasion, superior vena cava syndrome. Left upper quadrant pain may result from an enlarged spleen. The extent of disease in the spleen is correlated with the presence of disseminated disease. However, the mechanism of spread to the spleen is not clear. HD, unlike NHL, rarely involves gastrointestinal-associated lymphoid tissues such as Waldeyer's tonsillar ring (nasopharyngeal, palatine, and lingual tonsils) and Peyer's patches. Hepatic extension or bile duct obstruction may cause jaundice. Adenopathy in the retroperitoneal area may cause gastrointestinal and genitourinary dysfunction, abdominal pain, and ascites. Extension of lymph node regions into the viscera may involve other sites, such as pulmonary parenchyma from mediastinal or bronchopulmonary nodes, or a vertebral body from retroperitoneal or paravertebral nodes. Disease may progress to the bone marrow or bone but rarely to the central nervous system other than spinal cord compression from paravertebral lymph nodes. Patients with HD often have a functional deficit in T cell-mediated immunity at the time of diagnosis and before therapy that persists in patients who are cured (DeVita et al., 1993). This deficit is increased by treatment, especially radiation therapy with some recovery after completion of treatment.

Histopathology

Diagnosis of HD requires the presence of Reed-Sternberg cells in the microscopic examination of tissue. These large, often multinucleated cells constitute a small fraction of the cells present in malignant tissues examined. Reed-Sternberg cells may also be found in other malignant and benign conditions such as mononucleosis, Dilantin-induced lymphadenopathy, non-Hodgkin's lymphoma, lymphoid hyperplasia, and nonlymphoid malignancies including melanoma and carcinomas (Kaufman & Longo, 1995). Immunohistochemical and genetic marker techniques have been inconclusive in the search for the origin of the neoplastic cells of HD even though HD clearly arises in the lymphoreticular system (Kaufman & Longo, 1995; Urba & Longo, 1992; Variakojis & Anastasi, 1993).

The Rye classification system established in 1966 categorizes four histologic subtypes of HD based solely on the characteristics of the nonmalignant background of the malignant lymph node rather than on the malignant cells themselves (Lukes, Butler & Hicks, 1966) (see Table 15-1). With the success of current treatment on the prognosis of HD, the histologic subtype has minor impact on therapy.

Nodular Sclerosing HD

NSHD is the most common subtype in the United States and occurs in adolescents and young adults and is not common after 50 years of age (DeVita et al., 1993). Females have a somewhat higher incidence than males and the natural history of NSHD is less favorable than that of lymphocyte predominant HD (LPHD). Approximately one-third of patients experience B symptoms. The mediastinal and supraclavicular nodes are frequently involved.

Lymphocyte Predominant HD

LPHD frequently presents in early stage (I or II) and is often diagnosed in the fourth or fifth decade of life. Fewer than 10 percent have systemic symptoms. Two types have been described, diffuse and nodular, but there is little clinical or biologic justification for separating these (Kaufman & Longo, 1995). Prognosis is usually favorable.

Mixed Cellularity HD

Numerous Reed-Sternberg cells are present in MCHD. This subtype accounts for 15 to 30 percent of HD and is the most common subtype in HIV-infected individuals. Peak incidence is at ages 30 to 45 years and 40 to 55 years. Male to female incidence is 1.5 to 1.0. MCHD is more likely to involve retroperitoneal nodes and less likely to be localized compared to NSHD. More than 50 percent of patients have stage III or IV disease and most have B symptoms. Extranodal abdominal extension is common.

Lymphocyte Depleted HD

LDHD is the least common subtype in the United States and accounts for less than 5 percent of ini-

Table 15-1 • Rye Classification of HD

Histologic Subtype	Incidence (%)	Characteristics
Nodular sclerosing (NSHD)	40–60	Most common type HD. Most often seen in late adolescence or early adulthood. One-third present with B symptoms. Frequently involves mediastinum and supraclavicular nodes.
Lymphocyte predominant (LPHD)	10–15	Patient generally presents in stage I or II. Often in 4th or 5th decade. <10% have B symptoms. Most favorable prognosis.
Mixed cellularity (MCHD)	15–30	Many Reed-Sternberg cells. Most common type in HIV-related HD. Males > females. Generally occurs in middle-age adult. >50% present with stage III or IV disease. Most have B symptoms.
Lymphocyte depleted (LDHD)	<5	Often in elderly men. Present in advanced stage. 20% of HIV-related HD. Seen in relapse in heavily treated patients. Most unfavorable prognosis.

tial diagnosis of HD. Patients are most often elderly men, present with advanced-stage disease and B symptoms. This subtype has a tendency to involve retroperitoneal nodes and extralymphatic sites. Twenty percent of HIV-infected patients with HD present with this histologic type. LDHD may be seen as an evolution from MCHD or LPHD in relapsed heavily pretreated patients (Kaufman & Longo, 1995).

Histology varies with age. Nodular sclerosing HD is more common in young adults with mixed cellularity, more common in the middle-aged adult, and lymphocyte depleted is more common in elderly adults. Up to 50 percent of older patients with HD present with mixed cellularity and lymphocyte depleted histologies. They present at a later stage, making age an independent prognostic factor.

Prognosis

Prognosis is related to patient factors such as gender, age, and intercurrent disease, and HD factors such as stage, histology, volume of disease, systemic symptoms (B symptoms), number and location of sites, serum markers, and splenic involvement. Women have a slightly better prognosis than men (Hoppe et al., 1992). Effects on the reproductive system may have some influence on treatment decisions. Pelvic irradiation is a major factor in decision-making for women since oophoropexy does not completely protect the ovaries. Menopausal symptoms may occur following pelvic irradiation in women over 30 years. Fertility in men is greatly affected by alkylating agents, which result in sterility in most men receiving high doses of these chemotherapy agents. Children have a better prognosis than adults. However, factors such as growth impairment and secondary malignancies related to radiation therapy present special issues in the management of HD. Intercurrent disease with increasing age may affect the aggressiveness of staging and treatment. Pregnancy has no known effect on the natural history of the disease; however, pregnancy profoundly influences treatment. The most important prognostic factor influencing treatment recommendations and outcome is clinical and pathologic staging. Unfavorable prognostic factors include: mediastinal disease greater than one-third the diameter of the chest; B symptoms, especially when more than one symptom is experienced; extranodal disease; multiple involved sites; and mixed cellularity histology (Urba & Longo, 1992).

Staging and Treatment

Some controversy continues between medical oncologists and radiation oncologists concerning optimal treatment of HD. This is in part due to the over 20 percent failure rate of treatment and the considerable late effects of both radiation therapy and chemotherapy. Patients who relapse after radiation therapy alone for early-stage disease can often be successfully treated with chemotherapy.

Staging

After pathologic diagnosis of HD is established with biopsy, the extent of the disease must be determined through staging. Careful staging is required for optimal treatment choices and to allow comparison of treatment protocols. Staging classification for HD is based on a number of assumptions: (1) HD spreads in contiguous lymphatics; (2) extended field (nodal treatment beyond the involved field) radiation therapy is the treatment of choice in early disease; and (3) combination chemotherapy should be reserved for patients with advanced disease (Lister et al., 1989).

Staging includes: (1) clinical staging (CS), based on initial biopsy and clinical staging studies determined without staging laparotomy and (2) pathological staging (PS), based on subsequent biopsies including those performed during staging laparotomy.

The Ann Arbor-Cotswolds modification staging system is applied to both HD and NHL (see Table 15–2) (Lister et al., 1989). Stage I and II disease are confined to one side of the diaphragm. Stage I is defined as involvement of a single lymph node region (e.g., cervical, axillary, inguinal, mediastinal) (I) or localized extranodal (E) lymphoid site such as spleen, thymus, Waldeyer's ring (I_E). Stage II disease involves two or more lymph node regions (II) and may include localized extralymphatic involvement on the same side of the diaphragm (II_E). Stage III disease involves lymph node regions or lymphoid structures on both sides of the diaphragm. Stage III_1 indicates disease limited to the upper abdomen (spleen, splenic hilar, celiac, or portal nodes) and stage III_2 is disease limited to the lower abdomen (paraaortic, pelvic, or inguinal nodes). Splenic involvement (III_S) may precede widespread hematogenous dissemination. Stage III localized extranodal disease may be indicated by III_E. Stage IV includes diffuse or disseminated disease of one or more extralymphatic organs or tissues with or without associated lymph node involvement. Patients with liver and bone marrow involvement are classified as stage IV.

Table 15-2 • Cotswolds Modification of the Ann Arbor Staging Classification

Stage	Relation to Diaphragm	Characteristics
Stage I	One side of diaphragm	I: One lymph node region
		I_E: One localized extranodal lymphoid site
Stage II	One side of diaphragm	II: ≥2 lymph node regions
		II_E: Localized extranodal involvement
Stage III	Both sides of diaphragm	III: Lymph node regions or lymphoid structures
		III_1: Disease limited to upper abdomen
		III_2: Disease limited to lower abdomen
		III_S: Splenic involvement
		III_E: Localized extranodal involvement
Stage IV	Disseminated	IV: Diffuse or disseminated disease of one or more extranodal sites with or without associated lymph node involvement
Systemic symptoms		A: No systemic symptoms
		B: Systemic symptoms (fever, night sweats, weight loss)
Bulky disease		X: Bulky disease

Patient Evaluation

The pathologically proven extranodal site of HD may be identified by H (hepatic), L (lung), M (bone marrow), O (osseous), P (pleura), and D (dermal). Stages I, II, III, and IV can be classified into A and B categories. If no systemic symptoms are present, the letter A is used. The letter B indicates the presence of systemic symptoms of fever (≥38°C), drenching night sweats, or unexplained weight loss of greater than 10 percent of body weight. Bulky disease is designated as X and is described as widening of the mediastinum by more than one-third or the presence of a tumor mass with a maximum dimension greater than 10 cm.

Patient Evaluation

Because the extent of the disease influences treatment decisions, a careful assessment of the patient is essential. Table 15–3 summarizes the evaluation of patients diagnosed with HD and NHL. The pathologic diagnosis of HD is most often made after surgical excision of an easily accessible enlarged peripheral lymph node. Determination of staging studies is, in part, based on factors such as patient age and intercurrent disease. Specific patient symptoms may influence selection of imaging techniques. A complete history and physical examination are done. The patient is assessed for the presence of B symptoms and for palpable disease. Laboratory tests, radiographic evaluations, and bone marrow biopsies are completed as part of the staging work-up.

With the discovery and use of newer imaging techniques, lymphangiography is used less frequently than before. The use of the bipedal lymphangiogram (LAG) in staging is controversial and in some practices has largely been replaced with CT or MRI. Some clinicians believe that LAG and abdominal CT are complementary and that lymphangiography is the superior method of detecting retroperitoneal involvement and involved node-filling defects (Glatstein, 1993; Kaufman & Longo, 1995; Urba & Longo, 1992). The LAG is insensitive in detecting paraaortic involvement above the renal veins and in detecting splenic or mesenteric disease. In nodes that fill in the LAG, the dye is retained in those nodes for many months allowing ongoing assessment of node size and architecture with a simple flat plate x ray of the abdomen. The LAG defines nodal distribution, which may be valuable in planning abdominal or pelvic radiation therapy fields. However, this procedure is difficult for the physician to perform and to interpret.

A bone marrow biopsy is performed on every patient. Originally used to detect evidence of infiltration, a bone marrow biopsy can now detect involvement immunologically at the level of 1 cell in 100 or 1000, or molecularly at the level of 1 cell in 100,000 (Lister & Armitage, 1995). Additional biopsies of suspicious areas are also done to determine the stage of disease and treatment.

Laparotomy is another area of controversy in the staging of HD. In recent years the CT and MRI have been used extensively. The staging laparotomy includes splenectomy, liver biopsy, selected node biopsies, and open bone marrow biopsy. The spleen is the most common site of occult abdominal disease. Laparotomy is generally performed on patients with stage I or II disease above the diaphragm only if radiation therapy is the desired treatment and the pathological detection of intraabdominal disease would change the choice of

Table 15-3 • Evaluation of Patient with Hodgkin's Disease and Non-Hodgkin's Lymphoma

Evaluation	Rationale
Biopsy	Necessary for diagnosis of HD and NHL.
History and physical examination	Determine systemic (B) symptoms, palpable disease, and bone tenderness. Assess for alcohol intolerance, pruritus (especially HD), fatigue. Careful evaluation of Waldeyer's ring in NHL.
Erythrocyte sedimentation rate (ESR)	Important prognostically in HD. More often elevated in advanced stage disease. Can be used as a marker for recurrence in previously treated patients.
Serum copper	Nonspecific marker of disease activity. Elevated in HD and NHL. May be useful in monitoring response to therapy and early recurrence in HD and NHL.
Blood tests (CBC and differential, platelets, liver and kidney function tests, serum albumin, lactic dehydrogenase (LDH), calcium)	Abnormal CBC and platelets may indicate bone marrow involvement. Absolute lymphocytopenia may indicate more advanced HD. Elevated alkaline phosphatase may be secondary to hepatic parenchyma (rare if no B symptoms), bone marrow, or bone involvement. Elevated LDH correlates with poorer prognosis.
X rays	Chest x ray (CXR) positive for mediastinal, paratracheal, or hilar nodes in ⅔ of patients with HD.
CT of chest	More sensitive than CXR. Evaluate mediastinal, pulmonary, parenchymal, and pericardial involvement. Intrathoracic disease present in 85% at diagnosis of HD (Liebenhaut, 1993) but in only 20% of NHL. Also used for treatment planning.
MRI of chest	May be more sensitive than CT in detection of chest wall involvement and distinguishing between posttreatment residual and tumor recurrence.
CT of abdomen and pelvis	Evaluate adenopathy. Abdominal CT may detect gross splenic, liver, celiac axis, splenic hilar, and porta hepatic lymph node involvement in nodes larger than 1 cm.
Bipedal lymphangiogram	Controversial as a routine procedure. Evaluates abnormal internal node architecture. Not usually used in NHL evaluation.
Gallium scan	Useful in gallium-avid disease. Often useful in detecting disease sites in original staging. High sensitivity in detecting residual disease after treatment, especially in the mediastinum.
Bone marrow biopsy	Routine staging procedure in almost all patients. Rarely positive in HD unless advanced disease. Positive in 50% of NHL.
Exploratory (staging) laparotomy	Controversial as a routine procedure. Should only be performed if the information will influence treatment. Generally not indicated for NHL.

treatment. When the treatment plan for any reason includes the use of full-dose chemotherapy as part or all of the initial treatment of early stage HD, regardless of the presence or absence of disease below the diaphragm, staging laparotomy is contraindicated (Kaufman & Longo, 1995). In addition to high expense, staging laparotomy can result in both acute and late complications. Although there is a less than 1 percent mortality rate of staging laparotomy, risks include wound infections, adhesions, small bowel obstruction, delayed therapy, increased incidence of infection after splenectomy, and a possible higher incidence of secondary leukemia (Leibenhaut, 1993; Stupp et al., 1994; Zinzani et al., 1994). Laparotomy delays initial therapy from 4 to 7 weeks and splenectomy results in lifelong increased risk of overwhelming sepsis, most often caused by encapsulated gram-positive bacteria (usually pneumococcus). Evidence exists that survival of patients treated with radiation therapy alone is no better in surgically staged patients than in clinically staged patients with careful follow-up (Kauf-

man & Longo, 1995; Leibenhaut, 1993). Laparotomy is being used selectively by some clinicians for patients with certain poor prognostic factors that predict the likelihood of occult disease in the abdomen (e.g., B symptoms, bulky mediastinal disease, equivocal findings on CT or lymphangiography) and in young women whose ovaries will be surgically relocated for protection during pelvic irradiation (Cox, 1994; Zinzani et al., 1994). However, the reduced use of pelvic irradiation has made oophoropexy unnecessary in most patients (DeVita et al., 1993). Other clinicians recommend laparotomy for all patients who are candidates for radiation therapy alone or radiation therapy and limited chemotherapy (Glatstein, 1993; Leibenhaut, 1993; Sombeck et al., 1992).

Treatment of Hodgkin's Disease

Treatment of HD has achieved an outstanding level of success in this disease that historically was fatal. The goal of treatment is the highest possible cure rates with minimal risk of significant treatment complications. HD is a complex disease and may present in many different ways. Many disease factors as well as patient factors must be considered in treatment decisions. Treatment is primarily based on staging (see Table 15–4). Radiation therapy has been the treatment of choice in stages I and II HD without massive mediastinal disease (i.e., mass larger than one-third of the thorax diameter). With a large mediastinal mass, both radiation therapy and chemotherapy are routinely used. Multiagent chemotherapy alone in other stage I and II HD may show equivalent outcomes, but results in systemic toxicity.

Advanced disease requires systemic therapy. Chemotherapy or combined radiation therapy and chemotherapy have generally being administered in advanced disease, stages III and IV. Factors to be considered in combined modality therapy include: selection of chemotherapy agents, sequence of therapy, radiation dose, volume of radiation portals, and overlapping toxicities. There is much controversy concerning treatment of complex, advanced disease. Most complications of treatment are found in patients treated with both radiation therapy and full-dose chemotherapy or extended chemotherapy for more than 6 months (DeVita & Hubbard, 1993). Complications can be minimized with careful selection of therapy.

Decisions to use chemotherapy are also based on other factors including concurrent disease such as HIV, age of patient, or altered immune status. The most common chemotherapy combinations in the treatment of HD are nitrogen mustard, vincristine, procarbazine, prednisone (MOPP) and doxorubicin, bleomycin, vinblastine, dacarbazine (ABVD). Some current protocols alternate MOPP and ABVD primarily to reduce the emergence of resistant clones and to reduce toxicities. Urba and Longo (1992) list unfavorable prognostic factors for advanced disease as B symptoms, age over 45 years, mediastinal width greater than 45 percent of chest diameter, involved bone mar-

row, liver, pleura, or multiple sites of disease, low hematocrit, high lactate dehydrogenase (LDH), and high ESR.

Radiation Therapy in the Treatment of Hodgkin's Disease

Radiation therapy is the most effective single modality for treatment of patients with HD. Patients who have recurrent disease after treatment with radiation therapy have a relatively high probability of successful salvage treatment with chemotherapy. Patients treated with the single modality of radiation therapy rather than combined therapy with chemotherapy have a lower risk of late morbidity than when both modalities are used in initial treatment. For example, the 7 to 10 percent risk of acute leukemia in patients with HD is almost entirely related to the use of chemotherapy (Cox, 1994).

Technical Considerations

The aim of treatment is to eradicate the disease with a minimum risk of late sequelae. Radiation therapy for HD is primarily administered with a 6 to 10 MV linear accelerator photon beam. Treatment is delivered to large opposing fields shaped specifically for each patient according to anatomy and distribution of disease. Cobalt-60 has been used and is approximately equivalent to a 4 MV linear accelerator photon beam. Because of the size of the cobalt source itself, field edges (penumbra) with Cobalt-60 are not as clearly defined as with the linear accelerator. Beam shaping to precisely fit the field shape is most often accomplished with the use of divergent Cerrobend blocks placed near the head of the machine. Newer machines with built-in multileaf collimators to shape fields are used in some institutions.

Fractionated radiation therapy is most often given at a daily dose of 1.8 Gy delivered 5 days per week to a tumoricidal dose of 35 to 44 Gy. When very large fields are treated, daily fractions may be reduced to 1.5 Gy if the patient cannot tolerate higher fractions. Dose to subclinical disease is generally 30 to 35 Gy.

Treatment planning is often very complex, in part due to the large fields (often with varying thicknesses within the same field) as well as complex calculations of dose distribution within the treatment volume. To encompass large fields, treatment must often be done at extended distances, which requires both supine and prone positioning of patients. Position changes require changes in arm position as well as movement of

Table 15-4 • Treatment of HD by Stage

Stage	Treatment
Stage I and II	Radiation therapy (extended field) or total nodal irradiation (infrequently)
Stage I and II with large mediastinal disease	Chemotherapy followed by radiation therapy
Stage III and IV	Chemotherapy alone or chemotherapy plus radiation therapy

tissues within the treatment volume. This is an especially important consideration when additional portals will be treated immediately adjacent to the initial ones. A field separation, or gap, is calculated to avoid overlapping of fields below the skin surface resulting in high doses in the overlapped region. This is especially important in critical tissues such as the spinal cord (see Figure 15-2).

Field margins in areas of known disease should be relatively generous, especially in the mediastinum to reduce failure of disease control in these sites (Cox, 1994). Treatment margins in clinically uninvolved sites do not need to be as generous.

Radiation Treatment Fields in HD

Three treatment volumes are generally considered in HD: the mantle, paraaortic region, and pelvis. Radiation treatment for HD is very complex, with radiation fields designed specifically for each patient depending upon both patient factors and tumor factors. Treatment with radiation therapy may include involved sites, extended fields (mantle plus paraaortic nodes), or total nodal irradiation (TNI) (extended field plus pelvic nodes). Many studies have demonstrated that extended field irradiation, which includes contiguous lymph node chains, has superior results compared to involved field irradiation in which only the known sites of disease are treated. Extended fields

are based on the principle of involved fields as well as prophylactic treatment to areas of expected subclinical disease (Cox, 1994; Hoppe et al., 1992; Kaufman & Longo, 1995). Doses to these sites may be lower with a minimum of 30 to 35 Gy. Cox (1994) cites studies suggesting that the treatment of most patients with supradiaphragmatic stages IA and IIA HD should minimally include bilateral cervical, axillary, mediastinal, and hilar lymph nodes above the diaphragm as well as the paraaortic lymph nodes to the bifurcation of the aorta. The spleen should also be included in the treatment field. However, if the patient's spleen was removed, the splenic pedicle nodes are also treated (see Figure 15–3).

In less favorable early stage HD, such as IB or IIB, or in stage IIIA, total nodal irradiation (TNI) may be recommended. In addition to the above nodes, TNI includes iliac and inguinal nodes. These areas may be encompassed in two large, irregularly shaped fields, the mantle and the subdiaphragmatic region, or the "inverted Y" field. For patients with IIIA HD without bulky disease, multiagent chemotherapy alone is the treatment of choice (DeVita et al., 1993). With bulky IIIA disease, combined modality radiation therapy and chemotherapy are superior to either modality alone.

Supradiaphragmatic Irradiation

Mantle, literally meaning cloak, is used to describe the field that encompasses the major lymph node regions (neck, axilla, and mediastinum) above the diaphragm. This field typically extends from the lower mandible to just above the level of the insertion of the diaphragm (see Figure 15–4). Total lung volume in the field must be carefully considered. When mediastinal disease is very large, an increased amount of lung is in the treatment fields. Preirradiation chemotherapy to reduce the size of tumor or shrinking field irradiation (i.e., reducing field size as tumor size decreases) may be used to reduce the amount of normal lung treated in the portals. The effects of lung irradiation must especially be considered in patients who will also receive the drug bleomycin, which is also toxic to the lung.

Blocking in the mantle fields generally includes lung blocks, posterior occipital and spinal cord blocks, anterior larynx block, and anterior and posterior humeral head blocks. Cord dose is generally limited to 36 to 38 Gy and if mediastinal disease is present, the entire cardiac silhouette is treated to 15 Gy followed by shielding of a portion of the pericardium and heart (Hoppe et al., 1992).

Figure 15-2 • Two adjoining fields are separated at the skin surface to avoid overlap of fields below the surface resulting in a high dose to the spinal cord.

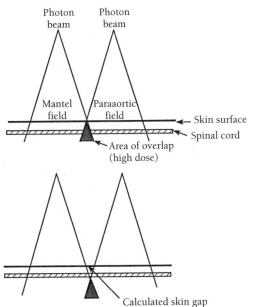

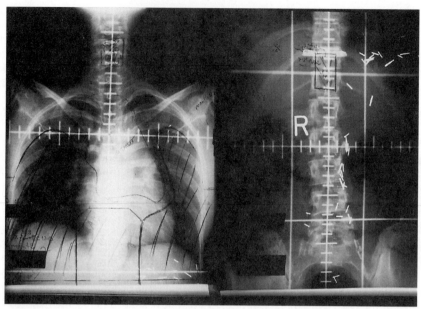

Figure 15-3 • Mantle and paraaortic fields in a 22-year-old female with stage IIA nodular sclerosing Hodgkin's disease presenting with left supraclavicular painless, enlarged lymph node and asymptomatic mediastinal disease. Splenectomy was performed. Staging laparotomy was negative.

Figure 15-4 • Diagram to illustrate large, individualized, irregular field (mantle) for irradiation of the supradiaphragmatic lymph nodes in patients with HD. Parallel opposed anterior and posterior fields are used; a block for the larynx may be used in the anterior field and a narrow block may be used in the posterior field to protect the cervical spinal cord. From Cox JD (1994). Lymphomas and leukemias. In JD Cox (Ed.), *Moss' Radiation Oncology: Rationale, Technique, Results* (7th ed., p. 809). St. Louis: Mosby.

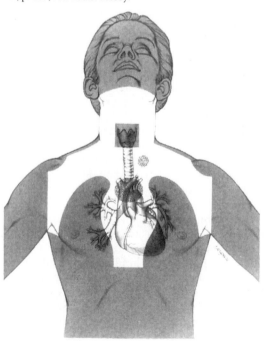

The effects of radiation dose to the heart must be considered especially in patients who will also receive doxorubicin, a cardiotoxic chemotherapy agent.

Subdiaphragmatic Irradiation

Treatment of the subdiaphragmatic region, the "inverted Y," includes paraaortic nodes and bilateral ilioinguinal node regions. The full "inverted Y" field extends from the diaphragm to the inguinal areas (see Figure 15–5). However, this full field is rarely treated. Instead, subtotal nodal irradiation is done with the lower border drawn at the level of the L4 to L5 interspace (paraaortic/splenic pedicle field) or below the bifurcation of the aorta including the common iliac nodes ("spade field") (Hoppe et al., 1992). The field includes the entire spleen if the spleen has not been removed. Kidneys are localized to determine inclusion in the fields. Pelvic fields are carefully blocked to minimize the amount of bone marrow irradiation in the sacral and pelvic regions. Oophoropexy with ovaries placed in front of or behind the uterus during staging laparotomy will help protect ovaries during the treatment course when a midline block is used during pelvic irradiation. The radiation dose can be reduced to approximately 8 percent of that received by the iliac nodes (Reddy et al., 1989). Testicular shielding may reduce testicular dose from 10 percent to less than 3 percent.

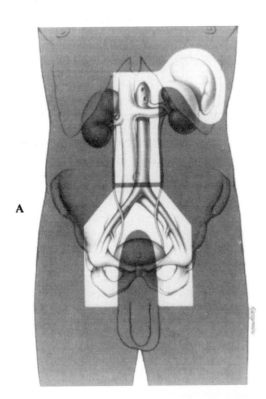

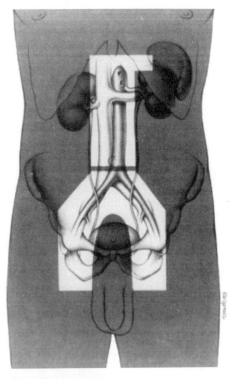

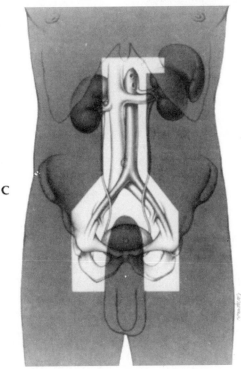

Figure 15-5 • Large, irregular field for irradiation of the infradiaphragmatic lymph nodes. (A) The spleen must be included if splenectomy has not been done; otherwise it is necessary to include the lymph nodes of the splenic pedicle, which should have been marked with clips at laparotomy (B and C). It is usually desirable to separate the paraaortic-splenic irradiation sequence from the pelvic irradiation sequence (A and B) to improve bone marrow tolerance. The paraaortic-splenic treatment may be interspersed with or immediately following the supradiaphragmatic treatment. If irradiation is to be given simultaneously to the paraaortic (plus spleen) and pelvic lymph nodes, it should follow the supradiaphragmatic treatment only after an interval of 2 to 4 weeks. From Cox JD (1994). Lymphomas and leukemias. In JD Cox (Ed.), *Moss' Radiation Oncology: Rationale, Technique, Results* (7th ed., p. 810). St. Louis: Mosby.

Pelvic irradiation is used much less frequently today because stages I and II supradiaphragmatic HD can be treated without pelvic irradiation. TNI has a limited role in stage III HD (DeVita et al., 1993). Treatment of both supra- and subdaphragmatic fields generally must be separated by 2 to 4 weeks to allow bone marrow recovery.

Total Body Irradiation

Total body irradiation (TBI) alone or with systemic combination chemotherapy has been used to destroy malignant cells in the bone marrow prior to bone marrow transplant. This procedure is followed by autologous, syngeneic, or allogeneic bone marrow transplant. Fractionated doses of radiation to a total of 12 to 16 Gy are generally given.

Results of Radiation Therapy Alone in Treatment of Stage I and II HD

Early stage HD (i.e., stages I and II) treated with radiation therapy alone results in approximately 75 percent long-term disease-free survival (Zinzani et al., 1994) and for supradiaphragmatic stages IA and IIA results in 14-year disease-free survival of 93 and 82 percent respectively (Urba & Longo, 1992).

Relapse of HD and Salvage Therapy

After appropriate treatment, 70 to 80 percent of patients with HD will have a complete response to treatment. Approximately 20 percent of patients will recur, most often outside of the radiation therapy portals. Most relapses after radiation therapy occur in unirradiated sites within 2 years after treatment (Erickson, 1994). Approximately 40 percent of patients with advanced disease who received chemotherapy will recur in sites of previous disease, usually lymph nodes. Relapse after radiation therapy is treated with chemotherapy with rates of complete remission and long-term survival of 50 to 80 percent (Urba & Longo, 1992).

The pattern of relapse of HD is most often related to the size of the initial mass, stage, and type of therapy. Relapse in a nodal region is related to the initial size at diagnosis with higher relapse rates in areas of large amounts of disease. Patients who received nodal irradiation to the mantle and high paraaortic nodes may recur in the next contiguous nodal group—the pelvic iliac nodes—which was not included in the original treatment. Patients treated with radiation alone or with combined radiation and chemotherapy are more likely to recur in sites that were not irradiated.

The risk of relapse after radiation therapy in stages I and II HD can be reduced by combining radiation with chemotherapy. However, for most patients, this constitutes overtreatment and considerably increases the risk of long-term side effects (Urba & Longo, 1992).

Seventy-five to 80 percent of patients with advanced stage HD with systemic symptoms will have complete remission with chemotherapy. One-third of these patients will have relapse and will require salvage therapy. Chemotherapy or large-field radiation therapy may be used as salvage therapy and one-third of patients will achieve complete remission. Improved results of salvage therapy may occur with high-dose chemotherapy with or without radiation and autologous bone marrow transplantation or peripheral blood stem cell transplantation. The rate of complete response after initial relapse is approximately 50 percent (DeVita & Hubbard, 1993).

Post HD Treatment Evaluation

Complete remission is the most important initial outcome of treatment for HD. One month after the last cycle of chemotherapy or radiation therapy is complete, all known sites of disease should be evaluated radiographically or if accessible, pathologically. Gallium scans are very useful in detecting residual disease when the HD was initially gallium-avid. The first 2 years after complete remission, patients are seen every 3 months. During the next 3 years the interval is extended to every 4 to 6 months and after 5 years, once per year.

Non-Hodgkin's Lymphoma

Non-Hodgkin's lymphoma (NHL) exhibits a variety of complex presentations and spread. The site(s) of disease, pathology, age over 60, performance status, elevated serum LDH, and extent of disease all influence prognosis and treatment. Lymphoma may arise in both nodal and extranodal lymphoid tissue. Examples include lymph nodes, spleen, bone marrow, Waldeyer's tonsillar ring, gastrointestinal tract (particularly stomach and small bowel), and other tissues in which lymphocytes circulate.

Epidemiology

The incidence of non-Hodgkin's lymphoma (NHL) increased approximately 60 percent in the United States from 1973 to 1989 (Weisenburger, 1994). With exception of the very young, higher incidences have been reported in the major cate-

gories of males and females, blacks and whites, all
adult age groups but especially in the elderly, and
those living in rural areas. Patients with acquired
immunodeficiency syndrome (AIDS) have an increased incidence of NHL. However, many of
these NHLs occur in young men and this increasing trend did not become apparent until the early
to mid-1980s, later than the overall trend, which
also demonstrated increases in older men and
women (Weisenburger, 1994). Therefore, factors
in addition to AIDS are contributing to the overall
increase in NHL. AIDS is estimated to account for
10 to 15 percent of all new NHL cases in the future
(Gail et al., 1991).

Cancer statistics from the American Cancer
Society (1997) estimate 53,600 new cases of non-
Hodgkin's lymphoma and 23,800 deaths in 1996.
Incidence in males compared to females is ap-
proximately 1.4 to 1.0. Caucasians are slightly
more likely to be affected than non-Caucasians.
The incidence of NHL gradually increases with
age, with a small peak in adolescence.

Etiology

The etiology of NHL is unknown. Development of
NHL has been associated with viruses, altered immunologic states (either suppression or stimulation), chemical exposure, and radiation exposure.

Similar to Hodgkin's disease, viral etiology
has been suspected. Infection with the Epstein-
Barr virus (EBV) is endemic throughout the
world. It is associated with a variety of lymphoproliferative diseases, both benign and malignant,
including infectious mononucleosis, Burkitt's
lymphoma, and high-grade B cell NHLs (Pallesen
et al., 1993). The EBV is associated with 98 percent of African Burkitt's lymphoma, which is endemic in Africa, but only 15 to 20 percent of
nonendemic Burkitt's (Longo et al., 1993). EBV
infection has also been associated with the development of NHL in immunocompromised patients
but does not appear to be sufficient alone for
transformation to lymphoma (Priest et al., 1993).
Approximately 5 percent of high-grade B cell malignancies found in patients with immunodeficiency diseases exhibit markers of EBV infection.
In the majority of B cell lymphomas, there is little
evidence linking EBV to the etiology. EBV markers have been found in several peripheral T cell
lymphomas but efforts to implicate them in etiology have been unsuccessful (Pallesen et al., 1993).
Other viruses including human T cell leukemia/
lymphoma virus 1 (HTLV-1) and HIV have been
associated with NHL.

Non-Hodgkin's lymphomas may develop in
association with acquired or inherited immune
system abnormalities such as autoimmune disorders, immune suppression in organ transplant recipients, genetic immune deficiency syndromes
(e.g., severe combined immunodeficiency syndrome), and AIDS. In patients receiving renal
transplant, the risk of developing NHL is 40 to 100
times greater than in the general population
(Lundquist, 1994). Posttransplant lymphomas
have a higher incidence of extranodal disease and
central nervous system involvement than NHLs in
the general population.

Environmental toxins such as pesticides, solvents, and occupational exposure to wood dust
and cotton dust have been implicated in NHL
(Weisenburger, 1994). Other associated factors
include: a higher incidence with increased economic status, urban population, and certain geographic locations. Weisenburger (1994) describes
a small increased risk in patients with long-term
use of hair dyes and tobacco.

Ionizing radiation exposure is associated with
an increase in NHL in survivors of the atomic
bomb in Hiroshima exposed to more than 1 Gy.
Patients treated for HD with both radiation therapy and chemotherapy have an increased risk of
developing secondary large cell lymphomas, especially those involving the gastrointestinal tract
(Longo et al., 1993). A recent study of primary
gastric NHL by Wotherspoon and associates
(1991) demonstrated the presence of *Helicobacter
pylori* (*H. pylori*) infection in 92 percent of the patients indicating that *H. pylori* may be an important predisposing factor for the development of
gastric NHL.

HIV and NHL

Human immunodeficiency virus (HIV) is associated with the development of NHL. In 1985, the
clinical definition of AIDS was changed to include
any patient with a positive HIV antibody test and
an intermediate or high-grade B cell lymphoma.
The incidence of NHL in patients with AIDS continues to increase possibly in part as a result of
longer survival of patients with AIDS. NHL associated with AIDS currently has a 100-fold relative
risk compared to the non-AIDS population and is
predicted to continue to increase and to account
for as many as 10 to 15 percent of all new NHL
cases (Weisenburger, 1994).

Characteristics of NHL associated with AIDS
differ from lymphoma in non-AIDS patients in
several ways: younger age, aggressive histologic
subtypes, more common B symptoms, more

advanced stage at diagnosis, more common extra-nodal disease, increased incidence of CNS lymphoma, and reduced tolerance of chemotherapy-induced myelosuppression, increasing risk of infection (Priest et al., 1993). The central nervous system is the most common site of NHL in the patient with AIDS.

Histopathology

Histopathology of NHL is difficult and controversial. NHLs are malignancies arising from B or T lymphocytes and rarely, from the monocyte/histiocyte line. B cell origin is found in 80 percent of lymphomas and most patients present with bone marrow or lymph node disease. NHL pathologic subtypes correspond to different stages of normal lymphocyte transformation (see Figure 15–6). Malignant cells may be found in lymph nodes, organs, bone marrow, and peripheral blood. Patients with B cell lymphoma may have abnormalities in immunoglobulin secretion, either increased or decreased. T lymphocytes in T cell lymphoma may have increased activation of lymphokines or macrophages. The natural history of a lymphoma depends primarily on its histological subtype.

The first accepted classification was the Rappaport system in 1956 based on pattern of malignant growth in the lymph nodes (follicular and diffuse) and degree of differentiation of the predominant cell type (Rappaport & Winter, 1956) (see Table 15–5).

New immunologic techniques allowed recognition of T and B cells; Lukes & Collins introduced a new classification system in 1974. T lymphocytes are found in large concentrations in the paracortical regions of the lymph nodes, in the periarterial lymphoid sheaths of the spleen, and in small concentrations in follicles (Medeiros & Jaffe, 1993). B lymphocytes are concentrated in the lymph node follicles, medullary cords, and spleen follicles. Approximately 70 percent of lymphomas are B cell and 20 percent are T cell with B cell lymphomas demonstrating a better prognosis.

The Working Formulation of Non-Hodgkin's Lymphoma for Clinical Use was developed in an attempt to create a common language that would allow clinicians to translate from one system to another in the 6 major classification systems of NHL, allowing comparisons of clinical therapeutic trials (National Cancer Institute, 1982). The Working Formulation system identifies 20 subtypes of NHL on the basis of morphology, clinical features, and prognosis (Hoppe et al., 1992). Follicular (nodular) lymphoma is considered to have a better prognosis than diffuse NHL, and major morphologic differences identified by Lukes and Collins (1974) are used. The Working Formulation system does not directly incorporate modern immunologic or immunogenetic concepts. Multiple histologic types occurring in the same patient is not uncommon. Composite lymphoma describes disease in which 2 or more distinctly different, well-delineated lymphomas occur in a single site (Medeiros & Jaffe, 1993).

The Working Formulation uses the categories of low grade, intermediate grade, and high grade to predict for survival. These categories correlate with degree of differentiation and aggressiveness of NHL. Ten-year survival rates reported by Simon et al. (1988) in an NCI study were 45 percent for low grade, 26 percent for intermediate grade, and 23 percent for high grade. The progression of NHL from low-grade to high-grade histology is relatively common in B cell lymphomas.

Low-Grade Lymphoma

The Working Formulation low-grade category of NHL includes the following malignant lym-

Figure 15-6 • B and T lymphocyte maturation (differentiation).

Mantle zone			Follicle Follicular (germinal) center cells				Mature cell
							→ Plasma cell
B cell →	Small cleaved →	Large cleaved →	Small noncleaved →	Large noncleaved →	Immunoblast (B cell) →		
							→ Memory (B cell)
Less differentiated			→				*More differentiated*
			Interfollicular Zone				
Uncommitted T cell	→	Convoluted T cell	→	Immunoblast T cell	→		Committed T cell

Table 15-5 • Histopathologic Classification of Malignant Lymphomas (ML)

Working Formulation for Malignant Lymphomas (1982)	Rappaport Classification (1956)	Lukes and Collins Classification (1974)
LOW GRADE		
ML, small, lymphocytic	Diffuse lymphocytic, well-differentiated	Small lymphocytic and plasmacytoid lymphocytic
ML, follicular, predominantly small cleaved cell	Nodular, poorly differentiated lympho-cytic	Small cleaved FCC, follicular only or follicular and diffuse
ML, follicular, mixed, small cleaved and large cell	Nodular, mixed lymphocytic-histiocytic	Small cleaved FCC, follicular; large cleaved FCC, follicular
INTERMEDIATE GRADE		
ML, follicular, predominantly large cell	Nodular histiocytic	Large cleaved or noncleaved FCC, follicular
ML, diffuse, small cleaved cell	Diffuse lymphocytic, poorly differen-tiated	Small cleaved FCC, diffuse
ML, diffuse, mixed small and large cell	Diffuse mixed lymphocytic-histiocytic	Small cleaved, large cleaved or large noncleaved FCC, diffuse
ML, diffuse large cell	Diffuse histiocytic	Large cleaved or noncleaved FCC, diffuse
HIGH GRADE		
ML, large cell immunoblastic	Diffuse histiocytic	Immunoblastic sarcoma, T cell or B cell type
ML, lymphoblastic	Lymphoblastic convoluted/ nonconvoluted	Convoluted T cell
ML, small noncleaved cell (Burkitt's)	Undifferentiated, Burkitt's and non-Burkitt's	Small noncleaved FCC
MISCELLANEOUS		
Composite		
Mycosis fungoides (cutaneous T-cell lymphoma)		
Histiocytic		
Extramedullary plasmacytoma		
Unclassifiable		

FCC = follicular center cell.

phomas: (1) small lymphocytic; (2) follicular small cleaved; and (3) follicular mixed, small cleaved, and large cell. These lymphomas are generally indolent, occur in older adults, and are considered curable only in stages I and II (Mendenhall & Lynch, 1995). Long-term survival is expected with or without aggressive treatment in stage III and IV disease. Presentation is usually a generalized lymphadenopathy and rarely involves extranodal extension other than liver and bone marrow. Low-grade lymphomas rarely occur in sanctuary sites such as testis or central nervous system. Low-grade lymphomas are thought to be responsive to immunoregulation. Patients may have a history of lymph nodes waxing and waning over a period of years prior to diagnosis. Death from low-grade lymphomas is generally due to progression of tumor and replacement of hematopoietic and lymphoid tissues that result in

clinical effects and/or transformation to a high-grade lymphoma.

All follicular NHL subtypes, including the intermediate-grade follicular, large cell type, have rearrangement of immunoglobulin genes within the malignant cells. Translocation of chromosomes 14 and 18 occurs in 85 to 95 percent of cases of follicular lymphomas (Lister & Armitage, 1995; Medeiros & Jaffe, 1993). The BCL-2 protooncogene on chromosome 18 is translocated to the chromosome 14 region of the immunoglobulin gene in follicular NHL. Protooncogenes are normal cellular genes involved in the control of cell proliferation or differentiation. When structurally or functionally altered, they have the potential to contribute to tumor induction or progression. It is thought that the BCL-2 gene affects programmed cell death and that overexpression results in decreased cell death. The BCL-2 gene is believed to become deregulated resulting in proliferation, possibly acquired additional genetic abnormalities, and ultimately, resulting in follicular lymphoma (Horning, 1993).

Intermediate-Grade Lymphoma

Intermediate- and high-grade lymphomas are considered aggressive lymphomas. Four intermediate-grade lymphomas, one follicular and three diffuse, are described in the Working Formulation: (1) follicular, large cell; (2) diffuse, small cleaved cell; (3) diffuse mixed, small and large cell; and (4) diffuse large cell. Follicular, large cell lymphoma has a more aggressive clinical course than low-grade follicular lymphomas. Disease is generally advanced at the time of diagnosis. The diffuse subtypes in this category are more aggressive and are primarily found in adults frequently presenting with stage I or II disease. Nodal and extranodal progression to the gastrointestinal tract, skin, and bone is common. Involvement of sanctuary sites may occur.

High-Grade Lymphoma

High-grade lymphomas in the Working Formulation are: (1) large cell, immunoblastic; (2) lymphoblastic; and (3) small noncleaved cell (Burkitt's, non-Burkitt's). All three are characterized by an aggressive clinical course and anaplastic malignant cells. Systemic B symptoms are more common, and extranodal and sanctuary sites are more commonly involved than in other lymphomas. High-grade lymphomas are not believed to be subject to immunoregulation. Almost all childhood NHLs are high grade.

Staging Classification

The Ann Arbor staging system was originally designed for HD, which generally spreads in an orderly, contiguous manner. The Ann Arbor-Cotswolds staging classification is most often used for NHL even though it does not take into account prognostic factors such as bulk of disease and patient's age (see Table 15–2). This classification system is based on distribution of nodal involvement, extralymphatic spread, and B symptoms. NHL includes heterogeneous subtypes, and the Ann Arbor-Cotswolds system is somewhat limited in its usefulness in separating prognostic groups of NHL.

Presentation

Histology is a primary determinant of presenting symptoms in non-Hodgkin's lymphoma. Painless,

peripheral lymphadenopathy is the presenting symptom in more than two-thirds of patients. Even though the most common site is the cervical lymph nodes, many patients present with multiple sites. Lymph nodes generally feel rubbery and mobile and may wax and wane in size over months (Priest et al., 1993). Unlike HD, which tends to spread to contiguous axial nodes, NHL is more likely to involve noncontiguous and more peripheral lymph node regions. Approximately 20 percent present with B symptoms, which are more common with more aggressive histology. Pruritus, common in HD, is rare in NHL. Mediastinal disease is much less common than in HD but occurs in 20 percent of NHL. Retroperitoneal lymphadenopathy is common especially in indolent NHL and may be large. Patients with NHL are much more likely to have bone marrow and mesenteric lymph node involvement than in HD. Waldeyer's ring, rarely involved in HD, is frequently involved in NHL (see Table 15–6).

Approximately 20 to 30 percent of patients with NHL will first be diagnosed with extranodal organ involvement (Weisenburger, 1994). The most frequent extranodal sites are the stomach, intestines, and skin. Increasing incidence in the brain, other areas of the nervous system, and the eye have occurred. T cell lymphocytic lymphomas may involve the skin, while B cell lymphomas infrequently exhibit cutaneous involvement. Lymphocytic lymphomas commonly involve the viscera, particularly lymphoreticular organs such as bone marrow, liver, and spleen. Bone marrow involvement occurs in 50 percent of patients with NHL and is highly dependent upon the histologic type. Hepatic and splenic involvement is common.

NHL frequently presents in the gastrointestinal (GI) tract, which has large amounts of lymphoid tissue. However, the most commonly involved GI organ, the stomach, does not contain lymphoid tissue. Gastric lymphoid tissue is acquired in response to localized infection of the stomach with *H. pylori*. Most primary lymphomas arising in the stomach are of the mucosa-associated lymphoid tissue (MALT) type and are almost always associated with infection by *H. pylori* (Wotherspoon et al., 1991). MALT malignant lymphomas are B cell lymphomas and have also been identified in GI tract, lung, salivary gland, and thyroid. Most patients with gastric lymphoma will have disease limited to stage I_E or II_E.

Waldeyer's ring makes up approximately 15 percent of extranodal lymphomas. Most often they are aggressive histologically and of B cell origin

Table 15-6 • Presentation of Hodgkin's Disease and Non-Hodgkin's Lymphoma

Category	Hodgkin's Disease	Non-Hodgkin's Lymphoma
Age	Bimodal peak	Median 60–65
B symptoms	30%	20%
Stage at presentation	May be localized	85% advanced stage
Spread	Contiguous nodes	Often not contiguous
Nodes involved	Axial most frequently	Peripheral involvement common (>67%)
Mediastinal involvement	85%	20%
Extranodal organ involvement	Infrequent	20–30%
Bone marrow involvement		40–50% of follicular 10% of diffuse
Other	Pruritius more common	Pruritus uncommon
Initial site	Cervical nodes most frequent (80%)	
CNS involvement	Rare	Frequent with AIDS
GI tract involvement	Rare	Not uncommon
Waldeyer's ring	Rare	Not uncommon

and are generally treated with limited-field radiation therapy.

Involvement of the central nervous system with lymphoma is a serious problem and generally indicates a poor prognosis whether lesions are primary or metastatic. Central nervous system lymphomas are increasing in incidence, particularly in patients with AIDS and organ transplant-related immunosuppression. Aggressive (diffuse) B cell lymphomas are the most common.

Patient Evaluation

Patient evaluation is similar to that for HD (see Table 15–3). Treatment decisions are based on histology and stage of disease with histology being the more useful determinant of prognosis and therapy. NHL is more often diagnosed in advanced stage with only 15 percent presenting in stage I or II.

A complete history and physical examination is performed including assessment for B symptoms and palpable disease. Mirror examination of the oral cavity and pharynx is important to assess Waldeyer's ring for involvement of disease.

Laboratory blood tests may be abnormal but changes may be nonspecific to NHL. Blood counts are normal in 90 percent of patients at diagnosis (Priest et al., 1993). Routine lab tests are completed. Anemia and thrombocytopenia generally indicate progressive bone marrow involvement, hypersplenism, and myelosuppressive therapy. Lymphopenia may occur but is less common than lymphocytosis, often indicating circulating malignant cells. Increased LDH levels in lymphoma may serve as an indicator of tumor extent.

Routine chest x rays are done with approximately 25 percent showing abnormalities. Chest CT may also be done. Bone scan is generally reserved for patients with diffuse, aggressive lymphomas who are symptomatic. Gallium scans, especially with newer techniques, can detect gastrointestinal, abdominal, and pelvic involvement in patients with diffuse subtypes of NHL. These scans are extremely sensitive in detecting mediastinal disease.

In a recent study by Newman and associates (1994) positron emission tomography (PET) scan was compared to CT scan in 16 patients, 11 with NHL and 5 with HD, in imaging thoracoabdominal lymphoma. In this small study, 54 foci of abnormal uptake were detected with PET in 13 patients in whom 49 corresponding sites were detected with CT. Three patients with HD had negative findings with PET, CT, and staging laparotomy. PET was found to be successful in detecting disease in patients with HD and low-, intermediate-, and high-grade lymphomas and could depict disease in lymph nodes as small as 1.0 cm. PET imaging continues to be investigated but appears to be a useful method for imaging HD and NHL. With further study, PET may prove to be an important tool for staging and monitoring HD and NHL.

Patients with NHL are often diagnosed in late stage and have positive lymphangiograms. However, patients with NHL commonly have disease detected in other sites and a positive LAG infrequently contributes to advancing the stage of disease. Therefore, LAG is rarely used in the staging of NHL (Priest et al., 1993).

Bone marrow biopsy is an essential diagnostic procedure in NHL. Marrow involvement is common in NHL and indicates stage IV disease. Staging laparotomy may be considered for the 15 percent of patients who, after clinical and radiographic evaluation, are considered to have stage I or II disease. The likelihood of upstaging with follicular histology is greater than with diffuse histology. If laparotomy results will potentially make a major change in treatment decisions, it should be performed. Generally only a small number of patients have staging laparotomy with NHL (Cox, 1994; Priest et al., 1993).

Radiation Therapy in the Treatment of NHL

Treatment of NHL is less successful than that for HD. While 30 to 50 percent of intermediate- and high-grade NHLs can be cured, low-grade NHLs are generally indolent with a long natural history and have transient responses to treatment. With NHL, it is often necessary to irradiate large areas of the body including a variety of sensitive normal tissues. Limited disease low-grade lymphomas are generally treated with involved-field irradiation. More advanced disease is primarily treated with chemotherapy. Aggressive NHL is generally treated with chemotherapy and involved-field radiation therapy (see Table 15–7). Whole-brain irradiation is the mainstay of treatment of CNS lymphomas.

NHL confined to one side of the diaphragm is generally treated with high-dose radiation therapy to the involved site(s). Total nodal irradiation (TNI) is not standard in the United States. Stage I localized diffuse lymphomas can be cured in 50 to 80 percent of patients and stage II disease is cured in 25 to 40 percent (Cox, 1994). Radiation doses for stage I disease, either follicular or diffuse histologic subtype, are generally a minimum of 40 Gy. An additional 10 Gy may be used to treat extranodal or large stage I disease. NHLs of bone and brain require the highest doses of radiation therapy, 50 to 60 Gy. Total doses may be decreased if chemotherapy is used during or before radiation therapy. Treatment portals usually include regional lymphatics, which drain the disease site(s).

While no therapy is curative with low-grade NHL, a variety of therapies can induce an initial response. Many treatment options for these nonaggressive stages III and IV NHL exist, including no treatment, single-agent adjuvant chemotherapy, combination chemotherapy, combination chemotherapy plus radiation therapy to bulky disease, low-dose total-body irradiation, total nodal irradiation and combination chemotherapy, and chemotherapy with TBI and bone marrow transplant. The clinical course of low-grade NHL generally includes a series of remissions and relapses with the duration of remissions progressively shorter after each relapse. In spite of the long natural history, these lymphomas generally result in death of the patient within 10 to 12 years of diagnosis.

Table 15-7 • Treatment of Non-Hodgkin's Lymphoma

Stage/Histology	Treatment
Stage I and II follicular	Radiation therapy: Involved field.
Stage I and II diffuse	Chemotherapy and involved field radiation therapy. Radiation therapy: Extended field. Controversial. Chemotherapy alone: Controversial.
Stage III and IV follicular (asymptomatic)	Controversy: Aggressive treatment vs. careful follow-up and treat when symptomatic. Chemotherapy. Controversy: Total nodal irradiation after CR with chemotherapy.
Stage III and IV unfavorable histology	Chemotherapy. Possible radiation therapy after chemotherapy. Possible total body irradiation. Possible BMT.
Recurrent or progressive follicular	Chemotherapy. Consider BMT with chemotherapy and TBI conditioning.
Follicular conversion to high-grade lymphoma	Combination chemotherapy.
Cutaneous T cell lymphoma	Topical chemotherapy in early stage with or without total skin electrons. Systemic chemotherapy for advanced disease.

Data from Lister TA & Armitage JO (1995). Non-Hodgkin's lymphomas. In MD Abeloff, JO Armitage, AS Lichter, & JE Niederhuber (Eds.), *Clinical Oncology* (pp. 2109–2147). New York: Churchill Livingstone; and Wasserman TH & Glatstein E (1992). Non-Hodgkin's lymphoma. In CA Perez & LW Brady (Eds.), *Principles and Practice of Radiation Oncology* (2nd ed., pp. 1329–1344). Philadelphia: JB Lippincott.

In patients with limited disease (stages I and II) follicular or diffuse histologies, radiation therapy alone results in prolonged remissions in a significant number of patients. Untreated intermediate- and high-grade lymphomas progress rapidly. However, these lymphomas may be curable when treated. Aggressive subtypes have a tendency to spread systemically early in the course of the disease. Based on this observation, many investigators now advocate the addition of combination chemotherapy to radiation therapy in localized, aggressive NHL (Lister & Armitage, 1995; Longo et al., 1989). Chemotherapy dose may be reduced if adjuvant radiation is given.

In extensive (stages III and IV) follicular low-grade lymphoma, an 80 to 90 percent response rate and long-term survival can be achieved with a variety of treatments including single- or multi-agent chemotherapy, combined modality treatment and total body irradiation (TBI) (Horning, 1993). The incidence of transformation from low-grade histology to intermediate- or high-grade histology increases over time and occurs in 40 to 45 percent of patients with and without initial treatment of their lymphoma (Horning, 1993; Lister & Armitage, 1995). Prognosis after disease progression is poor.

Whether stage II follicular NHL may also be managed with radiation therapy alone is controversial. Some investigators use total lymphoid radiation therapy while others recommend involved-field radiation therapy plus chemotherapy or chemotherapy alone (Lister & Armitage, 1995; Wasserman & Glatstein, 1992).

Stage III and IV diffuse and stage IV follicular NHL are generally treated with combination chemotherapy. In stage III follicular lymphoma, some investigators suggest treatment with high-dose TNI will result in prolonged disease-free survival in a significant number of patients (Wasserman & Glatstein, 1992). Aggressive treatment of NHL with chemotherapy relies on multidrug regimens, the standard being cyclophosphamide, doxorubicin, vincristine, and prednisone (CHOP). Survival at 4 years is estimated at 40 to 50 percent (Stupp et al., 1994). CHOP allows high-dose intensity and minimizes drug resistance (see Table 15–8 for other examples of drug combinations). Doxorubicin or mitoxantrone should be part of the drug combination for best results (Ballester et al., 1993). Some patients with poor prognostic factors may benefit from high-dose chemotherapy with autologous bone marrow or peripheral stem-cell rescue. NHL is more common in elderly adults, and aggressive chemotherapy regimens may have

Table 15-8 • Examples of Drug Combinations Used in Treatment of Non-Hodgkin's Lymphoma

CHOP	Cyclophosphamide, doxorubicin, vincristine, prednisone
CHOP-Bleo	CHOP, bleomycin
COP-BLAM	Cyclophosphamide, vincristine, prednisone, bleomycin, doxorubicin, and procarbazine
mBACOD	Methotrexate, bleomycin, doxorubicin, cyclophosphamide, vincristine and dexamethasone
BACOP	Bleomycin, doxorubicin, cyclophosphamide, vincristine, prednisone
Pro-MACE-MOPP	Cyclophosphamide, etoposide, doxorubicin, nitrogen mustard, procarbazine, high-dose methotrexate with leucovorin rescue, and prednisone

to be adjusted to less aggressive doses. Involved field radiation therapy may need to be added.

Non-Hodgkin's Lymphoma in the Elderly

Several factors may influence treatment and response in the elderly. The wishes of the elderly patient may be different from those of the young when a treatment regimen is being considered. Physiological changes in the elderly play a role as well. Significant immune function changes occur with increasing age. Decreased bone marrow cellularity results in more severe myelosuppression, and alterations in hepatic and renal function also occur with age. Elderly patients with NHL present more frequently with poor performance status, increased incidence of intercurrent disease, more aggressive histology and higher stage than younger patients (Goss, 1993). Non-Hodgkin's lymphomas are very responsive to treatment with radiation therapy and chemotherapy. However, many treatment trials do not include patients over 70 years old. Some trials require up to a 50 percent chemotherapy dose reduction in older patients. Decreased response and survival have been reported in elderly patients (Goss, 1993).

Salminen (1995) analyzed 98 NHL patients 70 years old or older. Eighty-two percent of patients had intermediate- or high-grade histopathology. Age and performance status were independent prognostic factors in NHL patients. Chemotherapy dose was reduced by 30 to 50 percent in patients with intercurrent illness or poor performance status.

Treatment in the elderly is complicated by reduced regenerative ability of the bone marrow, higher incidence of lung and cardiac toxicity, and diminished renal and hepatic excretion of many drugs. Myelotoxicity has been reduced with the use of hematopoietic growth factors. Patients treated with radiation therapy and chemotherapy combinations did not have fatal complications during treatment. However, 13 patients (13 percent), many with intercurrent diseases or other poor prognostic factors, had fatal complications during chemotherapy. Treatment deaths (other than due to lymphoma) have been reported in several series as 1 to 7 percent in patients younger than 60 to 70 years and 7 to 30 percent in patients over 60 to 70 years of age (Salminen, 1995). Relative survival of patients with NHL who are older than 65 years is significantly worse than younger patients. Additional investigations of innovative combinations of radiation therapy and chemotherapy in older patients with NHL seem warranted.

Survival of patients with low-grade lymphoma is believed by some investigators to be adversely affected by age over 60 years, perhaps due to a higher incidence of intercurrent disease (Ballester et al., 1993). In aggressive NHL in patients over 60, the influence of age is controversial. Ballester and colleagues (1993) conclude that advanced age is a poor prognostic factor only when associated with other negative parameters such as intercurrent disease and poor performance status.

Cutaneous T Cell Lymphoma

Cutaneous T cell lymphoma (CTCL), commonly known as mycosis fungoides, involves cutaneous infiltration of T cells in early stages of the disease. Treatment may be given with total skin electrons (TSE) and topical chemotherapy or photopheresis. Systemic chemotherapy may be used for treatment of more advanced disease.

When TSE is used, the patient is treated with 36 Gy over a period of 8 to 10 weeks with low-energy electrons (e.g., 4 MeV, 6 MeV). Six fields are used while the patient stands in 6 different positions in an effort to irradiate all skin surfaces possible. Boost fields are used for areas that cannot be irradiated in the 6 positions such as soles of feet, top of head, and perineum.

Treatment of Non-Hodgkin's Lymphoma

Intensive radiation therapy or intensive chemotherapy of NHL may not be possible due to ad-

vanced age or intercurrent illness. Most patients with NHL present with advanced disease.

Radiation Therapy

Many tumor and patient factors are considered when a dose is prescribed for treatment of NHL. A minimum of 35 Gy is used for sites of known disease. Most often doses are higher, 40 to 50 Gy, especially for diffuse lymphomas. Follicular lymphomas are often treated with 40 Gy. Palliative treatment may be given with 25 Gy.

Technical Considerations

Treatment volume is based on the primary site with adequate margins and the lymphatic regions draining that area. Most often contiguous lymphatics on the same side of the diaphragm are included. Technical considerations of treatment are similar to those used in HD (see Technical Considerations under HD).

Supradiaphragmatic Irradiation

The full mantle field may be treated as in HD or modified into a minimantle field. Mediastinal recurrence is rare if the mediastinum was not originally involved. In cases in which mediastinal extension is unlikely, the minimantle field, which does not include the mediastinal nodes, may be used (Wasserman & Glatstein, 1992). The full mantle must be used when mediastinal extension of disease is possible, such as with positive supraclavicular disease, or when upper abdominal disease is present. Elimination of the mediastinum in the field decreases radiation complications of heart and lung injury and reduces the amount of bone marrow irradiated.

Preauricular lymph nodes are frequently involved in NHL especially when cervical nodes or Waldeyer's ring are involved. Lateral opposing fields are used. When Waldeyer's ring is treated, the whole region and lymph nodes draining the area are included in the radiation therapy fields (see Figure 15–7). Other areas in the head and neck region require specific individualized treatment plans.

Central nervous system lymphomas are generally treated with radiation therapy to the whole brain to a dose of greater than 50 Gy.

Subdiaphragmatic Irradiation

Whole-abdominal radiation for massive disease may be delivered to anterior and posterior fields extending from the diaphragm to the iliac crests. Fifteen Gy is delivered in 2 weeks followed by lat-

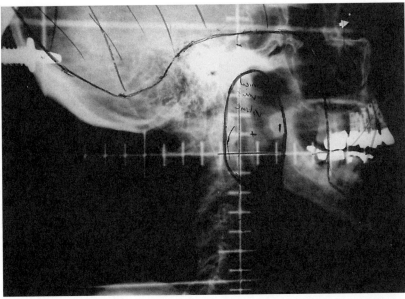

Figure 15-7 • Lateral head and neck field for treatment of a 77-year-old male with stage IB$_E$ NHL of Waldeyer's ring (nasopharynx). The primary tumor received 41.4 Gy through parallel opposed lateral fields and 30.6 Gy to the supraclavicular region.

eral fields to an additional 15 Gy in 2 weeks. When the whole abdomen is irradiated, the right lobe of the liver is shielded to reduce the dose to this organ. The kidneys are shielded to keep the renal dose to less than 25 Gy (see Figure 15–8). Daily doses to this large field generally are not greater than 1.5 Gy. The paraaortics may be given an additional 15 Gy through anterior and posterior fields. The total dose to the central abdomen may be 40 to 45 Gy over 5 to 7 weeks (see Figure 15–9).

Pelvic fields are generally treated with anterior and posterior fields either with abdominal irradiation or with separate pelvic fields after abdominal treatment. Blood counts, tumor size, and location are the primary determining factors in whether these fields will be treated simultaneously or separately. Midline pelvic adenopathy may develop in NHL. When the pelvis is treated, midline blocks must be placed at or below the symphysis pubis. Ovarian function cannot be preserved in young women with NHL.

Total Body Irradiation

Autologous bone marrow transplant (ABMT) has been used successfully over the past decade with and without total body irradiation (TBI) in the treatment of HD and NHL. Because lymphocytes are highly sensitive to radiation and may be disseminated in HD and NHL, TBI may be effective. The mechanism of action of TBI is unclear. A linear accelerator is used with various set-up tech-

niques to deliver fractionated radiation to the whole body. For example, in some institutions, the patient stands a distance from the machine and is treated with both anterior and posterior fields. In other institutions, the patient lies on a stretcher a distance from the machine and is treated with right and left lateral fields. TBI may be used in preparation for bone marrow transplant or palliation in advanced lymphoid malignancies

Figure 15-8 • Outline of kidneys, almost all of which will be blocked, on simulation film for abdominal treatment in a 46-year-old male with stage IIA diffuse small cleaved lymphoma (positive iliac and inguinal nodes). Whole-abdominal radiation was given followed by a boost to the inverted Y (see Figure 15-9).

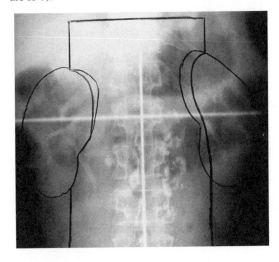

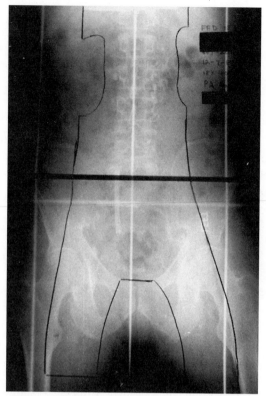

Figure 15-9 • Inverted Y boost field of patient in Figure 15-8 after 15 Gy to the whole abdomen in which the kidneys and right lobe of the liver were shielded. Total dose given was 40 Gy in 36 fractions.

(Wasserman & Glatstein, 1992). For bone marrow transplant preparation, TBI is used in conjunction with high-dose chemotherapy. For example, radiation may be delivered 3 times per day in 1.1 Gy per fraction to a total of 13.2 Gy (Demirer et al., 1995). Marrow is infused immediately after the last dose of TBI. Primary dose limiting toxicity for TBI is hepatotoxicity and interstitial pneumonitis.

Palliative TBI doses may be given in a number of fractionation schedules, for example, 1.5 Gy over 5 weeks delivered in 0.1 to 0.15 Gy fractions 2 to 3 times per week. Significant leukopenia or thrombocytopenia from prior treatment may reduce tolerance to this palliative treatment.

Relapse of NHL and Salvage Therapy

Few patients with relapsed NHL can be cured with conventional doses of chemotherapy or radiation therapy. High-dose chemotherapy given with or without total body irradiation and bone marrow or peripheral blood stem cell transplantation can be effective in obtaining disease-free survival for 20 to 50 percent of patients with relapse (Press et al., 1995). Salvage chemotherapy may include drug combinations such as mesna, ifosfamide, mitoxantrone, and etoposide (MINE) followed by etoposide, methylprednisolone, cytarabine, and cisplatin (ESHAP). Radiation therapy is frequently given to involved fields. Radiation therapy is an essential component of palliative therapy to provide pain relief and reduce compression of tissues by the tumor mass.

Post NHL Treatment Evaluation

Follow-up frequency and extent generally depend on the risk of recurrence. Patients who did not have a complete response may require more frequent CT scans to detect progression of disease than patients who had a complete response to treatment.

Radioimmunodetection and Radioimmunotherapy in HD and NHL

Normal cells as well as cancer cells are affected with current standard cancer therapies. Monoclonal antibodies (MoAb) can be used to selectively target cancer cells but are generally unable to kill these cells by immunologic mechanisms. New advances have allowed clinical trials to be done with selective cancer targeting of HD and NHL using MoAb-labeled radioisotopes to detect or treat the malignant disease. Radioimmunodetection has been investigated as a means to detect disease for accurate staging and early recurrence using low doses of radioisotopes. Baum and colleagues (1994) reported good imaging of soft tissue and bone tumor sites in various subtypes of lymphoma as well as detection of previously unknown sites of disease. No adverse reactions or toxicities were reported in this promising imaging technique.

With radioimmunotherapy (RIT) also called radiolabeled antibody therapy, monoclonal antibodies (Ab) labeled with higher doses of radionuclides are designed to selectively kill tumor cells while sparing normal tissues. Antibodies are proteins that recognize and attach to antigens such as tumor-associated antigens (e.g., CEA, AFP, ferritin, CA-125). A radioactive substance (e.g., iodine-131, yttrium-90) is attached to the antibody. The half-life of the isotope should be long enough to deliver an adequate dose to the tumor. RIT has been more effective in the radiosensitive hematologic malignancies, lymphomas and leukemias, than in solid tumors (Jurcic & Scheinberg, 1994). The radioactive labeled Ab should clear rapidly from the circulation, selectively target the tumor cells, and not be translocated to a non-tumor site, causing normal tissue irradiation. This is a particularly critical issue with radiometals where the free isotope may localize in bone marrow or bone. Myelotoxicity is the dose-limiting factor in RIT and in some studies, high-dose RIT has been followed by autologous bone marrow rescue. Macklis and associates (1994) report objective responses with RIT in greater than 50 percent of patients treated for refractory HD and NHL in spite of relatively low total dose per cycle of RIT (generally less than 15 Gy).

In a phase II trial, Press and associates (1995) recently used radiolabeled ^{131}I first to detect and then to treat areas of disease in relapsed B cell lymphoma. Complete responses were achieved in 16 of 21 patients. Autologous bone marrow reinfusions or peripheral blood stem cell transplants were performed to counteract severe myelosuppression in all patients. Promising results with multiple RIT clinical trials have led researchers to continue to investigate methods of optimizing radiolabeled antibodies and integrating them with conventional treatment.

Oncologic Emergencies in HD and NHL

Radiation therapy can be used to treat several oncologic emergencies related to HD and NHL to reduce symptoms. Because they are highly radiosensitive, these tumors often decrease in size rapidly in response to radiation. Mediastinal adenopathy generally becomes symptomatic in an insidious manner but may evolve rapidly and result in superior vena cava (SVC) syndrome. Venous drainage of the upper thorax is obstructed by the enlarged mediastinal nodes causing distention of the neck and chest veins, facial edema and plethora, and arm edema. Airway obstruction, hoarseness, cough, and dyspnea are common in this syndrome. Radiation therapy and/or chemotherapy can rapidly improve symptoms.

Spinal cord compression and increased intracranial pressure related to HD and NHL require immediate treatment. Radiation can be used to rapidly reduce the size of the tumor and reduce symptoms.

Although tumor lysis syndrome is most often related to tumor breakdown by chemotherapy, radiation therapy may also contribute to tumor lysis syndrome. Onset is usually very rapid and can result in death because of acute renal failure. Tumor lysis syndrome may be prevented with adequate hydration and high doses of allopurinol.

Side Effects of Radiation Therapy for HD and NHL

Sequelae of treatment are very important given the long-term survival and cure rates in HD and NHL (see Table 15–9). Side effects in combined therapy are more difficult to separate due to the effects of chemotherapy and radiation therapy on many of the same tissues. Side effects of radiation therapy depend on factors such as dose, volume of tissue irradiated, and specific site of irradiation. Most of the complications of HD and NHL irradiation occur in the mantle field. Doses of radiation administered in treatment of HD and NHL are frequently less than doses delivered for other types of cancer. Therefore, side effects in areas receiving lower doses are likely to be less severe though otherwise similar in type of effect. Specific detailed nursing management of radiation side effects can be reviewed in other chapters of the book related to specific sites of irradiation. For example, side effects from treatment of Waldeyer's ring are similar to those from other head and neck irradiation, and are less severe.

Acute Side Effects

Large volumes of tissue affecting numerous organs are often irradiated in patients with HD and NHL. Acute side effects include changes in blood counts, mild skin reaction, occipital hair loss, sore throat, possible altered sense of taste, xerostomia, esophagitis with dysphagia, fatigue, nausea, vomiting (infrequent), and diarrhea (rare). Early satiety has also been reported (Zinzani et al., 1994). Symptomatic management is generally administered.

Bone Marrow

Hematopoietic stem cells are among the most radiosensitive cells in the body. Limited amounts of bone marrow are irradiated locally in many fields and may alter blood counts. In the adult, distribution of active bone marrow is approximately 40 percent in the pelvis and 25 percent in the thoracic and lumbar vertebrae. Peripheral blood count changes related to radiation therapy are a result of effects on the blood forming organs and not an effect on circulating blood cells (Cox, 1994). Irradiation of large amounts of bone marrow may result in leukopenia, granulocytopenia, thrombocytopenia and anemia. Recovery of marrow after irradiation depends on patient age, dose of radiation, previous treatment affecting bone marrow, and volume of marrow in the radiation

Table 15-9 • Early and Late Effects of Radiation Therapy for HD and NHL

Site	Early Effects	Intermediate/Late Effects
HEAD AND NECK		
Mucosa	Mild mucositis	
Salivary glands	Xerostomia	Xerostomia, dental caries
Tongue, taste buds	Changes in taste	
Thyroid		Hypothyroidism
CHEST		
Lung	Radiation pneumonitis	Radiation pneumonitis, pulmonary fibrosis
Heart		Pericarditis, pancarditis, myocardial infarction
Esophagus	Mild esophagitis	
Hair	Occipital alopecia	
ABDOMEN		
Spine		Lhermitte's sign
		In children, significantly damages growth in axial spine.
Small bowel	Diarrhea	Small bowel obstruction
PELVIS		
Ovaries		Ovarian failure especially if >25
Testes		Azoospermia
Bone marrow	Thrombocytopenia, leukopenia	Immunologic dysfunction
		Herpes zoster, sepsis
		Myelodysplastic syndrome/secondary leukemia
General	Nausea and vomiting	
All sites	Fatigue	Carcinogenesis

fields. After total nodal irradiation, suppression of marrow may last for longer than a year. Knox et al. (1994) found that filgrastim (G-CSF) given to patients during subdiaphragmatic irradiation after mantle irradiation significantly increased the total white blood cell and absolute neutrophil cell (ANC) counts.

Skin

Skin reactions are generally mild to moderate erythema possibly with tanning. Skin reactions may be worse in patients who have received radiosensitizing chemotherapy (e.g., doxorubicin) that enhances skin reactions.

Mantle fields that extend to the mandible cause temporary occipital alopecia, a side effect that is often very disturbing to patients, especially those with short hair. Patient education prior to mantle irradiation must include information regarding this side effect.

Head, Neck, and Chest

Patients treated in the head and neck region (e.g., for Waldeyer's ring NHL) experience sore throat and significant taste loss as well as unpleasant tastes at approximately 30 Gy. They may continue to experience mild taste intensity impairment for 6 to 19 months after radiation therapy (Schwartz et al., 1993). The mechanisms of taste affected by radiation are unclear and radiation-induced salivary dysfunction alone is not likely to account for taste impairments.

Xerostomia increases risk of dental caries, periodontal disease, mucositis, difficulty eating, and altered taste. Dental prophylaxis is necessary with frequent cleaning and regular administration of fluoride solution. Dry mouth is also a problem when the mantle field is treated because the submandibular salivary glands are included in the treatment volume.

When the mediastinum is irradiated the patient will most likely experience a mild esophagitis with mild dysphagia.

Fatigue

Many patients undergoing cancer treatment experience significant amounts of fatigue possibly related to both physical and psychological factors. Fatigue may be an issue any time large radiation fields are treated such as the mantle, abdominal, and inverted Y fields. A study of patients treated for Hodgkin's disease with radiation demonstrated that most patients experienced a decreased energy level, which improved 6 to 18 months after treatment with one-third of these patients continuing to experience reduced energy (Fobair et al., 1986). Patients who receive combination therapy may experience fatigue related to both radiation therapy and chemotherapy (see Chapter 8).

Gastrointestinal

Nausea with or without vomiting may accompany radiation therapy especially when the stomach or significant amounts of intestine are in the field or when large volumes of tissue are treated. Patients may also experience gastritis when the stomach is irradiated. Early satiety as well as nausea, vomiting, and gastritis often contribute to reduced nutritional intake.

Diarrhea is an uncommon side effect. Factors that contribute to this low incidence of diarrhea include reduction in size of radiation fields after relatively low doses (both daily fraction and total dose) to large areas, blocking as much bowel as possible, and the use of lateral fields.

Intermediate and Late Side Effects

In the last 30 years, the long-term survival for HD and NHL has improved dramatically, making late effects a very important consideration of treatment. Goals of long-term follow-up include early detection of disease recurrence and late complications of treatment. Late complications may be related to direct injury to tissues caused by radiation therapy and/or chemotherapy, surgery (if applicable), or from persistent immunologic deficits related to the disease or treatment. Intermediate and late side effects of radiation include sepsis, immunologic impairments (herpes zoster), hypothyroidism, xerostomia, cardiac injury, pulmonary injury (pneumonitis and fibrosis), Lhermitte's sign, alteration in fertility, carcinogenesis, and psychosocial issues and concerns.

Sepsis

Infection is a risk for patients treated for HD and NHL and may be treatment-related or disease-related. Splenectomy or splenic irradiation increases the risk of life-threatening sepsis, especially with gram-positive encapsulated organisms. These infections are especially severe in children and young adults who receive chemotherapy. Jockovich et al. (1994) describes contributing factors to postsplenectomy sepsis as impaired humoral re-

sponsiveness, modified production of specific antibodies, and treatment- and disease-related immunologic changes. Late death from sepsis occurs in 0.5 percent of patients (Leibenhaut, 1993). Pneumococcal vaccination and possibly *Haemophilus influenzae* vaccination before the start of treatment may be recommended. Patients who have had a splenectomy should immediately report fevers more than 38°C. Prophylactic antibiotics may be recommended especially prior to invasive medical procedures.

Immunologic Impairments

Immunologic impairments due to disease and treatment may persist for years (Erickson, 1994). Fifteen to 20 percent of patients treated for Hodgkin's disease develop herpes zoster within the first 2 years after treatment. Acyclovir may be used to treat the herpes zoster.

Hypothyroidism

Hancock and associates (1991) reviewed 1677 patients with HD treated with radiation therapy that included the thyroid region and found the actuarial risk of hypothyroidism was 44% at 25 years after irradiation. The risk of thyroid dysfunction is higher in patients under 16 years of age (Tarbell et al., 1990). Decreased thyroid function is most often identified during the second and third years after treatment. Hypothyroidism can be detected by an increase in TSH and is treated with thyroid replacement therapy.

Xerostomia

Xerostomia is an early side effect that may persist long after treatment has been completed. The degree of xerostomia depends on the total dose and the volume of salivary glands included in the treatment fields. Treatment of Waldeyer's ring includes the parotid and the submandibular glands. Xerostomia is more problematic after this treatment than after mantle irradiation. Mantle fields generally include treatment of the submandibular salivary glands but not the parotid glands. Dental evaluation prior to treatment and ongoing dental care including fluoride is needed for all patients with xerostomia.

Cardiac Injury

Patients undergoing mantle irradiation for HD have a dose-dependent increased risk for cardiac injury including acute pericarditis, pericardial fibrosis, pancarditis (pericardial and myocardial fibrosis), valvular defects, conduction defects, and coronary artery disease. Since the 1970s, changes in treatment techniques have resulted in reduced doses to the heart in many patients. Hancock, Tucker, and Hoppe (1993c) followed 2232 consecutive HD patients treated from 1960 through 1991 and found an excess of heart disease-related deaths in patients who had cardiac irradiation greater than 30 Gy. A 3.1 to 3.2 increased risk of fatal myocardial infarction following mantle irradiation has been reported (Hancock et al., 1993c; Kaufman & Longo, 1995). Other factors influencing increased risk were age less than 20 years old at the time of irradiation, minimal protective cardiac blocking, and increased time since treatment.

Infrequently (less than 5 percent) acute, delayed, or chronic radiation pericarditis results from mantle irradiation. Onset of symptoms usually occurs 4 to 12 months after treatment but may occur years after irradiation. Symptoms such as pleuritic chest pain, friction rub, and fever may initially be managed with analgesics and nonsteroidal anti-inflammatory drugs. The patient may also have asymptomatic pericardial effusion, constrictive pericarditis, or tamponade (Benoff & Schweitzer, 1994). Constrictive pericarditis or tamponade occurs in approximately 1 percent of patients after mantle irradiation and may require surgery. The differential diagnosis includes recurrent Hodgkin's disease.

Other infrequent cardiac complications, especially after high-dose mediastinal irradiation, include myocardial and endocardial fibrosis, valvular fibrosis, and conduction abnormalities. Increased incidence of coronary artery disease has been reported following mediastinal radiation especially in patients irradiated at a young age (Benoff & Schweitzer, 1994; Hancock et al., 1993a). Regimens such as ABVD that include the cardiotoxic drug, doxorubicin, may increase toxicity to the heart when used in conjunction with mantle irradiation (Horning et al., 1994).

Pulmonary Injury

Injury to the lungs secondary to irradiation is related to the volume of lung in the field, total dose, fractionation, and type of radiation. Initial changes in tissue in the first 2 months after treatment include injury to small vessels and capillaries causing increased capillary permeability and alveolar exudates. At 2 to 9 months, changes include obstruction of capillaries by platelets, fibrin, and collagen with hyperplasia of type II pneumocytes and alveolar wall infiltration. Fibrosis is a late change. Mild early and intermediate pneumonitis may resolve (Horning et al., 1994). Man-

tle irradiation includes a considerable portion of the pulmonary parenchyma in the irradiated volume and may result in a mild radiation pneumonitis generally appearing 6 to 12 weeks after completion of the course of treatment. If symptomatic, the patient will experience symptoms such as cough, fever, and pleuritic chest pain, which subside over 4 to 6 months. Another clinical sign of pneumonitis includes a rapid pulse rate at rest. Chest x ray may show infiltrates corresponding to the treatment portals. Less than 5 percent of patients will be symptomatic (Tarbell et al., 1990). Radiation pneumonitis is managed symptomatically with a few patients being treated with a course of corticosteroids.

Signs of pulmonary fibrosis outlining the irradiated field on x ray are frequently observed after mantle irradiation but are not generally associated with symptoms. Gustavsson and colleagues (1992) describe mild perfusion and ventilation defects after 35 to 43 Gy mantle irradiation that were clinically insignificant in the majority of patients.

Several chemotherapy agents, including bleomycin, cyclophosphamide, methotrexate, and procarbazine, are known to be toxic to the lungs. Mah and associates (1994) conducted a prospective study to assess the incidence of lung changes determined by computed tomography related to mantle-type radiation therapy fields combined with multiagent chemotherapy. Results indicated that the addition of adriamycin, bleomycin, vincristine, DTIC (ABVD) or cyclophosphamide, adriamycin, vincristine (CAV) to radiation therapy reduced lung tolerance to radiation by 3 to 14 percent.

Neurologic Sequelae

Lhermitte's sign is the most common neurologic complication due to radiation therapy for HD and NHL and is characterized by numbness, tingling, or "electric shock-like" sensations extending into the arms and legs with neck flexion. Transient demyelinization of the spinal cord in the radiation field may be responsible for this effect, which occurs in 10 to 15 percent of patients 1½ to 3 months after mantle irradiation. Lhermitte's sign usually resolves over 2 to 6 months without treatment. These symptoms are not associated with permanent sequelae. Spinal cord transverse myelitis can occur months to years after irradiation if mantle and paraaortic fields overlap at the cord. However, extreme care is taken to avoid this complication.

Gonadal Dysfunction

Infertility may be induced by both radiation therapy and chemotherapy. Gonadal dysfunction is a concern in younger patients treated for HD and NHL not only because of reproductive issues in both men and women but also because of the effect on gonadal endocrine function in women. The incidence of gonadal dysfunction is markedly lower in patients treated for NHL than in patients treated for HD (Bokemeyer et al., 1994). Pelvic irradiation may affect fertility in both men and women. Shielding the testes reduces azoospermia and allows recovery of sperm counts (see Figure 15–10). Direct or scatter radiation in men of more than 2 Gy to the gonads results in sterility. Cumulative cyclophosphamide dose significantly affects sperm counts and high doses may result in permanent sterility.

Ovarian irradiation of 2 to 10 Gy may result in ovarian failure and sterility in women depending upon the age at the time of treatment. Premenopausal women over the age of 30 years may experience menopausal symptoms due to scat-

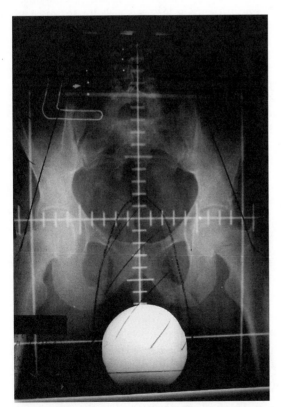

Figure 15-10 • Pelvic field in a 33-year-old male with stage IIIA mixed cellularity HD. Clam shell shielding is used to reduce scatter radiation to the testes.

tered radiation even after oophoropexy in HD. Scattered radiation is higher in women who are treated in the pelvic region. This scattered radiation may not be sufficient to cause menopausal symptoms in younger women. Madsen and associates (1995) studied pregnancies in 36 women age 10 to 40 years who had normal menstrual function when diagnosed with HD and who received mantle and paraaortic irradiation of 40 to 44 Gy. Scatter radiation dose to the ovaries was calculated to be 3.2 Gy. There were 38 pregnancies in 18 of the women. All children were normal. Premature menopause was experienced by one of the 36 women.

Alkylating agents often cause amenorrhea during treatment. When pelvic irradiation is combined with chemotherapy, the risk of impaired menstrual function and fertility may also occur in women under 30 years of age. Aisner and colleagues (1993) studied 221 patients of reproductive age successfully treated for HD with radiation therapy, chemotherapy, or both to determine the outcome of pregnancies. Ninety-four patients (43 females and 51 males) actively attempted conception resulting in 84 pregnancies and 68 living children. Of patients treated with both chemotherapy and radiation therapy, frequency of pregnancy in female patients and partners of male patients was lower than in the general population. Female patients had a higher rate of pregnancy than did partners of male patients. When compared with pregnancies in these patients before treatment and pregnancies in general, there were no apparent increases in complications of pregnancy, spontaneous abortions, or congenital abnormalities after treatment.

Gastrointestinal Complications

Sequelae of paraaortic field irradiation is rare. According to DeVita and colleagues (1993), small bowel obstruction occurs in 2.5 percent of patients, a finding similar to that seen with laparotomy without radiation therapy. Wide-field irradiation is limited by normal tissue tolerance in the abdomen. Doses used in subdiaphragmatic large-field treatment infrequently cause late radiation enteritis with bloody diarrhea, steatorrhea, or bowel obstruction.

Carcinogenesis

Carcinogenesis is a late effect that may occur after treatment for HD and NHL. Some question has arisen concerning whether second malignancies are treatment-related or a possibly genetic predisposition of the patient (Stupp et al., 1994). Second malignancies have been extensively studied in HD but less so in NHL. Age at diagnosis is a factor. Biti and associates (1994) have reported an increase in second malignancies in patients older at diagnosis of HD and as time since treatment increased.

Secondary acute leukemia occurs in both HD and NHL but is a higher risk in HD. Alkylating chemotherapy is known to be leukemogenic. The leukemogenic effects of radiation therapy are more difficult to determine. The occurrence of leukemia after treatment with radiation therapy alone is very rare (Cox, 1994; Hoppe et al., 1992). However, if radiation is used in combination with alkylating agent chemotherapy, leukemia risk is especially increased when chemotherapy is used for prolonged periods. Peak incidence is 4 to 9 years after treatment. The role of radiation therapy in increasing the risk of leukemia is controversial. Some investigators believe that the risk of leukemia after treatment of NHL with combined chemotherapy and radiation therapy is similar to the risk of chemotherapy alone (Ellis & Lishner, 1993). Others believe that second malignancies in general are more frequent after chemotherapy, especially when associated with subtotal or total nodal irradiation (Biti et al., 1994). Ellis and Lishner (1993) describe an increased risk of leukemia in patients with NHL as 10 to 105 times greater than that of the general population and list possible contributing factors as intrinsic susceptibility, impaired cellular immunity exacerbated by therapy, and effects of treatment especially chemotherapy.

Patients with HD are at increased risk of developing diffuse, aggressive lymphomas. Many of these involve the GI tract or retroperitoneum. The development of treatment-related solid tumors in HD has been attributed to either chemotherapy or radiation therapy with a latent period of 7 to 10 years. For more than 20 years after radiation therapy, there is increased risk of radiation-induced solid tumors, especially lung cancer and breast cancer (Kaufman & Longo, 1995). Hancock, Tucker, and Hoppe (1993b) reported a high risk of breast cancer in women under 30 years of age treated for HD with most of the tumors arising at the edge or within the mantle field. They recommend that younger women treated with mantle irradiation begin screening with mammograms no later than 10 years after the treatment.

Data concerning the risk of developing solid tumors after NHL have not been conclusive. Most studies have suggested that the risk of solid tumors is similar to that of the population in general but a few authors have suggested that bladder (also associated with cyclophosphamide) and lung (also associated with smoking) carcinomas occur relatively more frequently in patients treated for NHL (Ellis & Lishner, 1993).

Psychosocial Issues

Many patients with HD and NHL survive for many years after diagnosis and potentially face numerous psychosocial issues. The diagnosis of cancer has a powerful impact and creates circumstances that force patients to confront their own mortality. Treatment is often difficult and not only requires time away from work and routine activities but also may necessitate dependence on others. Insurance and expense may also be issues in patients with HD and NHL. After treatment is completed, there is the ongoing fear of recurrence and possible long-term side effects of treatment. Fobair et al. (1986) studied psychosocial problems in 403 long-term survivors of HD and identified difficulties in the areas of sense of well-being, family relationships, and employment. Persistent energy loss was a factor for most patients, especially for those who were older. Depression was noted in 18 percent and was correlated with energy loss, decreased sexual interest, poor body image, altered work patterns, and other problems. Moderately high divorce rates (32 percent), problems with infertility (18 percent), and less interest in sexual activity (20 percent) were reported. Work difficulties were reported by 42 percent. Patient education, individual counseling, and support groups may be helpful to patients during and after treatment.

Total Body Irradiation

Total body irradiation in preparation for bone marrow transplant is associated with a number of early and late side effects. Patients often experience nausea and vomiting. However, newer antiemetic medications such as ondansetron have effectively minimized this side effect (Ozsahin et al., 1994). An elevated systemic temperature of >38°C may occur with or without chills for 24 hours after irradiation. Headache, xerostomia, mild skin erythema, and diarrhea have also been reported. Ocular symptoms may include decreased lacrimation or ocular dryness, photophobia, and conjunctival edema. Decreased progenitor cells of plasma cells and lymphocytes reduce the effectiveness of the immune system.

The lungs are the dose-limiting organs in TBI. Interstitial pneumonitis (IP) and fibrosis can occur after lung irradiation. Graft versus disease is a major risk factor in the development of IP. Interstitial pneumonia has resulted in death weeks to months after total body irradiation (TBI).

Veno-occlusive disease (VOD) of the liver is an early life-threatening condition related to BMT conditioning with TBI and high-dose chemotherapy and is responsible for 5 to 10 percent of deaths that occur in conditioning (Ozsahin et al., 1994). Occlusion of small hepatic veins is related to hepatocytic damage. Etiology of VOD is not understood but risk factors include pretherapy hepatic disease, use of cytosine arabinoside, and radiation therapy.

Eyes cannot be adequately shielded during TBI and cataracts may result. Cataracts occur less frequently with fractionated than with single-dose radiation. Fife and colleagues (1994) reported the probability of cataract development requiring surgery after a single-dose regimen was 5 percent at 2 years, 39 percent at 5 years, and 58 percent at 10 years. Changes in endocrine function have been reported after conditioning for BMT with radiation and chemotherapy. Ovarian failure occurs in women over 25 years of age and in all but a very few women under age 25 (Ozsahin et al., 1994). Most men become azoospermic after TBI.

Treatment-induced myelodysplastic syndrome (MDS) and secondary leukemia, an infrequent complication after ABMT, may be influenced by the intensity and timing of chemotherapy, particularly alkylating agents, and dose and extent of radiation therapy. Preparation for ABMT with high-dose chemotherapy with or without TBI and prior, often prolonged, therapy for HD and NHL may play a role in inducing neoplastic transformation (Miller et al., 1994). However, it is impossible to determine the relative roles of each prior treatment. In their study of 262 patients who underwent ABMT for NHL, Stone and associates (1994) found that the two most predictive factors for development of posttransplant MDS were the use of pelvic irradiation and the interval between first treatment for NHL and subsequent ABMT procedure. Patients who developed MDS had a 31-month elapsed time since first therapy compared to 14 months in the group that did not develop MDS. Pretreatment factors found to increase the risk of developing MDS were age over 38 years and platelets less than 252,000. Etiology of MDS is uncertain but several factors have been considered (Miller et al., 1994; Stone et al., 1994). The high-dose therapy itself may damage rather than destroy some bone marrow stem cells. Failure of transplantation may result from failure to eliminate the lymphoma from

the patient or may arise from infused marrow rather than residual malignant host cells (Lister & Armitage, 1995). Chemotherapy and/or radiation therapy that is often administered well before the transplant may also play a role in the etiology of MDS.

Alkylating agents and TBI severely affect ovarian function. Although not life-threatening, these effects have implications for quality of life. In a prospective study Chatterjee and colleagues (1994) evaluated pituitary-gonadal function in 15 postmenarchal women ages 17 to 30 years of age with hematological malignancies who received bone marrow transplant (BMT). All patients had evidence of gonadal insufficiency prior to BMT preparation, possibly related to combination chemotherapy. All patients received chemoradiotherapy conditioning prior to transplant resulting in further injury and ovarian failure. Three to 4 months posttransplant, all patients were amenorrheic and experienced menopausal symptoms such as hot flashes (53 percent), dyspareunia (53 percent), diminished libido (40 percent), cystitis-like symptoms (25 percent), and insomnia (40 percent). Acute damage most often appears to be absolute and irreversible, and progressive depletion of the follicular compartment and interstitial fibrosis of the ovary have been demonstrated. Degree of recovery is uncertain. The anterior pituitary gland secretions appear unaffected. Table 15–9 summarizes early and late effects of irradiation in different regions of the body.

Radiation Effects in Children

As survival rates in children with cancer have increased, more attention has been paid to long-term complications of treatment, which influence quality of life and long-term survival. These complications may not be evident until many years after successful treatment. Multimodality treatment may also influence complications. Cardiac injury may be related to radiation therapy and to some chemotherapy agents (e.g., doxorubicin). Heart injury resulting from radiation therapy has most often occurred after mantle irradiation for mediastinal HD and is dependent upon the radiation dose to the heart. Complications include acute pericarditis, chronic pericarditis, coronary artery disease with myocardial infarction, valvular defects, and pericardial and myocardial fibrosis (Green, 1993; Hancock et al., 1993c). Hancock and associates (1993a) reviewed 635 children and adolescents treated with mantle irradiation for HD. Cardiac deaths occurred 3 to 22 years after 42 to 45 Gy to the mediastinum. Twelve cardiac deaths occurred, 7 from acute myocardial infarction, 3 from valve or congenital heart disease, and 2 from radiation pericarditis or pancarditis (pericardial and myocardial fibrosis). Risk of death from acute myocardial infarction was comparable for radiation therapy alone or radiation therapy combined with chemotherapy. Combined treatment was an increased risk for other cardiac deaths. No cardiac deaths occurred in patients who did not receive mediastinal irradiation or only lower mediastinal irradiation. Risk of cardiac injury and death have implications for low-dose radiation and combined modality treatment in children with HD needing treatment to the mediastinum.

Pulmonary function is also affected by radiation therapy and several chemotherapy agents (e.g., bleomycin, methotrexate). Green (1993) found that 20 percent of patients with HD irradiated to one or both lungs experienced symptomatic pneumonitis with a median onset of 3 months after completion of radiation. Symptoms often improve rapidly with corticosteroids. Interference with alveolar and chest wall development in irradiated areas may occur in young children. Late effects on lung include reduced diffusing capacity and small decreases in alveolar volume. Children treated with bleomycin in addition to radiation to the lung may experience more severe pulmonary reactions.

Radiation of the abdomen in children with HD or NHL may deliver dose to the extrarenal artery and the upper pole of the kidney parenchyma resulting in impaired renal function. Chemotherapy agents such as cisplatin (CDDP), BCNU, nitrosurea, ifosfamide, and methotrexate are also nephrotoxic.

Radiation therapy in children causes premature closure of irradiated epiphyses of growing long bones with resultant cessation of further growth.

Beaty and associates (1995) reviewed 499 children and adolescents treated for HD and found 25 second malignancies: 19 solid tumors, 5 leukemias, and 1 NHL. Twenty-three of the second malignancies occurred in patients 10 years old or older at diagnosis indicating a higher risk in patients treated as adolescents. Females were at increased risk. No differences were found between groups treated with radiation therapy alone, chemotherapy alone, or combined therapy.

Resources

The nursing literature has limited information specifically regarding radiation therapy in the treatment of HD and NHL. One recent publication by Gomez (1995) is a teaching resource for patients receiving mantle irradiation. Articles by Erickson (1994) and Lundquist (1994) are among the very few specifically related to HD and NHL in the nursing literature.

The National Cancer Institute (NCI) provides up-to-date information regarding HD and NHL through the PDQ (Physician's Data Query) database. Information is available for both patients and health care professionals through CancerFax and through the Internet through CancerNet. CancerLit is also available for current bibliographies. Other cancer databases on the Internet also contain information on HD and NHL.

Conclusions

HD and NHL are generally very treatable diseases. HD has an especially good prognosis. However, treatment is often difficult and risk of relapse and sequelae of treatment are frequently challenging. Nurses who care for these patients must understand the natural history of the diseases as well as treatment and side effects. Nurses have an essential role in patient education and minimizing and managing side effects of treatment.

References

Aisner J, Wiernik PH, & Pearl P (1993). Pregnancy outcome in patients treated for Hodgkin's disease. *Journal of Clinical Oncology, 11*, 507–512.

American Cancer Society. (1997). *Cancer Facts and Figures—1997.* Atlanta: American Cancer Society.

Ballester OF, Moscinski L, Spiers A, & Balducci L (1993). Non-Hodgkin's lymphoma in the older person: A review. *Journal of the American Geriatric Society, 41*, 1245–1254.

Baum RP, Niesen A, Hertel A, Adams S, Kojouharoff G, Goldenberg DM, & Hor G (1994). Initial clinical results with technetium-99m-labeled LL2 monoclonal antibody fragment in the radioimmunodetection of B-cell lymphomas. *Cancer, 73*, 896–899.

Beaty O, Hudson MM, Greenwald C, Luo X, Fang L, Wilimas JA, Thompson EI, Kun LE, & Pratt CB (1995). Subsequent malignancies in children and adolescents after treatment for Hodgkin's disease. *Journal of Clinical Oncology, 13*, 603–609.

Benoff LJ, & Schweitzer P (1994). Radiation therapy-induced cardiac injury. *American Heart Journal, 129*, 1193–1196.

Biti G, Cellai E, Magrini SM, Papi MG, Ponticelli P, & Boddi V (1994). Second solid tumors and leukemia after treatment for Hodgkin's disease: An analysis of 1121 patients from a single institution. *International Journal of Radiation Oncology, Biology, Physics, 29*, 25–31.

Bokemeyer C, Schmoll HJ, van Rhee J, Kuczyk M, Schuppert F, & Poliwoda H (1994). Long-term gonadal toxicity after therapy for Hodgkin's and non-Hodgkin's lymphoma. *Annals of Hematology, 68,* 105–110.

Carbone PP, & Kaplan HS (1971). Report of the committee on Hodgkin's disease staging classification. *Cancer Research, 31,* 1860–1861.

Chatterjee R, Mills W, Katz M, McGarrigle HH, & Goldstone AH (1994). Prospective study of pituitary-gonadal function to evaluate short-term effects of ablative chemotherapy or total body irradiation with autologous or allogeneic marrow transplantation in post-menarcheal female patients. *Bone Marrow Transplantation, 13,* 511–517.

Cox JD (1994). Lymphomas and leukemias. In JD Cox (Ed.), *Moss' Radiation Oncology: Rationale, Technique, Results,* (7th ed., pp. 795–826). St. Louis: Mosby.

Demirer T, Petersen FB, Appelbaum FR, Barnett TA, Sanders J, Deeg HJ, Storb R, Doney K, Bensinger WI, Shannon-Dorcy K, et al. (1995). Allogeneic marrow transplantation following cyclophosphamide and escalating doses of hyperfractionated total body irradiation in patients with advanced lymphoid malignancies: A phase I/II trial. *International Journal of Radiation Oncology, Biology, Physics, 32,* 1103–1109.

DeVita VT, Hellman S, & Jaffe ES (1993). Hodgkin's disease. In VT DeVita, S Hellman, & SA Rosenberg (Eds.), *Cancer Principles and Practice of Oncology,* (4th ed., pp. 1819–1858). Philadelphia: JB Lippincott.

DeVita VT, & Hubbard SM (1993). Hodgkin's Disease. *New England Journal of Medicine, 328,* 560–565.

Ellis M, & Lishner M (1993). Second malignancies following treatment in non-Hodgkin's lymphoma. *Leukemia and Lymphoma, 9,* 337–342.

Erickson JM (1994). Update on Hodgkin's disease. *Nurse Practitioner, 19,* 63–68.

Fajardo LF (1994a). Effects of ionizing radiation on lymph nodes. *Frontiers of Radiation Therapy and Oncology, 28,* 37–45.

Fajardo LF (1994b). Lymph nodes and cancer. *Frontiers of Radiation Therapy and Oncology, 28,* 1–10.

Fife K, Milan S, Westbrook K, Powles R, & Tait D (1994). Risk factors for requiring cataract surgery following total body irradiation. *Radiotherapy and Oncology, 33,* 93–98.

Fobair P, Hoppe RT, Bloom J, Cox R, Varghese A, & Spiegel D (1986). Psychosocial problems among survivors of Hodgkin's disease. *Journal of Clinical Oncology, 4,* 805–814.

Gail MH, Pluda JM, Rabkin CS, Biggar RJ, Goedert J, Horm JW, Sandik EJ, Yarchoan R, & Broder S (1991). Projections of the incidence of non-Hodgkin's lymphoma related to acquired immunodeficiency syndrome. *Journal of the National Cancer Institute, 83,* 695–701.

Gallucci BB, & McCarthy D (1995). The immune system. In PT Rieger (Ed.), *Biotherapy: A comprehensive review.* (pp. 15–42). Boston: Jones and Bartlett.

Glatstein E (1993). The vanishing lymphangiogram in Hodgkin's disease: The last of the Mohicans? *International Journal of Radiation Oncology, Biology, Physics, 25,* 567–568.

Gomez EG (1995). A teaching booklet for patients receiving mantle field irradiation. *Oncology Nursing Forum, 22,* 121–126.

Goss PE (1993). Non-Hodgkin's lymphomas in elderly patients. *Leukemia and Lymphoma, 10,* 147–156.

Green DM (1993). Effects of treatment for childhood cancer on vital organ systems. *Cancer, 71,* 3299–3305.

Gustavsson A, Eskilsson J, Landberg T, Larusdottir H, Svahn-Tapper G, White T, & Wollmer P (1992). Long-term effects on pulmonary function of mantle radiotherapy in patients with Hodgkin's disease. *Annals of Oncology, 3,* 455–461.

Hancock SL, Cox RS, & McDougall IR (1991). Thyroid diseases after treatment of Hodgkin's disease. *The New England Journal of Medicine, 325,* 599–605.

Hancock SL, Donaldson SS, & Hoppe RT (1993a). Cardiac disease following treatment of Hodgkin's disease in children and adolescents. *Journal of Clinical Oncology, 11,* 1208–1215.

Hancock SL, Tucker MA, & Hoppe RT (1993b). Breast cancer after treatment of Hodgkin's disease. *Journal of the National Cancer Institute, 85,* 25–31.

Hancock SL, Tucker MA, & Hoppe RT (1993c). Factors affecting late mortality from heart disease after treatment of Hodgkin's disease. *Journal of the American Medical Association, 270,* 1949–1955.

Hessol NA, Katz MH, Liu JY, Buchbinder SP, Rubino CJ, & Holmberg SD (1992). Increased incidence of Hodgkin's disease in homosexual men with HIV infection. *Annals of Internal Medicine, 117,* 309–311.

Hoppe RT, Glatstein E, & Wasserman TH (1992). Hodgkin's disease. In CA Perez, LW Brady (Eds.), *Principles and Practice of Radiation Oncology,* (2nd ed., pp. 1307–1328). Philadelphia: JB Lippincott.

Horning SJ (1993). Low-grade lymphoma 1993: State of the art. *Annals of Oncology, 5* (Suppl. 2), 23–27.

Horning SJ, Adhikari A, Rizk N, Hoppe RT, & Olshen RA (1994). Effect of treatment for Hodgkin's disease on pulmonary function: Results of a prospective study. *Journal of Clinical Oncology, 12,* 297–305.

Jockovich M, Mendenhall NP, Sombeck MD, Talbert JL, Copeland EM, & Bland KI (1994). Long-term complications of laparotomy in Hodgkin's disease. *Annals of Surgery, 219,* 615–624.

Jurcic JG, & Scheinberg DA (1994). Recent developments in the radioimmunotherapy of cancer. *Current Opinion in Immunology, 6,* 715–721.

Kaufman D, & Longo DL (1995). Hodgkin's disease. In MD Abeloff, JO Armitage, AS Lichter, and JE Niederhuber (Eds.), *Clinical Oncology* (pp. 2075–2107). NY: Churchill Livingstone.

Knox SJ, Fowler S, Marquez C, & Hoppe RT (1994). Effect of filgrastim (G-CSF) in Hodgkin's disease patients treated with radiation therapy. *International Journal of Radiation Oncology, Biology, Physics, 28,* 445–450.

Leibenhaut MH (1993). The changing role of staging laparotomy in the management of Hodgkin's disease. *Cancer Treatment and Research, 66,* 1–20.

Lister TA, & Armitage JO (1995). Non-Hodgkin's lymphomas. In MD Abeloff, JO Armitage, AS Lichter, and JE Niederhuber (Eds.), *Clinical Oncology* (pp. 2109–2147). New York: Churchill Livingstone.

Lister TA, Crowther D, Sutcliffe SB, Glatstein E, Canellos GP, Young RC, Rosenberg SA, Coltman CA, & Tubiana M (1989). Report of a committee convened to discuss the evaluation and staging of patients with Hodgkin's disease: Cotswolds meeting. *Journal of Clinical Oncology, 7,* 1630–1636.

Longo DL, DeVita VT, Jaffe ES, Mauch P, & Urba WJ (1993). In VT DeVita, S Hellman, & SA Rosenberg (Eds.), *Cancer Principles and Practice of Oncology,* (4th ed., pp. 1859–1927). Philadelphia: JB Lippincott.

Longo DL, Glatstein E, Duffey PL, Ihde DC, Hubbard SM, Fisher RI, Jaffe ES, Gilliom M, Young RC, & DeVita VT (1989). Treatment of localized aggressive lymphomas with combination chemotherapy followed by involved-field radiation therapy. *Journal of Clinical Oncology, 7,* 1295–1302.

Lukes RJ, Butler JJ, & Hicks BB (1966). Natural history of Hodgkin's disease as related to its pathologic picture. *Cancer, 19,* 317–344.

Lukes RJ, & Collins RD (1974). Immunologic characterization of human malignant lymphomas. *Cancer, 34,* 1488–1503.

Lundquist DM (1994). An update on non-Hodgkin's lymphomas. *Nurse Practitioner, 19,* 41–54.

Macklis RM, Beresford BA, & Humm JL (1994). Radiobiologic studies of low-dose-rate ^{90}Y-lymphoma therapy. *Cancer, 73,* 966–973.

Madsen BL, Giudice L, & Donaldson SS (1995). Radiation-induced premature menopause: a misconception. *International Journal of Radiation Oncology, Biology, Physics, 32,* 1461–1464.

Mah K, Keane TJ, VanDyk J, Braban LE, Poon PY, & Hao Y (1994). Quantitative effect of combined chemotherapy and fractionated radiotherapy on the incidence of radiation-induced lung damage: A prospective clinical study. *International Journal of Radiation Oncology, Biology, Physics, 28,* 563–574.

Medeiros LJ, & Jaffe ES (1993). Pathology of non-Hodgkin's lymphomas. In GA Pangalis & A Polliack (Eds.), *Benign and Malignant Lymphadenopathies: Clinical and Laboratory Diagnosis,* (pp. 187–246). USA: Harwood Academic Publishers.

Mendenhall NP, & Lynch JW (1995). The low-grade lymphomas. *Seminars in Radiation Oncology, 5,* 254–266.

Miller JS, Arthur DC, Litz CE, Neglia JP, Miller WJ, & Weisdorf DJ (1994). Myelodysplastic syndrome after autologous bone marrow transplantation: An additional late complication of curative cancer therapy. *Blood, 83,* 3780–3786.

Mueller N, Evans A, Harris NL, Comstock GW, Jellum E, Magnus K, Orentreich, N, Polk BF, & Vogelman J (1989). Hodgkin's disease and Epstein-Barr virus: Altered antibody pattern before diagnosis. *New England Journal of Medicine, 320,* 689–695.

National Cancer Institute (1982). The nonHodgkin's lymphoma pathologic classification project: NCI sponsored study of classification of nonHodgkin's lymphoma: Summary and description of a working formulation for clinical use. *Cancer, 49,* 2112–2135.

Newman JS, Francis IR, Kaminski MS, & Wahl RL (1994). Imaging of lymphoma with PET with 2-[F-18]-fluoro-2-deoxy-D-glucose: Correlation with CT. *Radiology, 190,* 111–116.

Ozsahin M, Pene F, Cosset JM, & Laugier A (1994). Morbidity after total body irradiation. *Seminars in Radiation Oncology, 4,* 95–102.

Pallesen G, Hamilton-Dutoit SJ, Rowe M, & Young LS (1991). Expression of Epstein-Barr virus latent gene products in tumor cells of Hodgkin's disease. *Lancet, 337,* 320–322.

Pallesen G, Hamilton-Dutoit SJ, & Zhou X (1993). The association of Epstein-Barr virus (EBV) with T cell lymphoproliferations and Hodgkin's disease: Two new developments in the EBV field. *Advances in Cancer Research, 62,* 179–239.

Parker SL, Tong T, Bolden S, and Wingo PA. (1997). Cancer statistics. *Ca-A Cancer Journal for Clinicians, 47,* 5-27.

Press OW, Eary JF, Appelbaum FR, Martin PJ, Nelp WB, Glenn S, Fisher DR, Porter B, Matthews DC, Gooley T, & Bernstein ID (1995). Phase II trial of ^{131}I-B1 (anti-CD20) antibody therapy with autologous stem cell transplantation for relapsed B cell lymphomas. *Lancet, 2,* 336–340.

Priest ER, Williams SF, & Golomb HM (1993). In GA Pangalis & A Polliack (Eds.), Benign and malignant lymphadenopathies: Clinical and laboratory diagnosis (pp. 65–81). Langhorne, PA: Harwood Academic Publishers.

Rappaport HW, & Winter J (1956). Follicular lymphoma: a reevaluation of its place in the scheme of malignant lymphoma based on a survey of 253 cases. *Cancer, 9,* 792–821.

Reddy S, Saxena VS, Pellettiere EV & Hendrickson FA (1989). Stage I and II non-Hodgkin's lymphomas: Long-term results of radiation therapy. *International Journal of Radiation Oncology, Biology, Physics, 16,* 687–692.

Salminen EK (1995). The outcome of ≥ 70-year-old non-Hodgkin's lymphoma patients. *International Journal of Radiation Oncology, Biology, Physics, 32,* 349–353.

Schwartz LK, Weiffenbach JM, Valdez IH, & Fox PC (1993). Taste intensity performance in patients irradiated to the head and neck. *Physiology and Behavior, 53,* 671–677.

Simon R, Durrleman S, Hoppe RT, Bonadonna G, Bloomfield CD, Rudders RA, Cheson BD & Berard CW (1988). The non-Hodgkin lymphoma pathologic classification project: Long-term follow-up of 1153 patients with non-Hodgkin lymphomas. *Annals of Internal Medicine, 109,* 939–945.

Sombeck MD, Mendenhall NP, Kaude JV, Tores GM, & Million RR (1992). Correlation of lymphangiography, computed tomography, and laparotomy in the staging of Hodgkin's disease. *International Journal of Radiation Oncology, Biology, Physics, 25,* 425–429.

Stone RM, Neuberg D, Soiffer R, Takvorian T, Whelan M, Rabinowe SN, Aster JC, Leavitt P, Mauch P, Freedman AS, & Nadler LM (1994). Myelodysplastic syndrome as a late complication following autologous bone marrow transplantation for non-Hodgkin's lymphoma. *Journal of Clinical Oncology, 12,* 2535–2542.

Stupp R, Samuels BL, & Ultmann JE (1994). Management of lymphoma in the 1990s: Introduction to the proceedings of the fifth international conference on malignant lymphoma. *Annals of Oncology 5,* 1–3.

Tarbell NJ, Thompson L, & Mauch P (1990). Thoracic irradiation in Hodgkin's disease: Disease control and long-term complications. *International Journal of Radiation Oncology, Biology, Physics, 18,* 275–281.

Urba WJ, & Longo DL (1992). Hodgkin's disease: Medical progress. *New England Journal of Medicine, 326,* 678–687.

Variakojis D, & Anastasi J (1993). Unresolved issues concerning Hodgkin's disease and its relationship to non-Hodgkin's lymphoma. *American Journal of Clinical Pathology, 99,* 436–445.

Wasserman TH, & Glatstein E (1992). Non-Hodgkin's lymphoma. In CA Perez, LW Brady (Eds.), *Principles and Practice of Radiation Oncology,* (2nd ed., pp. 1329–1344). Philadelphia: JB Lippincott.

Weisenburger DD (1994). Epidemiology of non-Hodgkin's lymphoma: Recent findings regarding an emerging epidemic. *Annals of Oncology, 5,* 19–24.

Wotherspoon AC, Ortiz-Hidalgo C, Falzon MR, & Isaacson PG (1991). *Helico-bacter pylori*-associated gastritis and primary B-cell gastric lymphoma. *Lancet, 2,* 1175–1176.

Zinzani PL, Barbieri E, Gherlinzoni F, Frezza G, Mazza P, Pica A, Ammendolia I, Bendandi M, Neri S, & Miniaci G (1994). Radiotherapy in early stage Hodgkin's disease. *Leukemia and Lymphoma, 13,* 285–289.

16
Lung Cancer

JOY MILLER KNOPP

Lung cancer remains the most frequent cause of cancer death in men and, in the last decade, has surpassed breast cancer as the most frequent cause of cancer death in women. Although progress has been made in recent years in improving long-term survival in lung cancer patients, only small gains have been made in 5-year survival rates, which have reached 13 percent in all patients, regardless of stage at diagnosis (Parker et al., 1997). Today, lung cancer is not considered to be a single disease entity, but rather several diseases characterized by histopathologic type, which determines patterns of spread, treatment options, and prognosis (Salazar et al., 1993).

Because bronchogenic carcinoma is a major oncologic problem, oncology nurses need to understand the pathophysiologic mechanisms that contribute to this disease. Nurses caring for lung cancer patients face significant challenges in dealing with different treatment modalities—surgery, radiation, chemotherapy, and/or biologic therapy—and with the natural progression of the disease (Schmitt, 1993). Most patients who have lung cancer will receive radiation therapy at some point during the course of their disease. Radiation treatment strategies in this disease depend upon its histopathologic type, extent (stage), and general well-being of the patient. This chapter describes the current state of knowledge and some promising newer treatment options. Numerous clinical trials that are under way or recently completed may establish new approaches to radiation therapy, and allow better integration with surgery and chemotherapy. Nursing interventions that minimize the symptoms of radiation therapy and thereby enhance the individual's quality of life are reviewed. Continuity of care issues provide a framework for long-term planning and for identifying potential problems. Late effects of therapy are discussed, because these must be anticipated

so that appropriate interventions and follow-up may be determined.

To understand the complications of radiation therapy related to the pulmonary system, one must first have a basic understanding of normal anatomy and physiology.

Anatomy of the Lung

Figure 16–1 illustrates the general anatomy of the thorax. The right lung consists of three lobes, the upper, middle, and lower. The oblique or major fissure separates the lower and the upper and middle lobes, and the horizontal or minor fissure divides the upper and middle lobes. The left lung consists of two lobes, upper and lower, divided by a single fissure. The trachea enters the mediastinum through the superior inlet of the thoracic cavity and bifurcates at the level of the fifth thoracic vertebrae. The hila of the lungs contain the bronchi, pulmonary arteries and veins, branches of the pulmonary plexus, bronchial arteries, veins, and lymphatics. The bronchi are lined with cilia that beat toward the pharynx to clear away foreign material. Irritation initiates the cough reflex to remove unwanted material. The respiratory unit consists of the bronchiole, alveolar ducts, atria, and alveoli. In the lungs there are approximately 300 million alveoli. Gaseous exchange occurs in the extremely thin alveolar walls, which consist almost entirely of capillaries. The alveolar gases being in close proximity to pulmonary blood allows the necessary diffusion to occur (Emami & Perez, 1992).

The lungs have a rich lymphatic supply. The lymphatic vessels drain the interstitial connective tissue and empty into several groups of nodes: the intrapulmonary nodes (along the secondary bronchi), the bronchopulmonary (hilar) nodes,

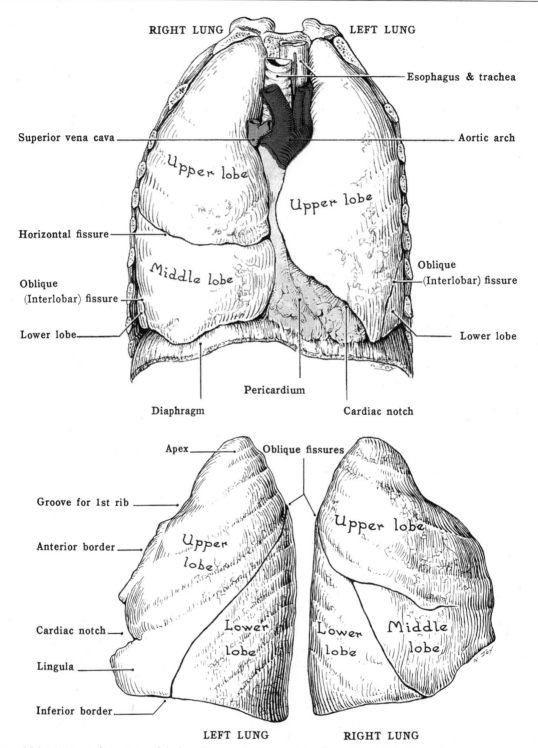

Figure 16-1 • Anatomical structures of the lung. Reprinted with permission from Grant J & Boileau C (1972). *Grant's Atlas of Anatomy* (6th ed.). Baltimore: Williams and Wilkins.

the mediastinal nodes, and the supraclavicular and scalene nodes. The intrapulmonary nodes are located peripherally along the segmental and sub-segmental bronchi. The bronchopulmonary nodes consist of the interlobar nodes, found along the lobar bronchi, and the hilar nodes, which are adjacent to the main bronchi. The mediastinal lymph nodes are subdivided into superior and inferior groups; the superior mediastinal lymph nodes are located above the carina (bifurcation of trachea) and consist of the upper paratracheal, tracheal (azygos), and aortic nodes; the inferior group are those in the subcarinal and lower mediastinal areas: paraesophageal, subcarinal, and nodes in the pulmonary ligaments. These distinctions become significant when planning radiation treatment fields, as they must include all potentially involved nodes and spare noninvolved tissue (Emami & Perez, 1992).

Physiology of Respiration

Guyton (1991) divides the process of respiration into four major categories: (1) pulmonary ventilation—inflow and outflow of air between atmosphere and alveoli; (2) diffusion of oxygen and carbon dioxide between alveoli and blood; (3) transport of oxygen and carbon dioxide in blood and body fluids to cells; and (4) regulation of ventilation.

Muscles of Breathing

Inflow and outflow of air is mediated by chest wall and diaphragmatic expansion and contraction. The movement of the diaphragm either lengthens or shortens the chest cavity, and the elevation or depression of the ribs regulates the anteroposterior chest cavity diameter.

When the diaphragm contracts, the chest cavity is pulled downward, increasing its length; relaxation of the diaphragm allows it to move upward with the elastic recoil of the lungs. With labored breathing, the abdominal muscles are also used, and their contraction forces abdominal contents against the base of the diaphragm, supplementing this upward movement.

With expiration, the ribs are pulled downward via their posterior attachment to the spinal column. With inspiration, the sternum is lifted upward and the ribs extend more horizontally, increasing the anterior-posterior diameter of the chest by approximately 20 percent. Normal breathing, however, is related almost entirely to the movement of the diaphragm. With dyspnea the external intercostals, sternocleidomastoids, scapular elevators, scalene, and erectus muscles of the spine are used to supplement inspiration, and the abdominals, internal intercostals, and posterior inferior serratus muscles assist expiration.

Pressures in the Lung

The compression and distention in the lungs caused by the respiratory muscles changes the pressure in the alveoli. Negative pressure with respect to the atmosphere during inspiration causes air to flow into the lungs. During expiration intraalveolar pressure rises and forces air out.

The membranes of the intrapleural space absorb fluids and gas, thereby creating a partial vacuum. The negative pressure of fluid in the intrapleural space is generally 10 mm Hg; this pressure allows the visceral pleura of the lungs to cling to the parietal pleura of the chest wall. The lungs are physically attached to the body only at the hila. As the chest cavity expands and contracts, this adherence allows the lungs to expand and contract as well. There are a few millimeters of a mucopolysaccharide fluid in the intrapleural space, which permits the sliding of the visceral pleura over the partial pleura as the lungs move up and down in the chest cavity (Guyton, 1991).

Lung Recoil and Surfactant

The lungs have a tendency to collapse based on their elastic properties and recoil away from the chest wall. Elastic fibers in the lung are stretched during inspiration and attempt to shorten. Alveoli also have a tendency to collapse from the surface tension of fluid within them.

Surfactant is a lipoprotein mixture secreted by alveolar type II pneumocytes in alveolar epithelium. The major component of surfactant is a detergent-like phospholipid known as phosphotidylcholine. This highly saturated phospholipid reduces surface tension within the alveoli and prevents alveolar collapse. Surfactant creates a layer between the fluid and air in the alveoli preventing the development of the high surface tension of a water-air interface (Coultas et al., 1987; Guyton, 1991; Shapiro et al., 1984). Without surfactant, pressures as high as 20 to 30 mm Hg are necessary to maintain open alveoli as the contractile force created by water tension tends to cause collapse. As alveoli become smaller, they have an even greater proclivity for collapse. Surfactant can reduce this surface tension, and the pressure required to maintain open alveoli can be reduced to only 3 to 5 mm Hg. Surfactant also plays an important role in maintaining the size of alveoli: large alveoli develop higher surface tension and become smaller, while with surfactant, small alveoli become larger as their surface tension decreases. The effect of radiation on surfactant may result in the development of pneumonitis as will be discussed later.

Energy of Respiration

Normal breathing requires only 3.5 percent of total energy. In pulmonary disease that alters compliance, increases airway resistance, or increases viscosity, as much as a third or more of total energy expended is devoted to respiration. This results in significant lifestyle changes for the individual (Guyton, 1991).

Epidemiology of Lung Cancer

Prior to the 20th century, lung cancer was uncommon, but in this century it has become a major worldwide problem. In the United States, approximately 178,100 new cases of lung cancer and 160,400 deaths from lung cancer were estimated for 1996 (Parker et al., 1997). Although the incidence of lung cancer is presently declining among middle-aged men, from a high of 87 per 100,000 in 1984 to 80 in 1991, it is increasing among women, from 37.7 per 100,000 in 1987 to 42 per 100,000 in 1991. Epidemiologic research has convincingly established that cigarette smoking is a cause of lung cancer, accounting for the majority of lung cancer cases. A study by Thun and associates (1995) examined changes in smoking-specific death rates from the 1960s to the 1980s. They found that premature mortality (the difference in all-cause death rates between smokers and nonsmokers) doubled in women and continued unchanged in men from the 1960s to the 1980s. Lung cancer surpassed coronary heart disease as the single largest subset of smoking-attributable deaths among white middle-class smokers. Other remediable causes of lung cancer, including exposure to occupational agents and indoor air pollutants, have been identified and are listed on Table 16–1.

Cigarette smoke, containing at least 43 carcinogens and the highly addictive substance nicotine, is the major initiator and promoter of lung cancer (Novello et al., 1991). Active and passive smoking probably accounts for more than 80 percent of cases of bronchogenic cancer. This risk of lung cancer is related to the cumulative number of cigarettes smoked; in persons with similar pack-per-year consumption, however, the duration of smoking appears to be more important than the number of cigarettes smoked per day. Other factors that influence cancer risk are smoking practices (size of puff, depth of inhalation, time of breath holding, amount of cigarette smoked) and type of cigarette smoked (tar content, filtered vs. nonfiltered). Of late, smoking in men has decreased; they are not initiating the habit as often, and are stopping at an earlier age. Women, however, are beginning to smoke in higher numbers than in the past, and are beginning to smoke in their teenage years. In addition, the marked increase in cigarette production and tobacco consumption in developing countries, contributes to this problem globally.

The focus of health care professionals should be on both prevention and reduction of smoking. Smoking cessation can be supported through the use of nicotine replacement, self-help "quit kits," and counseling. Educational tools are numerous, and can be obtained through the American Lung Association, American Cancer Society (ACS), and the National Cancer Institute (NCI). In the past 19 years, the Great American Smokeout, a well-known ACS event, encouraged smokers to quit for just 24 hours. The increase in "no smoking" areas in public areas discourages smoking and also reduces exposure to passive smoke. There are a number of dietary studies currently under way focusing on the prevention of lung cancer, but it is

Table 16-1 • Etiology of Lung Cancer Other than Smoking

AMBIENT AIR POLLUTION
Polycyclic hydrocarbons (from fossil fuels)
Metals (nickel and silver)
Radionuclides
Diesel exhaust
Asbestos fibers

INDOOR AIR POLLUTION
Tobacco smoke (second-hand)
Radon
Building materials
Combustion devices
Personal care and other household products

OCCUPATIONAL HAZARDS
Arsenic
Asbestos
Chloromethyl ethers
Nickel

Data from Samet JM (1993). The epidemiology of lung cancer. *Chest, 103,* 20S–29S.

not yet clear how dietary interventions can modify lung cancer risk.

Histologic Types of Lung Cancer

There are four major histologic types of bronchogenic tumors: squamous (epidermoid) carcinoma, adenocarcinoma, large cell carcinoma, and small cell lung cancer (SCLC). The first three are usually classified as non-small cell lung cancer (NSCLC). It is important to distinguish the different types, especially NSCLC from SCLC, since they have significant differences in presentation, natural history and response to therapy. Both types of lung cancer most likely originate from a common pluripotent stem cell (Feld et al., 1995).

Approximately 80 percent of patients with lung cancer will have NSCLC and 20 percent will have SCLC. Squamous cell cancers most often occur centrally near the main stem bronchi and produce obstruction with associated pneumonitis. Since these cancers remain localized and are amenable to local resection, patients generally have longer survival rates than other cell types. Adenocarcinomas and large cell carcinomas are more often located peripherally to the bronchi. These tumors tend to metastasize widely and frequently spread to the brain, adrenals, and bone.

Small cell tumors are usually located in the central regions of the lung, often at the hila, and are associated with early invasion of the surrounding structures, particularly the blood vessels. The rich supply of vessels and lymphatics in the lungs allows the disease to metastasize rapidly. Patients with SCLC usually have widespread disease at the time of diagnosis (Glover & Miaskowski, 1994). Metastases will often be found in regional lymph nodes, lung, abdominal lymph nodes, liver, adrenal gland, bone, central nervous system, and bone marrow.

The location of the primary tumor and invasion of specific structures may result in predictable symptoms. Any of the histopathologic types of lung carcinoma may occur in the extreme apex of either lung resulting in symptoms of shoulder pain, dysesthesias, and Horner's syndrome. There is also evidence of chest-wall invasion with destruction of the adjacent ribs or vertebrae (Pancoast's syndrome). Right-sided tumors more frequently invade or obstruct the superior vena cava, leading to swelling of the face, neck, and arms and evidence of collateral circulation over the anterior chest wall.

Other systemic presentations of lung cancer include paraneoplastic syndromes. These are seen more frequently in patients with SCLC and may include clubbing, ectopic hormone production (adrenocorticotropic hormone, calcitonin, human chorionic gonadotropin, antidiuretic hormone, parathormone), and a variety of neuromuscular syndromes. Hypercalcemia and parathyroid hormone syndromes are seen most frequently with squamous cell tumors. Effective treatment of the primary tumor may result in remission of symptoms.

The long natural history of lung cancer prior to clinical manifestations contributes to the usual late stage at diagnosis. Often occurring in concert with long-standing chronic obstructive pulmonary disease (COPD), lung cancer usually presents as a large mass with lymph node involvement. Emami and Perez (1992) report that cough is the most frequent presenting symptom. Individuals with COPD may ignore a change in a chronic cough, which further contributes to delay in diagnosis. Other presenting symptoms include chest pain, dyspnea, fever, pain from invasion of the pleura or chest wall, and symptoms of more advanced disease, such as weakness, malaise, and anorexia. Table 16–2 lists the clinical features of lung cancer due to local, regional, and metastatic spread.

Table 16-2 • Signs and Symptoms Associated with Lung Cancer at Presentation

LOCAL-REGIONAL
Shortness of breath
Cough
Hemoptysis
Fever associated with pneumonia
Chest pain
Shoulder pain
Superior vena cava syndrome
Horner syndrome
Pancoast syndrome
Ipsilateral supraclavicular and other neck nodes

SYSTEMIC
Weight loss
Fatigue
Cachexia

ORGAN-SPECIFIC
Bone pain
Headache
Neurologic findings
Hepatic and/or abdominal pain

Reprinted with permission from Feld R et al. (1995). Lung. In MD Abeloff, et al. (Eds.), *Clinical Oncology* (pp. 1083–1152). New York: Churchill Livingstone.

Work-Up and Staging

A chest radiograph is generally the first and probably the single most valuable tool in the diagnosis of lung cancer (Feld et al., 1995). Except for the rare occult tumor, most lung cancers are detected by an abnormal chest x ray. Radiographs can reveal peripheral nodules, a definitive mass, hilar and mediastinal changes suggestive of regional lymphadenopathy, and/or pleural effusions. Areas of segmental, lobar, or lung collapse suggest an endobronchial obstruction. Computed tomography (CT) of the thorax can further determine the extent of the primary tumor and regional lymph node status, and may also be used in radiation treatment planning. In addition, CT of the upper abdomen is valuable in the search for hepatic or adrenal metastasis. CT of the brain to rule out brain metastasis at diagnosis is usually performed in patients with SCLC, and in patients with adenocarcinoma and large cell carcinoma. When a thorough clinical evaluation is completed, more than half of all patients with bronchogenic carcinoma are found to have distant metastasis.

The most widely used staging system for lung cancer is the TNM system adopted by the American Joint Committee for Cancer Staging and End Results Reporting. The TNM International Staging system is shown in Table 16–3. Feld (1995) points out that there may not be such an orderly spread of disease from proximal to distal nodes and beyond. The mediastinal nodes may better serve as a marker of disease rather than an effective barrier to spread. Thus, the presence of mediastinal nodal involvement should be regarded as an indicator of other mediastinal (and quite possibly distant) disease. However, the absence of apparent nodal involvement does not rule out the presence of metastatic disease. The failure patterns in treated

Table 16-3 • International Staging System: TNM Classification

T1	A tumor 3 cm or less in greatest dimension, surrounded by lung or visceral pleura, and without evidence of invasion proximal to a lobar bronchus at bronchoscopy. A tumor more than 3 cm in greatest diameter or a tumor any size that invades the visceral pleura or has associated atelectasis or obstructive pneumonitis extending to the hilar region. At bronchoscopy the proximal extent of demonstrable tumor must be within a lobar bronchus or at least 2 cm distal to the carina. Any associated atelectasis or obstructive pneumonitis must involve less than an entire lung.
T2	A tumor more than 3 cm in greatest dimension, or a tumor of any size that either invades the visceral pleura or has associated atelectasis or obstructive pneumonitis extending to the hilar region. At bronchoscopy, the proximal extent of demonstrable tumor must be within a lobar bronchus or at least 2 cm distal to the carina. Any associated atelectasis or obstructive pneumonitis must involve less than an entire lung.
T3	A tumor of any size with invasion of the chest wall (including superior sulcus tumors), diaphragm, or the mediastinal pleura or pericardium without involving the heart, great vessels, trachea, esophagus, vertebral body, or a tumor in the main bronchus within 2 cm of the carina without involving the carina, or associated atelectasis or obstructive pneumonitis of the entire lung.
T4	A tumor of any size with invasion of the mediastinum or involving the heart, great vessels, trachea, esophagus, vertebral body or carina, or the presence of malignant pleural effusion.

NODAL INVOLVEMENT (N)

N0	No demonstrable metastasis to regional lymph nodes.
N1	Metastasis to lymph nodes in the peribronchial or the ipsilateral hilar region, or both, including direct extension.
N2	Metastasis to ipsilateral mediastinal lymph nodes and/or subcarinal lymph nodes.
N3	Metastasis to contralateral mediastinal, contralateral hilar, ipsilateral or contralateral scalene, or supraclavicular lymph nodes.

DISTANT METASTASIS (M)

M0	No distant metastasis
M1	Distant metastasis

STAGE GROUPING

Stage I	T1–2, N0, M0
Stage II	T1–2, N1, M0
Stage IIIa	T3, N0–2, M0
	T1–3, N2, M0
Stage IIIb	T4, any N, M0
	Any T, N3, M0
Stage IV	Any T, any N, M1

Data from Mountain CF (1986). A new international staging system for lung cancer. *Chest, 89,* 225S.

patients is high, which accounts for the tendency of radiation oncologists to include most or all of the mediastinal lymph nodes in the target volume of radiation.

Treatment

The appropriate treatment for bronchogenic cancer is based on consideration of several prognostic factors: histology, tumor extent, and the patient's physical condition. Surgery, radiation therapy, and chemotherapy are generally the considered treatment options, the first two of these having a long history of collaboration in the management of localized disease.

Non-Small Cell Lung Cancer

Surgery

While complete surgical resection offers the best chance for cure, only 20 to 25 percent of lung cancer patients qualify for curative surgery. Surgical candidates include those with localized, non-small cell (stage I and II) and occasionally those with localized (IIIa) disease, particularly in instances of squamous cell tumors. The procedure of choice (lobectomy, pneumonectomy, segmental or sleeve resection) is usually that which will excise all existing disease and provide maximum conservation of normal lung tissue. The different surgical approaches are schematically shown in Figure 16–2. The presence of distant or extrathoracic metastasis indicates inoperability.

Preoperative CT scanning allows the selection of appropriate surgical candidates. It is a useful way to avoid thoracotomy in selected patients who underwent this debilitating procedure in the past and were later found at surgery to be unresectable. When initial staging evaluation, including CT assessment, determines that the lesion is resectable, the patient must also be assessed for "operability." A high percentage of patients with lung cancer generally are chronic smokers and have significant cardiopulmonary compromise unrelated to the cancer (Ruckdeschel, 1995). There has been an increasing interest in limited surgical procedures such as segmented or wedge resection for patients with marginal pulmonary function. Small cell lung cancer is not considered a surgically treatable disease due to the high incidence of distant metastases.

The response and survival of surgically treated patients depend on their preoperative performance status and extent of disease. According to Mountain and associates (1987), if patients are clinically staged, surgery will control about 45 percent of patients with stage I, 25 percent of patients with stage II, and perhaps 10 percent of patients with stage IIIa disease. Patients having a complete resection (surgical complete responders) and who have squamous histology respond more favorably to treatment than those with nonsquamous histology. However, in many cases, surgical resection is limited because the primary tumor invaded adjacent structures or organs, or spread to mediastinal/supraclavicular lymph nodes.

Radiation Therapy

PREOPERATIVE RADIOTHERAPY

As discussed, results for well-selected patients with early stage disease who undergo surgery are good. Patterns of treatment failure suggest good local control, which negates the benefit of additional therapy. Most studies failed to demonstrate that preoperative radiation therapy is beneficial on either operability or survival (Damstrup & Skovgaard-Poulsen, 1994). On the contrary, the number of postoperative complications and their severity generally increase. Similarly, a review of trials by Payne (1994) found that postoperative radiation of early stage disease showed no benefit.

Preoperative radiation may be used before complete surgical resection particularly when tumors are located near a vital organ (Payne, 1994). Likewise, preoperative radiation may be used for the treatment of surgically operable Pancoast tumors. Pancoast (1932) described the association of apical NSCLCs with the constellation of arm or shoulder pain, Horner's syndrome, and rib erosion. These tumors can involve not only the ribs but also the chest wall, brachial plexus, vertebral bodies, and subclavian vessels. Radiation is given to the tumor and regional lymph nodes, either alone or in combination with chemotherapy. After a time interval, restaging is done and surgical treatment is undertaken if systemic metastatic involvement is not evident. Postoperative radiation may also be administered, as these tumors are often marginally resected (Shaw et al., 1993).

Lung cancer patients with limited pulmonary function or otherwise nonoperable early stage disease may be candidates for curative treatment with radiation therapy. Because radiation toxicity may lead to serious compromise in pulmonary reserve, alternative beam arrangements may be used to spare the uninvolved lung parenchyma. When

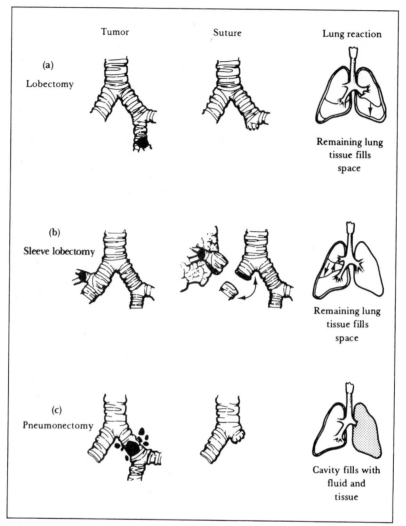

| | Tumor | Suture | Lung reaction |

Figure 16-2 • Different approaches to lung resection. (A) Lobectomy, resection of a pulmonary lobe, (B) sleeve lobectomy, resection of the cancerous lobe with a segment of the main bronchus, followed by an end-to-end anastomosis, and (C) pneumonectomy, entire lung removal. Reprinted with permission from Elpern EH (1993). Lung cancer. In SL Groenwald et al. (Eds.), *Cancer Nursing, Principles and Practice* (3rd ed.). Boston: Jones and Bartlett.

this is not possible, low-dose radiation may be used, but is unlikely to be curative. It is difficult to compare the results of patients treated with radiation versus surgery for early stage lung cancer due to different staging methods. One method is a clinical-radiological schema usually without mediastinoscopy while the other is a surgical-pathological one with accurate assessment of nodal involvement. It is known that tumors smaller than 4 to 6 cm are easier to eradicate than larger ones. Newer technical advances, such as portal imaging and three-dimensional treatment planning, may allow for reduction in normal tissue treated, thus allowing larger curative doses (Bezjak & Payne, 1993).

POSTOPERATIVE RADIOTHERAPY

In cases of complete resection of NSCLC with positive hilar and/or mediastinal nodes, postoperative radiation is known to decrease local recurrences. An improvement in survival, however, has not been well established, although some retrospective studies have shown survival benefit (Salazar et al., 1993). The Lung Cancer Study Group, in a 1986 prospective trial, showed that while postoperative radiation decreased local relapses, there was no significant increase in overall survival. More prospective, case-controlled studies are needed to evaluate improvement in survival.

In cases of incomplete resection or regional lymph node metastasis, postoperative radiation is almost always recommended. It is usually given immediately after surgery rather than awaiting recurrence of disease.

DEFINITIVE RADIATION THERAPY

A significant number of lung cancers will be assessed as inoperable at presentation. Emami and Perez (1992) reported that only 20 percent of new lung cancer cases are surgically curable. If disease is limited to the chest, radiation therapy is indicated. High doses (6000 to 6600 cGy) are necessary for a reasonable probability of eradicating the primary tumor. High-dose thoracic radiation is a prolonged treatment course with significant acute, subacute, and late side effects, a 30 percent risk of local relapse, and only 5 to 10 percent long-term survival rate (Bezjak & Payne, 1993). Thus, selection of therapy is often based on known prognostic factors such as good performance status and no evidence of weight loss. As in other areas of oncology, a clear and realistic goal of treatment, cure or palliation, must be established at the outset.

When control is the goal of treatment, smaller radiation doses are used to lessen the treatment side effects. There is justification for treatment even without significant improvement in survival since the minimal morbidity associated with therapy may preclude or delay the development of the more debilitating sequelae of locally recurrent disease (Kinsella, 1987). Airway obstruction, pneumonia, bleeding, fistula formation, and vocal cord paralysis may accompany recurrence. The improved quality of life achieved by preventing or delaying local recurrence justifies the treatment regimen.

Pleural mesothelioma, a rarely curable neoplastic disease often caused by asbestos exposure, typically causes dyspnea and nonpleuritic chest wall pain. The efficacy of radiation, like that of other treatments, is not clear in the definitive treatment of patients with pleural mesothelioma. The use of radioactive colloids such as phosphorus-32 in chromic phosphate instilled into the pleural space has been studied (Brady, 1981). The exact response rate is unknown but in one series, all 6 patients were alive at 12 months or longer after instillation of isotopes.

PALLIATIVE RADIATION THERAPY

Radiation therapy plays a larger role in treatment of problems caused by lung cancer, either by the tumor itself or its metastases. Common symptoms of the primary tumor are hemoptysis, cough, dyspnea, obstruction of major airways, chest pain, hoarseness due to vocal cord palsy, and sometimes obstruction of the superior vena cava or other major vessels. Localized metastases may produce bone pain. Mediastinal tumors may cause venous obstruction or esophageal compression. Brain involvement may produce neurologic deficits, and spinal cord compression may lead to paralysis. Radiation therapy often benefits patients with these grave symptomatic metastases, as it often can be delivered to the problem site without causing other untoward side effects. Palliative treatment is generally given in a shorter time course.

Local progression of disease such as tumors involving the carina and/or trachea can affect the airways, causing a major problem. Patients generally receive maximal external beam radiation and are candidates for laser resection followed by endobronchial brachytherapy with the use of iridium-192. While standard clinical indications and dosage schedules have not been established, endobronchial brachytherapy has been widely shown to effectively reduce symptoms of hemoptysis, dyspnea, and cough (Aygun & Blum, 1995). Bone metastases from lung cancer are frequent and multiple. The main goals of bone radiation are relieving pain, preventing impending pathologic fractures, assisting with orthopedic fixation in cases of impending or completed pathologic fractures, maintaining activity and function, and preventing or alleviating compression syndromes, especially of the spinal cord.

The syndrome of superior vena cava obstruction (SVCO) is well known in the disease progression of lung cancer, occurring in approximately 5 percent of patients. The superior vena cava vessel is thin-walled with low venous pressure and encased in a rigid compartment bordered anteriorly by the sternum at the level of the anterior-superior mediastinum (Figure 16–3). In addition, it is very near the right main bronchus and is encircled by important lymph node chains that drain the right and lower left thoracic cavities. Obstruction of the superior vena cava occurs by external compression or invasion by a right main bronchial lesion, by enlargement of surrounding lymph nodes, or in rare instances, by intraluminal thrombosis (Markoe, 1987; Roswit et al., 1953). Signs and symptoms of SVCO may be subtle or striking, depending on the degree of obstruction and the rapidity in which the obstruction develops (Figure 16–4; see also Color Plate 6). Patients most often complain of shortness of breath or dyspnea (50 to 70 percent) and facial swelling (39 to 43 percent). Thoracic vein distention (31 to 67 percent) and neck vein distention (58 to 67 percent) are the most common physical findings,

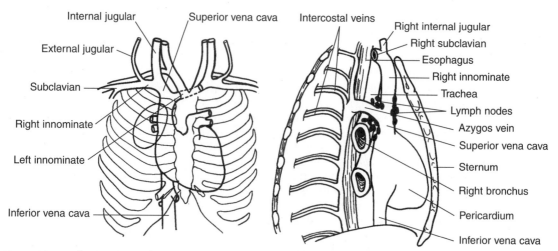

Figure 16-3 • Schematic representation of the frontal (*left*) and sagittal (*right*) sections of the thorax. Redrawn from Lokich J & Goodman R (1975). Superior vena cava syndrome. *Journal of the American Medical Association, 231,* 58–61. Copyright 1975, American Medical Association.

followed by facial edema (35 to 60 percent) (Armstrong et al., 1987; Bell et al., 1986; Perez et al., 1978). The classification of SVCO as a true oncological emergency is controversial, since it often develops and progresses slowly. It should be detected before an acute, life-threatening presentation occurs. It is usually possible to make a histologic or cytologic diagnosis before treatment.

Radiation remains the major treatment modality for most patients with SVCO. Portals are designed after consideration of both the pathological diagnosis and extent of disease. Mediastinal, hilar, and adjacent pulmonary parenchymal lesions are included. For solid tumors with an upper lobe lung lesion and mediastinal adenopathy, supraclavicular lymph nodes are usually treated. In patients with SVCO, those with SCLC have a more rapid, complete response than patients with NSCLC when treated with radiation therapy (Perez et al., 1978). Patients with SCLC are usually treated with systemic chemotherapy and concomitant thoracic radiation if the disease is limited to the chest (Komaki & Cox, 1995). Current recommendations are that the radiation schedule include higher daily fractions of 300 to 400 cGy for 2 to 4 days, followed by conventional daily dose fractions of 180 to 200 cGy. Total dose is determined by the histological picture and the extent of disease. Patients with SCLC, which is more radiosensitive, generally receive a total dose of 2000 to 4000 cGy. Less sensitive tumors such as squamous cell lung carcinoma or adenocarcinomas require a total dose of 5000 to 6000 cGy (Carabell & Goodman, 1985; Sculier

et al., 1986). Generally, corticosteroids have not been shown to contribute to more rapid relief of symptoms. With radiation therapy, 85 to 90 percent of patients have symptom relief within 3 weeks.

Chemotherapy Combine with Radiation

Persistent or recurrent intrathoracic disease and distant metastases are significant problems in locally advanced NSCLC treated with radiation. Over the years, various drugs, either as single

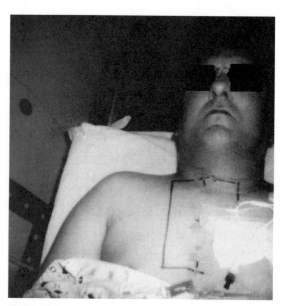

Figure 16-4 • A patient with classic superior vena cava syndrome signs.

agents or in combinations, have been investigated. Response rates exceeding 50 percent are now commonly reported in selected studies of induction cisplatin-based chemotherapy combinations in stage IIIa and IIIb disease. As a result, there has been increasing interest in evaluating multimodality programs in stage III NSCLC. The use of neoadjuvant chemotherapy, where two or three cycles of chemotherapy are given prior to radiation, are being evaluated (Salazar et al., 1993). Advantages include enhancing reoxygenation of hypoxic cells, which in turn increases radiosensitivity. Drug complications, however, may interrupt the radiation therapy course.

It is clear that as the intensity of the combined chemotherapy/radiation regimens increases, treatment-related toxicity will be a major factor. Byhardt (1995) suggests that decisions will need to be made as to "acceptable" levels of acute and late toxicities. A recent phase I trial in regionally advanced, unresectable NSCLC patients compared (1) standard radiation therapy, (2) induction chemotherapy followed by standard radiation therapy, and (3) twice-daily radiation therapy (Sause et al., 1995). One year survival (percent) and median survival (months) were as follows: (1) standard radiation therapy—46 percent; 11.4 months; (2) chemotherapy plus radiotherapy—60 percent; 13.8 months; and (3) hyperfractionated radiation therapy—51 percent; 12.3 months. Tannock (1994) suggests that even if small gains in survival are achieved, it is not certain whether they are of sufficient magnitude to recommend induction chemotherapy in routine clinical practice. He suggests the need for further research analyzing both the effects on quality of life of combined versus single modality treatment and the economic implications (expressed in cost per quality-adjusted life-year gained) for combined modality treatment.

Because of poor local control rates and the high rate of metastasis, recent trials have used radiosensitizers and the combination of radiation with chemotherapy. A review of study results done by Shaw et al. (1993) failed to show that two radiosensitizers, misonidazole and levamisole, improved local control and survival in comparison with standard radiotherapy only. In addition, intraoperative radiation therapy failed to show benefit in local control or survival with either incompletely resected or unresectable NSCLC.

Small Cell Lung Cancer

The disseminated nature and chemoresponsiveness of SCLC makes the use of systemic chemotherapy a primary treatment for this type of lung cancer. However, local failure commonly occurs with chemotherapy alone. The role of thoracic radiotherapy in small cell carcinoma is predominantly that of consolidation. A review by Arriagada and associates (1995) showed that chest radiation decreased the risk of thoracic recurrences and promised a gain in long-term survival of approximately 5 to 10 percent in patients with limited disease. In cases in which there has been limited or partial response, radiation therapy often may convert this into a complete response.

Thoracic radiation is now standard treatment in limited SCLC and may benefit some patients with disseminated disease. However, the total radiation dose, volume fractionation, and method of integration with chemotherapy are all controversial and the subject of many studies. These treatment factors can clearly influence hematological, pulmonary, and esophageal toxicities compared with the use of chemotherapy alone. The optimal radiation dose level, while not established, is thought to be at least 4500 to 5000 cGy (Turrisi, 1993). It is not clear, however, that a larger dose, by itself, will result in better survival or local control, particularly if the larger total dose is achieved at the price of interruption in treatment.

The use of upper hemibody irradiation for control has been discontinued due to severe toxicity and little improvement in response rates or survival. The current recommendation is to treat the primary tumor with a 1.5 to 2 cm free-margin, the hilum and subcarinal nodes, and bilateral mediastinal nodes up to the thoracic inlet. It is unknown whether treatment of supraclavicular nodes has any influence on long-term survival rates (Feld et al., 1995). Arriagada and associates (1995) favor the use of early chest radiation over late radiation due to the emergence of chemoresistant cells and tumor repopulation. In a review of studies by Salazar and associates (1993), early chest radiation alternating with chemotherapy appears to yield better tolerance, and in some studies, the response rates appear to be excellent (Bunn et al., 1987; Perez et al., 1984; Perry et al., 1987; Turrisi et al., 1987).

Prophylactic cranial radiation has been widely advocated in SCLC treatment due to the high incidence of central nervous system metastases (>50 percent). This concept is also being applied to both adenocarcinoma and large-cell anaplastic carcinomas. However, several studies have shown a reduction in brain metastasis but no effect on survival (Hazuka & Turrisi, 1993). Neurotoxicities commonly associated with whole-brain radiation include impaired mentation, apraxic gait, and urinary incontinence. They typically occur 6 to 18 months after completing therapy (Abner, 1993).

Radiation Treatment Delivery

As previously noted, most patients with lung cancer will receive radiation therapy. The overall poor prognosis in lung cancer creates difficulty in determining optimum treatment regimens as well as evaluating late effects of radiation. Patients who are most often referred to radiation oncology departments are those with incomplete resections or whose conditions are inoperable by disease or performance status.

Large doses of radiation are required to eradicate lung cancers. Using Fletcher's technique (1973) to determine dose-response curves, it is believed that doses in the range of 8000 to 10,000 cGy are needed to sterilize 100 percent of bronchogenic carcinoma. Most clinical trials report the use of doses ranging from 4000 to 6500 cGy. This represents a compromise between tumor dose requirement and normal tissue tolerance.

The treatment is most commonly given using a pair of opposed anterior and posterior beams. By using CT scanning, treatment area and portal size can be established together with computerized dose planning for the tumor and spinal cord shielding. Figure 16–5 illustrates a large lung field including the tumor and lymphatics, specifically the supraclavicular, hilar, and mediastinal node chains. Treatment fields may need to be modified where pulmonary function testing shows severe chronic obstructive pulmonary disease. In curative doses, the tumor dose exceeds the tolerance of the spinal cord, and part of the treatment is given with an alternate field arrangement that will spare the spinal cord. Figure 16–6 illustrates the small-field plan. Coverage of a centrally placed tumor and mediastinum can be achieved by an arrangement of obliquely angled beams. This technique avoids the problem of underdosing the mediastinum, which would otherwise result from employing a lead shield over the posterior beam to protect the spinal cord. A number of beam-modifying devices are often used to facilitate homogenous radiation of the tumor, such as shielding (layers of lead or metal alloys that absorb radiation to parts of the field that need not be treated), attenuators/compensators (thinner layers of lead that decrease the dose in selected parts of the field, i.e., the upper chest, where body thickness is least and tissues at midplane would otherwise receive

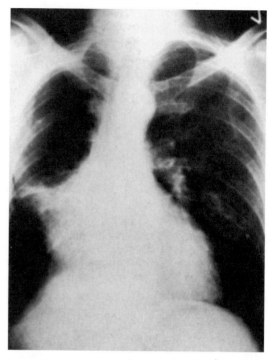

Figure 16-5 • Typical large lung radiation treatment field. From Strohl R (1992). Ineffective Breathing Patterns. In KH Dow & LJ Hilderley (Eds.), *Nursing Care in Radiation Oncology* (p. 166). Philadelphia: WB Saunders.

an unintended high dose), and wedges (wedge-shaped attenuators). These planning techniques are important when the prescribed dose exceeds the tolerance of irradiated normal tissues.

The usual plan of treatment involves daily fractions in the range of 180 to 200 cGy for a continuous 5- to 6-week treatment course. Another regimen is the split-course higher-dose (300 cGy) fractionation, which involves 10 fractions over 2 weeks of daily therapy, then 2 plus weeks off, followed by an additional 7 or so fractions over 1½ weeks for a total of 5100 cGy. This regimen allows for tumor regression during the hiatus. Smaller fields may be used after the break to decrease complications. No reported study has shown an increased survival with this approach, but there are several factors that may necessitate its use. Extremely ill patients may find the continuous 5 to 6 weeks of conventional therapy difficult to manage. In addition, early discharge from the hospital has created tremendous transportation and home care problems that may make a split-course regimen more tolerable. Late effects of therapy are the same for both treatment courses. Salazar and colleagues (1976) report that acute reactions are minimized

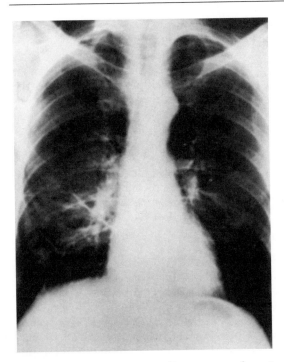

Figure 16-6 • Radiation response of lung tumor as shown in Figure 16-5. From Strohl R (1992). Ineffective Breathing Patterns. In KH Dow and LJ Hilderley (Eds.), *Nursing Care in Radiation Oncology* (p. 167). Philadelphia: WB Saunders.

with the split-course technique approach. For the acutely ill individual, this plan of care may allow treatment to be completed.

Patients with locally advanced lesions have been treated with large doses on a once weekly basis. In this hypofractionated plan, patients receive 500 cGy per week for a total dose of 6000 cGy in a 12-week time frame. The spinal cord is protected after 3000 cGy. Although hypofractionation seems to promote much better acute tolerance and convenience, it can increase the potential for late complications such as pulmonary fibrosis and osteoradionecrosis of bone structures (Salazar et al., 1993).

Radiobiologically, the use of larger than conventional doses is an approach to deal with hypoxic tumor cells that are less radiosensitive. In a large mass, large radiation fractions destroy more neoplastic cells, allowing better oxygenation of the tumor core and rendering it more radiosensitive for the next treatment. The treatment course of 12 weeks is long, but for the debilitated patient, being treated only once weekly is well tolerated. Late effects have been difficult to evaluate because of the generally poor prognosis of these patients (Salazar et al., 1983, 1984). Controversy does

exist about hypofractionated therapy, however. Emami and Perez (1992) report that in patients with inoperable tumors, 29 percent of those treated with conventional therapy were free of tumor at autopsy, compared with 18 percent of those treated once weekly. The best response (40 percent tumor-free) was achieved in a group receiving three large fractions of 400 to 1000 cGy followed by conventional daily fractions.

Multiple daily fractions delivered between a 4- to 6-hour interval have been advocated. Tumor cell kinetic studies have shown short potential doubling times in human NSCLCs. Accelerated radiation attempts to overcome this rapid cellular proliferation by shortening the overall treatment time, and thereby lessening the opportunity for tumor cell repopulation. CHART (continuous hyperfractionated accelerated radiotherapy) is being studied in numerous trials. The Radiation Therapy Oncology Group (RTOG) randomized phase 2 trial evaluated a dose range from 6000 to 8000 cGy, with 7000 cGy yielding the best 1-year survival rate of 58 percent (Cox et al., 1991).

Many ongoing studies using doses greater than 6000 cGY show that these high doses can be administered safely with results and survival equivalent to trials of hyperfractionation or combined chemoradiotherapy. A review by Emami and colleagues (1994) suggests that higher doses of radiation to the tumor may result in improved local control in inoperable NSCLC. These studies use new technology (CT planning using 3-D displays), which allows for conforming the radiation dose more precisely to the shape of the tumor volume while minimizing the dose to critical normal tissues, such as the lungs, spinal cord, and heart (Hazuka & Turrisi, 1993). The role for very high dose (greater than 6000 cGy) hyperfractionation, including CHART, is currently being evaluated in ongoing studies.

Nursing Management

Pathophysiology of Acute Radiation Toxicity

The trachea and lungs are composed of a variety of tissues that generally tolerate moderate doses of radiation. The acute pathological effect of radiation is related to both vascular and airway injury. It is difficult to attribute changes to one specific injury. Rubin (1984) believes that radiation damage results from parenchymal stem cell hypoplasia, and alterations of vasculature and fibroconnective tissues. While these events are certainly contributory, the late effects of radiation are believed to derive principally from arterio-capillary fibrosis, which predominates in late irreparable injury.

The ciliated epithelium may appear normal after a total dose in the range of 5000 to 6000 cGy in 6 weeks. However, cilia cease to function early in the radiation treatment course. Dry, irritated mucosa results from a decrease in mucous production, and patients may report an increase in nonproductive coughing (Komaki & Cox, 1995).

Radiation-induced lung damage has two distinct clinical phases: pneumonitis and pulmonary fibrosis. Fibrosis will be discussed under the section on late side effects.

Pneumonitis

Engelstadt (1940) reported four stages in the development of radiation-induced pneumonitis. In the first stage, leukocytes infiltrate the mucosa, and the bronchial mucosa becomes hyperemic with increased transudate. Edema of the mucosa does not generally cause clinical symptoms with conventional daily doses (Engelstadt, 1940). Cameron and associates (1969) reported that in patients with tumor-related airway obstruction, edema may occur after 2 or 3 doses of radiation. Komaki and Cox (1995) report that this edema has not been found to cause additional clinical symptoms.

The second stage in the development of pneumonitis is a period of normal function that lasts 2 to 3 weeks. The degenerative or third stage is reported between 1 and 3 weeks and up to 6 months after a single large fraction and several weeks after conventional doses. Acute radiation pneumonitis is characterized by swelling and sloughing of endothelial cells of small vessels. The damage to the vascular walls allows fluid to accumulate in interstitial tissues and alveoli. Fibrosis of the septa, interstitial fibrosis, and thrombosis with vascular sclerosis all contribute to decreased compliance and lung volume. With conventional doses of radiation, septal cells will proliferate and clear the alveoli by scavenging the accumulated debris. Interstitial and alveolar exudates are absorbed, and repair of sublethal damage then begins (Englestadt, 1940; Komaki & Cox, 1995).

The final stage of acute radiation pneumonitis is regeneration. The microvasculature of the airways and alveoli is reepithelialized. Interstitial fibrosis and progressive vascular sclerosis, however, may occur in doses larger than 4500 cGy.

Role of Surfactant in Development of Pathology

The role of surfactant production and radiation-induced lung damage have been explored. Shapiro and colleagues (1984) reported that in vitro type II alveolar pneumocytes are damaged by radiation. This results in membrane receptor-mediated surfactant release. According to Rubin (1984), this response occurs within minutes to hours after exposure to radiation and is related to radiation effect on the lamellar bodies of the alveolar type II cells. According to Coultas et al. (1987), radiation releases existing surfactant stored in lamellar bodies, increasing surfactant in alveolar spaces and depleting it in lung tissue. Nine days after radiation, surfactant levels return to normal levels. By 2 weeks after radiation, surfactant turnover is reduced. Three weeks after radiation, surfactant levels rise again (Coultas et al., 1987; Rubin, 1984; Rubin et al., 1986). Figure 16–7 illustrates the dramatic sequential changes in the alveolar type II cells.

The increase in surfactant in the alveoli contributes to alveolar septal thickening along with vascular congestion and infiltrating mononuclear

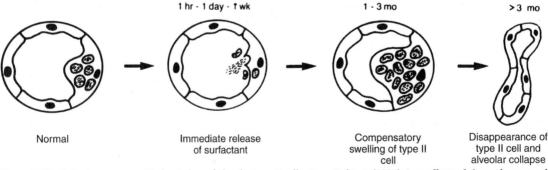

| 1 hr - 1 day - 1 wk | 1 - 3 mo | >3 mo |

| Normal | Immediate release of surfactant | Compensatory swelling of type II cell | Disappearance of type II cell and alveolar collapse |

Figure 16-7 • Radiation pneumonitis due to loss of alveolar type II cells. From Rubin P (1984). Late effects of chemotherapy and radiation therapy; A new hypothesis. *International Journal of Radiation Oncology, Biology, Physics, 10,* 5–34. Copyright 1984 by Elsevier Science Inc.

cells. This congestion contributes to the development of radiation pneumonitis.

Clinical Manifestations of Pulmonary Toxicity

There are usually minimal pulmonary side effects noted within the first month following thoracic radiation. There may be an increase in nonproductive cough during radiation treatment due to a decrease in mucous production, resulting in irritation of the larger bronchioles and bronchi (McDonald et al., 1995). Symptoms of pneumonitis usually occur 1 to 3 months after completion of radiation.

The degenerative and regenerative phases are clinically evident. Dyspnea and cough (occasionally productive of a thick, white sputum), fever, and night sweats characterize the degenerative phase. Physical examination of the chest during this phase is often surprisingly unrevealing. Evidence of consolidation is sometimes found in the region corresponding to pneumonitis, and a pleural friction rub or pleural fluid may be detected. Usually the symptoms resolve within 2 to 3 months, despite persistent radiographic abnormalities. Frequently, the only clinical manifestations of radiation pneumonitis are the radiographic changes, usually an infiltrate on chest film, conforming to the treatment field. If the volume of lung irradiated to a dose above 2500 to 3000 cGy is very large, the clinical signs and symptoms of pneumonitis may appear in 3 to 6 weeks (Komaki & Cox, 1995). An accelerated phase of the syndrome may develop within a period of days after concomitant chemotherapy. Pneumonitis can be very severe and produce acute respiratory distress, with significant cough, dyspnea, and fever. Tachycardia is a frequent clinical sign; patients can be taught to assess for pneumonitis by checking for a rapid pulse rate at rest. Careful treatment planning which limits doses to normal lung tissue can minimize pneumonitis and fibrosis. Symptoms from pulmonary radiation are the exception rather than the rule.

Generally, the acute symptomatic phase of pneumonitis is relatively short. Patients who become symptomatic are often treated with steroids; the usual dose is 30 to 60 mg of prednisone (approximately 1 mg/kg) per day for 2 to 3 weeks with a slow taper over 3 to 4 weeks or more (McDonald et al., 1995). Corticosteroids may reverse the symptoms of radiation pneumonitis in some patients within hours, but they do not prevent or reverse the fibrotic phase. In the presence of secondary infection, antibiotics may be necessary. In severe cases, the use of oxygen, bronchodilators, and sedatives help control coughing. The acute phase of pneumonitis is followed by an intermediate phase, during which the histologic changes described continue, but in which clinical symptoms are generally not as apparent.

Prevention is clearly the ideal goal in the management of pulmonary toxicities from radiation. Strict attention to chemotherapeutic and cumulative radiation dosages must be ensured when concomitant treatment is given. A review of the dose-escalation studies of the Radiation Therapy Oncology Group has confirmed the much greater importance of the volume of lung irradiated over the dose given, once the radiation is in a therapeutic range (above 5000 cGy). There has been no greater frequency of acute or late pulmonary toxicity demonstrated with increasing total doses from 6000 to 7400 cGy (Komaki & Cox, 1995).

Acute Side Effects

Dyspnea

Patients with lung cancer may experience some degree of dyspnea during their therapy, which is related to both disease and treatment factors. Dyspnea is a subjective sensation of difficult or uncomfortable breathing (Gift, 1990). The self-report is an essential aspect. Dyspnea is not a clinical sign, such as tachypnea, which can be documented by an observer; it is a subjective sensation that only the individual who experiences it can identify. Patients with increased anxiety, anger, depression, and cognitive disturbances report more respiratory symptoms (Dales et al., 1989).

Coy and Kennelly (1980) report that 15 to 40 percent of patients with lung cancer report dyspnea at diagnosis. Cancer therapy and its complications, such as infection and anemia, may enhance dyspnea. Knowledge of the pretreatment disease state and lung function, information on prior surgical procedures such as lobectomy and pneumonectomy, and the proposed radiation dose and volume of tissue to be treated help the nurse to predict the degree of dyspnea. Roberts and colleagues (1993) examined the phenomenon of dyspnea during the last weeks of life as it is experienced by patients with cancer and understood by nurses providing care. Findings suggested an inadequate assessment of dyspnea by nurses, as well as suboptimal management. It is essential to remember that the nurse's assessment of the severity of dyspnea may not correlate well with the patient's experience of distress, which may be either under- or overinterpreted.

A guide to the assessment of dyspnea and respiratory distress is presented in Table 16–4. Brown and associates (1986) described the experience of dyspnea in patients, who were interviewed using the American Thoracic Society Questionnaire, Grade of Breathlessness Scale, Dyspnea Visual Analog scale, and Karnofsky Performance Status. Patients used the term "short of breath" to describe the experience of dyspnea. Other terms used were fatigue, tightness, suffocating, and drowning. Emotions experienced during dyspneic episodes were anger, helplessness, depression, loss of strength, agitation, anxiety, nervousness, and fear. Brown (1988) describes scales such as the Dyspnea Interview Schedule, which documents the effects of dyspnea on activities of daily living.

The Baseline Dyspnea Index is used to determine the level of dyspnea at the start of therapy. A Transitional Dyspnea Index measures alterations in this baseline that might be related to disease or therapy.

PRETREATMENT TEACHING

Receiving radiation treatment may be a difficult experience for patients with lung cancer. Peck and Boland (1977) reported that 54 percent of patients were concerned about being alone in the room. Even a large treatment room may seem claustrophobic to the individual who is short of breath. Patients need information about the length of treatment and the fact that they can be seen and heard during treatment. Reassuring patients about the length of remaining treatment time may be helpful. Extremely anxious individuals may benefit from bringing a tape recorder to the treatment room with them. Listening to recordings of favorite music or relaxation tapes during treatment provides a time sense and end point for daily treatment.

PRETREATMENT INTERVENTIONS

The necessity of lying flat for treatment may also be distressing for individuals with dyspnea. Inter-

Table 16-4 • Assessment of Dyspnea and Respiratory Distress

PRETHERAPY DISEASE STATE	MEDICATIONS
Extent of lung damage	Narcotics
Prior respiratory disease (COPD, infection)	Sedatives
Prior therapy and influence on respiratory status (pneumonectomy, lobectomy, chemotherapy)	Bronchodilators
	SIGNS AND SYMPTOMS OF RESPIRATORY DISTRESS
PULMONARY FUNCTION	Air hunger
Respiratory rate and rhythm	Cough
Pulmonary function test	Dyspnea
Laboratory data	Edema cyanosis
$PaCO_2$	Signs and symptoms of infection: fever, chills, pain, and change in
PaO_2	sputum
HCO_3	NUTRITIONAL STATUS
Hgb	
Hct	MENTAL STATUS
Use of accessory muscles for breathing	PSYCHOLOGICAL ASPECTS
Skin color	Anxiety
Presence and degree of dyspnea	Environment
Orthopnea	Family issues
Auscultation of lungs and airway for breath sounds	Coping strategies
	Activities of daily living
STATUS OF COUGH	Understanding of disease process
Frequency	
Productivity	
STATUS OF SPUTUM	
Color	
Odor	
Consistency	
Amount	
Time of day	

Data from Brown (1988); Brown et al. (1986); Foote et al. (1986); Gift (1990). From Strohl R (1992) Ineffective Breathing Patterns. In KH Dow & LJ Hilderley (Eds.), *Nursing Care in Radiation Oncology* (p. 168). Philadelphia: WB Saunders.

ruption of therapy may be necessary. Allowing the patient to sit up at intervals during treatment might be required, especially in the initial phase of radiation treatment. Patients may actually need to start treatment in a sitting position if orthopnea is severe. Frequent reassurance may be required for the anxious, dyspneic individual. While the role of oxygen in patients with COPD, lung cancer, and related dyspnea is not clear, Schwartzstein and colleagues (1987) report that blowing oxygen on the face may have some effect in alleviating dyspnea. Humidified room air or a fan may be helpful in lessening air hunger as well.

INTERVENTIONS DURING RADIATION THERAPY

Physical activity, like crying and smoking, can increase dyspnea. Emotional factors such as anxiety, familial discord, and concerns about the future often precipitate dyspnea. Environmental factors such as wind, pollen, crowding, and poor weather may also contribute to dyspnea. Brown and associates (1986) report self-care activities used by patients to manage dyspnea. Immediate coping strategies included leaning forward on the edge of a chair with support of a table for the arms and upper body; moving slower; use of inhalers, postural modifications, medication, and pursed-lip breathing. The bracing of the arms appears to increase ventilatory capacity, improving the function of the accessory respiratory muscles (Gift, 1990).

Long-term adaptive strategies include seeking help with daily activities, such as bathing, eating, and dressing. Advanced planning of activities might include a change in timing or effort. Social and emotional strategies that may be helpful include attempting to accept the situation, avoiding being alone, use of prayer or meditation, keeping a positive attitude and remaining calm. Teaching patients relaxation techniques may be helpful in alleviating anxiety. Interestingly, in two investigations, only 10 percent of patients reported receiving instruction from health professionals related to dyspnea (Brown et al., 1986; Foote et al., 1986).

Clearly the nurse has an important role in teaching the patient to manage sequelae from chest radiation and to manage the problem of dyspnea. Table 16–5 presents specific nursing interventions for acute side effects of chest radiation.

Cough

Cough may be an extremely debilitating symptom leading to loss of appetite, sleep, and strength. As the cilia of the columnar epithelium and the mucus secreting glands cease to function, the bronchial mucosa becomes edematous, hypervascular, dry,

---

Table 16-5 • Specific Nursing Interventions for Acute Side Effects of Chest Irradiation

COUGH AND SHORTNESS OF BREATH
Instruct patient to drink 2–3 liters per day unless contraindicated.
Instruct patient and family to keep environment ventilated, free of smoke odors, calm; avoid crowds and people with infections.
Instruct in use of oxygen at home, importance of humidification, amount, safety techniques.
Instruct in use of medications as prescribed—bronchodilators, expectorants, etc.

FATIGUE
Teach patient to alter his/her daily schedule to allow for rest periods.
Carefully monitor blood counts with RBC transfusions when indicated.

PHARYNGITIS/ESOPHAGITIS/ANOREXIA
Assess patient's nutritional status by frequent weights and dietary intake records.
Instruct patient about protein calorie packing of food and small frequent feedings of soft, nonirritating food as well as avoidance of tobacco and alcohol.
Counsel regarding use of commercial nutritional supplements to give patient more protein and calories.
Refer patient to dietitian as indicated.
Assess patient for need of megestrol acetate to improve appetite and adequacy of food intake.
Provide analgesic/antacids as needed.
Assess for symptoms of herpetic or fungal infection.

SKIN
Teach patient skin care guidelines including avoiding trauma to skin, using skin care products only given out in department, avoiding sun.
Assess for signs and symptoms of dry and moist desquamation, providing care as needed with use of topical agents and dressings to alleviate discomfort, manage drainage, and promote healing.
Assess for use of chemotherapeutic agents or other drugs that may increase skin sensitivity.

Data from Emami and Perez (1992); *Manual for Radiation Oncology Nursing Practice and Education* (1992); Brown et al. (1986); and Gift (1990).

and irritated. Secretions turn thick and sticky and tend to accumulate distally due to narrowing of the edematous bronchi. A nonproductive cough can persist for many months after chest radiation. Increased hydration, humidification, and cough suppressants are all measures that may be helpful.

Fatigue

For patients with lung cancer, fatigue is often associated with dyspnea, and is known to be a common side effect during thoracic radiation. The actual mechanism has not been clearly defined, but appears to be related to the presence of excess toxic metabolites and waste products of cell destruction. Studies clearly show that increased levels of fatigue occur as radiation therapy progresses and the cumulative doses are increased (Haylock & Hart, 1979; Kobashi-Schoot et al., 1985; King et al., 1985). Compounding factors may include anemia, pain, malnourishment, medications, chemotherapy, and frequency of treatment visits.

Fatigue that is directly related to radiation itself is usually self-limited. As noted by one study, however, it may take several months to completely recover. King and associates (1985) found that during the first week of treatment, fatigue was experienced by 60 percent of patients. By the third week of therapy, 93 percent of patients reported fatigue, which persisted in 46 percent of patients 3 months after completion of treatment. Chapter 8 describes measures to minimize or alleviate fatigue.

Pharyngitis

The epithelial cells of the pharynx are highly radiosensitive and are frequently within the treatment area for lung cancer. Pharyngitis can occur approximately 2 to 3 weeks from the start of treatment. For some patients the pharyngitis spontaneously resolves after a few weeks, but for others it persists until the end of treatment. Patients may report a "lump" or "fullness" in their throats and have difficulty swallowing foods. It is common to hear patients say that although their throat is not painful, the food "just doesn't go down." Other patients may complain of a mild to severe sore throat.

Nursing interventions may include teaching the patient to gargle with warm saline before and after meals. Liquid narcotic-based analgesics are sometimes needed to control pain and should be taken 30 to 60 minutes before meals. Many patients may benefit from a local anesthetic/antacid/antihistamine mixture, e.g., equal parts of

Dyclone 0.5%/Maalox elixir/Benadryl powder. Another frequently recommended admixture is called Rothwell's Solution, containing nystatin suspension 14.5 ml, tetracycline syrup 24 ml, hydrocortisone powder 120 mg, and Benadryl powder, 650 mg. Dietary interventions include a soft, bland diet with the addition of commercially available high-caloric supplements. In general, patients find that thicker, soft foods and fluids are easier to swallow than clear fluids such as water or juice. Small frequent meals and snacks are advantageous, as well as avoidance of irritants such as tobacco and alcohol.

Esophagitis

Mediastinal radiation may lead to the inflammation and denudation of the surface epithelium of the esophagus. Dysphagia resulting from acute desquamation of the esophageal mucosa may develop as treatment progresses. Edema of the tissues can induce a stenosis observed several months after the treatment or a necrosis leading to fistula. The latter is a very rare complication in the absence of tumor progression, or prior surgery involving the esophagus (Van Houtte et al., 1994). Coarse foods and extremely hot or cold foods and liquids can further traumatize the mucosa. Patients may report epigastric pain or discomfort, esophageal reflux, and pain with swallowing certain or all foods. Esophagitis usually occurs approximately 2 to 3 weeks after the start of radiation therapy and may occur sooner if concurrent chemotherapy is administered. This symptom may last through the remainder of the treatment and up to 2 weeks after completion of therapy (Iwamoto, 1992). Chronic esophagitis may indicate a herpetic or fungal infection.

Measures to relieve esophagitis include antacids prior to meals and as needed. Rothwell's Solution as described previously is a beneficial analgesic for patients as well, and may reduce the incidence of candidiasis. Dietary measures such as those discussed for pharyngitis will be helpful and should be included in patient teaching.

Anorexia

All of the above symptoms, dyspnea, fatigue, pharyngitis, and esophagitis, as well as pain, contribute to anorexia. More than 50 percent of patients with lung cancer have been reported as experiencing some weight loss during the 6 months prior to diagnosis (DeWys et al., 1980). Anorexia has been reported in 60 percent of patients by the fourth week of treatment (King et al., 1985). Brown (1993) found that male gender, increased age, and current smoking status were positively associated with cancer-related weight loss 4 to 6 weeks postradiotherapy. Interestingly, Larson and associates (1993) found that patients over the age of 65 did not show any significant difference in caloric intake or in meeting their energy requirements. A review by Sarna and colleagues (1993) found that, historically, variables predictive of treatment response and survival in adults with lung cancer have been good performance status, minimal symptom distress, and minimal weight loss. Patients need to be aware that preventing weight loss is important to maximize the benefit of lung cancer treatment.

Nursing management of anorexia includes helping the patient to control other contributing factors such as fatigue, pain, and pharyngitis to minimize the detrimental effects on appetite (Tait & Aisner, 1989). Frequent, small meals rather than three large meals can be less overwhelming for the patient to consume. Nutrient-dense meals should be provided so that the patient will be able to obtain the necessary calories and proteins in a small volume of food. Commercial nutritional supplements can be used in the daily dietary plan to boost protein and calorie intake. The use of megestrol acetate has been shown to improve appetite and adequacy of food intake, which positively affected weight gain (Tchekmedyian et al., 1992). A dose of 800 mg in a single daily dose as an appetite stimulant is beneficial to many patients. If the patient has lost greater than 5 to 10 percent of usual body weight and continues to experience nutritional problems, a dietitian should be consulted for expert advice and planning to meet the patient's individual nutritional needs (Iwamoto, 1992).

Skin

Radiation may induce an acute skin reaction (erythema, moist desquamation) or late damage (fibrosis, telangiectasia); however, these reactions are rarely observed for lung cancers treated with megavoltage equipment (Van Houtte et al., 1994). Chapter 8 describes measures for skin care.

Late Side Effects

Lung Fibrosis

Lung fibrosis develops during the regenerative phase and is generally considered to be a late effect. McDonald and associates (1995) describe the progression to fibrosis, which typically takes 6 to 24 months to evolve, even though histologic and biochemical changes are evident sooner. The slowly progressive arteriolar fibrosis and interstitial fibrosis contribute to a delayed parenchymal destruction, via both direct cellular effects and the effect of decreased circulation. Fibrosis can occur without previous pneumonitis, but once pneumonitis occurs, fibrosis is almost certain to take place. The degree of blood flow impairment, preexisting vascular compromise, demand for collateral circulation, and capacity for vascular regeneration will determine the extent of fibrosis. In combined modality treatment, the late effects of thoracic radiation are exacerbated by the additional effects of chemotherapy. These late effects begin with swelling of small vessel endothelial cells leading to partial obstruction and decreased blood flow.

Radiation produces blistering of the capillary endothelial cells resulting in a generalized inflammatory response. With extensive lung damage, symptoms may develop from the resultant fibrosis. Abscess formation, infection, fever, chills, dyspnea, orthopnea, and clubbing may result. In an extreme case, progressive pulmonary capillary disease led to right-sided heart failure. Such severe cases are usually the result of large-field radiation (McDonald et al., 1995). Arteriovenous shunting may be a major cause of dyspnea and cyanosis. Treatment planning that avoids treating large volumes of normal lung tissue to a high dose obviates many of these severe sequelae.

Areas of fibrosis seen within the treated volume are generally asymptomatic (Englestadt, 1940; Fryer et al., 1978; Komaki & Cox, 1995; Rubin, 1984). The symptoms related to pulmonary fibrosis are proportional to the lung parenchyma involved and the patients' preexisting pulmonary reserves. A few patients will develop a picture of chronic debilitation due to respiratory compromise. Clinical assessment should include evaluating for dyspnea, rales, cough, and decreased exercise tolerance. Regular chest films and pulmonary function tests can monitor for pulmonary insufficiency. Chest x rays may show linear streaking radiating from the area of previous pneumonitis, and that may extend outside the irradiated area, with concomitant regional contraction, pleural thickening, and tenting of the diaphragm (McDonald et al., 1995). Supportive care, such as with bronchodilators and oxygen, is warranted. Unless the symptoms are severe, it is preferable to avoid long-term use of corticosteroids with their potentially adverse effects.

Predictive biochemical assays for late radiation effects are being studied. Rubin et al. (1986) explored the role of assays of surfactant as predictors of late effects. In rabbit studies, there was a strong correlation with surfactant release at 7 and 28 days, with lethality several months later. Markers of tissue damage detectable in the subclinical phase, before permanent damage occurs, could allow for modification of treatment before tissue is irreparably damaged. Functional changes such as alterations in breathing rates and pneumonitis do not represent early changes since irreversible changes have already occurred (Rubin et al., 1986). Biochemical, histological, and ultrastructural techniques need to be developed to predict late effects.

WR-2721, a radioprotective agent, was found to protect against late effects in murine studies. Protection against radiation damage was greater for fibrosis than for pneumonitis but occurred for both late effects (Travis et al., 1984; Travis et al., 1985). Further studies are needed to determine the role of such radiation protectors in humans. See Chapter 5 for additional information on chemical modifiers.

Quality of Life

Since the intent of lung cancer treatment is more often palliative than curative, emphasis needs to be placed on the patient's subjective experience (Elpern, 1993). Since it is important to include appropriate end points of palliation in lung cancer trials, both quality of life and survival should be assessed (Tannock, 1994). McNeil and associates (1978) found that some patients with operable lung cancer preferred radiation therapy to surgery (thus avoiding the risk of perioperative mortality), despite a lower probability of long-term survival. Other patients with lung cancer might agree to receive more toxic therapy in return for a small increase in the probability of long-term survival. Clearly, the modest gains seen in combined modality treatment for lung cancer may not be of sufficient magnitude to recommend adoption in routine clinical practice (Tannock, 1994).

Quality of life has been defined as a multidimensional construct, including the central dimensions of physical, psychological, and social well-being. These include functional status, specific symptoms from the disease or treatment, anxiety or depression secondary to the disease or treatment, and disruptions in normal social activities (Bernhard & Ganz, 1995; Fergusson & Cull, 1991). Research areas to be addressed include development of a systematic database on the psychosocial concerns of lung cancer patients, development and evaluation of quality-of-life instruments in lung cancer patients in all phases of disease and treatment, and longitudinal description of quality-of-life patterns during the course of treatment (Bernhard & Ganz, 1995). These data would provide better information for providing patient care, planning intervention programs, and optimally utilizing resources.

Follow-Up Care

The issue of smoking in the individual with lung cancer is often a difficult topic to address. The patient may believe that since a cancer has developed there is no reason to stop smoking. However, even patients with advanced disease may benefit from smoking cessation. Improved ventilation, appetite, and taste can enhance quality of life in advanced disease. Smoking during treatment will increase mucosal irritation. Respiratory compromise related to disease and treatment are exacerbated by the effects of tobacco. The pulmonary effects of radiation therapy including cough, esophagitis, and dysphagia are worsened by smoking. One must also address the role that smoking has played for the patient in coping with anxiety and stress. Alternative coping strategies may need to be introduced.

If prognosis in individuals with lung cancer improves, it can be predicted that more cases of radiation pulmonary fibrosis will be detected. Patients need to understand the concept of late radiation effects and the importance of routine follow-up exams. Methods to predict late effects in normal tissues are necessary. Quality assurance and meticulous treatment planning control the dose-related contributions to late effects by minimizing treatment error and areas of overdose (Withers, 1986).

Continuity of Care

The nurse caring for a patient with lung cancer who is receiving radiation treatment must coordinate care with other health professionals in a variety of settings. Inpatients who have been newly diagnosed or treated with surgery will often be discharged to home before treatment begins. A coordinated effort between inpatient and community health nurses facilitates continuity of care and avoids duplication of services. Wound care, pulmonary rehabilitation, nutritional support, psychosocial issues, and pain management will be ongoing concerns at home. When radiation treatment begins, the community health nurse may coordinate transportation to the radiation oncology facility. Transportation of the patient who is oxygen-dependent can be an anxiety-provoking situation. Coordination of efforts and a well-prepared outpatient setting can allay patients' fears. Identification of a service responsible for primary needs, such as oxygen and pain medications, is crucial to prevent the patient from receiving multiple prescriptions from a variety of physicians (Foote et al., 1986; Larkin & Benson, 1991; Schreiber, 1991; Wood & Ryan, 1991).

In all settings of care, the nurse's role as patient and family educator is essential. Patients and families are usually responsible for management of symptoms. Tasks such as wound care, suctioning, coughing, and deep breathing may be necessary. Caring for an anxious, dyspneic individual is an arduous task and the nurse must first assess the patient's and family's resources and their ability to manage the required activities. Teaching must begin during hospitalization with continued reinforcement by the ambulatory and home care nurses. A consistent plan of teaching should be developed to allay anxieties and facilitate learning. The patient, family, and nurse must become partners in this process. This coordinated effort will facilitate mastery of the complex aspects of care necessary in the clinical management of individuals with lung cancer.

Summary

In the radiation oncology setting, the ultimate goal is to maximize the quality of life for persons with lung cancer using innovative treatment strategies and comfort measures. A major role of nursing is to help patients predict the sequelae of therapy and to manage the consequences of disease and treatment. Respiratory symptoms such as dyspnea and cough related to malignant disease and its treatment have the potential to disrupt the individual's life in a significant way. Nursing interventions that help the patient to conserve energy and alleviate symptoms can assist the patient in maintaining quality of life. Nurses caring for such patients must understand the etiology of these problems to make them comprehensible to the patient. As patient survival increases, the issues related to late effects will assume more importance. Education and support of patients and their families will provide them the knowledge and skills necessary to cope with treatment and its effects.

The need for more effective strategies for the prevention and early detection of lung cancer remains abundantly clear. The recent decrease in incidence of lung cancer in men is a positive trend, possibly indicating that programs to encourage smoking cessation are becoming effective. Nurses must continue to play a leading role in the prevention and early detection of lung cancer by development of and involvement in smoking cessation programs and the education of the public in general.

References

Abner A (1993). Prophylactic cranial radiation in the treatment of small cell carcinoma of the lung. *Chest, 103,* 445S–448S.

Armstrong BA, Perez CA, Simpson JR, & Wederman MA (1987). Role of radiation in the management of superior vena cava syndrome. *International Journal of Radiation of Oncology, Biology, Physics, 13,* 531–539.

Arriagada R, Pignon JP, & Le Chevalier T (1995). The role of chest radiation in small cell lung cancer. *Cancer Treatment and Research, 72,* 255–271.

Aygun MD & Blum JE (1995). Treatment of unresectable lung cancer with brachytherapy. *World Journal of Surgery, 19,* 823–827.

Bell DR, Woods RL, & Levi JA (1986). Superior vena caval obstruction: A 10-year experience. *Medical Journal of Australia, 145,* 566–568.

Bernhard J & Ganz PA (1995). Psychosocial issues in lung cancer patients. *Cancer Treatment and Research, 72,* 363–390.

Bezjak A & Payne D (1993). Radiotherapy in the management of non-small cell lung cancer. *World Journal of Surgery, 17,* 741–750.

Brady LW (1981). Mesothelioma: The role for radiation. *Seminars in Oncology, 8,* 329–334.

Brown JK (1993). Gender, age, usual weight, and tobacco use as predictors of weight loss in patients with lung cancer. *Oncology Nursing Forum, 20,* 466–472.

Brown M (1988). Measuring dyspnea. In MF Stromborg (Ed.). *Instruments for Clinical Nursing Research.* Norwalk, CT: Appleton & Lange.

Brown M, Carrier V, Janson-Bjerklie S, & Dodd M (1986). Lung cancer and dyspnea: The patient's perception. *Oncology Nursing Forum, 13,* 19–25.

Bunn PA, Jr., Lichter AS, Makuch RW, Cohen MH, Veach SR, Mathews MJ, Anderson AJ, Edison M, Glatstein E, & Minna JD (1987). Chemotherapy alone or chemotherapy with chest radiation therapy in limited stage small cell lung cancer. *Annals of Internal Medicine, 106,* 655–662.

Byhardt RW (1995). Turning up the heat on non-small cell lung cancer: Is the toxicity of concurrent cisplatin-based chemotherapy and accelerated fractionation acceptable? *International Journal of Radiation Oncology, Biology, Physics, 31,* 431–433.

Cameron SJ, Grant IWB, Lutz W, & Pearxon JG (1969). The early effects of radiation on ventilatory function in bronchial carcinoma. *Clinical Radiology, 20,* 12–18.

Carabell SC & Goodman RL (1985). Superior vena caval syndrome. In VT DeVita, S Hellman, S Rosenberg (Eds.). Cancer: *Principles and Practice of Oncology.* (3rd ed.). Philadelphia: JB Lippincott.

Coultas PG, Ahier RG, & Anderson RL (1987). Altered turnover and synthesis rates of lung surfactant following thoracic radiation. *International Journal of Radiation Oncology, Biology, Physics, 13,* 233–237.

Cox JD, Azarnia N, Byhardt RW, Shin KH, Emami B, & Perez CA (1991). N2 (Clinical) non-small cell carcinoma of the lung: prospective trials of radiation therapy with total doses 60 Gy by the Radiation Therapy Oncology Group. *International Journal of Radiation Oncology. Biology, Physics, 20*, 7–12.

Coy P & Kennelly GM (1980). The role of curative radiotherapy in the treatment of lung cancer. *Cancer, 45*, 678–702.

Dales RE, Spitzer WO, Schechter MT, & Suissa S (1989). The influence of psychological status on respiratory symptom reporting. *American Review of Respiratory Disease, 139*, 1459–1463.

Damstrup L, & Skovgaard-Poulssen H (1994). Review of the curative role of radiotherapy in the treatment of non-small cell lung cancer. *Lung Cancer, 11*, 153–178.

DeWys WD, Begg C, Lavin PT, Band PR, Bennett JM, Bertino JR, Cohen MH, Douglass HO Jr., Engstrom PF, Ezdinli EP, Horton J, Johnson GJ, Moertel CG, Oken MM, Perlia C, Rosenbaum C, Silverstein MN, Skeel RT, Sponzo RW, & Tormey DC (1980). Prognostic effect of weight loss prior to chemotherapy in cancer patients. *American Journal of Medicine, 69*, 491–497.

Donaldson SS (1984). Nutritional support as an adjunct to radiation therapy. *Journal of Parenteral and Enteral Nutrition, 8*, 302–310.

Elpern EH (1993). Lung cancer. In SL Groenwald et al. (Eds.). *Cancer Nursing, Principles and Practice* (3rd ed.). Boston: Jones and Bartlett.

Emami B, Graham MV & Purdy JA (1994). Three-dimensional conformal radiotherapy in bronchogenic carcinoma: considerations for implementation. *Lung Cancer, 11*, S117–S128.

Emami B & Perez C (1992). Carcinoma of the lung. In C Perez & L Brady (Eds.). *Principles and Practice of Radiation Oncology* (2nd ed.). Philadelphia: JB Lippincott.

Emami B (1992). Mediastinum and trachea. In C Perez & L Brady (Eds.). *Principles and Practice of Radiation Oncology* (2nd ed.). Philadelphia: JB Lippincott.

Englestadt RB (1940). Pulmonary lesions after roentgen and radium radiation. *American Journal of Roentgenology, 43*, 676–681.

Feld R, Ginsberg RJ, Payne DG, & Shepherd FA (1995). Lung. In MD Abeloff et al. (Eds.), *Clinical Oncology* (pp. 1083–1152). New York: Churchill Livingstone.

Fergusson RJ & Cull A (1991). Quality of life measurements for patients undergoing treatment for lung cancer. *Thorax, 46*, 671–675.

Fletcher GH (1973). Clinical dose-response curves of human malignant epithelial tumors. *British Journal of Radiology, 46*, 1–12.

Foote M, Sexton D, & Pawlik L (1986). Dyspnea: A distressing sensation in lung cancer. *Oncology Nursing Forum, 13*, 25–33.

Fryer CJ, Fitzpatrick PJ & Rider WD (1978). Radiation pneumonitis: experience following a large single dose of radiation. *International Journal of Radiation Oncology, Biology, Physics, 4*, 931–936.

Grant JC (1972). *Grant's Atlas of Anatomy*, (6th ed.). Baltimore: Williams and Wilkins.

Gift A (1990). Dyspnea. *Nursing Clinics of North America, 25*, 955–965.

Glover J & Miaskowski C (1994). Small cell lung cancer: pathophysiologic mechanisms and nursing implications. *Oncology Nursing Forum, 21*, 87–97.

Guyton A (1991). *Textbook of Medical Physiology*, (8th ed.). Philadelphia: WB Saunders.

Haylock JJ & Hart LK (1979). Fatigue in patients receiving localized radiation. *Cancer Nursing, 2*, 461–469.

Hazuka MB & Turrisi AT (1993). The evolving role of radiation therapy in the treatment of locally advanced lung cancer. *Seminars in Oncology, 20*, 173–184.

Iwamoto RR (1992). Altered Nutrition. In KH Dow & LJ Hilderley (Eds.), *Nursing Care in Radiation Oncology*, (pp. 69–95). Philadelphia: WB Saunders.

King KB, Nail L, Kreamer K, Strohl R, & Johnson J (1985). Patients' description of the experience of receiving radiation therapy. *Oncology Nursing Forum, 12*, 55–61.

Kinsella T (1987). Review of status of radiotherapy in the management of lung cancer. *Oncology, 1*, 30–31.

Knox LS (1983). Nutrition and cancer. *Nursing Clinics of North America, 18*, 97–109.

Kobashi-Schoot JA, Hanewald GJ, van Dam FS, & Bruning PF (1985). Assessment of malaise in cancer patients treated with radiotherapy. *Cancer Nursing, 8*, 306–313.

Komaki R & Cox JD (1995). The lung and thymus. In JD Cox (Ed.) *Moss' Radiation Oncology: Rationale, Technique, Results* (7th ed.). St. Louis: Mosby.

Larkin M & Benson L (1991). Ineffective airway clearance. In J McNally, E Somerville, C Miaskowski, & M Rostad (Eds.). *Guidelines for Cancer Nursing Practice* (2nd ed.). Philadelphia: WB Saunders.

Larson PJ, Lindsey AM, Dodd MJ, Brecht ML, & Packer A (1993). Influence of age on problems experienced by patients with lung cancer undergoing radiation therapy. *Oncology Nursing Forum, 20*, 473–480.

Lokich JJ & Goodman R (1975). Superior vena cava syndrome. *Journal of the American Medical Association, 231*, 58–61.

Lung Cancer Study Group. (1986). Effects on postoperative mediastinal radiation on completely resected stage II and stage III epidermoid cancer of the lung. *New England Journal of Medicine, 315*, 1377–1381.

Manual for Radiation Oncology Nursing Practice and Education (1992). Pittsburgh: Oncology Nursing Society.

Markoe AM (1987). Radiation oncologic emergencies. In CA Perez, LW Brady (Eds). *Principles and Practice of Radiation Oncology*. Philadelphia: JB Lippincott.

McDonald S, Missaillidou D, & Rubin P (1995). Pulmonary complications. In MD Abeloff et al. (Eds.). *Clinical Oncology* (pp. 789–807). New York: Churchill Livingstone.

McDonald S, Rubin P, Phillips TL, & Marks LB (1995). Injury to the lung from cancer therapy: clinical syndromes, measurable endpoints, and potential scoring systems. *International Journal of Radiation Oncology, Biology, Physics, 31*, 1187–1203.

McNeil BJ, Weichselbaum R & Pauker SG (1978). Fallacy of the five-year survival in lung cancer. *New England Journal of Medicine, 299*, 1397–1401.

Morgan GW & Breit SN (1995). Radiation and the lung: A reevaluation of the mechanisms mediating pulmonary injury. *International Journal of Radiation Oncology, Biology, Physics, 31*, 361–369.

Mountain CF, Lukeman JM, Hammar SP, Chamberlain DW, Coulson WF, Page DL, Victor TA, & Weiland LH (1987). Lung cancer classification: the relationship of disease extent and cell type to survival in a clinical trials population. *Journal of Surgical Oncology, 35*, 147–156.

Mountain CF (1986). A new international staging system for lung cancer. *Chest, 89*, 225S.

Novello AC, Davis RM, & Giovino GA (1991). The slowing of the lung cancer epidemic and the need for continued vigilance (editorial). *Ca-A Cancer Journal for Clinicians, 41*, 133–135.

Outcome Standard for Cancer Nursing Practice (1987). Kansas City: American Nurses' Association.

Pancoast HK (1932). Superior pulmonary sulcus tumor. *Journal of the American Medical Association, 99*, 1391–1396.

Parker SL, Tong T, Bolden S, & Wingo PA (1997). Cancer statistics. *Ca-A Cancer Journal for Clinicians, 47*, 5–27.

Payne DG (1994). Is preoperative or postoperative radiation therapy indicated in non-small cell cancer of the lung? *Lung Cancer, 10*, S205–S212.

Peck A, & Boland J (1977). Emotional reactions to radiation treatment. *Cancer, 40*, 180–184.

Perez CA, Einhorn L, & Oldham RK (1984). Randomized trial of radiotherapy to the thorax in limited small cell carcinoma of the lung treated with multi-agent chemotherapy and elective brain radiation: a preliminary report. *Journal of Clinical Oncology, 2*, 1200–1208.

Perez CA, Presant CA, & Van Amburg AL (1978). Management of superior vena cava syndrome. *Seminars in Oncology, 5*, 123–133.

Perry MC, Eaton WL, Propert KJ, Chahinian AP, Skarin A, Carey RW, Ware JH, Kreisman H, Zimmer B, & Faulkner C (1987). Chemotherapy with or without radiation therapy in limited small cell carcinoma of the lung. *New England Journal of Medicine, 316*, 912–918.

Roberts DK, Thorne SE, & Pearson C (1993). The experience of dyspnea in late-stage cancer patients' and nurses' perspectives. *Cancer Nursing, 16*, 310–320.

Roswit B, Kaplan G, & Jacobson HG (1953). The superior vena cava obstruction in bronchogenic carcinoma. *Radiology, 61*, 722–737.

Rubin P (1984). Late effects of chemotherapy and radiation therapy: A new hypothesis. *International Journal of Radiation Oncology, Biology, Physics, 10*, 5–34.

Rubin P, Finkelstein J, Siemann P, Shapiro D, Van Houtte P, & Penney D (1986). Predictive biochemical assays for late radiation effects. *International Journal of Radiation Oncology, Biology, Physics, 12*, 469–476.

Ruckdeschel JC (1995). Carcinoma of the lung. In RE Ravel (Ed.), *Conn's Current Therapy* (pp. 156–162). Philadelphia: WB Saunders.

Salazar OM, Van Houtte P, & Rubin P (1993). Lung cancer. In P Rubin, *Clinical Oncology, a Multidisciplinary Approach for Physicians and Students* (7th ed.). Philadelphia: WB Saunders.

Salazar OM, Van Houtte P, & Rubin P (1983). Once-a-week radiation for locally advanced lung cancer. *International Journal of Radiation Oncology, Biology, Physics, 9*, 923–930.

Salazar OM, Van Houtte P, & Rubin P (1984). Once-a-week radiation therapy for locally advanced lung cancer: Final report. *Cancer, 54*, 719–725.

Salazar OM, Rubin P, Brown JC, Feldstein ML, & Keller B (1976). The assessment of tumor response to radiation of lung cancer: Continuous vs. split-course regimens. *International Journal of Radiation Oncology, Biology, Physics, 1*, 1107–1118.

Samet JM (1993). The epidemiology of lung cancer. *Chest, 103*, 20S–29S.

Sarna L, Lindsey AM, Dean H, Brecht ML, & McCorkle R (1993). Nutritional intake, weight change, symptom distress, and functional status over time in adults with lung cancer. *Oncology Nursing Forum, 20*, 481–489.

Sause WT, Scott C, Taylor S, Johnson D, Livingston R, Komaki R, Emami B, Curran WJ, Byhardt RW, & Turrisi AT (1995). Radiation Therapy Oncology Group (RTOG) 88-08 and Eastern Cooperative Oncology Group (ECOG) 4588: Preliminary results of a phase III trial in regionally advanced, unresectable non-small cell lung cancer. *Journal of the National Cancer Institute, 87*, 198–205.

Schmitt R (1993). Quality of life issues in lung cancer. *Chest, 103*, 51S–55S.

Schreiber J (1991). Impaired gas exchange. In J McNally, E Somerville, C Miaskowski, & M Rostad (Eds). *Guidelines for Cancer Nursing Practice*. (2nd ed). Philadelphia: WB Saunders.

Schwartzstein RM, Lahive K, Pope A, Weinberger S, & Weiss W (1987). Cold facial stimulation reduces breathlessness induced in normal subjects. *American Review of Respiratory Disease, 136*, 58–61.

Sculier JP, Evans WK, Feld R, DeBoer G, Payne DG, Schepherd TA, Pringle JK, Yeoh JS, Quirt IC, & Curtis JE (1986). Superior vena caval obstruction syndrome in small cell lung cancer. *Cancer, 57*, 847–851.

Shapiro LD, Finkelstein J, Rubin P, Penney D, & Siemann D (1984). Radiation induced secretion of surfactant from cell cultures of type II pneumocytes: An in vitro model of radiation toxicity. *International Journal of Radiation Oncology, Biology, Physics, 10*, 375–378.

Shaw GS, Bonner JA, Foote RL, Martenson JA, Frytak S, Deschamps C, & McDougall JC (1993). Role of Radiation Therapy in the Management of Lung Cancer. *Mayo Clinic Proceedings, 68*, 593–602.

Tait N & Aisner J (1989). Nutritional concerns in cancer patients. *Seminars in Oncology Nursing, 5*, 58–62.

Tannock IF (1994). New perspectives in combined radiotherapy and chemotherapy treatment. *Lung Cancer, 10*, S29–S51.

Tchekmedyian NS, Hickman M, Siau J, Greco FA, Keller J, Browder H, & Aisner J (1992). Megestrol acetate in cancer anorexia and weight loss. *Cancer, 69*, 1268–1274.

Thun MJ, Day-Lally CA, Calle EE, Flanders WD, & Heath CW (1995). Excess mortality among cigarette smokers: changes in a 20-year interval. *American Journal of Public Health, 85*, 1223–1230.

Travis EL & DeLuca AM (1985). Protection of mouse lung by WR-2721 after fractionated doses of radiation. *International Journal of Radiation Oncology, Biology, Physics, 11*, 521–526.

Travis EL, Parkins CS, Holmes SJ, Down JD, & Fowler JF (1984). WR-2721 protection of pneumonitis and fibrosis in mouse lung after single doses of x-rays. *International Journal of Radiation Oncology, Biology, Physics, 10*, 243–251.

Turrisi AT (1993). Incorporation of radiotherapy fractionation in the combined-modality treatment of limited small cell lung cancer. *Chest, 103*, 418S–422S.

Turrisi AT, Glover DJ, & Mason BA (1987). Concurrent twice daily multifield radiotherapy and platinum-etoposide chemotherapy for limited small cell lung cancer update 87 (abstract). *Proceedings of the American Society of Clinical Oncology, 6*, 172.

Van Houtte P, Danhier S, & Mornex F (1994). Toxicity of combined radiation and chemotherapy in non-small cell lung cancer. *Lung Cancer, 10*, S271–S280.

Withers HR (1986). Predicting late normal tissue responses. *International Journal of Radiation Oncology, Biology, Physics, 12*, 693–698.

Wood H & Ryan JE (1991). Ineffective breathing pattern. In J McNally, E Somerville, C Miaskowski, M Rostad (Eds.). *Guidelines for Cancer Nursing Practice* (2nd ed.). Philadelphia: WB Saunders.

Pediatric Cancers–The Special Needs of Children Receiving Radiation Therapy

CATHERINE COMEAU LEW

In the past two decades major advances have occurred in the diagnosis and treatment management of childhood cancer. In the United States, the current cure rate of all childhood cancers combined is between 66 and 90 percent (Bleyer, 1993; Robison, 1993). It is estimated that approximately two-thirds of the children up to 15 years of age with cancer are surviving their disease (Lampkin, 1993). The dramatic change in prognosis for most childhood and adolescent cancers has provided a growing population of long-term survivors. With survivorship comes an increased appreciation for the short- and long-term consequences of therapy. A multidisciplinary approach is needed to assist the child and family to deal with the physical and psychosocial issues related to their disease and treatment and to make a healthy transition to adulthood.

The improved prognosis of many childhood cancers results from advancements in tumor classification, diagnosis, immunology, genetics, pathology, molecular biology, surgery, chemotherapy, radiation therapy, and diagnostic radiology. The ability to integrate knowledge from laboratory investigations into clinical research and practice has enabled physicians to subclassify patients at diagnosis according to risk group, assign appropriate intensive therapy to maximize the chance of cure, and minimize acute and late toxicities (Link et al., 1993). The collaborative efforts of research and participation in clinical trials of disease-specific treatment regimens are expanding our understanding of disease, its biological characteristics, and the effectiveness of available treatment modalities. With intensification of treatment come toxicities that may impede the delivery of the treatment protocol. Optimal management of the side effects and toxicities of therapy is essential for providing supportive care for the pediatric patient.

The role of radiation therapy in the management of childhood cancers is being redefined. The potential late effects on skeletal, soft tissue, and organ development, neuropsychological function, and risk of second malignancies have focused attention on developing treatment strategies that will minimize these effects. Improved chemotherapeutic agents and drug combinations have eliminated the need for radiation in some situations and have changed the radiotherapeutic approach in others. To provide treatment care for children with cancer it is imperative to understand the biological, physiological, and psychological characteristics that distinguish children from adults. Awareness of child and adolescent growth and development and concepts of illness can guide the development of nursing interventions, strategies for teaching, and methods of assisting children to adapt to intrusive procedures.

This chapter presents an overview of the epidemiology of childhood cancers and the role of radiation therapy in the treatment of childhood malignancies. It describes the short- and long-term physiological effects of treatment. The growth and development needs of children at different ages and special considerations for caring for the child undergoing radiation therapy are discussed.

Epidemiology of Childhood Cancer

On a world-wide basis, cancer plays a relatively minor role in morbidity and mortality among children (Robison, 1993). In industrialized societies, where improvements in sanitation and nutrition have reduced the consequences of infection and malnutrition, childhood cancers play a relatively more important role. Approximately 7,800 new cases of childhood cancer were reported in the United States in 1992 (Halperin et al., 1994a). In the United States cancer is now second among causes of death in children aged 0 to 14 years, accounting for a total of 1,611 reported deaths in 1993 (Parker et al., 1997). Leukemia, tumors of the central nervous system, and endocrine tumors account for 76 percent of cancer-related deaths in this age group, notwithstanding improvements in five-year survival in the first two groups (Parker et al., 1997). Data from a decade earlier suggested that the incidence of all three of these tumor types rose significantly from 1973 to 1988 (Bleyer, 1993).

The distribution of tumor types and cancer-related mortality differs markedly in the pediatric age group from that seen in adult populations, where tumors of the lung, colon and rectum, breast, and prostate predominate (Parker et al., 1996). In children, the predominant tumors are leukemias and lymphomas (48 percent), tumors of the central nervous system (20 percent), and tumors of the sympathetic nervous system, soft tissues, bone, eye, and germ cells (Pizzo et al., 1993; Table 17–1). Carcinomas are relatively rare in children. Other distinguishing features of tumors in children include high growth rates and the influences of age, sex, genetics, race, and geography on their incidence and behavior (Pizzo et al., 1993; Table 17–2).

Age is an important variable for several reasons. The predominant type of cancer changes with age. Some tumors have bimodal peaks and may occur in both early childhood and adolescence (Table 17–1). A histologically similar tumor may behave differently at different ages (Pizzo et al., 1993). The highest incidence of pediatric malignancies occurs between birth and 5 years of age (Bleyer, 1993). Many of these early tumors—Wilms' tumor, testicular germ cell tumors, acute lymphoblastic leukemia, retinoblastoma, sacrococcygeal teratoma, medulloblastoma, glioma, rhabdomyosarcoma, and hepatoblastoma—are

Table 17-1 • Incidence of Childhood Cancers

Malignancy	Rate (per million/y)	Ratio: Sex (M/F)	Ratio: Race (W/B)	Peak Age (y)
LEUKEMIA				
Acute lymphocytic	24.7	1.3	2.4	2–5
Acute nonlymphocytic	5.0	1.2	1.0	<2
LYMPHOMAS				
Non-Hodgkin's	9.3	2.9		6–16
Hodgkin's	7.5	3.0	1.6	>10
CENTRAL NERVOUS SYSTEM TUMORS				
Gliomas	13.4	>1.0	1.1	Constant
Medulloblastoma	4.9	1.6	0.8	5–10
Ependymoma	2.1	>1.0	2.6	<5
SOLID TUMORS				
Neuroblastoma	8.0	1.4	1.6	<3
Wilms' tumor	6.9	0.9	0.9	<5
Retinoblastoma	3.0	<1.0	0.8	<3
Rhabdomyosarcoma	3.7	>1.2	0.9	Bimodal: 2–6 and 14–18
Ewing's sarcoma	2.1	>1.0	>1.0	10–18
Osteosarcoma	3.1	>1.0	1.2	10–18
Primary hepatic	1.6	>1.3		Bimodal: <2 and >14
Germ cell teratoma	0.4	0.3	0.8	Bimodal: <2 and >14

From Pizzo P, Poplack D, Horowitz M, Hays D, & Kun L (1993). Solid tumors of childhood. In V DeVita, S Hellman, & S Rosenberg (Eds.), *Cancer Principles and Practice of Oncology* (4th ed., pp. 1738–1791). Philadelphia: JB Lippincott. Used with permission of the publisher.

Table 17-2 • Predominant Pediatric Cancers by Age and Site

Tumors	Newborn (<1 y)	Infancy (1–3 y)	Children (3–11 y)	Adolescents and Young Adults (12–21 y)
Leukemia	Congenital leukemia AML AMMoL CML, juvenile	ALL AML CML, juvenile	ALL AML	AML ALL
Lymphomas	Very rare	Lymphoblastic	Lymphoblastic Undifferentiated	Lymphoblastic Undifferentiated (Burkitt's, Hodgkin's)
SOLID TUMORS				
Central nervous system	Medulloblastoma Ependymoma Astrocytoma Choroid plexus papilloma	Medulloblastoma Ependymoma Astrocytoma Choroid plexus papilloma	Cerebral astrocytoma Medulloblastoma Astrocytoma Ependymoma Craniopharyngioma	Cerebellar astrocytoma Astrocytoma Craniopharyngioma Medulloblastoma
Head and neck	Retinoblastoma Rhabdomyosarcoma Neuroblastoma Multiple endocrine neoplasia	Retinoblastoma Rhabdomyosarcoma Neuroblastoma	Rhabdomyosarcoma Lymphoma	Lymphoma Rhabdomyosarcoma
Thoracic	Neuroblastoma Teratoma	Neuroblastoma Teratoma	Lymphoma Neuroblastoma Rhabdomyosarcoma	Lymphoma Ewing's Rhabdomyosarcoma
Abdominal	Neuroblastoma Mesoblastic nephroma Hepatoblastoma Wilms' (>6 mos)	Neuroblastoma Wilms' Hepatoblastoma Leukemia	Neuroblastoma Wilms' Lymphoma Hepatoma	Lymphoma Hepatocellular carcinoma Rhabdomyosarcoma
Gonadal	Yolk sac tumor of testis (endodermal sinus tumor) Teratoma Sarcoma botryoides Neuroblastoma	Rhabdomyosarcoma Yolk sac tumor of testis Clear cell sarcoma kidney	Rhabdomyosarcoma	Rhabdomyosarcoma Dysgerminoma Teratocarcinoma, teratoma Embryonal carcinoma of testis Embryonal cell and endodermal sinus tumors of ovary
Extremity	Fibrosarcoma	Fibrosarcoma Rhabdomyosarcoma	Rhabdomyosarcoma Ewing's	Osteosarcoma Rhabdomyosarcoma Ewing's sarcoma

ALL, acute lymphoblastic leukemia; AML, acute myelogenous leukemia; AMMoL, acute myelomonocytic leukemia; CML, chronic myelogenous leukemia.
From Pizzo P, Poplack D, Horowitz M, Hays D, & Kun L (1993). Solid tumors of childhood. In V DeVita, S Hellman, & S Rosenberg (Eds.), *Cancer Principles and Practice of Oncology* (4th ed., pp. 1738–1791). Philadelphia: JB Lippincott. Used with permission of the publisher.

of embryonal cell origin. This suggests that prenatal factors may interfere with the developing fetus and result in oncogenesis. Tumors of the hematopoietic and lymphopoietic systems, such as Hodgkin's disease, bone cancers, acute leukemia, and most central nervous system tumors peak in incidence after the age of 5, suggesting that postnatal environmental factors play a role in their origin (Altman & Schwartz, 1983; Synder, 1986). The predominant pediatric tumors by age and site are found in Table 17–2.

Age also influences the biologic behavior and prognosis of certain tumors. For example: Leukemia in children less than 2 years or greater than 10 years of age is associated with a relatively poor prognosis. Acute leukemia in infancy has the highest frequency of poor prognostic features: high leukocyte count, hepatosplenomegaly, CNS involvement, and thrombocytopenia. Leukemic disease in this age group is associated with the worst outcome (Reaman, 1993). Age and stage play a similar but inverse role in neuroblastoma. Neuroblastoma in children less than 1 year of age has an overall disease-free survival of 75 percent, and in infants with stage IV disease the survival range is 40 to 90 percent (Rosen et al., 1984; Reaman, 1993).

Sex is another factor that influences the incidence of pediatric cancer. Pediatric cancers are more common in males, with the highest risk ratios occurring in Hodgkin's and non-Hodgkin's lymphoma and in medulloblastoma (Table 17–1). Females are affected more frequently by germ cell teratomas (Pizzo et al., 1993).

Geographic and Racial Variations

The prevalence of certain malignances varies with geographic location. Retinoblastoma has a high incidence in India and Central America, whereas it accounts for only 1 percent of childhood cancers in the United States. Burkitt's lymphoma accounts for more than half of the childhood cancers in Uganda but is rare outside of Africa. Acute leukemia occurs more commonly in the industrialized countries of the West than in North Africa, the Middle East, or Asia (Poplack, 1993). The influence of race within a geographic region is demonstrated by the higher incidence of acute leukemia, Ewing's sarcoma, and testicular cancers among white as compared to black children in the United States. The overall incidence of cancer among children in the United States is 20 percent higher in whites than in blacks (Pizzo et al., 1993).

Drugs Influencing Carcinogenesis

Several pharmaceutical agents have been implicated as transplacental carcinogens. Adenocarcinoma of the vagina and cervix has been noted in daughters of women given the estrogen *diethylstilbestrol* to prevent miscarriage (Mulvihill, 1993). *Phenytoin* has been associated with the development of neuroblastoma and other neoplasms in the offspring of mothers who received the drug during pregnancy. This effect may be mediated by suppression of T cell function (Mulvihill, 1993). *Androgenic steroids*, administered during pregnancy for treatment of Fanconi's anemia or aplastic anemia, may foster development of primary liver neoplasms in children, and *immunosuppressive regimens* prescribed for children with renal transplants appear to increase the risk of malignancy (Snyder, 1986).

Recent growth in the numbers of long-term survivors of pediatric malignancies has brought an appreciation of the role that chemotherapeutic agents play in the development of secondary neoplasms. Antineoplastic drugs identified with the risk of second tumors include teniposide, epipodophyllotoxin, cyclophosphamide, procarbazine, nitrogen mustard, chlorambucil, and CCNU (Tucker, 1993; Halperin et al., 1994b).

Ionizing Radiation and Radiation Carcinogenesis

Exposure to radiation is an established cause of childhood cancer. Studies of Japanese atomic bomb survivors showed most graphically that children who were less than 15 years old at the time of exposure developed acute leukemia at a frequency that was 20-fold greater than normal (Miller, 1986). Secondary malignancies also may arise in children previously treated with radiation therapy. The occurrence of radiation-induced sarcomas and the development of second primary neoplasms have been carefully documented in long-term follow-up studies on late effects of radiation in children (Bucholtz, 1992a; Halperin et al., 1994b; Tucker, 1993). The most common treatment-related tumors are sarcomas of soft tissue and bone, leukemias, and cancers of the brain, thyroid, and breast (Kun & Moulder, 1993; Tucker, 1993). In comparison to age-matched populations, children who develop a first malignancy have a 6- to 15-fold increased risk for developing a second cancer (Halperin et al., 1994). Age is an important variable in determining the risk of secondary tumors.

In children, the most commonly observed secondary neoplasms occur in tissues undergoing rapid cell proliferation (Halperin et al., 1994b). It has been suggested that the relative risk for development of secondary tumors is higher in children with genetically determined disorders, such as heritable retinoblastoma, Li-Fraumeni syndrome, neurofibromatosis, and xeroderma pigmentosum (Kun & Moulder, 1993). The immune dysfunction associated with other cancers, such as Hodgkin's disease, also may add to the risk of secondary tumors following radiation therapy (Tucker, 1993). The relative risk for development of thyroid cancer increases 53-fold, compared to the general population, in children who have been treated for neuroblastoma, Wilms' tumor, Hodgkin's disease, and non-Hodgkin's lymphoma (Tucker, 1993).

Genetics

Some genetic disorders, chromosomal disorders, congenital malformations, and inherited immunodeficiency disorders are associated with an increased risk of cancer in children (Tables 17–3 and 17–4). Acute leukemia has a well-defined association with the chromosomal anomalies found in Down's syndrome (Waskerwitz & Leonard, 1986). There are certain patterns of cancer within families that support the theory of *oncogenesis*.

Table 17-3 • Ecogenetics in Tumors of the Young

Environmental Agent	Genetic Trait	Tumor or Outcome
Ionizing radiation	Ataxia-telangiectasia with lymphoma	Radiation toxicity
	Retinoblastoma	Sarcoma
	Nevoid basal cell carcinoma syndrome	Basal cell carcinoma
Ultraviolet radiation	Xeroderma pigmentosum	Skin cancer, melanoma
	Cutaneous albinism	Skin cancer
	Hereditary dysplastic nevus syndrome	Melanoma
Stilbestrol	Turner's syndrome	Adenosquamous endometrial carcinoma
Androgen	Fanconi's pancytopenia	Hepatoma
Iron	Hemochromatosis	Hepatocellular carcinoma
Tyrosine	Tyrosinemia	Hepatocellular carcinoma
Monosaccharides	Glycogen storage disease type I	Hepatic adenoma
Epstein-Barr virus	Purtilo X-linked lymphoproliferative syndrome	Burkitt's and other lymphomas
Papillomavirus type 5	Epidermodysplasia verruciformis	Skin cancer
Hepatitis B virus	Virus integration site	Hepatocellular carcinoma

From PA Pizzo, M Horowitz, D Poplack, D Hays & L Kun (1993). Solid tumors of childhood. In V DeVita, S Hellman, & S Rosenberg (Eds.), *Cancer Principles and Practice of Oncology* (p. 1741). Philadelphia: JB Lippincott. Used with permission.

The *Li-Fraumeni syndrome*, for example, is characterized by loss of genetic material or mutations on chromosome 17 (p53 gene) and has a correlation with the increased incidence of breast cancer in the mothers of children treated for osteogenic sarcoma and rhabdomyosarcoma (Mulvihill, 1993). The interaction between certain genetic disorders and radiation therapy in promoting secondary tumors is discussed in the preceding section.

Cancer genetics is now a burgeoning field that is beyond the scope of this chapter. It has become

Table 17-4 • Childhood Cancers Associated with Congenital Syndromes or Malformations

Syndrome or Anomaly	Tumor
Aniridia	Wilms' tumor
Hemihypertrophy	Wilms' tumor, hepatoblastoma, adrenocortical carcinoma
Genitourinary abnormalities (including testicle maldescent)	Wilms' tumor, Ewing's sarcoma, nephroblastoma, testicular carcinoma
Beckwith-Wiedemann syndrome	Wilms' tumor, neuroblastoma, adrenocortical carcinoma
Dysplastic nevus syndrome	Melanoma
Nevoid basal cell carcinoma syndrome	Basal cell carcinoma, medulloblastoma, rhabdomyosarcoma
Poland's syndrome	Leukemia
Trisomy 21 (Down's syndrome)	Leukemia, retinoblastoma
Bloom's syndrome	Leukemia, gastrointestinal carcinoma
Severe combined immune deficiency disease	EBV-associated B-lymphocyte lymphoma/leukemia
Wiscott-Aldrich syndrome	EBV-associated B-lymphocyte lymphoma
Ataxia-telangiectasia	EBV-associated B-lymphocyte lymphoma, gastric carcinoma
Retinoblastoma	Wilms' tumor, osteosarcoma, Ewing's sarcoma
Fanconi's anemia	Leukemia, squamous cell carcinoma
Multiple endocrine neoplasia syndromes (MEN-I, -II, -III)	Adenomas of islet cells, pituitary, parathyroid, and adrenal glands
	Submucosal neuromas of the tongue, lips, eyelids
	Pheochromocytomas, medullary carcinoma of the thyroid
	Malignant schwannoma, nonappendiceal carcinoid
Neurofibromatosis (von Recklinghausen's syndrome)	Rhabdomyosarcoma, fibrosarcoma, pheochromocytomas, optic glioma, meningioma

Pizzo PA, Poplack D, Horowitz M, Hays D, & Kun L (1993). Solid tumors of childhood. In V DeVita, S Hellman, & S Rosenberg (Eds.), *Cancer Principles and Practice of Oncology* (4th ed., pp. 1738–1791). Philadelphia: JB Lippincott. Used with permission of the publisher.

quite clear that children with certain genetic disorders require lifelong monitoring for development of malignancies. Surveillance is important in all children who have had a malignancy, whether they have been treated with surgery only or with antineoplastic chemotherapy or radiation therapy.

Radiation Therapy and Its Role in the Management of Childhood Cancers

Radiation therapy has an important role in the management of many pediatric malignancies. The indications for its use, the specific timing and techniques employed, and its role are frequently dictated by multidisciplinary and clinical trial protocols. The management of childhood malignancies requires careful integration of disciplines—surgery, chemotherapy, radiation therapy—to ensure maximal benefit and minimal toxicity.

The role of radiation therapy in the treatment of many childhood cancers, such as Wilms' tumor, leukemia, Hodgkin's disease, non-Hodgkin's lymphoma, and bone and soft tissue tumors, has been under constant redefinition. Many of the above tumors now can be stratified into good and bad prognostic groups, based on immunologic typing, molecular analysis, histologic features, clinical staging, and presentation (Pizzo et al., 1993). Treatment protocols now are customized to adjust the intensity of therapy to match a child's prognostic group and clinical presentation. Aggressive combined-modality treatment protocols have proved to be a two-edged sword in children. Along with improved overall long-term survival has come a growing list of grave complications, such as altered growth and development of muscle, bone, and soft tissue, neuropsychological sequelae, endocrine deficiencies, and second malignancies (Kun & Moulder, 1993; Pizzo et al., 1993). Defining appropriate treatment regimens is of paramount importance in reducing the long-term complications of treatment in children.

The complexities of managing children with malignancies demand the coordinated participation of many pediatric specialties and support services. In complex cases, the assistance of oncologists, surgeons, anesthesiologists, nurses, diagnostic specialists, laboratory scientists, and pharmacists often is needed during the treatment phase. When long-term treatment- or disease-related problems are anticipated, appropriate subspecialty referrals should be made. Individual circumstances may require the involvement of specialists in endocrinology, neurology, neuropsychology, cardiology, pulmonary medicine, vision and hearing, dentistry, orthopedics, nutrition, or social services.

Radiation and Surgery

Radiation therapy may be given as a definitive treatment with curative intent to a localized tumor that has either been biopsied or subtotally excised. Preoperatively, radiation may be used alone or in combination with chemotherapy to reduce a tumor's size, so that the tumor is more easily resected or limb function is preserved (Pizzo et al., 1993). In some situations, it may be preferable to use radiation therapy postoperatively, to enhance local control after complete resection of a tumor. In the latter case, radiation therapy is delivered to the surgical site to eradicate residual microscopic foci of disease or peripheral extension of the disease beyond the operative margins (Kun & Moulder, 1993).

Intraoperative radiation therapy has potential applications in pediatric cancers, such as large retroperitoneal sarcomas or locally resected malignant lesions of long bones (Kun & Moulder, 1993). The rationale for this technique is to eradicate residual microscopic disease through delivery of local, immediate treatment to the operative bed. The shortcomings of this procedure are the dose-limiting toxicities to surrounding tissues, organs, and peripheral nerves and the limited availability of the technology (Kun & Moulder, 1993).

Brachytherapy

Brachytherapy is the direct application to a tumor of a temporary or permanent radioactive source, such as iridium 192, iodine 125, or radioactive colloidals (phosphorus-32). This technique offers the advantage of delivering a high dose of radiation to a specific tumor volume, with rapid fall-off in dose to adjacent tissue (Hassey-Dow, 1992). The types of brachytherapy available are intracavitary, interstitial implants, plaques, radiation needles, and wires. The pediatric experience with these techniques has been limited. Plaques have been used for treatment of retinoblastoma, intracavitary interstitial brachytherapy has been used for soft tissue sarcomas, vaginal rhabdomyosarcomas, and gliomas, and seed implants have been used for infantile subglottic hemangiomas, brain tumors, sarcomas, neuroblastomas, hepatoblastomas, and pancreatic carcinomas (Curran et al., 1988; Kun & Moulder, 1993; Halperin et al., 1994c; Healey et al., 1995).

Combined Modality Therapy

One of the fundamental approaches in the treatment of pediatric malignancies is the coordinated use of radiation and chemotherapy, so that the actions of each can potentiate antitumor effects selectively (Kun & Moulder, 1993). The advantages of chemotherapy are that it offers a systemic means of eliminating distant micrometastases outside the radiation field. When given before radiation, chemotherapy may decrease the size of the tumor, and, when given in combination with radiation, it may act to sensitize tumor cells, thereby enhancing the response to radiation (Hirshfield-Bartek, 1992; Phillips, 1994). The advantages of radiation are that it can reduce the size of the tumor mass and improve the blood supply to the tumor so that cellular uptake of chemotherapy can be enhanced (Phillips, 1994).

Drug-radiation interactions can be classified into three categories: *independent, enhancing*, and *protective*. In *independent* interactions, the drug and radiation do not act together on the same cell populations. Radiation may be used for local control in areas of the body where chemotherapy alone is inadequate. A common example would be the treatment of children with high-risk leukemia with C2 whole-brain radiation as a supplement to systemic and intrathecal chemotherapy. In this instance, radiation therapy affects "sanctuary sites" in the central nervous system that chemotherapy alone cannot reach. This type of interaction also has been termed *spatial cooperation* (Phillips, 1994).

In *enhanced* interactions, radiation and chemotherapy act together on the same cell populations. Phillips has recognized three types of enhanced interactions: *additive, supraadditive*, and *subadditive* (Phillips, 1994). In *additive* interactions, the combined effect of the two modalities theoretically equals the sum of the individual effects. Additive effects have been noted in certain pediatric solid tumors, such as Wilms' tumor, rhabdomyosarcoma, and Ewing's sarcoma (Kun & Moulder, 1993). In *supraadditive* reactions, the combined effect of radiation and chemotherapy is greater than sum of each modality's individual effects. In theory, *subadditive* effects may be observed, if there is a negative interaction that reduces the combined effect of the two modalities to a level that is less than the sum of their individual effects (Phillips, 1994).

Protective interactions occur when a chemical agent decreases the effect of radiation on cells. Ideally, this effect would occur in normal cells, but not in the targeted tumor cells. An example of this type of interaction is the use of sulfhydryl agents to reduce injury to irradiated tissues (Phillips, 1994).

The timing of the administration of chemotherapy and radiation therapy can affect the efficacy and toxicity of combined modality treatment. *Neoadjuvant* chemotherapy is administered before radiation with the intent of eliminating micrometastases and reducing the number of cells in the primary tumor. With *concurrent* therapy both modalities are administered simultaneously or in rapidly alternating courses. *Adjuvant* chemotherapy is administered after radiation therapy, with or without surgery, primarily to sterilize micrometastases outside the treatment field (Phillips, 1994). The interactions of chemotherapy and radiation therapy are complex. Children receiving combined modality treatment require careful monitoring for bone marrow suppression, pneumonitis, pericarditis, hemorrhagic cystitis, impaired wound healing, increased susceptibility to infection, and altered nutritional status caused by injury to the gastrointestinal mucosa. The late effects of combined modality therapy on normal tissues have become a topic of increasing interest and concern and are summarized in Table 17–5.

Total Body Irradiation

Total body radiation (TBI) is an important component of the preparative regimen for bone marrow transplantation for several malignancies. These neoplasms include acute lymphoblastic leukemia (ALL) in second or subsequent remission, ALL-Ph chromosome positive, acute myelogenous leukemia, chronic myelogenous leukemia, myelodysplasia, multiple myeloma, Hodgkin's, disease, non-Hodgkin's lymphoma, and sarcomas (Tarbell et al., 1994). TBI provides three important benefits: (1) myeloablation, to create a space within the bone marrow to allow engraftment of the donor marrow; (2) immunosuppression of the host, to prevent graft rejection; (3) eradication of residual malignant cells in the patient (Tarbell et al., 1994). The use of fractionated TBI has improved both host tolerance and cell kill. This assumes particular importance in children, for whom the effects on growth and developing organs are a concern (Halperin et al., 1994d).

Important aspects of treatment delivery include administration of a uniform dose of radiation to the entire body, provision of adequate lung shielding, and attention to the radiation time–dose

Table 17-5 • Radiation Dose Toxicity Levels for Subacute and Late Visceral Effects

Organ	Toxicity	Whole Organ Irradiation			Partial Organ Irradiation				Chemotherapy Effect
		5–10% Incidence	Dose*	>25–50% Incidence	Volume	<5–10% Incidence	Dose*	>25–50% Incidence	
Lung	Subacute pneumonitis or late fibrosis	18–20 Gy 15–18	(CTx−)† (CTx+)‡	24–25 Gy 21–24	<30% of one lung	25–30 Gy <20	(CTx−)† (CTx+)‡	45–50 Gy >35	++
Heart	Subacute pericarditis Late cardiomyopathy	35–40 45–50 30–40	(CTx−) (CTx+)	>50 >60 >50	<50% <25%	40–50 <40 30–40	(CTx−) (CTx+)	60–70 >70 >50	+/− +++
Liver	Subacute hepatopathy	25–30 20–25	(CTx−) (CTx+)	>40 >35	<60%	NA§		NA	+
Kidney	Subacute or late nephropathy Late hypertension	18–20 16–18 Similar to subacute levels	(CTx−) (CTx+)	24–28 22–26	>50% >50%	20–24 20–25		>30 >35	+ +/−
Small bowel	Subacute enteropathy	15–25		>40	<50%	20–25		>60	+
Brain	Late necrosis	54–60		>65	<50%	Equal to whole brain		>60	+
Spinal cord	Subacute-late	40–45		>50	<15%	45–50		>55	−

* Dose assumes conventional fractionation (150–200 cGy once daily, 5 days per week).
† (CTx−) implies without prior, concurrent, or subsequent chemotherapy.
‡ (CTx+) implies interaction with one or more chemotherapeutic agents in any sequence.
§ NA not applicable.

From Kun L & Moulder J (1993). General principles of radiation therapy. In P Pizzo & D Poplack (Eds.), *Principles and Practice of Pediatric Oncology* (2nd ed., pp. 273–302). Philadelphia: JB Lippincott. Used with permission of the publisher.

interval. The major complications of TBI are infection, interstitial pneumonitis, veno-occlusive disease, nephrotoxicity, graft-versus-host disease, tumor recurrence (Tarbell et al., 1994). TBI also may enhance the cardiac toxicity of cyclophosphamide and anthracyclines and produce an increased incidence of arrhythmias, pericarditis, and cardiomyopathies (Halperin et al., 1994d; Tarbell et al., 1994).

Stereotactic Procedures

Conventional radiation therapy plays an important role in the management of pediatric brain tumors. Despite the therapeutic benefits of brain irradiation, this therapy has been associated with a variety of long-term sequelae that are of particular significance to children. These neurotoxicities include cranial nerve damage, memory and intellectual deficits, pituitary and hypothalamic dysfunction, demyelinization of brain tissue, and secondary malignancies (Dunbar & Loeffler, 1994; Lew & LaVally, 1995; Sheline et al., 1980). Other risk factors that may contribute to these problems are young age, hydrocephalus, tumor location, postsurgical neurologic status, high doses of radiation therapy, large radiation treatment fields, and use of intrathecal chemotherapy (Mulhern, 1994).

Several innovative treatment approaches have been developed specifically to address the issue of treating brain tumors. These stereotactic technologies share the primary objective of delivering therapeutic doses of radiation to the site of disease while minimizing damage to surrounding normal tissue. The *gamma-knife*, using cobalt-60 as its energy source, directs multiple point sources of gamma irradiation to converge on the tumor volume. *Linear accelerators* have been modified to use stereotactic technique (three-dimensional CT/MRI planning and stereotactic head immobilization devices) to deliver precise beams of radiation in noncoplanar arcs to the treatment target volume. The *cyclotron* uses high-energy proton beams as its source of irradiation.

Stereotactic radiation therapy (SRT) offers an alternative to conventional radiation therapy. The specific advantages of this technique are accurate delivery of focal treatment to the target area, significant reduction of radiation dose to non-target tissue, and precise immobilization and three-dimensional planning. The biological advantages of SRT are that it allows for the use of conventional fractionation schedules, reduces brain and cranial nerve damage, and permits treatment in critical brain regions that might be considered inoperable because of their central location or involvement of adjacent sensitive tissues (brain stem, optic tract, internal capsule, motor and speech areas) (Dunbar & Loeffler, 1994).

SRT offers a desirable alternative to the treatment of pediatric brain tumors. Its use is generally restricted to lesions that have small tumor volumes (<5 cm), are radiographically distinct, and are noninfiltrating and noninvasive (Loeffler et al., 1993). It has been suggested that tumors fitting the above selection criteria include: low-grade gliomas, pituitary adenomas, craniopharyngiomas, meningiomas, low-grade astrocytomas, optic nerve gliomas, retinoblastomas, and recurrent lesions in the setting of prior conventional radiation (Loeffler et al., 1992; Loeffler et al., 1993). Long-term follow-up studies are needed to establish the efficacy of SRT, to identify the long-term sequelae of treatment, and to evaluate outcome, particularly in the areas of neuropsychological and endocrine function.

Palliation

Radiation therapy may play a palliative role in children with incurable metastatic disease. Under these circumstances, radiation is administered to alleviate symptoms, such as bone pain, pain caused by tumor impingement on nerves, respiratory compromise due to airway obstruction, neurologic deficit due to compressing lesions in the brain or spinal cord, or to manage organ dysfunction caused by tumor invasion.

Oncologic Emergencies

Oncologic emergencies can arise in pediatric patients from one of three situations: a space-occupying lesion causes pressure or obstruction; leukemia or a solid tumor creates a metabolic or hormonal problem; cytopenias arise from the effects on the bone marrow of the disease or treatment (Lange et al., 1993).

In the situations of superior vena cava syndrome (SVC) or superior mediastinal syndrome (SMS), tracheal compression and respiratory compromise present true medical emergencies. The clinical signs and symptoms of SMS are: cough, hoarseness, dyspnea, orthopnea, and chest pain. Examination of the patient may reveal the following findings: mental status changes, lethargy, distorted vision, ear fullness, swelling of the face and neck, plethora, cyanosis of the face, neck and upper extremities, wheezing, stridor, engorgement of veins in the neck and chest (Lange et al., 1993). Chest x rays will demonstrate a mass in the anterior mediastinum with or without pleural and pericardial effusions. Non-Hodgkin's lymphoma, Hodgkin's disease, T cell leukemia, dysgerminomas, and seminomas may present with SVC or SMS. The diagnosis and evaluation of SVC and SMS must be expeditious but carefully considered, since children with these syndromes often are not sufficiently stable to tolerate invasive procedures requiring general anesthesia. Pleurocentesis, pericardiocentesis, lymph node aspiration or biopsy, computed tomography of the chest, bone marrow biopsy, examination of peripheral blood may achieve the required diagnosis.

Radiation treatment options for SVC and SMS are weighed very cautiously, as there is a risk of postirradiation respiratory deterioration. This phenomenon, as it was described by Lange and associates, appears to be unique to children and adolescents, perhaps because of the greater compressibility of the respiratory structures in younger patients and the limited capacity of relatively narrow airway lumens to accommodate edema (Lange et al., 1993). In some situations, chemotherapy agents, such as steroids, cyclophosphamide, vincristine, and/or anthracyclines might be preferable to radiation for the management of SVC or SMS (Lange et al., 1993).

Neurologic emergencies may be the presenting manifestations of tumors in children, or they may arise from recurrent or metastatic malignancies, dysfunction of other organ systems, or as a consequence of treatment. Examples of the latter are cerebral edema, thrombosis, and hemorrhage (Lange et al., 1993). Since the causes of this type of emergency are varied, the diagnostic evaluation must include a careful history, neurological examination, and imaging with CT scan and/or MRI.

Another common type of neurologic emergency in pediatric patients involves the spinal cord and its surrounding structures. Four percent of children with cancer develop spinal cord dysfunction related to tumor compression, with sarcomas accounting for 43 to 63 percent of malignant spinal cord disease; and neuroblastoma, lymphoma, and leukemias accounting for the rest (Lange et al., 1993). Other etiologies for back pain and spinal cord dysfunction include tumor involvement of surrounding bony structures and treatment-related myelitis.

After the nature and extent of central nervous system disease have been determined, effective treatment plans can be formulated. In some situations, neurosurgical intervention, such as emergency shunts or spinal cord decompression and laminectomy, may be warranted. Emergency radiation may play a role in the management of rapidly progressing brain tumors, such as brain stem gliomas, or metastatic disease to the brain or spine (commonly caused by neuroblastoma, lymphoma, or rhabdomyosarcoma). Radiation therapy may be used in combination with steroids to treat tumors with known radiosensitivity. Local irradiation also may follow decompression surgery or be used with chemotherapy to provide disease control.

Treatment Planning

The primary goal of therapeutic radiation is to achieve a *therapeutic balance* between providing an effective tumoricidal treatment dose and minimizing the risks of acute and late complications. This requires careful simulation and treatment planning, accurate localization of tumor volume, and proper immobilization. Accuracy in defining the target volume often requires the use of computerized tomography (CT), magnetic resonance imaging (MRI), positron emission tomography (PET), and radiography (Halperin et al., 1994e). In determining the treatment approach, several factors must be taken into consideration. These include the tumor histology, the natural history of the disease, tumor size, site, potential for microscopic extension, involvement of local or adjacent lymph nodes, the extent of disease as determined at the time of surgery, and tumor location with respect to normal tissue structures (Kun & Moulder, 1993). The treatment plan is generated by the radiation oncologist with the collaboration of the dosimetrist and radiation oncology therapists at the simulation facility.

One of the major priorities in treating children is to reproduce the treatment position accurately on a consistent daily basis. The high degree of precision, immobility, and reproducibility essential for daily treatment is influenced by several factors: the child's age; level of emotional maturity; degree of physical comfort; the coping style of the child and parent; previous experiences with invasive procedures; level of anxiety; clinical condition; requirement for sedation or anesthesia. The groundwork for treatment planning and daily therapy should be established prior to the planning session with a thorough assessment of the child and family. It is especially important to create an atmosphere of trust with the parents and to assess the child's understanding of treatment and his/her previous reactions to illness, hospitalization, treatments, and novel situations.

The parents' and child's first impressions of the planning session experience need to be positive and supportive. Children and parents often benefit from the expertise of a child life specialist. Working closely with the oncology team, the child life specialist can assist with the psychological preparation for treatment planning and daily treatment. The preplanning session should serve as an opportunity to explain the treatment to the parents, to elicit parents' support for behaviors expected of the child during treatment, to familiarize the child with the treatment setting and personnel, to provide a gradual exposure to treatment position and daily routine, and to determine whether or not sedation or anesthesia will be required. Play therapy creates opportunities for the child to become familiar with treatment procedures and equipment, to work through fears and anxieties, and to rehearse the treatment position. It is important to explain to children what they might expect in terms of sights, sounds, smells, and touch and to provide explanations that are simple and meaningful. Intervention strategies might include a demonstration using a miniature radiation therapy machine and doll, observation of another child going through a similar procedure, and role playing using a parent, staff member, or doll to enact the sequence of events to take place. The child should be encouraged to practice lying in the treatment position, with the required behavior and rules simply but clearly stated. Positive reinforcement with praise, stickers, and small rewards can be used to strengthen desirable cooperative behaviors and motivation (Bucholtz, 1994; Slifer et al., 1994; Lew & Lavally, 1995).

Story-telling, fantasy, and distraction techniques such as music, stories on tape, counting, blowing bubbles, and mobiles, can provide helpful tools for capturing the child's attention, reducing anxiety, and gaining cooperation during planning and treatment. Patient education materials are available in the form of instructional videotapes and printed materials. The latter include coloring books about radiation therapy, pamphlets, and written materials developed by individual treatment centers and the National Cancer Institute. Parents can help by encouraging the child to practice his or her role at home before the first planning and treatment sessions. Well-conducted studies support the use of behavioral training techniques for desensitizing children and teaching motion control. These techniques are most helpful with preschoolers and with older children with developmental delays, physical handicaps, or anxiety related to previous painful experiences and

are effective for reducing the need for anesthesia and limiting the costs of treatment (Slifer et al., 1994).

Practice sessions for treatment planning and simulation should be scheduled in advance so that the child and family have sufficient opportunity to rehearse the routine, get comfortable with procedures, and have time to review the overall treatment plan with the radiation oncologist. If anesthesia or sedation will be required, additional preparation is needed in the form of preoperative evaluation and consent, preoperative teaching, and review of NPO and sedation guidelines with the parents. The additional time required for anesthesia and recovery must be incorporated into the work schedule of nurses, radiation therapists, and physicians.

Many children have venous access devices, such as Broviac or Hickman catheters, or subcutaneous ports. These must be accessed with the same degree of rigor that is required for similar devices in adults. The use of EMLA Cream (Astra Pharmaceuticals, Westborough, MA) has made insertion of intravenous catheters and accessing of ports a less traumatic experience for children by providing a topical anesthetic effect. To avoid adverse negative associations, invasive or potentially painful procedures should not be performed in the simulation or treatment rooms (Bucholtz, 1994).

Immobilization Devices

Physical comfort is fundamental for ensuring immobility and cooperation from children during radiation treatments. Standard measures include padding of sensitive pressure points, pain control with analgesics, warmth, and respect for body integrity and privacy (Bucholtz, 1994). A large variety of immobilization devices can be used, including custom-made head holders, frames, plaster of Paris casts, vacuum bags filled with styrofoam beads, and molded devices fashioned from thermoplastics or polyurethane foams (Halperin et al., 1994e; Lew & Lavally, 1995). Standard accessory devices include foam pillow supports, firm head and neck supports, head stabilizers for prone positioning that have cut-outs for the eyes and nose, and safety straps. Immobilization devices must be designed to accomplish their desired effects without compromising circulation, ventilation, or access to airways or intravenous devices.

Treatment planning sessions vary in length from 20 minutes to 3 hours depending upon the treatment field, the need to perform special imaging studies, such as CT or MRI, and the need for sedation or anesthesia to ensure immobility. The requirement for sedation or anesthesia at the time of planning doesn't necessarily carry through to the later stages of treatment. The comfort, confidence, and clinical status of many children often will improve sufficiently to eliminate the need for anesthesia as treatment proceeds.

Overview of the Major Childhood Cancers

Neuroblastoma

Neuroblastoma is a tumor thought to be derived from the paraspinal sympathetic ganglia or adrenal medulla. It represents 8 percent of cancers diagnosed in children less than 15 years of age and accounts for one-third of all malignancies in children under 1 year of age (Reaman, 1993). The most common sites of primary involvement are the abdomen, paraspinal ganglion, thorax, and pelvis. Two-thirds of children over the age of 1 year present with metastatic disease, most often to regional lymph nodes, or via a hematogenous route to bone marrow, bone, liver, and subcutaneous tissue (Brodeur & Castleberry, 1993; Tarbell et al., 1990).

The use of several nonstandardized staging systems has made the literature on treatment of neuroblastoma difficult to interpret (Brodeur & Castleberry, 1993; Lukens, 1994). The International Neuroblastoma Staging System has been proposed as the standard for future clinical trials (Brodeur et al., 1993). The management of neuroblastoma is based upon age, clinical stage, degree of surgical resectability, and estimated risk of recurrence. Surgery plays a role in defining the local extent of tumor and the degree of lymph node involvement and is sometimes used as a "second look" procedure. Early stage I disease should be surgically excised, if possible, since the disease-free survival is greater than 90 percent (Brodeur & Castleberry, 1993). Children with unresectable localized tumors are generally treated with combination chemotherapy, delayed surgical resection, and radiation therapy (Brodeur & Castleberry, 1993). Chemotherapy has been the principal approach in the management of unresectable local tumor, metastatic, and recurrent disease. Agents that have demonstrated activity against advanced or recurrent neuroblastoma include cyclophosphamide, cisplatin, doxorubicin, teniposide, VM-26, etoposide, and VP-16. The drug combinations currently showing the most clinical activity are cyclophosphamide plus doxorubicin and cisplatin plus teniposide (Brodeur & Castleberry, 1993).

Radiation therapy has been shown to be of benefit in children with regional lymph node metastases and in newborns with Evans stage IV-S disease in respiratory distress caused by hepatomegaly. Radiation may be used alone or in combination with laminectomy to treat neuroblastoma causing spinal cord compression, but this use is associated with a high risk of skeletal growth abnormalities, and data support the use of chemotherapy as an alternative (Hayes et al., 1989). Total body irradiation (TBI) is being employed as part of the preparative regimen in autologous bone marrow transplantation protocols (Brodeur & Castleberry, 1993).

Wilms' Tumor

Wilms' tumor, which is a primary tumor of the kidney, accounts for approximately 5 percent of childhood cancers. The majority of cases occur in children under 5 years of age (median age $3\frac{1}{2}$ to 4 years), and both sexes are affected equally (Green et al., 1993; Tarbell et al., 1990). Congenital anomalies known to be associated with Wilms' tumor include: aniridia, hemihypertrophy, malformations of the genitalia, rare congenital malformation syndromes, and neurofibromatosis (Green et al., 1993). Wilms' tumor commonly presents as an asymptomatic flank or abdominal mass, abdominal pain, hematuria, fever, and anorexia. Surgical staging is important in determining treatment and prognosis. Staging evaluation should include preoperative imaging, exploratory laparotomy, transperitoneal nephrectomy, lymph node sampling, and radiographic examination of the lungs. Staging and histopathology of the primary tumor are accurate predictors of prognosis and determine therapeutic approach (Lukens, 1994). Factors that influence prognosis adversely include unfavorable histology, distant metastasis, and lymph node involvement (Pizzo et al., 1993).

Radiation therapy is being used more conservatively because of the long-term consequences of treating young children with large abdominal fields. These include growth disturbances, risk of second tumors (thyroid, breast, sarcomas, leukemia, and lymphoma), and the risks of hepatic, pulmonary, and cardiac injury when chemotherapy and radiation are used in combination (Green et al., 1993). The role of radiation therapy now appears limited to NWTS stages III and IV disease (National Wilms' Tumor Study Committee,

1990). Surgery followed by adjuvant chemotherapy now produces a 95 percent cure rate for stage I patients with favorable histology, and radiation appears to provide little or no added benefit to patients with stage II disease treated with two- or three-drug regimens (Green et al., 1993; Lukens, 1994). Postoperative radiation is used for stage III and IV Wilms' tumors with favorable histology, but use of combination chemotherapy regimens can limit the radiation dose to 1000 cGy in stage III patients (Green et al., 1993). Postoperative radiation therapy is indicated in stages II–IV anaplastic Wilms' tumor, with doses ranging from 1260 to 3780 cGy, depending on the patient's age (Green et al., 1993). The clear-cell histologic variant of Wilms' tumor is associated with a relatively high rate of local-regional disease recurrence, and postoperative radiation and chemotherapy are indicated for all stages (Green et al., 1993). Whole-lung radiation is recommended for patients who present with pulmonary metastases, but at least one study has suggested that results with radiation are no better than with nephrectomy and chemotherapy, without radiation (Green et al., 1993).

Retinoblastoma

Retinoblastoma is the most common primary tumor of the eye occurring in childhood, and it accounts for 1 percent of pediatric tumors. It has many important features that distinguish it clinically. Retinoblastoma arises from the nuclear layer of the retina, and it may present as multifocal, bilateral, congenital, inherited, or acquired disease. Other features that make this tumor unique are its association with chromosomal abnormalities and the genetic susceptibility for oncogenesis in patients with the inheritable form of the disease (Donaldson et al., 1993). Bilateral disease is always heritable, and children of long-term survivors require careful monitoring, because they will have a 50 percent risk of developing retinoblastoma. Twelve percent of patients with sporadic unilateral disease also will have the heritable form, conferring a 5 percent risk of retinoblastoma in the first child of such patients (Donaldson et al., 1993). Patients with the *heritable* form have a high rate of secondary malignancies, occurring within and outside of the treatment field, with sarcomas being the most common tumor type. Second malignancies have developed in children who have not received radiation therapy (Donaldson et al., 1993). The most common clinical presentation of retinoblastoma in children

without a known family history is strabismus, leukoria (cat's eye reflex), and disturbance of vision (Tarbell et al., 1990).

The evaluation of retinoblastoma requires careful ophthalmologic examination of both eyes, bone marrow aspiration and biopsy, lumbar puncture for cerebrospinal fluid cytology examination, and computerized tomography of the head to determine the extent of orbital disease. The rapid growth of the tumor mandates prompt evaluation and treatment once the diagnosis is suspected.

The Reese and Ellsworth staging system has been widely accepted for staging intraocular disease. It predicts the likelihood of tumor control and preservation of vision, but it does not predict survival (Ellsworth, 1969). There is no accepted staging system for disease that extends beyond the globe. Poor prognostic signs include orbital invasion, extension to the central nervous system, and hematogenous spread. The primary goals in the selection of therapy for retinoblastoma are cure and preservation of vision in the affected eye, if possible. Enucleation is recommended for unilateral disease if the eye is blind, or if there is no reasonable expectation of preserving vision. Cryotherapy, photocoagulation, or radiotherapy are options for early-stage unilateral disease. When bilateral disease is present, the extent of disease must be determined in each eye independently. Since bilateral disease makes it difficult to predict how much vision will be preserved, it is now recommended that both eyes be treated with radiation. Patients who are so treated must be monitored for recurrence (Donaldson et al., 1993).

Radiation therapy is the treatment of choice for the majority of children with retinoblastoma. The use of external beam radiation therapy is indicated when the retinoblastoma is large, multifocal, close to the macula or optic nerve, or has seeded the vitreous. Therapy is now administered in small daily fractions of 180 to 200 cGy (total dose 4500 to 5400 cGy over 4.5 to 6 weeks) to minimize the long-term effects previously observed with large-fraction therapy (Donaldson et al., 1993). The treatment technique is critical, and anesthesia usually is required to ensure immobilization and fixed ocular position. Chemotherapy is now restricted to children with extraocular disease. Long-term follow-up is needed to monitor for tumor recurrence, treatment complications, and second tumors. Genetic counseling is important for those cases that are considered to be inherited.

Central Nervous System Tumors

Tumors of the central nervous system are the most common solid tumors in children and the second most common tumors in the pediatric age group. They are the third leading cause of death in children under the age of 16 (Shiminski-Maher & Wisoff, 1995). Pediatric brain tumors differ from those in adults in their cell type and site of origin. Whereas the majority of brain tumors in adults are supratentorial and are astrocytomas, the majority of pediatric brain tumors are infratentorial, and 40 percent are primitive neuroepithelial neoplasms (Heideman et al., 1993). The classification of brain tumors is complex because of the diversity of the phenotypically distinct cells capable of malignant transformation, the ability of these tumors to arise in different locations within the cranium and spinal axis, and the predominance of tumors at different ages (Levin et al., 1993). In children, tumors of the supratentorium include astrocytoma, glioblastoma, oligodendroglioma, sarcomas, neuroblastoma, and mixed gliomas. Pediatric infratentorial tumors include astrocytoma, medulloblastoma, ependymoma, and brain stem glioma. Pediatric tumors of the sellar and parasellar regions include craniopharyngioma and optic glioma (Levin et al., 1993).

The clinical presentation of brain tumors is governed principally by their location and growth rate. Tumors of the posterior fossa commonly present with signs and symptoms attributable to increased intracranial pressure, especially headache and vomiting. Involvement of the cerebellar hemispheres may produce ataxia and nystagmus, whereas involvement of the brain stem usually produces cranial nerve deficits and/or hemiparesis. Common manifestations of supratentorial tumors are hemiparesis, sensory deficits, seizures, and visual and intellectual disturbances. Tumors arising in the hypothalamic and pituitary region often produce visual field defects, endocrine disturbances, and nausea and vomiting caused by increased intracranial pressure. Many of the cardinal symptoms of brain tumors are difficult to detect in infants and small children, making early diagnosis a particular challenge. Irritability, anorexia, and developmental delay—all early signs of increased intracranial pressure—may be the principal manifestations. In school-age children, the initial signs may be nonspecific and subacute, and may include decreased academic performance, personality changes, fatigue, intermittent vaguely described headaches, difficulties with coordination, and visual changes (Heideman et al., 1993; Shiminski-Maher & Shields, 1995).

The role of radiotherapy in the management of pediatric brain tumors is dependent on the tumor histology, anatomic location, grade, pattern of spread, and degree of surgical resectability. For example, low-grade supratentorial astrocytomas may be cured by surgery alone, if the resection is complete. Higher grades of astrocytoma, grades 3 and 4, are managed by surgery and radiation therapy (Heideman et al., 1993; Tarbell et al., 1990). In situations where surgical morbidity and mortality limit this approach, radiation may serve as the definitive mode of treatment. It may also be used as an adjunct to chemotherapy and surgery. In tumors with known predisposition for seeding to the craniospinal axis, such as medulloblastoma or ependymoma, radiotherapy may include the entire craniospinal axis.

The techniques for delivering radiation therapy to the central nervous system are of critical importance, since sparing of uninvolved normal tissue is a paramount consideration. Stereotactic radiation techniques may be used for small (<5 cm), well-defined tumors in surgically inaccessible locations. Tumors that are amenable to this approach include pituitary adenomas, craniopharyngiomas, meningiomas, low-grade astrocytomas, optic nerve gliomas, and retinoblastomas. Another important application for stereotactic radiation is for recurrent tumor in patients who have been treated previously by conventional therapy (Dunbar & Loeffler, 1994; Lew & LaVally, 1995). Conventional radiotherapy treatment plans vary with the location and size of the tumor. A variety of head and spine immobilization devices and methods for sparing adjacent tissues, such as three-field, opposed laterals and arc rotation techniques may be used. Dose and fractionation schemes vary according to tumor volume and location, the age of the child, and tissue tolerance.

The use of radiation therapy for treatment of brain tumors in infants and very young children is now being reconsidered. Although surgery and chemotherapy may contribute to long-term sequelae, the effects of radiation therapy on the developing brain are thought to be especially deleterious. Irradiation of the developing brain can disrupt axon growth, dendrite arborization, and synapse formation. Brain development begins during the prenatal period and continues at a rapid pace during the first several years. Children under 5 years of age therefore are particularly vulnerable to CNS toxicity. The long-term manifestations of CNS irradiation are profound intellectual, cognitive, and social impairment, and neuroendocrine dysfunction (Heideman et al.,

1993; Moore, 1995). Postsurgical chemotherapy has been proposed as a method of delaying radiotherapy for some brain tumors in very young children until CNS maturation has taken place. The agents used and the intensity of treatment vary with the tumor type and are the subjects of current clinical trials.

Children who have received brain irradiation require careful long-term follow-up and management of treatment-related problems. The interval between radiation therapy and the appearance of sequelae varies with patient age, radiation dose, and the disease being treated. For example, this interval is apt to be shorter for a child treated for a brain tumor than for a child treated with C2 whole-brain radiation for leukemia (Moore, 1995). It is therefore necessary to establish the child's developmental baseline and to conduct regularly scheduled long-term follow-up evaluations. The services of endocrinologists, neuropsychologists, physical and occupational therapists, special needs teachers, and hearing and speech therapists may be required.

Rhabdomyosarcoma

Rhabdomyosarcoma is the most common soft tissue sarcoma of childhood, and represents 5 to 8 percent of all solid tumors in children less than 15 years of age. The cell of origin is a mesenchymal cell that initiates striated muscle differentiation. This tumor appears to have two age peaks of occurrence, in children between 2 and 6 years, and in adolescents between 14 and 18 years. Tumors occurring in the head and neck region and genitourinary tract are usually associated with the earlier age peak. Primary tumors of the male genitourinary tract, head and neck region, trunk, and extremities, are usually found during the adolescent period. Rhabdomyosarcoma is associated with several congenital disorders, including neurofibromatosis, Gorlin's basal-cell nevus syndrome, and fetal alcohol syndrome. Relatives of children with rhabdomyosarcoma appear to have an increased frequency of breast cancer, and there appears to be an increased incidence of rhabdomyosarcoma in the siblings of children with brain tumors and adrenal cortical carcinoma (Pizzo et al., 1993). Three histologic subtypes of rhabdomyosarcoma are recognized: embryonal, alveolar, and pleomorphic. These subtypes vary according to age and site and are useful for assigning prognosis. The alveolar subtype tends to occur in older children and young adults, is the most aggressive, and is associated with the poorest prognosis.

The clinical presentations of rhabdomyosarcoma are as varied as the sites in which they occur. Some of the more common presentations are: abdominal or retroperitoneal mass; biliary tract obstruction; orbital mass; ear pain and chronic otitis media caused by mass in the middle ear; nasopharyngeal mass causing airway obstruction, sinusitis, epistaxis, or dysphagia. In adolescents, the tumor often presents as a painless mass in the trunk, extremity, or scrotum. The most widely recognized staging system is the Intergroup Rhabdomyosarcoma Study system, which, unless there is dissemination, uses the magnitude of the surgery required for resection (Pizzo et al., 1993).

The overall goal of therapy for rhabdomyosarcoma is to achieve local control of the tumor while maintaining functional and cosmetic preservation of surrounding tissues. Surgery and radiation therapy are used principally to achieve local control of tumors, whereas chemotherapy has greatly enhanced disease-free survival, presumably by eliminating distant micrometastases. The relative roles of surgery and radiation therapy depend on the location and extent of the primary disease and whether the tumor can be removed in its entirety with surgery. In many cases, surgery will reduce the amount and extent of radiation required, and, in the case of bulky primary tumors, preradiation may make surgical resection feasible. For certain primary sites of tumor, such as the orbit, parameningeal region, vagina, and prostate, surgery usually is limited to initial biopsy of the tumor and regional lymph nodes and is followed by primary radiation and adjuvant chemotherapy. At other sites, such as the trunk, extremities, and scrotum, when the tumor is limited in size and more accessible, treatment may be limited to surgical resection and adjuvant chemotherapy, with radiation reserved for disease with unfavorable histology (alveolar cell type) or stage higher than I (Pizzo et al., 1993).

The timing of radiation therapy and chemotherapy has become an important issue in rhabdomyosarcoma. In at least two locations (cranial parameningeal and bladder or prostate), delay of radiation therapy has been correlated with persistent local tumor. For this reason, aggressive radiation therapy often must be administered simultaneously with or soon after chemotherapy, despite the enhanced risk of mucositis, skin reactions, and other toxicities (Raney et al., 1993). Brachytherapy offers an alternative to conventional external beam treatment of small rhabdomyosarcomas in certain locations, such as the head and neck, bladder, prostate, vagina, or extremity (Curran et al., 1988; Raney et al., 1993).

Chemotherapeutic agents with known activity against rhabdomyosarcoma include actinomycin D, chlorambucil, methotrexate, vincristine, adriamycin, cyclophosphamide and cisplatin, etoposide, and VP-16. Combinations of up to five of these agents have been employed in recent protocols. Chemotherapy usually is administered for up to 2 years after diagnosis. The regimens employed have considerable toxicity, and the management of children receiving them requires supportive management of myelosuppression, infections, mucositis, skin reactions, nutritional deficits, fluid and electrolyte imbalances, and pain (Raney et al., 1993).

Acute Leukemia

Acute leukemia is the most common malignancy in childhood, comprising one-third of all pediatric cancers in the United States (Poplack, 1993; Halperin et al., 1994f). Acute lymphoblastic leukemia (ALL) is the dominant type, accounting for 75 percent of these cases. ALL occurs most frequently between the ages of 2 and 10 years, with a peak incidence between 2 and 6 years of age. ALL, especially the T cell immunophenotype, is more common in boys, and its frequency in white children is twice that of non-whites. Acute non-lymphoblastic leukemia (ANLL) accounts for 20 percent of cases in childhood, and chronic myelogenous leukemia constitutes the remaining 5 percent (Poplack, 1993).

The etiology of childhood leukemia and its association with environmental, hereditary, and immune factors have been the focus of several recent investigations. Exposures to ionizing radiation, toxic chemicals, and alkylating agents have been implicated as risk factors for leukemia. There is an associated risk for the development of leukemia in certain genetic syndromes and chromosomal abnormalities, such as Down's syndrome, Bloom's syndrome, ataxia-telangiectasia, Klinefelter's syndrome, and the trisomy G syndrome. Immunodeficiency states that appear to confer an increased risk for leukemia in children include the Wiskott-Aldrich syndrome, congenital hypogammaglobulinemia, and severe combined immunodeficiency disease (Poplack, 1993).

The clinical presentations of ALL and ANLL may be similar, but the diseases differ significantly in their therapies and long-term prognosis. In acute leukemias, undifferentiated, immature myeloid or lymphoid cell precursors invade the bone marrow, peripheral blood, and extramedullary sites. The presenting symptoms and physical findings in the child with leukemia may include pallor, fatigue, anorexia, petechiae, bleeding, fever, infection, localized or generalized lymphadenopathy, splenomegaly, hepatomegaly, and bone pain. Many of these signs and symptoms are mediated by anemia, thrombocytopenia, and neutropenia, which are common early laboratory manifestations. The diagnostic evaluation for acute leukemia should include a detailed history and physical examination, bone marrow aspiration and biopsy, cerebrospinal fluid cytology, and chest x ray. Baseline laboratory studies should include a complete blood count and measurement of serum uric acid, electrolytes, and renal and hepatic function. Specialized studies, such as immunophenotyping of the blast cells, cytogenetic analysis, molecular genotyping, and FAB morphologic classification, often are performed because of their potential value for classifying the leukemia, assigning prognosis, and defining treatment (Poplack, 1993).

It has long been appreciated that certain parameters at presentation can be used to assign children with ALL to groups with low or high risk for recurrence. Children at low risk can be treated with lower intensity regimens that carry reduced potential for short- and long-term toxicity. Children at high risk for early recurrence, on the other hand, can be assigned to more aggressive regimens, since acceptance of a higher level of toxicity in return for the possibility of improved outcome seems justified. Although some risk criteria enjoy nearly universal acceptance, their application by large study groups has not been uniform, and this in turn has generated difficulties for those attempting to compare the outcomes of protocols on an intergroup level. A consensus group recently pooled data from four large study groups to delineate the most reliable risk criteria. Age <10 years at presentation and WBC count at diagnosis of <50,000/µl clearly define a standard-risk group of ALL patients, whereas children who do not meet these criteria fall into a high-risk group with a 4-year event-free survival of ≈65 percent. The consensus group has recommended uniform use of the above criteria in all future protocols (Smith et al., 1996). Other prognostic factors, such as DNA index, early response to therapy, cytogenetic abnormalities, and CNS disease at presentation should be monitored and reported for all patients and may be used by individual study groups to stratify risk (Smith et al. 1996).

Combination chemotherapy is the principal treatment modality for ALL. The ability to assign children accurately to risk categories has permitted adjustments in the intensity of the treatment regimens and allows treatment to be tailored accordingly. The treatment course is divided into four phases: induction, central nervous system prevention, consolidation, and maintenance. The optimal duration of maintenance therapy has not been established, and the length of maintenance treatment varies among centers from 2.5 to 3 years (Poplack, 1993).

One of the major obstacles to long-term treatment success in ALL is the development of recurrent disease. The central nervous system (CNS) and testes are considered sanctuary sites for leukemic infiltration and are the most common sites of disease relapse (Poplack, 1993). CNS leukemia is felt to result from leukemic metastases from hematogenous spread of circulating cells, or by direct extension from the cranial bone marrow (Poplack, 1993). Leukemic cells may infiltrate the deep arachnoid spaces, subglial regions, and brain parenchyma. The blood–brain barrier is thought to hinder the penetration of therapeutic concentrations of chemotherapeutic agents into these areas (Poplack, 1993; Halperin, 1994f). Patients known to be at increased risk for CNS leukemia are infants, children of black race, and children who present with high WBC counts, T cell immunophenotype, lymphadenopathy, or hepatosplenomegaly (Poplack, 1993).

CNS preventive therapies are directed at eradicating potential sites of leukemic infiltration. The optimal treatment approach is unknown and remains the focus of intense investigation in many treatment centers. The adverse effects of cranial irradiation and intrathecal chemotherapy are becoming more evident as data on late effects of treatment become available. CNS preventive therapy has been associated with CT scan abnormalities, impaired intellectual and psychomotor function, and neuroendocrine abnormalities (Poplack, 1993).

The search for purely chemotherapeutic approaches to CNS preventive therapy has centered on combinations of systemic methotrexate and intrathecal agents. Regimens may use triple intrathecal chemotherapy (methotrexate, cytosine arabinoside, hydrocortisone) alone, or combinations of systemic methotrexate and intrathecal methotrexate in different dosing schemes (Poplack, 1993).

Cranial irradiation is indicated for high-risk ALL, T cell immunophenotype, or CNS involvement at diagnosis, since it has been shown to be effective for controlling occult meningeal leukemia (Halperin et al., 1994f). The timing of cranial irradiation varies with institutional protocol. The treatment volume should encompass the entire intracranial subarachnoid space, the posterior retina and orbital apex, and the extension of the subarachnoid space along the optic nerves and into the spine to the bottom of the second cervical vertebra. Meticulous attention to detail is required during clinical setup to include all potential sites of disease involvement. The standard treatment regimen delivers a total cranial dose of 1800 cGy in ten 180 cGy fractions. *Hyperfractionated treatment*, which delivers 90 cGy twice a day in 20 treatments (total dose = 1800 cGy) is being studied as a means to reduce the incidence and severity of late CNS effects in children, particularly infants (Halperin et al., 1994f).

Children may develop several treatment-related side effects while they are receiving CNS preventive therapy. Acute neurotoxicities may be attributable to both cranial irradiation and chemotherapy, and they may include nausea, vomiting, headaches, meningismus, conjunctival irritation, lethargy, and irritability. *Somnolence syndrome* may occur from 5 to 7 weeks after cranial irradiation and may present with somnolence, lethargy, anorexia, fever, and irritability. These symptoms usually are self-limited and are managed with supportive care and symptomatic treatment (Poplack, 1993).

Non-Hodgkin's Lymphoma

Non-Hodgkin's lymphoma (NHL) comprises 10 percent of malignancies among white children in North America. In equatorial Africa, NHL accounts for 50 percent of all childhood malignancies, reflecting the high incidence of Burkitt's lymphoma. NHL, whether of B cell or T cell origin, usually presents in children as a diffuse, high-grade tumor with a widespread pattern of dissemination (Halperin et al., 1994g). T cell lymphomas account for 40 percent of NHL cases in children, whereas the corresponding percentage for adults is 20 percent (Poplack et al., 1993). Disease can occur in multiple sites that normally contain lymphoid tissue, such as lymph nodes, Peyer's patches, Waldeyer's ring, the thymus, and bone marrow. Common extranodal sites include skin, bone, and the orbit. The most common site of presentation of NHL is in the abdomen, where typically it is of the small noncleaved cell type. In 70 percent of patients with lymphoblastic lymphoma, the chest is the primary site of involvement, where the disease may present as a large mediastinal mass accompanied by dyspnea, dysphagia, pleural effusion, or superior vena cava syndrome (Poplack et al., 1993).

The etiology of NHL is unknown. There is a known risk-association between NHL and immunodeficiency states, both inherited and acquired, and certain chromosomal abnormalities. Environmental factors and certain infectious agents, notably herbicides, plants containing phorbol esters, chronic use of phenytoin, prior treatment for Hodgkin's disease with chemotherapy and radiation, Epstein-Barr virus, and malaria also appear to increase the risk of NHL (Poplack et al., 1993).

There are three principal clinical, histologic, and immunologic subgroups of NHL: lymphocytic, undifferentiated Burkitt's or non-Burkitt's, and diffuse histiocytic (large lymphoid cell variety). Intensive combination systemic chemotherapy is the mainstay of treatment for childhood NHL. Since the potential for dissemination is high in children, chemotherapy is required, regardless of disease histology or stage (Halperin et al., 1994g). Chemotherapy induces remissions in 85 to 95 percent of patients, achieving a 90 percent cure rate in children with early-stage disease and a 60 to 80 percent cure rate in children with extensive disease (Poplack et al., 1993). Treatment protocols for childhood NHL usually divide the disease into lymphoblastic and nonlymphoblastic types. Most protocols use multiple agents in short but intensive regimens that are highly specific to the institutions studying them (Poplack et al., 1993). Agents with demonstrated activity against NHL include adriamycin, methotrexate, vincristine, prednisone, 6-mercaptopurine, cyclophosphamide, cytosine arabinoside, l-asparaginase, VM-26, thioguanine, and hydroxyurea (Halperin et al., 1994g).

The role of radiation therapy in pediatric NHL is limited by the high success rates achieved with multiagent chemotherapy regimens. Intrathecal chemotherapy alone is highly effective in preventing CNS relapse, thereby eliminating the need for cranial irradiation. Radiation is used principally in emergency situations, such as superior vena cava syndrome, acute respiratory distress, spinal cord compression, orbital proptosis, and cranial nerve palsy (Poplack et al., 1993). In these cases, radiation generally is given in short courses or in hyperfractionation schedules. Radiation also may be used to treat overt disease in locations where there is a high likelihood of failure with chemotherapy alone. For example, patients who have central nervous system lymphoma or cranial nerve palsies at the time of diagnosis usually receive cranial irradiation as a part of their initial treatment. In patients with recurrent NHL, radiation frequently is used as a consolidative treatment to regions of local disease prior to or following bone marrow transplantation (Halperin et al., 1994g). Palliative radiation may be beneficial for treating painful areas of tumor in bone, or in the chest or abdomen.

Hodgkin's Disease

Hodgkin's disease is a malignancy of the lymphoid system, and it comprises 6 percent of all childhood malignancies in the United States (Halperin et al., 1994h). The illness appears to have bimodal age peaks in industrialized countries, the first occurring in the mid-to-late 20s and the second in late adulthood. Hodgkin's disease is rare in children, especially those under 5 years of age. In children over 15 years of age, it is more common in whites than in blacks. Among children less than 10 years of age there is a higher incidence in boys than girls (Leventhal & Donaldson, 1993; Poplack et al., 1993).

The etiology of Hodgkin's disease remains uncertain. Several causal relationships have been suggested. Hodgkin's disease has been found in increased frequency in children with certain immunodeficiency syndromes. Bacterial and viral etiologies have been proposed. Most notably, the development of Hodgkin's disease after infectious mononucleosis or Epstein-Barr virus infection has been described (Leventhal & Donaldson, 1993). An increased incidence of Hodgkin's disease has been noted in some families among siblings of the same gender, or among parents and children (Poplack et al., 1993). This increased risk might be related to the genetic or environmental influences on the host's level of immune competence (Liebhauser, 1993).

The majority of children present with disease above the diaphragm, principally with cervical, mediastinal, or supraclavicular nodal involvement (Poplack et al., 1993). An estimated 80 percent of children present with disease in one or both sides of the neck, and one-third have axillary lymphadenopathy. These nodes usually are firm and rubbery in texture and not painful (Donaldson & Link, 1991). Mediastinal involvement is detected in two-thirds of patients. Anteroposterior and lateral chest x rays and chest computed tomography are critical for calculating the extent of disease and degree of respiratory compromise. A less favorable prognosis is associated with masses that are more than one-third of the thoracic diameter (Leventhal & Donaldson, 1993). The presence of splenomegaly or hepatomegaly often indicates a more advanced stage of disease (Liebhauser, 1993).

Lymphangiography is a valuable technique for evaluating intrinsic lymph node architecture and distinguishing tumor involvement from reactive hyperplasia in enlarged lymph nodes. Its accuracy is 95 percent when correlated with histopathologic results. This study is reserved for children with negative CT scans to whom only radiation treatments will be given (Parker & Moore, 1993). Most younger children are treated with chemotherapy and low-dose involved-field radiation. The technical expertise required to perform lymphangiography in children and the expense of the procedure have led some institutions to favor the use of enhanced CT scans or MRI scans. CT scan of the abdomen is not as effective as lymphangiography for detecting splenic, hilar, mesenteric, celiac, or porta hepatis lymph nodes (Donaldson & Link, 1991; Baker et al., 1990). Primary disease below the diaphragm is rare and occurs in only 3 percent of cases (Leventhal & Donaldson, 1993).

The distribution of histologic subtypes differs in children from that found in adolescents and adults. Lymphocyte predominance and mixed cellularity are more common in younger children (<10 years of age). Nodular sclerosing disease is more prevalent in adolescents (77 percent) and adults (72 percent) than in younger children (44 percent) (Halperin et al., 1994h).

The diagnostic evaluation of children with Hodgkin's disease includes: CBC; erythrocyte sedimentation rate; serum copper; liver and renal function tests; thyroid function tests; diagnostic radiology studies (lymphangiography, CT scan, gallium scan, MRI); and bone marrow biopsy. There is considerable controversy about the need for staging laparotomy and splenectomy in children. These operations impose some surgical morbidity and increased susceptibility to bacterial infections, but many experts believe that these procedures afford valuable added information that is not obtainable by imaging alone (Gilchrist & Evans, 1985; Leventhal & Donaldson, 1993). The use of polyvalent pneumococcal, meningococcal, and *Haemophilus influenzae* type B vaccines, in addition to prophylactic antibiotic therapy with penicillin or erythromycin, may help to reduce the incidence of postsplenectomy infection. In children, staging laparotomy and splenectomy are reserved for cases where precise identification and localization of abdominal disease are needed to guide management decisions. One example of such a case would be the patient with clinical stage I disease for whom radiotherapy will be the primary treatment (Leventhal & Donaldson, 1993). If there is a possibility that a girl or young woman might require pelvic irradiation, the ovaries should be moved outside the anticipated field. It is more difficult to justify staging laparotomy and splenectomy when combined modality therapy is used. Recent data indicate that the use of chemotherapy and extended-field, low-dose radiation in all children with Hodgkin's disease, without the use of staging laparotomy, results in 85 percent survival, and the relapse-free survival rate for clinical stages I, II, and III is close to 90 percent (Jenkins & Doyle, 1987).

Treatment strategies for managing Hodgkin's disease in children are becoming more standardized and tailored to the age of the child, the extent of disease, and the presence or absence of unfavorable prognostic features at presentation. The complications of chemotherapy and radiation therapy make treatment decisions difficult and complex. There is a delicate balance between maximizing the disease-free survival and minimizing the late effects of treatment. The potential toxicities of current chemotherapeutic regimens (ABVD—doxorubicin, bleomycin, vincristine, DTIC; and MOPP—nitrogen mustard, vincristine, 6-mercaptopurine, and prednisone) include myelosuppression, increased susceptibility to infection, sterility, ovarian dysfunction, neurotoxicity, cardiac and pulmonary toxicity, and the risk for developing acute myelogenous leukemia. The potential complications of radiation therapy in children include impairment of growth and development in bone, muscle, and soft tissue, thyroid dysfunction, functional asplenia, cardiac and pulmonary toxicity, and the risk of second tumors (Green, 1993; Poplack et al., 1993). Host factors, especially age at the time of exposure to radiation, appear to influence the risk of second tumors. Early childhood and adolescence are considered high-risk periods. Long-term follow-up of these children reveals that increasing numbers of soft tissue sarcomas, bone tumors, melanomas, basal cell skin cancers, lymphomas, and carcinomas of the stomach, breast, thyroid and lung are occurring in young adults 15 to 19 years after radiation therapy. Increased risk for development of leukemia has been associated with both methods of treatment—chemotherapy and combined-modality treatment—and with splenectomy (Tucker, 1993). These issues underscore the importance of lifelong surveillance of patients previously treated for Hodgkin's disease, with emphasis on early detection of secondary malignancies and patient education about avoidance of tobacco consumption, the use of sunscreens, self-examination of the skin and breasts, and routine mammography screening.

The overall 5-year remission rate for children receiving combined-modality treatment is 90 percent for those with early-stage Hodgkin's disease and 80 percent for those with advanced stage IIIb and IV disease (Leventhal & Donaldson, 1993). Radiation therapy in doses ranging from 2000 to 2500 cGy to involved fields and chemotherapy have become the standard treatment approach (Donaldson & Link, 1991). Alternative treatment approaches are being studied at many cancer centers. These trials include the use of full-dose radiation (3500 to 4400 cGy) in fully grown adolescents with early-stage Ia, Ib, or IIa disease and favorable histology. For children who have not completed their growth, combined-modality treatment with lower radiation doses (1500 to 2500 cGy) delivered to less extensive volumes will be used. For prepubescent children and those with advanced-stage disease, chemotherapy and low-dose radiation therapy are recommended (Halperin et al., 1994h). The optimal chemotherapeutic regimens, number of cycles, and sequencing schedules for chemotherapy and radiation remain to be defined. The most common chemotherapy regimens currently used for Hodgkin's disease are MOPP: nitrogen mustard, Oncovin, prednisone, procarbazine; ABVD: adriamycin, bleomycin, dacarbazine; MOPP-ABVD; COPP: cyclophosphamide, Oncovin, procarbazine, prednisone; ChLVPP: chlorambucil, vinblastine, procarbazine, prednisone; OPPA/COPP: Oncovin, procarbazine, prednisone, adriamycin, cyclophosphamide, Oncovin, procarbazine, prednisone (Donaldson & Link, 1991).

The nursing care of children with Hodgkin's disease involves ongoing patient and parent teaching about disease, treatment and management of side effects, ongoing evaluation for acute side effects of treatment, and coordination of care with referring physicians, oncologists, and surgeons. The acute side effects seen during treatment can include temporary hair loss, changes in taste, xerostomia, skin erythema, particularly in the neck and shoulder region, nausea, vomiting, nutritional deficits secondary to inadequate food intake, and dehydration. Children receiving combined-modality treatment are susceptible to enhanced tissue and skin reactions, myelosuppression, and risk of infection. This warrants careful observation of counts and observation for signs and symptoms of infection, particularly chickenpox, herpes zoster, sepsis, pulmonary infections, oral herpes simplex, and candidal infections. Compliance with prophylactic antibiotic treatment in asplenic patients and dental prophylaxis (dental consult prior to treatment and nightly fluoride treatments) are mandatory for patients treated with mantle fields. It is important to discuss with patient and parents self-care practices, such as use of sunscreens, dental care, breast examination, sexual health, avoidance of smoking, and the importance of long-term follow-up.

Bone Tumors

The Ewing's sarcoma family of tumors contains tumors of bone or soft tissue origin, including Ewing's sarcoma, peripheral primitive neuroectodermal tumor (PPNET), and extraosseous Ewing's sarcoma (Horowitz et al., 1993). Ewing's sarcoma tumors have their origins from epithelial and neuronal elements. PPNET tumors are primitive round-cell tumors of soft tissue and bone with neuroectodermal features. Ewing's sarcomas and PPNETs share a common chromosomal translocation, t(11;22) (q24;q12) (Halperin et al., 1994i). Because many of their features are similar, and the tumors often are difficult to differentiate from one another by immunohistochemistry and electron microscopy, Ewing's sarcomas and PPNETs are grouped together in treatment protocols (Halperin et al., 1994i; Horowitz et al., 1993).

Ewing's sarcoma and PPNET are typically seen in the second decade of life and correlate with pubertal growth. They occur with equal frequency in males and females until the age of 13, when they become more prevalent in males. These tumors are rare in children of African or Chinese ancestry (Pizzo et al., 1993). Approximately 200 tumors of this type occur yearly in the United States (Halperin et al., 1994i).

The primary sites of involvement with Ewing's sarcoma and PPNET are, in descending order of frequency, the extremities, pelvis, chest wall, spine and paravertebral regions, and the head and neck (Horowitz et al., 1993). The presenting clinical signs and symptoms are determined by the site(s) of involvement and the extent of tumor. Pain, palpable mass, pathologic fracture, limitation of movement, and neurologic symptoms caused by spinal cord or peripheral nerve compression, may be presenting features (Halperin et al., 1994i). Tumor may involve the entire medullary cavity of a bone, or it may extend through the cortex into the adjacent soft tissues (Pizzo et al., 1993). A tumor mass accompanied by locally increased temperature, swelling and tenderness may be created by hemorrhage and necrosis within the Ewing's tumor (Horowitz et al., 1993). Metastatic disease is present in 20 percent of children at the time of diagnosis, with the most common sites being long bones and bone marrow (Halperin et al., 1994i).

CT scans and MRI are valuable for defining the extent of disease in marrow and soft tissue and for monitoring the response of the disease to treatment. Bone scans are used to define the extent of tumor, screen for metastases, and assess possible involvement of the epiphyseal plates, the occurrence of which can have important consequences for determining surgical and radiotherapeutic strategies.

The primary goals of treatment of the Ewing's family of sarcomas are preservation of function, control of the primary site of disease, and elimination of metastatic deposits (Horowitz et al., 1993). Systemic chemotherapy is given for local control and treatment of potential micrometastases. The current overall survival rates of 50 to 75 percent for patients without metastases at diagnosis has been attributed to the activity of multiagent regimens using cyclophosphamide, vincristine, and actinomycin D, with or without adriamycin (Halperin et al., 1994i). Newer trials will attempt to improve survival rates by adding ifosfamide and etoposide to these four agents (Horowitz et al., 1993).

The role of surgical resection in the combined-modality treatment approach to Ewing's sarcoma has been the subject of recent review (Horowitz et al., 1993). Surgical resection, when it is used, may follow neoadjuvant chemotherapy or radiation and chemotherapy. Surgery is considered an option for lesions that occur in dispensable bones (e.g., proximal fibula, rib, clavicle, iliac wings) that can be resected without significant functional deficit. Surgical removal of extremity lesions has been proposed for very young children (<7 years of age), for whom the long-term consequences of radiation therapy are likely to be impaired growth and functional loss. Newer surgical approaches incorporate neoadjuvant chemotherapy to reduce tumor volume prior to resection, limb sparing procedures, and the use of bone allografts and customized prostheses.

The role of radiation therapy in the treatment of Ewing's sarcoma is undergoing modification. Local control rates for primary sites treated with radiation and adjuvant chemotherapy now approach 75 to 90 percent (Horowitz et al., 1993). The treatment planning technique for Ewing's sarcoma uses CT and MRI to delineate the tumor and adjacent tissue. A variety of immobilization techniques are employed to help patients maintain proper body alignment. These include plaster casts, molds, and polymer casts. Extremity lesions require particular attention to detail. Special technical considerations may include maintaining a strip of unirradiated tissue to prevent the development of edema or fibrosis, excluding uninvolved epiphyseal plates and joint spaces, testicular shielding, and sparing the Achilles tendon (Horowitz et al., 1993). It is important to consider the close proximity of normal tissues and organs adjacent to the treatment field and minimize their exposure to radiation.

The optimum radiation dose for achieving local control has not been defined. Past studies have achieved local control of 80 to 90 percent of primary tumors with radiation doses of 4500 to 5000 cGy in 180 to 200 cGy fractions to the initial tumor volume and margins and a cone-down boost of 1000 to 1500 cGy (Horowitz et al., 1993). Newer studies will assess the role of hyperfractionated irradiation.

Developmental Aspects of Illness

It is important for the health care professional providing care for children with cancer to have an understanding of human growth and development. The child's concept of self, perception of illness, and psychosocial adjustment are influenced by his or her own personality and interactions with others in the home and treatment environments. Recognition of the developmental tasks and needs of children in each age group permits identification of problem issues, definition of special age-dependent needs, and helps the caregiver to assist the child and family to make a healthy adjustment to the illness. In the following section, the most common cancers found in each age group, the role of radiotherapy in their management, and suggested nursing interventions based on identified developmental needs will be presented.

Infancy—The Child from Birth to 12 Months

Cancer during the first year of life is relatively rare, with distribution frequencies of malignant tumors differing from those of older children. Neuroblastoma ranks first in frequency, accounting for more than 50 percent of cancers in the newborn, followed by Wilms' tumor, acute leukemia, and sarcomas (approximately 12 percent each), retinoblastoma (rare in neonates, but 9 percent of malignant tumors in infants), and tumors of the central nervous system (3 to 8 percent) (Reaman, 1993). Acute lymphocytic leukemia during infancy usually has a CALLA-negative phenotype and is associated with a poor prognosis.

Radiation therapy must be used judiciously in infants because of its potential for causing major long-term side effects on rapidly growing tissues and developing organ systems. The central nervous system is particularly vulnerable, and children treated with radiation for brain tumors at young ages have a high incidence of mental retardation (Reaman, 1993). The skeletal system, kidney, liver, and lung are also at risk for long-term side effects.

The indication for radiation therapy in infancy is determined by the natural history of the disease. In some situations, radiation may be administered in low-dose fractions, or as part of a split course of treatment (alternating or simultaneous courses of chemotherapy). Chemotherapy often plays an important role in debulking tumors to make them more amenable to surgery, or to permit the use of smaller fields of radiation. In children with brain tumors, radiation therapy is generally deferred until they are at least 24 to 36 months of age. Several promising clinical trials have used chemotherapy regimens in an attempt to defer the use of radiation. The agents used have included vincristine and cisplatin; vincristine, nitrogen mustard, and procarbazine; and cisplatin and VP-16 (Reaman, 1993).

Role of Radiation Therapy—Infancy to 6 Years

Radiation may play either a definitive role or serve as an adjunct to surgery and chemotherapy in the management of the tumors. The decision to treat with radiation therapy is dependent upon the patient's age, disease, tumor histology, clinical status, and whether or not the tumor can be cured with surgery and/or chemotherapy alone. The potential risk of inducing long-term complications in the child's musculoskeletal system, central nervous system, and visceral organs must be weighed against the likelihood of cure.

Nursing Interventions and Preparation for Treatment

The diagnosis of cancer during the first two years of life can be disruptive to the infant's process of growth and development. Although infants lack the ability to comprehend illness and treatment, they are sensitive to the emotional responses of their parents. Interruptions in the pattern of daily routine, intrusive procedures, and fear of being separated from parents can foster feelings of insecurity, stress, and distrust of strangers.

The goal of nursing is to facilitate a healthy adjustment to illness and treatment by establishing a trusting relationship with the child and parents. Interventions include assisting the parents to deal with their feelings about their child's diagnosis and treatment, providing teaching about treatment and management of anticipated side effects, and encouraging parental participation in their child's care. The developmental needs of the infant—comfort, nurturance, security, stimulation, and nutrition—should be supported at all times. Specific nursing interventions based on these developmental needs in infants are outlined in Table 17–6.

Infants and children under the age of 3 do not have the ability to maintain the degree of immobility required to provide accurate and reproducible daily radiation treatment. In this group of children, the need for sedation or anesthesia is an important consideration. Adequate preparation for parents is an essential part of decreasing their apprehension and helping them feel more confident about the treatment. The specifics of sedation, anesthesia, and parent teaching will be discussed in the section entitled "Special Considerations—Anesthesia for Infants and Toddlers."

Toddlerhood—The Child from 1 to 3 Years of Age

The most common malignancies during toddlerhood are: acute lymphocytic and acute non-lymphocytic leukemia; neuroblastoma; retinoblastoma; rhabdomyosarcoma; primary hepatic tumors; germ cell teratomas; and brain tumors (medulloblastoma, ependymoma, astrocytoma, and choroid plexus papilloma) (see Tables 17–1 and 17–2). The peak incidence for the majority of these tumors is in children less than 5 years of age (Pizzo et al., 1993).

Nursing Interventions—Preparation for Treatment

Before treatment begins, parents should be told what is involved in the treatment and what is expected of the child. The nurse should evaluate the child's coping skills by determining what

Table 17-6 • Preparation of Infants Receiving Radiation Therapy

Considerations	Interventions
DEVELOPMENTAL ISSUES	
Trust versus mistrust	Provide consistency in caregivers, and be attentive to comfort, nurturance, and security needs.
Object permanence/ separation anxiety	Assess parents' ability to be involved in their child's care during procedures and examinations. Parental participation should be encouraged if it provides a source of comfort and reassurance for the child.
Sensorimotor	Provide toys that are soft, cuddly, and colorful and that provide visual and auditory stimulation.
Comfort	Provide a quiet environment for waking after anesthesia. Foster a sense of security by providing touch, soothing voices, warmth.
Nurturance	Carefully monitor for nutritional disturbances, such as anorexia, dehydration, altered gastrointestinal function, hypoglycemia. During recovery, assess degree of alertness, cough, gag reflexes. Introduce clear liquids slowly. Instruct parents to introduce soft solid foods and fluids at home.
Parent teaching	Assess level of understanding of disease and treatment and identify learning needs. Incorporate parent teaching in child's plan of care. Review treatment plan with parents, and instruct them in guidelines for children receiving daily anesthesia and skin care. Identify treatment-related side effects and instruct parents in their management.

approaches have worked best in previous stressful situations and what has served as a source of comfort. The nurse should assess the child's response to illness and hospitalization, and identify potential problem areas, such as adjustment reactions, clinical problems related to disease and treatment, delayed developmental milestones, infection, sleep disturbance, poor nutrition, and metabolic abnormalities.

Preparation for the toddler should be done just prior to treatment. This can be accomplished by explaining to the child in simple terms what is going to be done. Rehearsing the treatment position in a safe environment, such as the playroom, or on a couch at home, may help the child assume and hold the correct position during radiation treatment (Wear et al., 1982). Demonstrations using inanimate objects, such as stuffed animals, are helpful. They allow the child to role play and learn the rules of the task ("Hold still!" "No wiggling!" "All done!"). This type of play also helps the child express fears or misconceptions about the treatment. It is important to observe what the child is communicating through verbal and nonverbal expression.

The imitative nature of toddlers also make them receptive to the concept of role playing. They may feel more confident and become more cooperative if they can observe their parent or another child go through a similar "treatment." Uncertainties and fears usually make the first day of radiation treatment the most difficult for the child and care providers. Older toddlers often adjust to the treatment routine in a few days.

Respect for toddlers' privacy is important. They are very fearful for their body and any procedures done to it. Children's sense of integrity is fostered by allowing them to wear their own clothes, covering untreated body areas with a blanket, and not removing dressings unless necessary.

Consistency in approach and detail are important. The toddler needs to feel safe and secure in his or her environment. Support for the child can be provided by having parents or staff talk to the child over the intercom during treatment, standing close to the child, holding the child's hand when repositioning the machine, and praising good behavior. Specific interventions for preparing a toddler for treatment, based on developmental needs, are listed in Table 17–7.

Special Considerations—Anesthesia for Infants and Toddlers

In pediatric radiotherapy, the key elements of treatment are accuracy, daily reproducibility, and cooperation on the part of the child. In very young children, usually those under the age of 4, it is often difficult to achieve the degree of cooperation and immobility required to deliver a technically precise treatment. In such instances, daily anesthesia will be required. A close cooperative relationship between the pediatric anesthesia team and the radiation therapists will help ensure the safe delivery of treatment.

The degree of cooperation in children between the ages of 2½ and 4 years is variable. Several factors may contribute to this—the child may have apprehensions about intrusive procedures based upon past experiences, be unable to comprehend the reasons for treatment, fear separation from parents, and feel overwhelmed by a strange environment. Some children in this age group may be persuaded to hold still for treatment with the proper advanced preparation. Specific suggestions and nursing interventions were discussed previously in this chapter. If cooperation cannot

Table 17-7 • Preparation of Toddlers Receiving Radiation Therapy

Considerations	Interventions
DEVELOPMENTAL ISSUES	
Trust	Provide consistency in caregivers and approach to child. Establish a daily routine.
Separation object permanence	Parents should accompany child for procedure. Talking or reading to child via intercom provides reassurance that they are nearby.
Security	Use transitional objects, such as a favorite toy or blanket, to accompany the child.
Limited reasoning	Inform child of procedure just before it happens, and explain that he will see, feel, hear. Provide simple explanations and commands.
Control mastery	Orient child to treatment room. Assist child to explore environment to see and touch objects in room. Praise good behavior, provide simple rewards. Set up rules and guidelines for acceptable behavior.
Initiative	Role playing—child may feel more comfortable if he can watch his parent or another child go through a similar procedure.
Body integrity	Protect privacy as much as possible. Allow child to wear his own clothes and uncover only those areas that need to be exposed. Maintain child's sense of integrity by protecting dressings, bandages, intravenous catheters.

be obtained by trying to talk the child through the procedure, then the use of anesthesia is important. Adequate sedation can greatly reduce the amount of fear and apprehension and allow for the treatment course to proceed more smoothly.

It is understandable that a certain degree of parental anxiety will be present. Parents often feel responsible for their children's illness and guilty about having to subject them to uncomfortable procedures. Feelings of powerlessness, inadequacy, and the need to be protective may emerge. The development of healthy coping mechanisms may be achieved by addressing parental concerns, clarifying misconceptions, providing information, and defining for parents the measures they can take to help their children. The radiation oncologist, nurse, anesthesiologist, child life specialist, psychologist, and radiation therapist are also valuable resources for parents and children. Sufficient time should be allotted to review preanesthesia instructions and the radiation therapy treatment plan to prepare the child and parent for treatment. Sample instructions for parents may be found in Table 17–8.

ANESTHESIA FOR RADIATION THERAPY

Anesthesiologists providing care for children receiving treatment for malignancies face a unique challenge: provision of daily or even twice-daily sedation and anesthesia under technically demanding conditions for sustained periods of up to 6 weeks. The shared goals of anesthesia and radiation therapy are to provide the necessary degree of immobility and sedation and to achieve precision, accuracy, and reproducibility in daily treatment. The approach to sedation and anesthesia varies with the available institutional resources. The expertise of pediatric anesthesiologists is desirable because of their knowledge of childhood illnesses and malignancies, their familiarity with the procedures and anesthetic agents that are appropriate for children, and their ability to intervene when complications occur. The desired elements of pediatric anesthesia include the following: assurance of immobility; rapid onset and brief duration of sedation; smooth recovery with limited disruption of the child's normal daily routines; repeated administration without the development of tolerance; and the assurance of airway patency despite treatment position (Schulman, 1994).

The selection of anesthetic technique is determined by the specifics of the patient's history, underlying malignancy, physical and laboratory findings, and discussion with the parents, child, and radiation team. General anesthesia may be accomplished with intravenous agents (e.g., sodium pentothal, ketamine, propofol, or methohexital sodium [Brevital]) or with inhalation agents (e.g., halothane, enflurane, isoflurane, or desflurane) (Schulman, 1994). A newer technique for administering general inhalation anesthesia is the use of the laryngeal mask airway (LMA), which is a silicone tube with an elliptical-shaped cuff that forms a low-pressure seal when inserted into the larynx and inflated. This device permits the delivery of anesthetic gasses and supports spontaneous ventilation in a variety of positions without the need for endotracheal intubation (Schulman, 1994).

Intravenous anesthetics are effective for use in pediatric radiation therapy. They may be given in short, repeated boluses, or via continuous infusion pumps. A secure route of administration is mandatory for prolonged courses of radiation therapy. Tunneled central venous catheters (e.g., Broviac

Table 17-8 • Instructions for Parents of Children Who Are Receiving Daily Anesthesia

For your child's radiation therapy treatment to be provided in the safest and most accurate way, the administration of anesthetics is required. An anesthesiologist, a doctor who specializes in anesthesia in children, will examine your child and ask you specific questions regarding his or her health history, illnesses, medications, allergies, and past surgical experiences. A consent for anesthesia will be obtained for treatment planning and before daily radiation therapy treatments.

We understand that this is a difficult period of time for you and your child and would like to help you as much as we can. You will meet with your radiation oncologist for an "on treatment visit" weekly. He/she is available at all times to address any questions you may have. Your primary nurse will be with you and your child each day. Please feel free to ask questions or discuss any concerns you may have.

The following guidelines are suggested for your child:

1. Treatments are daily—Monday through Friday at 8:00 AM—unless otherwise advised.
2. Your child should have no solid food or milk products for 8 hours prior to sedation. Clear liquids (apple juice, sugar water, white grape juice, popsicles, non-carbonated gingerale) may be given up to 4 hours prior to sedation. This is critical because it would be harmful to your child to vomit while under anesthesia.
3. All morning medications should be held until after the treatment. Bring them with you, and we will give them to your child once he or she is fully awake and alert.
4. Please inform us of any food/medication allergies your child might have, prescribed medications, or any difficulties he or she may be experiencing, such as fever, colds, congestion, vomiting, diarrhea, poor feeding, sleep disturbances.
5. Anesthesia will be given through the child's central line, port, peripheral IV, or by injection.
   A. For children receiving medication through their central lines: You may accompany your child into the treatment room and hold him during the administration of the anesthesia. Your child will fall asleep almost immediately. It is not uncommon for children to develop a "glassy-eyed" appearance, have eye movement, and become limp as the medication takes effect. Your child will then be placed on the treatment table, and monitoring equipment will be attached to him to evaluate his heart and respiratory status closely while the treatment is being delivered.
   B. For children who are receiving intramuscular shots: Emla cream will be provided to numb the skin area designated to receive the injection. If you would like, you may assist us in this procedure by holding your child while the medication is given. The medication will be given as a shot into either the upper arm muscle or the thigh. It takes 5 to 7 minutes to reach sedative effect. Your child will feel limp, develop a glassy-eyed appearance, and fall into a deep sleep. He or she will then be placed on the treatment table, and monitoring equipment will be attached. You will be asked to leave the room and rejoin your child in the recovery room.
      We will also respect your wish not to be associated with an uncomfortable procedure, if you choose not to. We appreciate how difficult it is to want to protect your child from pain yet know that this is essential for having the treatment done safely.
   C. The amount of anesthetic medication administered is determined by the child's weight, general health, and tolerance to the drug. It is not unusual to require a higher dose of anesthetic medication after several days of treatment. The decision of what particular medication to use will be made by the anesthesiologist before each daily treatment.

RECOVERY—WAKING-UP PERIOD

The length of time it takes a child to recover from the effects of the anesthesia will vary, depending on the child's response to medication, route of administration, dosage of medication required to maintain sedation for the treatment, and the child's degree of wellness. Your child will be closely monitored by the nurse and anesthesiologist with frequent assessment of vital signs and monitoring equipment (pulse oximeter, blood pressure cuff, EKG). In addition, intravenous fluids and antinausea medications may be administered during this time.

WHAT TO EXPECT

Your child will be sleepy, disoriented, glassy-eyed, and lethargic. Some children reach out with their hands and call out, although they are not really aware of their action. It is not unusual to have facial flushing, nausea, and dry heaving during the waking-up period. Your child will be closely watched by the nurses and the anesthesiologist until he or she is fully awake and ready to go home or back to the hospital unit. You will be permitted to hold your child once he or she has gone through the initial stages of anesthesia recovery. Because of the size of the room, we request that only one parent per child be in the recovery room at one time. The playroom is close by and serves as a waiting area for siblings and other family members.

If your child has a favorite toy, blanket, or stuffed animal, please bring this with you, as it will serve as an additional source of comfort and security.

Siblings are welcome to come and observe for portions of the procedure. Your child's nurse will be available to help you prepare your children for this experience, answer questions, and assist you with any specific questions you might have.

Before going home, your child will be encouraged to drink some clear liquids, such as water or apple juice. If your child has been nauseated, we would advise that fluids and foods be gradually introduced (such as juices, Jell-O, sherbet, toast, crackers, soups). Usually, by lunch time your child's appetite will have returned to normal.

It is not uncommon for children undergoing daily radiation therapy and anesthesia to have a decrease in energy and activity level. Your child may want to rest or nap in the afternoon. If you have concerns about your child, please do not hesitate to bring them to our attention.

or Hickman catheters) and subcutaneous ports, which often are already present for administration of fluids, chemotherapy and blood products, are now widely used for access during anesthesia.

The selection of intravenous anesthetic agent(s) is influenced by the underlying malignancy, the clinical status of the child, and many other factors. Children with brain tumors may have increased intracranial pressure, cranial nerve deficits, metabolic imbalances, centrally mediated respiratory depression, and/or cardiac arrhythmias, any of which might determine the agents to be used. The use of ketamine, for example, is contraindicated in children with increased intracranial pressure, because it may exacerbate this condition. Bulky tumors, such as Wilms' tumor and neuroblastoma, may compromise ventilation and may induce renin- or catecholamine-mediated arterial hypertension. In these situations, anesthetic agents that suppress ventilation and/or induce hypertension should be avoided. The chemotherapeutic agents in use also play a role in the selection of anesthetic agents. The anthracyclines, such as adriamycin and daunorubicin, are associated with cardiac toxicity in the form of cardiomyopathy and rhythm disturbances, such as supraventricular tachycardia, ventricular ectopy, and conduction disturbances. Bleomycin has been associated with pulmonary fibrosis and restrictive lung disease (Schulman, 1994).

SEDATION

The use of sedative agents such as chloral hydrate or Demerol compound (meperidine, chlorpromazine, and promethazine) intramuscularly is practiced at some centers as an alternative to general anesthesia. The limitations of the agents are the variability in absorption and onset of action, suboptimal sedative effects, prolonged somnolence, and increased potential for serious adverse reactions, such as respiratory or cardiac depression when multiple drugs or high doses of medications are used (Bucholtz, 1992b; Mitchell et al., 1982; Redner, 1987).

SCHEDULING

Arrangements for early-morning radiation treatments are recommended and should be coordinated with the anesthesia department and radiation therapists.

PREANESTHESIA EVALUATION

A complete daily evaluation of the child's health status is generally performed by the anesthesiologist. This includes confirmation of N.P.O. status,

medical history, review of systems, medication allergies, current medications, identification of potential risk factors such as debilitation, fluid and electrolyte disturbances, infection, recent chemotherapy and radiation therapy and related side effects, review of recent laboratory values, and family history of malignant hyperthermia. Parents should be instructed to withhold solid food and milk products from the child for 6 to 8 hours prior to anesthesia. Clear liquids (apple juice, popsicles, and sugar water) may be given up to 3 to 4 hours prior to anesthesia, depending on the anesthesiologist's recommendations.

PERSONNEL

The remote location of the radiation therapy department requires a high degree of self-sufficiency on the part of the anesthesiologist. Training in pediatric anesthesiology is an essential component of safe delivery of anesthesia. A registered nurse with experience in cardiopulmonary resuscitation, recovery room experience, and proficiency in airway management should be available to assist the anesthesiologist. An identified mechanism for obtaining assistance for emergencies should be in place. It is important that the radiation therapist review each child's case with the anesthesiologist to verify that the treatment position is optimal from both airway management and radiation treatment perspectives.

CONSENT

A separate consent for anesthesia should be obtained by the administering physician. Consent for daily radiation therapy treatment should be obtained by the radiation/therapist prior to initiating the treatment plan.

PREPARATION AND MONITORING

The daily radiation therapy treatment schedule should allot sufficient time to prepare the room for the anesthesia case and deliver the treatment. Due to the rapid onset of the anesthetics, the child should be medicated in the treatment room. As a source of comfort and security to the child, the parent (at the discretion of the anesthesiologist) might be permitted to hold the child during the administration of the medication. Once the sedative effect of the anesthesia has taken place, the child should be moved into the treatment position, monitors placed, and blow-by oxygen delivered.

The ability to monitor the child accurately during the actual radiotherapy treatment is critical. The use of closed-circuit television to focus directly on the child and the displays of monitoring equipment—electrocardiogram, pulse oximeter, blood pressure, and carbon dioxide analyzer—are essential (Murray, 1989). The ability to visualize chest movements during the treatment may be aided by the placement of a small piece of tape or face mask on the chest. Attentiveness to cardiorespiratory status, airway management problems, and adequate sedation are key components to safe delivery of anesthesia sedation.

ADMINISTRATION OF ANESTHETICS

Short-acting anesthetics may be administered intramuscularly, intravenously, or rectally. In pediatric oncology patients who have thrombocytopenia and leukopenia secondary to myelosuppression, intramuscular and rectal routes of administration are suboptimal due to the increased risk of infection, bleeding, hematoma formation, and rectal irritation. Intramuscular sites of drug administration should be rotated daily, using the arm or thigh muscles. EMLA Cream (Astra Pharmaceuticals, Westborough, MA) may be applied 1 hour prior to injection to the designated injection site to minimize local discomfort. The onset of drug action by this route is usually within 5 to 10 minutes. Administration of intravenous or inhalation anesthetics should be done in the treatment suite, because of the rapid onset of sedation and risk of respiratory depression.

Within the radiation treatment area and recovery room, it is necessary to have an oxygen source, suction equipment, an anesthesia machine and monitoring equipment, a pediatric code cart that contains airways and endotracheal tubes of appropriate size, Ambu bags, code drugs, and intravenous equipment. All equipment should be checked daily prior to the initiation of treatment. A system of communication such as intercom, direct telephone line, and code system must be in place to summon immediate medical support in the event of an emergency.

At the discretion of the attending anesthesiologist, parents may be present during the induction of anesthesia. Parents can provide reassurance and support by holding their child for intramuscular injections or the administration of medication through the central line, and then talking softly to the child as he drifts off to sleep. Parents should then leave the treatment room and wait to rejoin their child in the recovery area.

The recovery period usually lasts 30 to 90 minutes, depending on the drug(s) used and the route of drug administration. Careful monitoring of vital signs and observation for potential problems with airway secretions, laryngospasm, obstruction, vomiting, and cardiorespiratory depression should be maintained at all times. Extended periods of fasting predispose small children to hypoglycemia, and prolonged recovery from anesthesia warrants measurement of blood glucose and corrective replacement, if necessary. Hypothermia after anesthesia is another hazard for infants and small children with immature thermoregulation. Adequate warmth must be maintained during the recovery period. Once the child is fully awake, with vital signs stable, able to tolerate fluids, the child may be discharged from the radiation therapy unit.

The Preschool Child—Ages 3 to 6 Years

The preschool years are considered the period of development that occurs between the ages of 3 and 6. The most common malignancies during this period are acute leukemia, central nervous system tumors (medulloblastoma, astrocytoma, ependymoma), Wilms' tumor, and rhabdomyosarcoma. Acute lymphoblastic leukemia has a peak incidence between the ages of 2 and 6 years. Rhabdomyosarcoma is unique in that it has a bimodal incidence peak between 2 to 6 and 14 to 18 years. Children in the earlier age group develop tumors in the head and neck region or genitourinary tract, whereas adolescents may develop tumors in the male genitourinary tract, head and neck, trunk, and extremities (Pizzo et al., 1993; Tables 17–1 and 17–2). The role of radiation in the management of these tumors was discussed in the section entitled "Role of Radiation Therapy—Infancy to 6 Years" and is applicable to children of preschool age.

Nursing Interventions and Preparations for Treatment

There are certain factors that alter the child's ability to process information. These include the child's level of cognitive development, concept of illness, and coping mechanisms. At each stage of development, children reconstruct a concept of the world to understand and cope with it (Perrin & Garrity, 1981). They have a limited ability to process information and often will distort what they have been told. Information should be presented to children with honesty but with consideration for their limited cognitive abilities.

Individual differences in coping mechanisms also must be considered. Factors such as the quality of parent-child relationship, family dynamics, the meaning of the illness to the child and family, and prior exposure to intrusive procedures combine with age and developmental stage to govern the child's reaction to illness and treatment (Gordon & Cotanch, 1986). Each child is unique and must be approached according to individual needs. See Table 17–9 for suggested intervention in preparing preschoolers for treatment.

Preparing the preschool child for radiation treatment begins with talking to the parents. This provides an opportunity to identify their feelings about illness and treatment, to explain anticipated side effects, and to prepare parents for what will take place on a day-to-day basis. Parents are a valuable resource of information about the child's growth and development, understanding of illness, past experiences and difficulties with treatment, and approaches that have been supportive in the past. Involving parents in preparing their child for the procedure serves a dual purpose: it helps them to feel that they are playing an active role in fighting the disease and it provides emotional support to the child.

The main objective in preparing the preschooler should be to present information that is easy to understand and as nonthreatening as possible. The child will be concerned about whether the treatment is going to hurt or entail separation from parents, and may view the procedure as punishment for bad thoughts or misdeeds. Explanations should be honest, simple, brief, and should include a description of the behaviors required of the child during the procedure (Ritchie, 1979). ("We are going to take special pictures of you with a big camera. We will not use any needles or anything that will hurt you. It is very important for you to hold still, no wiggling. A safety belt, just like the one you wear in the car, will be put on you so you will feel nice and safe. You may bring your favorite toy with you. Mom and Dad are going to be watching you on TV. When the pictures are all done, you can go home.")

Information also may be provided with illustrations, storytelling, or through play. Play serves as a means of developing understanding and mastery. The child may benefit by rehearsing the event with the support of parents or by playing with models of equipment that will be used in the procedure (Wear et al., 1982). A miniature radiation therapy machine and stuffed animals or dolls can be used to demonstrate what will happen during radiation treatment and can provide an opportunity for the child to be in control through hands-on experience (Figure 17–1).

The child's verbal and nonverbal reactions to the presented information should be observed carefully. A preschooler may become overwhelmed or frightened by too much information. Anxiety may be expressed by avoidance, regression, aggression, or crying. For some children, role playing and direct explanation may create

Table 17-9 • Preparation of Preschoolers Receiving Radiation Therapy

Considerations	Interventions
DEVELOPMENTAL ISSUES	
Initiative versus guilt	Use parents' knowledge of child and previous response to procedures to develop approach to child. Identify coping mechanisms.
	Assess child's concept of illness, fears, understanding of radiation therapy.
	Encourage child's autonomy by permitting him to explore environment, ask questions.
	Set reasonable limits on behavior. Offer praise for good behavior and accomplishment of tasks.
Fear of unknown, limited comprehension	Determine readiness to learn.
	Provide simple explanations about what is going to happen, what child will see, feel, and is expected to do.
	Use a picture book to illustrate points.
	Practice the position that will be required for the procedure.
	Provide opportunity for role playing using miniature XRT machine. Start with an inanimate object, such as a toy or stuffed animal, then advance to a doll.
Imitative	Have the child observe another child receiving the same treatment.
Security	Encourage parents to accompany child to treatment room and inform child that they will be waiting close by.
	Parents may talk to child via intercom to offer encouragement.
	Encourage child to bring a favorite toy, stuffed animal, or security object to hold during treatment.
Body integrity	Talk to child during procedure. Explain things as they are about to occur, e.g., dimming lights, repositioning, placing markings on skin.
	Protect privacy as much as possible by limiting amount of clothing that needs to be removed.
Hero worship/fantasy	Explore child's sense of imagination. Use fantasy as a distraction technique while treatment is being given, e.g., astronaut buckling up for space shuttle, superhero becoming energized with special powers.
	Use story-telling to prepare child for treatment.

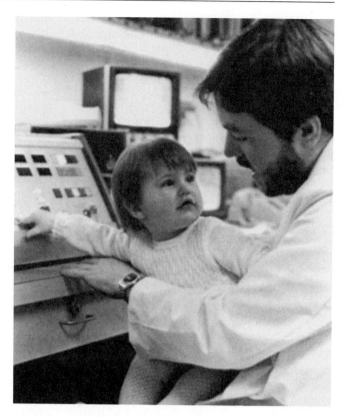

Figure 17-1 • Toddler and therapist—forming a trusting relationship. (Courtesy Norman C. Dow Photography.)

more anxiety (Ritchie, 1979). An alternative approach in this situation is to make up a story involving the child's favorite cartoon character or hero. Fantasy can be used to present information in a nonthreatening way, and the "adventure" becomes a means of providing simple understanding and support.

The School Age Child—Age 6 to 12 Years

During the school age years, there is a notable change in the relative incidence of cancers. Leukemia remains the most common malignancy in children less than 15 years, with its peak incidence occurring between the ages of 2 to 6 years. Tumors of the central nervous system are the second most frequent malignancies in children under 15 years (Heideman et al., 1993). The most common brain tumors during this period are medulloblastoma, gliomas of the optic nerve and optic chiasm, astrocytomas, ependymomas, and craniopharyngiomas (Pizzo et al., 1993). The incidence of medulloblastoma peaks between 5 and 9 years of age. Tumors of embryonic cell origin, such as Wilms' tumor and neuroblastoma, have peak occurrences at very early ages and are rare in chil-

dren over the age of 5 (Pizzo et al., 1993). The lymphomas, non-Hodgkin's and Hodgkin's disease, are the third most common malignancy and account for approximately 10 percent of cancers in children less than 15 years of age (Link, 1985). There is a gradual increase of lymphoma throughout childhood, with peak incidence occurring between 7 and 11 years. Hodgkin's disease is rare in children less than 10 years of age. In this age group the lymphocyte-predominant subtype is the most common form of Hodgkin's disease, whereas nodular sclerosing is the most common subtype in adolescents (Donaldson & Link, 1991). Rhabdomyosarcoma has its early peak occurrence between ages 2 and 6 and most commonly involves the head and neck region, genitourinary tract, and orbit (Pizzo et al., 1993).

Nursing Interventions and Preparation for Treatment

In preparing the school age child for radiation therapy, the developmental concepts previously discussed should be incorporated into the child's plan of care. Nursing interventions should be directed toward fostering the child's independence, promoting a positive self-image, providing an understanding of the disease and treatment, and assisting the child to develop effective coping strategies. Suggestions for preparing the school age child for radiation treatment, based on developmental tasks for this age group, are listed in Table 17–10.

Adolescence—Age 11 to 18 Years

The most common malignancies during adolescence are leukemia, lymphoma, Hodgkin's disease, and central nervous system tumors. Rhabdomyosarcoma, a highly aggressive soft tissue sarcoma, has its second peak occurrence during adolescence, at 14 to 18 years. This later peak is associated with tumors of the genitourinary tract in males and tumors of the head and neck region, trunk, and extremities (Pizzo et al., 1993; Tables 17–1 and 17–2). Of the primary bone tumors that occur during this period, osteogenic sarcoma and Ewing's sarcoma are the most common. In some studies a correlation between incidence of bone tumors and the skeletal growth and hormonal changes with puberty has been noted (Greene, 1982). Acute lymphoblastic leukemia in older children (>10 years) is associated with a less favorable prognosis than leukemia in younger children. Children in this high-risk category are treated with more intensive chemotherapeutic regimens and receive cranial radiation as part of their CNS preventive treatment (Poplack et al.,

1993). Hodgkin's disease is more prevalent in adolescents than in younger children. Its first disease-specific age peak occurs at 15 to 40 years of age. The nodular sclerosis subset is the most prevalent histopathologic subtype, occurring in 77 percent of adolescents (Donaldson & Link, 1991).

Developmental Tasks

Adolescence is a period of transition from childhood to adulthood. It is a turbulent period of development characterized by physical, social, and intellectual maturation. The developmental challenges are establishment of identity and self-image; development of a positive sexual role; development of peer relations with both sexes; attainment of autonomy and emotional independence from parents and other adults; development of career goals; assumption of social responsibility; preparation for family and married life; and establishment of values (Ettinger & Heiney, 1993; Rechner, 1990).

During early adolescence, the physical changes of puberty begin with an increase in individual growth and development of secondary sexual characteristics. Puberty ends with closure of the epiphyseal bone plates and completion of sexual maturation (Mercer, 1979). Puberty often is associated with feelings of awkwardness,

Table 17-10 • Preparation of School Age Children Receiving Radiation Therapy

Considerations	Interventions
DEVELOPMENTAL ISSUES	
Industry versus inferiority (Reasoning, mastery, sense of accomplishment)	Assess level of understanding of illness and treatment.
	Provide descriptions of behaviors required during procedure, sequence of events, length of time.
	Illustrate explanations with photographs, bodygram, or demonstration with miniature XRT machine.
	Provide opportunity to rehearse procedure or role-play event with miniature XRT machine.
	Orient to treatment room. Provide simple explanation of how machine works and equipment that will be used.
	Talk to child during treatment set-up. Reinforce behavioral expectations.
	Provide encouragement and empathetic support. Acknowledge child's participation in procedure; reinforce sense of accomplishment.
Body image	Discuss with child/parents the temporary side effects of treatment and what measures can be taken to minimize them.
	Explore child's feelings about changes in body image and offer suggestions about how to cope with changes in appearance, physical limitations, peer/family reactions.
	Respect child's need for privacy by limiting exposure of body.
Independence	Encourage self-care activities.
	Promote participation in school/social activities.
	Encourage family to establish daily routine and to maintain normal limit setting and behavioral expectations.
	Provide some flexibility in choices, e.g., schedule of daily treatment, route of blood drawing.
Security/trust	Provide consistency in caregivers and approach to treatment.
	Establish daily routine.
	Provide opportunities for child to verbalize concerns, frustrations, fears. Assist child to work through feelings with play, art.
	Refer for additional counseling, as needed.

uncertainty, and frustration as the individual tries to adjust to changes in body image. The development of a positive self-image is dependent on the adolescent's ability to overcome feelings of self-consciousness and attain peer acceptance.

Middle adolescence focuses on attainment of independence from parents and establishment of self-identity. The achievement of these goals is derived through peer and social interactions, which permit the individual to try out different roles, become more comfortable with his/her sexual identity, and establish a personal value system.

The latter phase of adolescence is devoted to establishing intimate relationships, making decisions about career goals, and working toward emotional and financial independence from parents. This phase is often marked by periods of conflict between parents and children. The adolescent frequently will challenge parental restrictions while seeking self-expression and independence.

The psychological growth of the adolescent progresses from the concrete, egocentric thoughts of childhood to more formal operational processes. The adolescent becomes capable of viewing things from multiple perspectives and considering alternative solutions while learning to feel more secure in self-identity. Physical and psychological maturation may occur at disparate rates in the individual. Information must be presented to adolescents with this in mind. Although physically mature, adolescents may be emotionally or intellectually immature, leading to feelings of confusion and uncertainty.

IMPACT OF ILLNESS

The diagnosis of a life-threatening illness affects the adolescent on several levels. It creates a disruption in lifestyle, peer relationships, school activities, and future goals (Hockenberry, 1986). The physical changes associated with treatment, such as hair loss, surgical scars, amputation, anorexia, weight gain, and musculoskeletal weakness, can lower self-esteem and contribute to feelings of self-consciousness and fear of peer rejection. Social isolation and withdrawal may result from the adolescent's inability to keep up with peers, difficulty dealing with the reactions of friends, and poor self-acceptance. Adolescents are painfully aware of body image. The issues of establishing intimate relationships, fertility, and physical changes that occur as a result of treatment need to be discussed openly and honestly.

The adolescent's initial response to illness may be anger, frustration, denial, withdrawal, or depression. The adolescent may resent the changes that illness and treatment impose and may fear loss of autonomy and independence. Illness heightens dependence on parents and diminishes control over one's life. Parent-adolescent conflicts may occur over issues such as overprotectiveness, noncompliance with treatments, decision making, information sharing, or disruption in family dynamics. Although adolescents may have the cognitive ability to understand the implications of having cancer and the need for treatment, they may not have the personal strength or sufficient life experience to help them contend with this new stress (Ettinger & Heiney, 1993; Leiken, 1993; Wells et al., 1990).

Nursing Interventions

The adolescent requires support to maintain a sense of autonomy, control, and self-image and to establish effective coping skills. It is important to maintain consistency in involvement and honesty in explanations, and to be available to listen to the adolescent's feelings and concerns. Measures that foster adolescents' sense of autonomy include respect for individuality, encouragement of participation in decision making, and acknowledgment of needs for privacy and confidentiality (Hockenberry, 1986). Sensitivity to the informational needs of adolescents is crucial when explanations about treatments and anticipated side effects are provided. The adolescent wants to know what to expect in terms of changes in physical appearance, constraints on physical and social activities, and needs opportunities to discuss fears related to disease and treatment (Fotchman & Foley, 1982). Strategies with demonstrated beneficial effect on adjustment to illness include taking a positive stance on illness; trying to maintain normalcy despite side effects; not letting others feel sorry for you; and sharing feelings in groups (Ettinger & Heiney, 1993). The development of new coping skills can be promoted by establishing a support network among peers and family and other adolescents sharing the experience of cancer and its treatment. Continued participation in school and special interests should be encouraged. School reentry programs can facilitate the transition from hospital to classroom by providing guidance for patients, classmates, and teachers. Psychological interventions, such as guided imagery, biofeedback hypnosis, and individual counseling also may enhance the adolescent's sense of self-control and reduce anxiety (Ettinger & Heiney, 1993). Radiation treatment schedules should provide some flexibility, so that these objectives can be met. Suggestions for preparing the adolescent for radiotherapy are listed in Table 17–11.

Table 17-11 • Preparation of the Adolescent Receiving Radiation Therapy

Considerations	Interventions
DEVELOPMENTAL ISSUES	
Identity, independence	Determine perceptions of illness and treatment. Clarify misconceptions.
	Explain rationale for treatment, procedures, behavioral expectations, and potential side effects.
	Encourage participation in decision-making by providing opportunities for the individual to express feelings, opinions.
	Encourage individual to take responsibility for self-care, e.g., skin care, medications, fluoride treatments, nutrition, physical activity.
	Promote continued participation in school and physical and social activities. Arrange treatment schedule to accommodate these needs.
Body image	Provide a supportive relationship that allows for open communication.
Self-concept	Reassure individual of staff's availability to him or her.
	Provide opportunities to discuss feelings about changes in body image, sexuality, physical limitations.
	Provide empathy and reassurance. Acknowledge concerns. Assist individual to establish effective coping skills and to adjust to alterations in body image and role.
	Encourage independence and participation in peer activities.
	Protect confidentiality and need for privacy during treatments and physical examinations.

Side Effects of Therapy

The acute side effects of radiation therapy by disease and treatment site are summarized in Table 17–12. The specific nursing interventions for management of side effects are discussed in detail in the chapters covering common clinical problems.

Improvements in the treatment of children and adolescents with cancer have led to an increase in the numbers of long-term survivors. In order to help these individuals meet the challenges of the future, an appreciation of the potential long-term complications of therapy is necessary. Table 17–13 provides a summary of the late effects of treatment for childhood cancer. Long-term follow-up of patients is essential for the early detection and management of health care problems. Parents and older children need to be counseled as to what problems they should look for, and be provided with the appropriate referrals to deal with specific issues. The overall objective is to prepare them to face the physical and psychosocial challenges of the future, and make a healthy adjustment as adults.

Summary

The role of radiation therapy in the management of childhood cancers is being redefined by a new appreciation of the benefits of combined-modality therapy and the unique long-term complications of radiation in children. The latter include late changes in skeletal and soft tissue development, neuropsychological dysfunction, and the occur-

rence of second malignancies in long-term survivors. Treatment strategies of the future will seek the optimal balance between the risks and benefits of surgery, chemotherapy, and radiation therapy.

The future will also bring increased sophistication in the manner in which radiation therapy is delivered. Treatments will be tailored to the disease and will be based on stage, tumor histology, clinical presentation, and prognostic factors. Treatment planning and simulation techniques that employ three-dimensional computer-guided plans will permit therapists to deliver high doses of radiation to the tumor volume while minimizing the dose to normal tissue. This has specific application in the areas of stereotactic radiosurgery and radioactive implants. The use of radiosensitizers, which increase the sensitivity of tumor cells to the effects of radiation, may improve the outcome of certain types of pediatric brain tumors.

Control of malignancies in pediatric patients must be achieved in ways that permit children to resume normal development when treatment is finished. The unifying objective of all current research efforts in this area is to bring us closer to this ideal.

Resources

Some of the most current resources available for children, their families, and medical professionals can be found in the following listings:

American Brain Tumor Association, Tel. (800) 886-2282.
American Cancer Society, 1599 Clifton Rd. N.E., Atlanta, GA 30329, Tel. (800) ACS-2345.

Table 17-12 • Acute Side Effects of Radiotherapy by Disease and Treatment Site

Disease	Treatment Site	Side Effects	Interventions
ACUTE LYMPHOCYTIC LEUKEMIA	Brain	Meningeal irritation Nausea, vomiting Potential dehydration Headache Skin sensitivity Alopecia Somnolence period— 4–8 weeks following XRT	Monitor for signs and symptoms of meningitis or neurological dysfunction. Assess fluid/electrolyte balance, nutrition, IV hydration, antiemetics, antipyretics as needed, skin care teaching—hats, sunscreens, moisturizers to scalp
BRAIN TUMORS Astrocytoma Craniopharyngioma Glioma	Brain—size of field and technique dependent on tumor	Nausea, vomiting Headache Alopecia Fatigue Skin sensitivity Cerebral edema Somnolence period— 4–8 weeks following XRT	Monitor for signs and symptoms of increased intracranial pressure, metabolic/endocrine imbalance, altered neurological function, shunt malfunction, post-op infection, hemorrhage, cerebral edema. Seizure precautions, if indicated. Monitor compliance with medications, e.g., steroids, anticonvulsants. Activity as tolerated. Physical/occupational therapy, as indicated. Nutritional counseling as needed.
Medulloblastoma Primary neuroectodermal tumor	Craniospinal field	Nausea, vomiting Headache Alopecia Fatigue Tracheal irritation Esophagitis Myelosuppression Skin sensitivity Somnolence period— 4–8 weeks following XRT	Monitor hematological status closely. Biweekly counts, increase frequency as needed. Monitor for myelosuppression, signs and symptoms of infection, altered nutritional status, dehydration, skin reaction. Encourage high-protein, high-calorie foods. Nutritional counseling as needed. Skin care teaching for parents: sunscreens, hats, moisturizers to scalp. Comfort measures for esophagitis: increased intake of nonacidic fluids, antacids, kaolin/pectin, diphenhydramine, lidocaine swish and swallow, nystatin as needed for oral thrush, antiemetics pretreatment daily and as needed, steroid taper. Baseline neuropsychological testing, hearing evaluation, and referral to subspecialties as needed (Physical Therapy, Occupational Therapy, Hearing/Speech, Social Service, Psychology).
HODGKIN'S DISEASE	Mantle	Parotitis Taste changes Xerostomia Dysphagia Esophagitis Fatigue Skin sensitivity Anorexia Nausea, vomiting Myelosuppression, especially if prior chemotherapy	Analgesics as needed for jaw discomfort. Monitor CBC, platelet counts closely for myelosuppression; gargles with warm water and salt solution; topical anesthetics as needed. Skin care teaching: observe for sensitivity reaction, desquamation. Loose, comfortable clothing. Observe for signs and symptoms of eating disturbances. Nutritional consultations, as needed. Encourage nonspicy, nonacidic foods/fluids. Small, frequent meals. Dental referral for cleaning, fluoride treatment, and repair of caries before therapy. Use of fluoride trays nightly. Antiemetics as needed.
	Paraaortics	Infertility—females Nausea, vomiting Myelosuppression	Oophoropexy at time of staging laparotomy. Antiemetics as needed. Monitor nutritional status. Encourage small, frequent meals, oral fluids. Monitor CBC, platelet counts for myelosuppression.
	Pelvis	Infertility Abdominal cramping Diarrhea Myelosuppression	Discuss issues of infertility, sexuality before therapy. Nutritional counseling: low-roughage/low residue foods. Encourage oral fluids. Antiemetics, antidiarrheals as needed.

Table 17-12 • Acute Side Effects of Radiotherapy by Disease and Treatment Site (*Continued*)

Disease	Treatment Site	Side Effects	Interventions
RETINOBLASTOMA	Eye	Conjunctivitis Skin sensitivity Alopecia (minimal)	Gently cleanse eye with saline. Artificial tears as needed. Skin care teaching. Long-term ophthalmology follow-up.

WILMS' TUMOR
NEUROBLASTOMA
	Abdomen
	
	Lung
		Abdominal cramping
		Nausea, vomiting
		Diarrhea
		Myelosuppression
		Skin sensitivity and
		  recall reaction
		  (actinomycin D)
		Pneumonitis
		Myelosuppression
		Esophagitis
			Monitor counts closely for potential problems with myelosuppression. Blood product support as needed. Observe nutritional status, difficulty with nausea/vomiting, diarrhea, cramping, diminished food/fluid intake. IV fluid hydration, nutritional support, antiemetics, antidiarrheals, as needed.

RHABDOMYOSARCOMA	Head and neck	Skin recall reaction
		  (actinomycin D,
		  doxorubicin)
		Mucositis—oropharynx,
		  nasal passages
		Orbital inflammation/
		  irritation
		Taste alteration
		Xerostomia
			Nutrition: soft foods, frequent nonacidic fluids. Baseline dental consultation and continued follow-up. Preventive fluoride treatments nightly. Oral hygiene: warm saline gargles, gentle toothbrushing. Gently clean nares with warm water. Saline nose drops. Humidifier/vaporizer at home. Oral analgesics as needed. Eye care: saline compresses, artificial tears. Baseline ophthalmology, ENT, and endocrine evaluations, with long-term follow-up.

	Pelvis Genitourinary tract	Cystitis Diarrhea Abdominal cramping Mucositis Skin recall reaction Proctitis Myelosuppression Alopecia	Monitor GU function for problems with burning, frequency, spasms, abdominal cramping, hematuria, hemorrhagic cystitis, rectal irritation, infection, pain on defecation. Obtain urinalysis and culture to rule out infection. Antispasmodics, antidiarrheals as needed. Rectal care: gentle washing with mild soap and water, sitz baths. Apply protective coating of Aquaphor, Lubriderm, or Eucerin lotions. Avoid constipation. Rectal procedures contraindicated. Frequent diaper changes. Monitor skin for sensitivity reaction: erythema, desquamation—treatment break may be indicated. Monitor CBC, platelets for myelosuppression. Nutrition: bland diet, low roughage. Encourage non-caffeinated fluids. Monitor for weight loss, dehydration.
	Extremity	Skin recall reaction Functional limitation Increased susceptibility to fracture	Monitor skin for erythema, desquamation. Skin care teaching: gentle washing of site, application of hydrophilic ointments several times per day. Sunscreens, loose, comfortable clothes. Avoid trauma to extremity. Advise of potential risk of home fracture. Physical and/or occupational therapy, as needed.

Table 17-13 • Late Effects of Treatment for Childhood Cancer

Organ System	Side Effect	Contributing Factors
CARDIOVASCULAR	Pericarditis Pericardial effusion Cardiomyopathy Dysrhythmias	Prior chemotherapy: cyclophosphamide, dactino- mycin, mithramycin, doxorubicin Radiation dose to whole heart >3000–3500 cGy Total body irradiation (TBI)

ENDOCRINE	Growth hormone deficiency
	Pituitary dysfunction
	Hypothyroidism
	Infertility
	Ovarian dysfunction
	Testicular dysfunction
		Cranial radiation dose/technique, location of
		  tumor
		TBI
		Prior lymphangiography with iodine-containing
		  dyes
		Radiation to head and neck
		Radiation to pelvis
		Chemotherapy: cyclophosphamide, nitrogen mus-
		  tard, busulfan, vinblastine, chlorambucil, procar-
		  bazine

GASTROINTESTINAL	Strictures Intestinal obstruction Malabsorption Vascular abnormalities Radiation enteritis Hepatic toxicity/fibrosis	Prior abdominal surgery Chemotherapy: doxorubicin, dactinomycin Prior hepatic infection

MUSCULOSKELETAL
  Spine
	Shortened stature
	Reduced sitting height
	Scoliosis
	Kyphosis
	Thyroid dysfunction
		XRT to children <6, or before puberty growth
		  spurt; medulloblastoma, Wilms' tumor, neuroblas-
		  toma, Hodgkin's disease involving large spinal
		  fields
		Structural changes resulting from surgery,
		  muscle/soft tissue contractures

HEAD/NECK	Asymmetry of facial bones/soft tissue
	Dental abnormalities: stunted tooth growth, incom-
	  plete calcification, delayed development of sali-
	  vary secretions
	Endocrine dysfunction
		Prior radiation to head and neck region, e.g.,
		  retinoblastoma, rhabdomyosarcoma, Ewing's sar-
		  coma, Hodgkin's disease
		Chemotherapy
		Total body irradiation

NERVOUS SYSTEM
  Brain
	Leukoencephalopathy
	Decreased intelligence
	Memory impairment
	Distractibility
	Impaired cognitive function
	Endocrinopathies
	  Thyroid
	  Pituitary dysfunction
	  Growth hormone deficiency
	Intracranial calcifications
	Lhermitte's syndrome
	Brain necrosis
		Age <5 years
		Cranial irradiation plus intrathecal methotrexate
		Prior cranial surgery, difficulties with ICP and infec-
		  tion
		Increased intracranial pressure
		Craniospinal irradiation
		XRT to hypothalamic–pituitary axis
		
		Brain XRT >2000 cGy
		Spinal irradiation >4000 cGy
		Radiation doses >5500–6000 cGy

EYE	Cataracts Corneal pain, necrosis Retinal damage Vascular occlusion Visual impairment	Radiation dose >200 cGy to lens Radiation dose >5000 cGy Radiation dose >5500 cGy Treatment of tumors of nasopharynx and orbit Treatment with corticosteroids

HEARING	Ototoxicity
	High or low frequency hearing loss
		Radiation therapy to head and neck tumors, brain
		  tumor involving XRT to middle ear
		Combined modality treatment: radiation plus oto-
		  toxic chemotherapeutic agents or antibiotics, e.g.,
		  cis-diaminedichloroplatinum

Table 17-13 • Late Effects of Treatment for Childhood Cancer (*Continued*)

Organ System	Side Effect	Contributing Factors
PULMONARY	Radiation pneumonitis (2–6 months after therapy) Pulmonary fibrosis	Whole-lung dose >2000–2500 cGy Mantle Hodgkin's field 3500–4000 cGy Chemotherapy: nitrosoureas, bleomycin, busulfan, cyclophosphamide, dactinomycin, methotrexate, doxorubicin Underlying pulmonary disease Previous infections
RENAL	Nephritis	Abdominal irradiation for Wilms' tumor, neuroblastoma, non-Hodgkin's lymphoma, Hodgkin's disease XRT dose >2500 cGy to kidney Chemotherapy—related to toxicity
	Bladder fibrosis, telangiectasis	Radiation dose to bladder >4000 cGy Cyclophosphamide Radiation to bladder

Data from Green D (1989). Effects of treatment for childhood cancer on vital organ systems. *Cancer, 71,* 3299–3305; Halperin E, Constine L, Tarbell N, & Kun L (1994). Late effects of cancer treatment. In E Halperin, L Constine, N Tarbell, & L Kun (Eds.), *Pediatric Radiation Oncology* (2nd ed., pp. 485–554). New York: Raven Press.

Association for Care of Children's Health, 7910 Woodmont Ave., Suite 300, Bethesda, MD 20814, Tel. (301) 654-6549.

Brain Tumor Foundation for Children, Tel. (770) 458-5554.

Brain Tumor Society, Rabena Calhoun, LICSW, Tel. (617) 783-0340 or (800) 770-8287.

Candlelighters Childhood Cancer Foundation, 7910 Woodmont Ave., Suite 460, Bethesda, MD 20814, Tel. (800) 266-2223.

Cancer Facts, National Cancer Institute—Cancer Information Services, PDQ, Physicians' Data Query—Computer database that contains cancer information, listings of research studies, clinical trials, directories of physicians and organizations involved in cancer care. Tel. (800) 422-6237.

Cancernet, cancernet@icicb.nci.nih.gov.

The Children's Brain Tumor Foundation, Tel. (914) 797-0301.

Christ G, Moynihan R, Loscalzo M, & Weinstein L (1993). Providing community resources for cancer patients. In V DeVita, S Hellman, & S Rosenberg (Eds.), *Cancer Principles and Practice of Oncology* (4th ed., pp. 2513–2528). Philadelphia: JB Lippincott.

Make-A-Wish Foundation of America, (602) 234-0960.

National Brain Tumor Foundation, 785 Market St., Suite 1600, San Francisco, CA 94103, Tel. (800) 934-CURE, Fax (415) 284-0209.

National Cancer Institute (NCI), 9000 Rockville Pike, Bethesda, MD 20892, Tel. (301) 496-4000.

Cancer Information Service, Tel. (800) 4-CANCER.

Office of Cancer Communications, Tel. (301) 496-5583—Physician Data Query.

National Institutes of Health, Publications Office, 9000 Rockville Pike, Bethesda, MD, Tel. (301) 496-4000. Professional materials, printed booklets for children and families.

Soghomonian Y (1993). Resources for children with cancer and for their families and physician. In P Pizzo & DG Poplack (Eds.), *Principles and Practice of Pediatric Oncology* (pp. 1253–1291). Philadelphia: JB Lippincott.

Taking Charge of Your Health: A guide to cancer prevention for men (women) who had cancer in childhood, Part 1. Meadows AT, Gallagher J, Jarrett P, Blumberg B. Source: Children's Hospital of Philadelphia, 34th and Civic Center Blvd., Philadelphia, PA 19104.

Taking Charge of Your Health: A guide to medical follow-up for adults who had cancer in childhood. Meadows AT, Gallagher J, Jarrett P, Blumberg B. Source: Children's Hospital of Philadelphia, 34th and Civic Center Blvd., Philadelphia, PA 19104.

References

Altman A & Schwartz A (1983). *Malignant Diseases of Infancy, Childhood and Adolescence*, (2nd ed., pp. 1–10). Philadelphia: WB Saunders.

Baker LL, Parker ER, Donaldson SS, et al. (1990). Staging of Hodgkin's disease in children: Comparison of CT and lymphangiography with laparotomy. *American Journal of Roentgenology, 154,* 1251.

Bleyer WA (1993). What can be learned about childhood cancer from "Cancer Statistics Review 1973–1988." *Cancer 71,* 3229–3236.

Brodeur GM & Castleberry RP (1993). In P Pizzo & DG Poplack (Eds.), *Principles and Practice of Pediatric Oncology*, (2nd ed., pp. 739–767). Philadelphia: JB Lippincott.

Brodeur GM, Pritchard J, Berthold F, Carlsen NLT, Castel V, Castleberry RP, et al. (1993). Revisions of the international criteria for neuroblastoma diagnosis, staging, and response to treatment. *Journal of Clinical Oncology, 11,* 1466–1477.

Bucholtz J (1992a). Radiation carcinogenesis. In K Hassey-Dow & L Hilderley (Eds.), *Nursing Care in Radiation Oncology* (pp. 342–357). Philadelphia: WB Saunders.

Bucholtz J (1992b). Issues concerning the sedation of children for radiation therapy. *Oncology Nursing Forum, 19,* 649–655.

Bucholtz J (1994). Comforting children during radiotherapy. *Oncology Nursing Forum, 21,* 987–994.

Curran WJ, Littman P, & Raney RB (1988). Interstitial radiation therapy in the treatment of childhood soft tissue sarcomas. *International Journal of Radiation Oncology, Biology, Physics, 14,* 169–174.

Donaldson SS, Egbert PR, & Lee W (1993). Retinoblastoma. In P Pizzo & DG Poplack (Eds.), *Principles and Practice of Pediatric Oncology,* (2nd ed., pp. 683–696). Philadelphia: JB Lippincott.

Donaldson S & Link M (1991). Hodgkin's disease: Treatment of the young child. *Pediatric Clinics of North America, 38,* 457–473.

Doyle K (1984). The young child. In S McIntire & A Cioppa (Eds.), *Cancer Nursing—A Developmental Approach.* New York: John Wiley and Sons.

Dunbar SF & Loeffler JS (1994). Stereotactic radiation therapy. In P Mauch & J Loeffler (Eds). *Radiation Oncology, Technology and Biology.* (pp. 237–251). Philadelphia: WB Saunders.

Ellsworth RM (1969). The practical management of retinoblastoma. *Transactions of the American Ophthalmological Society, 67,* 462–534.

Ettinger RS & Heiney SP (1993). Cancer in adolescents and young adults. Psychosocial concerns, coping strategies, and interventions. *Cancer 71,* 3276–3280.

Foley G & Yeaske P (1982). Common issues in pediatric cancer. In D Fochtman & G Foley (Eds.), *Nursing care of the child with cancer.* Boston: Little, Brown.

Gilchrist G & Evans R (1985).Contemporary issues in pediatric Hogkin's disease. *Pediatric Clinics of North America,* 32, 721–734.

Gordon A & Cotanch P (1986). Coping strategies for children with cancer. In M Hockenberry & D Coody (Eds.), *Pediatric Oncology and Hematology—Perspectives on Care.* (pp. 450–462). St. Louis: CV Mosby.

Green D (1989). Long-term complications of therapy for cancer in childhood and adolescence. Baltimore: The Johns Hopkins University Press.

Green D (1993). Effects of treatment for childhood cancer on vital organ systems. *Cancer 71,* 3299–3305.

Green DM, D'Angio, GJ, Beckwith JB, Breslow NE, Finklestein JZ, Kelalis P, & Thomas PR (1993). Wilms' tumor (nephroblastoma, renal embryoma). In P Pizzo & DG Poplack (Eds.), *Principles and Practice of Pediatric Oncology,* (2nd ed., pp. 713–737). Philadelphia: JB Lippincott.

Green P (1982). Malignant bone tumors. In D Fochtman & G Foley (Eds.), *Nursing care of the child with cancer.* Boston: Little, Brown.

Halperin E, Constine, L, Tarbell N, & Kun L (1994a). The cancer problem in children. In E Halperin, L Constine, N Tarbell, & L Kun (Eds.), *Pediatric Radiation Oncology.* (2nd ed., pp. 1–11). New York: Raven Press.

Halperin E, Constine L, Tarbell N, & Kun L (1994b). Secondary tumors. In E Halperin, L Constine, N Tarbell, & L Kun (Eds.), *Pediatric Radiation Oncology.* (2nd ed., pp. 555–575). New York: Raven Press.

Halperin E, Constine L, Tarbell N, & Kun L (1994c). Soft tissue sarcomas other than rhabdomyosarcomas; desmoid tumor. In E Halperin, L Constine, N Tarbell, & L Kun (Eds.), *Pediatric Radiation Oncology.* (2nd ed., pp. 341–358). New York: Raven Press.

Halperin E, Constine L, Tarbell N, & Kun L (1994d). Late effects of cancer treatment. In E Halperin, L Constine, N Tarbell, & L Kun (Eds.), *Pediatric Radiation Oncology.* (2nd ed., pp. 485–554). New York: Raven Press.

Halperin E, Constine L, Tarbell N, & Kun L (1994e). Stabilization and immobilization devices. In E Halperin, L Constine, N Tarbell, & L Kun (Eds.), *Pediatric Radiation Oncology.* (2nd ed., pp. 588–599). New York: Raven Press.

Halperin E, Constine L, Tarbell N, & Kun L (1994f). Leukemia. In E Halperin, L Constine, N Tarbell, & L Kun (Eds.), *Pediatric Radiation Oncology.* (2nd ed., pp. 12–39). New York: Raven Press.

Halperin E, Constine L, Tarbell N, & Kun L (1994g). Non-Hodgkin's lymphoma. In E Halperin, L Constine, N Tarbell, & L Kun (Eds.), *Pediatric Radiation Oncology.* (2nd ed., pp. 244–261). New York: Raven Press.

Halperin E, Constine L, Tarbell N, & Kun L (1994h). Hodgkin's disease. In E Halperin, L Constine, N Tarbell, & L Kun (Eds.), *Pediatric Radiation Oncology.* (2nd ed., pp. 215–243). New York: Raven Press.

Halperin E, Constine L, Tarbell N, & Kun L (1994i). Ewing's sarcoma. In E Halperin, L Constine, N Tarbell, & L Kun (Eds.), *Pediatric Radiation Oncology.* (2nd ed., pp. 262–286). New York: Raven Press.

Hassey-Dow K (1992). Principles of brachytherapy. In K Hassey-Dow & L Hilderley (Eds.), *Nursing Care in Radiation Oncology* (pp. 16–29). Philadelphia: WB Saunders.

Hayes FA, Green AA, & O'Connor DM (1989). Chemotherapeutic management of epidural neuroblastoma. *Medical Pediatric Oncology, 17,* 6.

Healey EA, Shamberger RC, Grier JE, Loeffler JS, & Tarbell NJ (1995). A 10-year experience of pediatric brachytherapy. *International Journal of Radiation Oncology, Biology, Physics, 32,* 451–455.

Heideman RL, Packer R, Albright L, Freeman C, & Rorke L (1993). Tumors of the central nervous system. In P Pizzo & DG Poplack (Eds.), *Principles and Practice of Pediatric Oncology,* (2nd ed., pp. 633–681). Philadelphia: JB Lippincott.

Hirshfield-Bartek J (1992). Combined modality therapy. In K Hassey-Dow & L Hilderley (Eds.), *Nursing Care in Radiation Oncology* (pp. 251–263). Philadelphia: WB Saunders.

Hockenberry M (1986). Impact of cancer. In M Hockenberry & D Coody (Eds.), *Pediatric Oncology and Hematology—Perspectives on Care.* (pp. 421–431). St. Louis: CB Mosby.

Horowitz M, DeLaney T, Malawer M, & Tsokos M (1993). Ewing's sarcoma family of tumors: Ewing's sarcoma of bone and soft tissue and the peripheral primitive neuroectodermal tumors. In P Pizzo & DG Poplack (Eds.), *Principles and Practice of Pediatric Oncology,* (2nd edition, pp. 795–821). Philadelphia: JB Lippincott.

Jenkins D & Doyle J (1987). Paediatric Hodgkin's disease—late results and toxicity. *International Journal of Radiation Oncology, Biology, Physics, 13,* 92.

Kun L & Moulder J (1993). General principles of radiation therapy. In P Pizzo & DG Poplack (Eds.), *Principles and Practice of Pediatric Oncology,* (2nd ed., pp. 273–302). Philadelphia: JB Lippincott.

Lampkin BE (1993). Introduction and executive summary. *Cancer 71,* 3199–3201.

Lange B, D'Angio G, Ross A, O'Neill J, & Packer R (1993). Oncologic emergencies. In P Pizzo & DG Poplack (Eds.), *Principles and Practice of Pediatric Oncology,* (2nd ed., pp. 951–972). Philadelphia: JB Lippincott.

Leikin S (1993). The role of adolescents in decisions concerning their cancer therapy. *Cancer 71*, 3342–3346.

Leventhal BG & Donaldson SS (1993). Hodgkin's disease. In P Pizzo & DG Poplack (Eds.), *Principles and Practice of Pediatric Oncology*, (2nd ed., pp. 577–594). Philadelphia: JB Lippincott.

Levin VA, Gutin PH, & Leibel S. (1993). Neoplasms of the central nervous system. In V DeVita, S Hellman, & S Rosenberg (Eds.), *Cancer Principles and Practice of Oncology* (4th ed., pp. 1679–1737). Philadelphia: JB Lippincott.

Lew CC (1992). Special needs of children. In K Hassey Dow & L Hilderley (Eds.), *Nursing care in radiation oncology* (pp.177-202). Phildelphia: WB Saunders.

Lew CC & LaVally B (1995). The role of stereotactic radiation therapy in the management of children with brain tumors. *Journal of Pediatric Oncology Nursing, 12*, 212–222.

Liebhauser P (1993). Hodgkin's disease. In G Foley, D Fochtman, & K Hardin-Mooney (Eds.), *Nursing Care of the Child with Cancer* (2nd ed., pp. 397–434). Philadelphia: WB Saunders.

Link MP, Stevens J, Friend SH, Israel MA, Knudson AG, & Sondel PM (1993). Laboratory–clinical interface. *Cancer 71*, 3219–3221.

Loeffler JS, Tarbell NJ, Dunbar SR, et al. (1992). The potential role of stereotactic radiotherapy in the management of intracranial lesions. *Proceedings from the Varian 14th Users' Meeting*, pp. 8–10.

Loeffler JS, Alexander E, Kooy HM, et al. (1993). Stereotactic radiotherapy: rationale, techniques, and early results. In A DeSalles & S Goetsch (Eds.). *Stereotactic Surgery and Radiosurgery*, (pp. 307–320). Madison, WI: Medical Physics Publishing.

Lukens JN (1994). Progress resulting from clinical trials. Solid tumors in childhood cancer. *Cancer, 74*, 2710–2718.

Mercer R (1979). Perspectives on the adolescent and adolescence. In R Mercer (Ed.), *Perspectives on adolescent health care*. Philadelphia: WB Saunders.

Miller B (1986). Aetiology and epidemiology. In P Voute, A Barrett, H Bloom, J Lemerle, & M Neidhardt (Eds.), *Cancer in Children—Clinical Management* (2nd ed.). Berlin: Springer-Verlag.

Mitchell A, Louik C, Lacouture D, Sloane D, & Shapiro S (1982). Risk to children from computed tomographic scan premedication. *Journal of the American Medical Association 247*, 2385–2388.

Moore IM (1995). Central nervous system toxicity of cancer therapy in children. *Journal of Pediatric Oncology Nursing, 12*, 203–210.

Mulhern RK (1994). Neuropsychological late-effects In D Bearison & R Mulhern (Eds.) *Pediatric Psychooncology* (pp. 99–121). New York: Oxford University Press.

Mulvihill JJ (1993). Childhood cancer, the environment, and heredity. In P Pizzo & DG Poplack (Eds.), *Principles and Practice of Pediatric Oncology*, (2nd ed., pp. 11–27). Philadelphia: JB Lippincott.

Murray W (1989). Anesthesia for external beam radiotherapy. In E Halperin, L Kun, L Constine, & N Tarbell (Eds.) *Pediatric Radiation Oncology*. New York: Raven Press.

National Wilms' Tumor Study Committee. (1991). Wilms' tumor: status report, 1990. *Journal of Clinical Oncology, 9*, 877–887.

Parker B & Moore S (1993). Imaging studies in the diagnosis of pediatric malignancies. In P Pizzo & DG Poplack (Eds.), *Principles and Practice of Pediatric Oncology*, (2nd ed., pp. 153–178). Philadelphia: JB Lippincott.

Parker SL, Tong T, Bolden S, & Wingo PA (1997). Cancer statistics, 1997. *Cancer, 47*, 5–22.

Phillips T (1994). Biochemical modifiers: drug-radiation interactions. In P Mauch & J Loeffler (Eds.) *Radiation Oncology, Technology and Biology*. (pp. 113–151). Philadelphia: WB Saunders.

Pizzo P, Horowitz M, Poplack D, Hays D, & Kun L (1993). Solid tumors of childhood. In V DeVita, S Hellman, & S Rosenberg (Eds.), *Cancer Principles and Practice of Oncology* (4th ed., pp. 1738–1791). Philadelphia: JB Lippincott.

Poplack DG (1993). Acute lymphoblastic leukemia. In P Pizzo & DG Poplack (Eds.), *Principles and Practice of Pediatric Oncology*, (2nd ed., pp. 431–481). Philadelphia: JB Lippincott.

Poplack DG, Kun L, Magrath I, & Pizzo P (1993). Leukemias and lymphomas of childhood. In V DeVita, S Hellman, & S Rosenberg (Eds.), *Cancer Principles and Practice of Oncology* (4th ed., pp. 1792–1818). Philadelphia: JB Lippincott Co.

Raney RB, Hays DM, Tefft M, & Triche TJ (1993). Rhabdomyosarcoma and the undifferentiated sarcomas. In P Pizzo & DG Poplack (Eds.), *Principles and Practice of Pediatric Oncology*, (2nd ed., pp. 769–794). Philadelphia: JB Lippincott.

Reaman GH (1993). Special considerations for the infant with cancer. In P Pizzo & DG Poplack (Eds.), *Principles and Practice of Pediatric Oncology*, (2nd ed., pp. 303–314). Philadelphia: JB Lippincott.

Rechner M (1990). Adolescents with cancer: getting on with life. *Journal of Pediatric Oncology Nursing, 7*, 139–144.

Redner A (1987). Radiation. In S Maul-Mellot & J Adams (Eds.), *Childhood Cancer—A Nursing Overview*, (pp. 103–123). Boston: Jones and Bartlett.

Ritchie J (1979). Preparation of toddlers and preschool children for hospital procedures. *Canadian Nurse*. Dec. 1979, 30–32.

Robison LL (1993). General principles of the epidemiology of childhood cancer. In P Pizzo & DG Poplack (Eds.), *Principles and Practice of Pediatric Oncology*, (2nd ed., pp. 3–27). Philadelphia: JB Lippincott.

Rosen E, Cassady JR, Frantz C, Kretschmar C, Levy R, & Sallan S (1984). Neuroblastoma: the Joint Center for Radiation Therapy/Dana Farber Cancer Institute/Children's Hospital experience. *Journal of Clinical Oncology, 2*, 9–732.

Schulman S (1994). Anesthesia in external beam radiotherapy. In E Halperin, L Constine, N Tarbell, & L Kun (Eds.), *Pediatric Radiation Oncology*. (2nd ed., pp. 576–587). New York: Raven Press.

Sheline GE, Wara WM, & Smith V (1980). Therapeutic irradiation and brain injury. *International Journal of Radiation Oncology, Biology, Physics, 6*, 1215.

Shiminski-Maher T & Shields M (1995). Pediatric brain tumors: Diagnosis and management. *Journal of Pediatric Oncology Nursing, 12*, 188–198.

Shiminski-Maher T & Wisoff JH (1995). Pediatric brain tumors. *Critical Care Nursing Clinics of North America, 7*, 159–169.

Slifer K, Bucholtz J, & Cataldo M (1994). Behavioral training of motion control in young children undergoing radiation treatment without sedation. *Journal of Pediatric Oncology Nursing, 11*, 55–63.

Smith M, Arthur D, Camitta B, Carroll A, Crist W, Gayon P, Gelber R, Heerema N, Korn E, Link M, Murphy S, Pui C, Pullen J, Reaman G, Sallan S, Sather H, Shuster J, Simon R, Trigg M, Tubergen D, Uckun F, & Ungerleider R

(1996). Uniform approach to risk classification and treatment assignment for children with acute lymphoblastic leukemia. *Journal of Clinical Oncology, 14,* 18–24.

Synder C (1986). *Oncology Nursing.* Boston: Little, Brown.

Tarbell NJ, Neuberger P, Pazola K, Sallan S, Schwenn M, & Shamberger R (1990). Cancers in Children. In R Osteen, B Cady, & P Rosenthal (Eds.). *Cancer Manual* (8th ed.; pp. 383–393). Boston: American Cancer Society.

Tarbell NJ, Chin LM, & Mauch PM (1994). Total body irradiation for bone marrow transplantation. In P Mauch & J Loeffler (Eds.) *Radiation Oncology, Technology and Biology.* (pp. 387–401). Philadelphia: WB Saunders.

Tucker M (1993). Secondary tumors. In V DeVita, S Hellman, & S Rosenberg (Eds.), *Cancer Principles and Practice of Oncology* (4th ed., pp. 2407–2416). Philadelphia: JB Lippincott.

Walker C, Wells L, Heincy S, Hymovich D, & Weeks D (1993). Nursing managment of psychosocial care needs. In G Foley, D Fochtman, & K Hardin-Mooney (Eds.), *Nursing Care of the Child with Cancer* (2nd ed., pp. 397–434). Philadelphia: WB Saunders.

Waskerwitz M & Leonard M (1986). Early detection of malignancy: from birth to twenty years. *Oncology Nursing Forum, 13,* 50–57.

Wear E, Covey J, & Brush M (1982). Facilitating children's adaptation to intrusive procedures. In D Fochtman & G Foley (Eds.), *Nursing Care of the Child with Cancer.* (pp. 61–80). Boston: Little, Brown.

Wells LM, Heiney SP, Swygert E, Troficanto G, Stokes C, & Ettinger RS (1990). Psychosocial stressors, coping resources, and information needs of parents of adolescent cancer patients. *Journal of Pediatric Oncology Nursing, 7,* 145–148.

Whaley L & Wong D (1983). *Nursing Care of Infants and Children.* (pp. 417–701). St. Louis: CV Mosby.

Wharam M (1983). Radiation therapy. In A Altman & A Schwartz (Eds.), *Malignant Diseases of Infancy, Childhood, and Adolescence* (2nd ed.). Philadelphia: WB Saunders.

18

Skin Cancer

JOSEPH D. GIULIANO

Skin cancer is the most common malignant neoplasm in the United States Caucasian population. The American Cancer Society estimates that in the United States more than 700,000 new skin cancers are diagnosed each year. Of these newly diagnosed cases, 40,300 are melanomas that result in approximately 7,300 deaths annually (Parker et al., 1997). Skin cancers, when detected early, hold an excellent prognosis. In addition, these malignancies are the most preventable of all cancers.

Most skin carcinomas are detected early and cured with surgery alone. Although limited, there is a role for radiotherapy in the management of skin cancers. This chapter discusses the radiotherapy treatment niche and outlines some specific techniques used in the treatment of skin neoplasms.

Radiation oncology nursing interventions focus on disease prevention and early detection. In addition, a discussion of the role of the nurse in caring for patients experiencing altered body image is included.

Anatomy of the Skin

The integumentary system including the skin and its derivatives provides the external protective covering of the body. The skin plays an important role in maintaining homeostasis and temperature regulation while protecting the body from injury and the introduction of infectious agents. The skin consists of two layers: the epidermis and the dermis (corium). (See Chapter 8.) The four avascular layers of the epidermis are made up of keratinized stratified squamous epithelium and are 0.05 to 0.15 mm thick. The outer most layer, the *stratum corneum* (horny layer), is the thickest layer and is comprised of dead cell material and keratin fibers. The next layer is the thin translucent band of cells called the *stratum lucidum* and is primarily made up of anuclear keratinocytes. The process of keratinization begins in the next layer, the *stratum granulosum*, where the thin layer of flattened cells produce the substance keratohyalin, a precursor of the protein, keratin. Mitotically active cells are found in the next two layers, the *stratum spinosum* and *basale*, which make up the *stratum germinativum* (the growing layer). Cells from these layers migrate and replace cells in the outermost stratum corneum where they lose their nuclei and flatten. About one-fourth of the cells in the stratum basale are specialized melanocytes, which produce the pigment melanin. In addition, Merkel cells, which are believed to be associated with sensory nerve endings and touch reception, are located in the deepest layer of the epidermis.

The dermis is 1 to 2 mm thick and borders the stratum generativum. The dermis is comprised mainly of a connective tissue matrix containing nerves, lymphatics, blood vessels, and elastin fibers. Skin derivatives including hair follicles, and sweat and sebaceous glands are found in the dermal layer.

Pathology and Epidemiology

The majority of skin cancers are basal (BCCa) or squamous cell carcinomas (SCCa) arising in squamous epithelium. Of the two cell types, basal cell carcinoma is more prevalent. The number of new cases of BCCa and SCCa of the skin exceed 500,000 each year and the number of deaths are 3,800 (Parker et al., 1996). This statistic illustrates how common skin cancer is, and its high cure rate. Other carcinomas arising in the skin include malignant melanomas, keratocanthomas, lymphomas (T cell lymphoma, mycosis fungoides), angiosarcomas, Kaposi's sarcoma, and metastases.

355

Individuals of Celtic background with fair skin and individuals in occupations involving prolonged exposure to the sun are at increased risk for developing skin cancer. Sun exposure, specifically exposure to UVB light, is the single most common cause of skin cancers (Kopf, 1988). In addition, chemical carcinogens such as coal tar, arsenic, and topical nitrogen mustard, as well as ionizing radiation, immunosuppression, and papillomavirus are also implicated as causes of skin cancer (Cohen et al., 1987). The development of squamous cell carcinomas have been associated with chronic skin irritation in the setting of thermal burns and syphilis. A variety of genetic conditions related to the development of skin cancer include xeroderma pigmentosa, albinism, phenylketonuria, and Gorlin syndrome.

In addition to carcinomas arising in epithelial cells, melanomas arise in melanocytes. Depending on the depth of their invasion into the skin, melanomas can carry a very poor prognosis. Merkel cell carcinoma is a rare neoplasm arising in touch receptors and is characterized by a propensity for regional spread despite adequate surgical resection and adjuvant treatment.

Prevention and Detection

Considering that nonmelanoma skin cancer is the most common neoplasm and is demonstrating a steady increase in incidence over the past decade, early detection and aggressive prevention are crucial. The nursing role provides an excellent opportunity to review basic skin cancer prevention and detection information with the patient and family. In the prevention of skin neoplasms, it is important to undertake a comprehensive review of prevention information, as given in Table 18-1

Table 18-1 • Strategies for Prevention of Skin Cancer

- Minimize skin exposure to the sun between 10 AM and 3 PM.
- Use protective clothing (i.e., hats, pants) during long exposures to sun.
- Use sunglasses.
- Use sunscreen with a minimum SPF of 15 (reapply every three hours and after swimming).
- Use sunscreens with benzophenones while taking thiazides, sulfonamides, and antineoplastic agents, because of photosensitivity.
- Avoid tanning parlors.
- Keep infants out of the sun.

From Berwick M, Bologna JL, Heer C, Fine JA (1991). The role of the nurse in skin cancer prevention, screening, and early detection. *Seminars in Oncology Nursing, 7,* 64–71.

(Berwick et al., 1991). In addition to preventive measures, it is important to teach patients and their families to assess for early signs in the changes of nevi and stress the need to perform a monthly, systemic body survey for new or changing lesions. In assessing nevi, patients should look for changes in color, shape, diameter, and irregular borders. If there is a family history of skin cancer or other risk factors, the patient should be referred to a dermatologist for regular skin surveys.

Diagnosis and General Management

Diagnosing skin neoplasms begins with a careful history and thorough physical exam including a complete body survey. Referral to a dermatologist with an appreciation for subtle changes in normal skin appearance is important. The history should include questions about topical medications used in the past, scars, chronic skin ulcerations, burns, and exposure to chemical agents and ionizing radiation. Premalignant lesions such as actinic keratoses may appear in sun exposed areas as multiple, red, rough (grain-of-sand appearance) papules 1 to 3 mm in size. Some early observable signs of skin neoplasms include the following changes in skin appearance and texture: papules with telangiectasia, firmness, and induration with irregular borders and scaling. Later signs include loss of skin markings, pinpoint or diffuse changes in pigmentation, and regular heaped-up borders of hyperkeratosis. Advanced lesions appear ulcerative with heaped-up irregular borders. Precursor lesions of malignant melanoma include dyplastic nevi that may be familial and covering large areas of the body or smaller isolated areas. Melanomas are asymmetric with irregular borders, color variegations, and a diameter generally greater than 6 mm (see Figure 18–1).

The excisional biopsy remains the standard for diagnosis of malignant neoplasms of the skin. In some cases, the biopsy can be therapeutic if microscopic evaluation reveals negative margins. Special immunoperoxidase staining techniques are employed to distinguish the type of neoplasm and to plan appropriate treatment. Based on a tumor's propensity for invasion of local structures and metastatic spread, a computerized tomograph study (CT scan) and/or other radiologic studies may be obtained to rule out regional involvement.

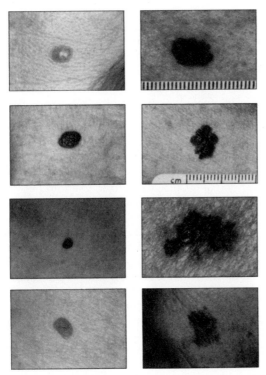

Figure 18-1 • Differences between noncancerous lesions (*left*) and melanoma (*right*) showing asymmetry, ragged borders, uneven color, and change in diameter.

Treatment Modes

Treatment of skin cancer is custom-tailored for the patient and is based on a variety of factors (see Table 18–2). The goal of treatment remains the same: to eradicate the disease and obtain local control while preserving function and cosmesis.

Surgery

Surgery remains the mainstay of treatment, with most basal cell carcinomas being cured using surgery alone. Overall, surgery and radiation therapy result in comparable rates of local control for basal and squamous cell carcinomas of the skin. The main advantage of surgical excision is that a good cure rate can be obtained in one outpatient procedure at a relatively low cost.

Table 18-2 • Factors Influencing Treatment Choices

Size of the lesion
Location
Histopathologic diagnosis
Nature of the lesion (primary or recurrence)
Patient's lifestyle and preferences
Performance status of patient

Curettage is a commonly used surgical technique that involves excising a tumor using spoon-shaped curettes. This technique is used in the setting of previously untreated superficial tumors. Chemical cautery can be used to obtain hemostasis and the resulting surgical defect heals in 3 to 4 weeks by secondary intention. Microscopic review of margins is not possible using this technique.

Cryotherapy, like curettage, is used for small, noninvasive tumors, which are usually precancerous lesions. Liquid nitrogen is used to freeze the tumor and surrounding tissue forming an eschar that heals by secondary intention.

Moh's micrographic surgery is a lengthy procedure performed by a specially trained dermatologic surgeon. The surgery is employed in areas where normal tissue is at a premium and in the setting of more aggressive or recurrent tumors. Multiple meticulous horizontal sections are excised and examined microscopically to map out areas of positive margins. This technique allows the surgeon to proceed conservatively along the path of positive margins, preserving normal tissue while obtaining a negative surgical margin. In addition to recurrent and aggressive carcinomas in tissue sensitive areas, Moh's surgery is indicated in areas of high-risk recurrence (nose, ear, temple, periorbital area) and in skin cancers with clinically ill-defined borders.

Chemotherapy

Chemotherapeutic agents have been used in treating recurrent and advanced skin cancers. Research into the use of chemotherapy agents alone, mainly cisplatin, 5-FU, bleomycin, and doxorubicin, have demonstrated unsatisfactory results with most patients experiencing progressing tumor (Sadek et al., 1990). Systemic retinoid therapy along with alpha-interferon is being used in clinical trials and shows promise in treating basal cell carcinomas (Lippman et al., 1988). Topical 5-FU, while having an extremely limited role in the treatment of most skin neoplasms, does show some promise in the treatment of some precancerous lesions like actinic keratoses (Schwartz, 1988).

Radiation Therapy

The role of radiotherapy in the management of skin cancer is limited to lesions less than 1 cm that are deemed inoperable or lesions that would result in a surgical defect unacceptable to the patient. Radiotherapy is also used in medically inoperable patients, such as the elderly, and in situations of recurrent disease, metastases, or a positive surgical margin. Radiation therapy is contraindicated in patients with xeroderma pigmentosum, epidermodyplasia verruciformis, and basal cell nevus syndrome because of the potential to induce tumors in the treatment field (Brady et al., 1987).

Orthovoltage x rays and megavoltage electrons are the best modalities for treating skin cancers. With the increased use of megavoltage, most radiation therapy departments use electron energies to treat skin carcinomas. Technical concerns in treatment planning focus on some unique considerations, such as the superficial nature of most skin cancers and the need for an adequate cosmetic result. In addition to the rapid dose fall-off, electron energies provide the advantage of uniform dose distributions from the surface to a prescribed depth, allowing for homogeneity even when treating over undulating surfaces. However, when using electron energies a bolus material (usually 1 to 1.5 cm) is used to increase the skin surface dose or to treat to an isodose line. The treatment volume and prescribed depth are dependent on the size of the lesion, its histopathologic characteristics, and the infiltrative nature of the tumor.

When orthovoltage x rays are used to treat skin cancers, half-value layers (HVL) of either aluminum or copper are used. The thickness of the HVL depends on the energy, skin to surface distance (SSD), and desired dose fall-off. Orthovoltage energies offer the advantage of delivering 100 percent of the dose to the skin surface; however, a slower dose fall-off requires care in preserving underlying structures.

A variety of treatment aids are used in treating skin cancers, especially when sensitive areas such as the eyes or nose are involved. Lead cutouts are frequently employed to delineate the treatment volume and protect surrounding structures. Stability of the area being treated is achieved using a variety of immobilization devices such as plastic masks or alpha cradles. In order to shield the radiosensitive anterior portion of the eye, lead eye shields are used when treating carcinoma of the eyelid or canthi. These shields are placed into the conjunctival sac after a local ophthalmic anesthetic is applied. In some cases, erythromycin ointment can be used to lubricate the eye for easy placement of the shield while preventing both infection and damage to the cornea. When treating nasal skin tumors, paraffin boluses are used to compensate for the curvature of the nose and ensure homogeneity of dose. In addition, a shield is placed over the eyes to protect them from scatter radiation. In areas of the body where there is less

subcutaneous tissue (e.g., dorsum of the hand) using external beam radiation therapy can increase the risk of radiation-induced necrosis. Therefore, radioactive molds of radium, gold, or radon seeds are fashioned and placed over the tumor.

The definitive radiation dose varies with tumor size and depth, location, histopathology, size of the treatment field, and dose fractionation. In general, treatment is delivered in 200 to 500 cGy fractions to a total dose of 3000 to 5000 cGy in 6 to 20 fractions for most basal cell carcinomas, and 5000 to 6000 cGy in 6 to 30 fractions over 10 to 35 elapsed days for squamous cell carcinoma (Brady et al., 1987).

Tumor response is influenced by the following factors: (1) the total dose; (2) dose fractionation (if one increases the size of the fraction there is an increase in late effects); and (3) the volume being treated (the same dose of radiation given to a small field may result in necrosis if used on a larger field). Overall local tumor control using primary radiation therapy or radiation after surgical failure is reported by Lovett and associates (1990) to be 86 percent (292 of 339 patients) with a 91 percent local control rate for BCCa and 75 percent for SCCa. The same study reports 97 percent and 91 percent local control rates for BCCa and SCCa, respectively, for lesions 1 cm or less. For lesions 1 to 5 cm, local control was 87 percent for BCCa and 76 percent for SCCa, and for tumors greater than 5 cm tumor control was 87 percent and 56 percent, respectively. Additional studies from Hahnemann University in Philadelphia (Brady et al., 1987) and Princess Margaret Hospital (Fitzpatrick, 1984) report comparable disease-free survival and local control statistics. The disease-free survival is not as favorable for recurrent squamous cell carcinoma because of its increased propensity for metastatic spread.

Other Skin Tumors

Melanoma

Cutaneous malignant melanoma (CMM) arises in melanocytes and accounts for approximately 1.5 percent (Rigel et al., 1987) of all skin cancers and has demonstrated a rapid doubling of its incidence over the past decade. There are three major forms of melanoma. The first is superficial spreading melanoma (SSM) with a horizontal growth pattern and flat scaly appearance. This lesion is the most common type and accounts for 60 to 70 percent of melanomas. Nodular melanoma (NM) represents 30 percent of melanoma cases and is characterized by an elevated dome-like appearance with a dark pigmentation and irregular borders. NM is an aggressive variant and usually invades deep into the dermis and can metastasize quickly. The third most common type is the lentigo malignant melanoma (LMM), which most commonly occurs as a premalignant lesion in elderly patients.

In staging melanomas, the most important characteristic and best known prognostic factor is depth of invasion (Clark et al., 1975). The American Joint Committee staging criteria for malignant melanoma are a combination of the Clark and Breslow staging systems (see Table 18–3).

Surgical resection remains the mainstay of treatment especially for lesions detected early. Surgery involves wide local excision with adequate margins and special attention is given to deep inva-

sion and possible lymph node metastases. In metastatic disease, a combination of surgery, radiotherapy, chemotherapy, and immunotherapy may be employed. Chemotherapeutic agents that have shown efficacy include dacarbazine (DTIC) and the nitrosoureas (BCNU, CCNU). There are several investigational protocols using interferon, tumor cell vaccines, and monoclonal antibodies (Wallack et al., 1995). Recently, the Food and Drug Administration (F.D.A.) approved the use of interferon-alpha as adjuvant therapy for the treatment of melanoma based on results of a multicenter, randomized clinical trial administered by the Eastern Cooperative Oncology Group (ECOG) (Kirkwood et al., in press).

Because melanoma is relatively radioresistant, higher-than-usual dose fractionation schemes are used to compensate for the ability of these cells to repair sublethal DNA damage. Overgaard (1980)

Table 18-3 • AJCC Staging for Malignant Melanoma

PRIMARY TUMOR

TX	Primary tumor cannot be assessed
T0	No evidence of primary tumor
Tis	Melanoma in situ, not an invasive lesion Clark's Level I: confined to epidermis with no invasion through basement membrane
T1	Tumor 0.75 mm or less in thickness and invades the papillary dermis Clark's Level II: penetrates basement membrane into papillary dermis
T2	Tumor more than 0.75 mm but not more than 1.5 mm in thickness and/or invades to papillary-reticular dermal interface Clark's Level III: Cells fill papillary dermis and abut the reticular dermis without invasion
T3	Tumor more than 1.5 mm but not more than 4 mm in thickness and/or invades the reticular dermis Clark's Level IV: Cells extend between bundle of collagen characteristic of reticular dermis
T3a	Tumor more than 1.5 mm but not more than 3 mm in thickness
T3b	Tumor more than 3 mm but not more than 4 mm in thickness
T4	Tumor more than 4 mm in thickness and/or invades the subcutaneous tissue and/or satellite(s) within 2 cm of the primary tumor Clark's Level V: Invasion into subcutaneous tissue
T4a	Tumor more than 4 mm in thickness and/or invasion of subcutaneous tissue
T4b	Satellite(s) within 2 cm of the primary tumor

REGIONAL LYMPH NODES

NX	Regional lymph nodes cannot be assessed
N0	No regional lymph node metastasis
N1	Metastasis 3 cm or less in greatest dimension in any regional node
N2	Metastasis greater than 3 cm in any regional node and/or in-transit metastasis
N2a	Greater than 3 cm in regional node(s)
N2b	In-transit metastasis
N2c	Both (N2a and N2b)

DISTANT METASTASIS

MX	Presence of distant metastasis cannot be assessed
M0	No distant metastasis
M1	Distant metastasis
M1a	Metastasis in skin or subcutaneous tissue or distant lymph nodes
M1b	Visceral metastasis

Note: In-transit metastasis involves skin or subcutaneous tissue more than 2 cm from the primary tumor not beyond regional nodes.
From Beahrs OH, Henson DE, Hutter RVP, & Myers MH (Eds.) (1992). Manual for staging of cancer, 4th ed. Philadelphia: JB Lippincott. Used with permission.

demonstrated that larger doses per fraction worked best in treating CMM. The preferred regimen was found to be 900 cGy in three fractions over 8 days. Radiotherapy is used frequently and effectively in treating metastatic disease to the brain, bone, and other sites that may be causing pain or other symptoms. Hyperthermia, when used in combination with radiation therapy, is effective on large cutaneous lesions with good palliative results (Emami, 1988). Stereotactic radiosurgery coupled with fractionated whole-brain irradiation is used to treat solitary or multiple metastatic melanoma brain lesions with good results (Somaza et al., 1993).

Keratocanthoma

Keratocanthoma is a malignant neoplasm of the skin that resembles squamous cell carcinoma histopathologically and with a rapid onset and progression. The natural history of this tumor results in serious scarring and tissue destruction making removal desirable. Surgical excision is usually curative. However, in areas where cosmesis is a challenge for the surgeon, such as around the eyes and nose, radiation therapy may be employed. The recommended treatment dose is 25 Gy delivered in five daily fractions. In most cases, the cosmetic results are excellent with rapid tumor regression and durable complete responses.

Merkel Cell Carcinoma

First identified in 1972, Merkel cell carcinoma, also known as cutaneous neuroendocrine carcinoma, is a very rare primary skin neoplasm that arises from the Merkel cell touch receptors. This tumor is characterized by recurrence after surgical resection, frequent regional lymph node involvement, and common distant metastasis. Overall, patients with Merkel cell carcinoma do better after combined surgery and radiation therapy. The radiation therapy port includes the entire surgical bed with a generous margin including areas of possible lymphatic involvement, especially in the head and neck region. For subclinical disease, 5000 cGy in standard fractions is used while 6000 to 7000 cGy is delivered when there is microscopic or gross residual disease.

Nursing Considerations

Changes in skin integrity and body image present the greatest concern for patients with skin cancer.

Body image is a part of the patient's self-concept and can be defined as that aspect of the perceived-self consisting of the images of the body including its contour and function (van der Velde, 1985).

A diagnosis of skin cancer brings with it concerns of loss of body function and changes in the normal shapes and contours of body parts. Many patients have undergone repeated surgeries, some involving the face, with protracted reconstructive procedures using skin grafts, flaps, and even prostheses. For some patients, radiation therapy may offer an alternative to disfiguring surgery, while for others it is another treatment modality that will alter their body image and produce untoward side effects. In this setting, the role of the radiation oncology nurse includes educating, counseling, and symptom management.

After an adequate and complete educational needs assessment, the nurse provides the patient with information acceptable to that patient's learning style. The nurse works in collaboration with the radiation oncologist who secures informed consent and discusses with the patient treatment alternatives, potential risks and benefits of treatment, and prognosis. The education process continues by encouraging the patient and family to ask questions and confirm that patient education is a fundamental right and an ongoing process.

Some of the feelings that may result from a disturbance in body image include: refusal of social contact, expressions of fear of rejection, hopelessness, denial, and even a marked grieving response. Assisting patients and their families with these psychosocial needs demands the skills and collaboration of a multidisciplinary team, including: psychologists, plastic surgeons, cosmetologists, psychiatric liaison nurses, social workers, counselors, nutritionists, and the radiation therapist. Many times the nurse is the first member of the team to discuss these feelings with the patient, and with the patient's consent, can act as a liaison or coordinator of services for the patient and family. The nurse should never underestimate the value of sitting with a patient or family member and listening intently, allowing them to verbalize and clarify their feelings. This, in addition to the work of other members of the team, can make a difference in the quality of a patient's life.

Symptom management affects body image and patient perceptions. The proper and timely management of side effects, such as skin reactions and pain, can influence the patient's and family's self-image and hopefulness. In addition, appropriate management of radiation skin reactions can minimize scarring and decrease the chances of developing necrotic nonhealing ulcerations (Sitton, 1992). Draining odiferous wounds that are not properly dressed and cared for can influence a patient's ability to perform important social and job functions and family contacts. Symptom management goes beyond the focus on a body part or function and profoundly influences a person's ability to function.

Summary

Skin neoplasms are the most preventable and curable of all cancers. The role of radiotherapy in the treatment of these neoplasms is limited to specific situations using specialized techniques. Nursing care for the patient and family includes education about prevention and symptom management with a particular emphasis on changes in body image.

References

Berwick M, Bolognia JL, Heer C, & Fine JA (1991). The role of the nurse in skin cancer prevention, screening, and early detection. *Seminars in Oncology Nursing, 7*, 64–71.

Brady LW, Binnick SA, Fitzpatrick PJ (1987). Skin cancer. In CA Perez & LA Brady (Eds.), *Principles and Practice of Radiation Oncology* (pp. 377–394). Philadelphia: JB Lippincott.

Clark WH, Ainsworth AM & Bernandino EA (1975). The developmental biology of primary human malignant melanomas. *Seminars in Oncology, 2*, 83–103.

Cohen EB, Komorowski RA, Clowry LJ (1987). Cutaneous complications of renal transplant recipients. *American Journal of Clinical Pathology, 88*, 32–37.

Emami B, Perey CA, Konefal J (1988). Thermoradiotherapy for malignant melanoma. *International Journal of Hyperthermia, 4*, 373–381.

Fitzpatrick PJ, Thompson GA, Easterbrook WM, Gallie BL, & Payne DG (1984). Basal and squamous cell carcinoma of the eyelids and their treatment by radiotherapy. *International Journal of Radiation Oncology, Biology, Physics, 10*, 449–454.

Kirkwood J et al. (1995). Randomized, multicenter clinical trial of alpha-interferon in stage IV melanoma. *Cancer* (in press).

Kopf AW (1988). Prevention and early detection of skin cancer: Melanoma. *Cancer, 62*, 1791–1795.

Lippman S, Shimm D, & Meyskens F (1988). Nonsurgical treatments for skin cancer, retinoids and alpha-interferon. *Journal of Dermatology, Surgery, Oncology 14*, 862–869.

Lovett RD, Perez CA, Shapiro SJ, & Garcia DM (1990). External irradiation of epithelial skin cancer. *International Journal of Radiation Oncology, Biology, Physics, 19*, 235–242.

Overgaard J (1980). Radiation therapy of malignant melanoma. *International Journal of Radiation Oncology, Biology, Physics, 6*, 41–44.

Parker SL, Tong T, Bolden S, Wingo PA (1996). Cancer statistics 1996. *Ca-A Cancer Journal for Clinicians 46*, 5–27.

Rigel DS, Kopf AW, & Friedman RJ (1987). The rate of malignant melanoma in the United States: Are we making an impact? *Journal of the American Academy of Dermatology, 17*, 1050–1053.

Sadek H, Azl N, Wendling JL, Cvitkovic E, Rahal M, Mamelle G, Guillame JC, Armand JP, & Avril MF (1990). Treatment of advanced squamous cell carcinoma of the skin with cisplatin, 5-fluorouracil, and bleomycin. *Cancer, 66*, 1692–1696.

Schwartz RA (1988). Skin cancer: Recognition and management. New York: Springer-Verlag.

Sitton E (1992). Early and late radiation-induced skin alterations, part II: Nursing care of irradiated skin. *Oncology Nursing Forum, 19*, 907–912.

Somaza S, Kondziolka D, Lunsford LD, Kirkwood JM, & Flickinger JC. (1993). Stereotactic radiosurgery for cerebral metastatic melanoma. *Journal of Neurosurgery, 79*, 661–666.

van der Velde CD (1985). Body images of one's self and of others: Developmental and clinical significance. *American Journal of Psychiatry, 142*, 527–537.

Wallack MK, Sivanandham M, Balch CM, Urist MM, Bland KI, Murray D, Robinson WA, Flaherty LE, Richards JM, & Bartolucci AA (1995). A phase III randomized, double-blind multi-institutional trial of vaccinia melanoma oncolysate—active specific immunotherapy for patients with stage II melanoma. *Cancer, 75*, 34–42.

III

Dimensions of Oncology Nursing
Practice in Radiation Oncology

Continuous Process Improvement: One Department of Radiation Oncology's Experience

ANNE E. LARA

"The kind of thinking that led to past success will not lead to future success."

Blanchard et al. (1996)

Reengineering, cross-functional work teams, restructuring, rightsizing, empowerment, coaching, continuous process improvement, and zapping are present-day buzzwords that describe 1990s organizational processes. General Motors, AT&T, DuPont, Proctor & Gamble, and Chrysler are among the corporations adopting or adapting to these emerging workplace philosophies. The health care industry has not escaped these workplace changes.

Hospitals across the country are exploring ways to integrate novel managerial strategies into daily operations. Radiation oncology department administrators are challenged to empower staff while reengineering daily operations in a customer-oriented, cost-effective manner. This chapter will explore one radiation oncology department's experience in meeting this challenge.

The Department

The Medical Center of Delaware's Department of Radiation Oncology is an American College of Radiology (ACR)–accredited hospital-based practice. Six radiation oncologists, five oncology certified registered nurses (including a master's prepared clinical nurse specialist and master's prepared nurse manager), fifteen radiation therapists, seven dosimetrists, three physicists, and seven secretaries make up the department staff. Ancillary staff consisting of a research nurse, social worker, and oncology data center registrar provide support to the department staff and patients receiving radiation therapy.

Organizationally, the chief therapist, the nurse manager, and the chief physicist share managerial responsibilities and report directly to an administrative vice president at the hospital. The chief therapist supervises the activities of the radiation therapists, the chief physicist coordinates treatment planning and physics services, and the nurse manager oversees nursing, dosimetry, and support staff processes (patient registration, scheduling, billing, filing, staffing, and so on).

An average of 150 patients receive treatment daily on one of four linear accelerators (two with 23 MEV capability and two with 6 MEV capability). Treatment planning is performed on one of two simulators using on-site CAT scan planning when clinically indicated. Patients requiring treatment for superficial skin lesions are treated on the department's orthovoltage unit or with hyperthermia. In addition, total body irradiation (TBI) is provided to patients undergoing bone marrow transplantation (BMT). Referrals to radiation oncology are made by medical oncologists, hematologists, surgeons, urologists, pulmonologists, and neurosurgeons. Patients are treated definitively, adjuvantly, or palliatively with radiation therapy.

There are five different types of patient appointments: new patient, simulation, on treatment, follow-up, and emergency. Prior to each patient's scheduled appointments, their demographic information must be entered into three different automated systems. Insurance coverage needs to be verified and authorized before treatment can be initiated. Physician dictation has to be transcribed and filed. Charts have to be assembled and maintained.

The Challenges and the Opportunities

A department of radiation oncology such as the one described poses many operational challenges for the manager. These challenges, however, provide stimulus for creativity, innovation, and change. They are opportunities to improve productivity and increase customer satisfaction. The sections that follow will describe how daily challenges foster opportunities for growth.

Continuous Improvement Through Process Teams

The processes mentioned above—staffing, registration, scheduling, chart maintenance, transcription, filing, and database entries—are integral components of the daily operations of the Department of Radiation Oncology. These operations support the critical patient care activities and are an important part of the foundation upon which customer satisfaction and cost efficiency are based. Measurement of both customer satisfaction and cost efficiency is accomplished through continuous process improvement (CPI), which focuses on processes and organized data collection and analysis, rather than on individual mistakes and quick solutions to problems.

Byham and Cox (1994) liken CPI to casting a spell. This spell can be used to explore problems and identify solutions. The five steps of their action spell are as follows:

1. Assess the situation and define the problem.
2. Determine the causes.
3. Target the solutions and develop ideas.
4. Implement ideas.
5. Make it an ongoing process.

With the action spell or CPI in mind, each departmental process provides an opportunity for exploration and improvement. The goal of exploration is to improve the process so that a measurable improvement in customer satisfaction and productivity is realized. Who better to assess the situation and define the problem than staff in-

volved in the processes? In an effort to improve productivity, decrease duplication, and minimize rework, process teams were formed using CPI principles and the "Empowerment Keys." Blanchard et al. (1996) describe these keys as follows:

1. Share information.
2. Create autonomy through boundaries.
3. Replace the hierarchy with self-directed teams.

Three process teams were formed to focus on issues of (1) filing, (2) scheduling, and (3) employee satisfaction. Team members targeted solutions, developed ideas, and implemented solutions. The goal of all efforts was to address customer-driven concerns. The following filing team activities demonstrate how CPI principles and staff empowerment strategies can result in increased productivity and customer satisfaction.

A Team in Action

In today's corporate world, a world of which health care is a large part, there are two types of organizations: pyramid and circular. Organizations that have a pyramid style of operating are characterized by limited job descriptions, tight control by supervisors, feedback and communication from the top down, slow change, and unmotivated employees. Circle organizations, by contrast, have the following characteristics: team focus, rapid change, cross-training of employees, decisions coming from the bottom up, rewards for innovation, focus on process, and action driven by customer satisfaction. Applying the characteristics of a circular organization, the filing process team embarked upon its challenge: how to get reports in the charts in a timely manner. Figure 19–1 depicts the department's adaptation of the circle style of organizational operations.

The team, facilitated by the nurse manager, met weekly for nine months. Preliminary team activities focused on defining the purpose, identifying meeting ground rules, and developing process flow charts. The team brainstormed ideas to identify process improvement ideas, which were then discussed. Those with the greatest potential for improvement were implemented department-wide.

The impact of such ideas was measured in a number of ways. One measurement involved recording the presence or absence of reports in the radiation chart. Run charts (bar graphs) were used to illustrate data collection results, as illustrated in Figures 19–2 and 19–3. Process checks are now conducted monthly in order to help determine

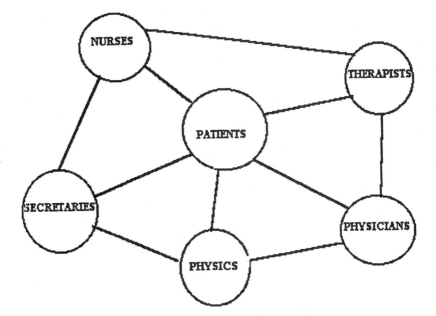

Figure 19-1 • The circle of interaction in radiation oncology.

Figure 19-2 • Sample graph of reports in the radiation chart.

Figure 19-3 • Sample bar graph to illustrate data collection results.

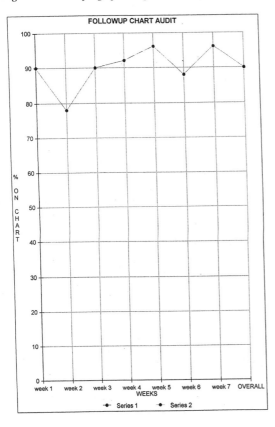

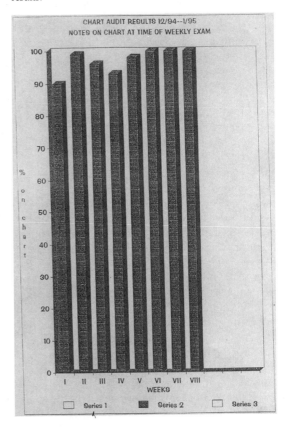

whether ongoing process improvements continue to be successful. An idea is considered successful if it increases the frequency with which reports are found on the radiation chart. For example, Figure 19–3 depicts an improvement in notes on the chart at time of weekly exam. Weeks I–IV were pre- or peri-implementation of improvement ideas; weeks V–VIII were postimplementation.

Staffing and Scheduling: A Managerial Opportunity

In addition to process team activities, staffing and scheduling issues presented another managerial opportunity. Before a manager can begin exploration of a project, however, she needs to be aware of her role and responsibilities—that are the functions of a manager.

Allen (1994) identifies six functions in the work of a manager as follows:

- establishing objectives
- organizing
- motivating
- developing people
- communicating
- measurement and analysis

The departmental processes of staffing and scheduling provide opportunities for a manager to exercise these six functions.

The staffing and scheduling objectives for a Department of Radiation Oncology are:

- to provide patient care in a safe and cost-effective manner
- to maintain skill level and competency of staff
- to foster continuity of patient care
- to develop empowered, motivated, team-oriented staff

In order to meet these objectives, a manager must organize daily operations to provide appropriate staffing, foster a positive work environment so that staff is motivated to provide exemplary patient care, provide ongoing education for staff, challenge staff to problem solve without managerial interference, serve as a role model in regard to communicating departmental or hospital-wide process changes to all members of the staff, and develop methods to measure and communicate success. The following discussion illustrates a number of these managerial activities.

Patient care teams are critical to daily department operations because it is these teams that pro-

vide safe patient-centered care. Teams are composed of a radiation oncologist, oncology nurse, secretary, therapist, and dosimetrist. Each team's objective is to provide comprehensive care in a manner that fosters patient continuity.

Teams function best when there is a one-to-one relationship among members—that is, one nurse, one physician, one secretary, one therapist, and one dosimetrist. When the number of one team member exceeds that of the others (for example, two physicians per one nurse), creative approaches that preserve the team concept and promote patient continuity need to be employed.

In this author's department, five oncology nurses (including the nurse manager and clinical nurse specialist) work with six radiation oncologists. When the number of physicians exceeds the number of nurses, how does a manager provide staffing that promotes patient care continuity? The solution to this concern involves using one primary nurse to work with two physicians, with the nurse manager or clinical nurse specialist providing backup or relief to the teams. For example, if a primary nurse is teaching a new patient about management of radiation-related side effects, the backup nurse may triage a patient problem for one of the primary nurse's patients under treatment.

Promoting continuing education for the staff has already been identified as a managerial objective. The manager not only needs to provide opportunities for education but also must maintain documentation of clinical competency and skill acquisition. Two examples of nursing critical skills checklist are depicted in Figures 19–4 and 19–5.

Productivity and Cost Efficiency: Empowerment and Outsourcing in Action

In an environment that purports to promote staff responsibility and accountability, employees must be given the tools to exercise these activities. Time management is an example of one of these tools. Prior to July 1994, all department staff were categorized as nonexempt and eligible for overtime when hours worked exceeded eight hours per day. As a result of this situation, the staff was forced to adhere to rigid working hours and overtime was high. Overtime hours were accrued on "busy" days, and staff were less productive yet obligated to put in time on less "busy" days. Nurses were frustrated by the fact that they had to sign in and sign out when starting and ending their work day.

GOAL: To demonstrate competency in caring for the patient being treated with a strontium 90 applicator.

Evaluator
Initials

1. Explains procedure to patient/family. _____
2. Obtains written consent. _____
3. Takes face photograph of patient. _____
4. Assists the physician to anesthetize the eye with two to three drops of tetracaine ophthalmic solution and to retract. _____
5. Assists the physician in the instillation of Strontium to the eye. _____
6. Measures the actual time of contact of Strontium using a stopwatch. _____
7. Returns the beta applicator to its storage box. _____
8. Places a patch over the eye. _____
9. Instructs the patient to keep the patch in place for one hour. _____
10. Gives subsequent treatment appointments to the patient. _____
11. Completes appropriate documentation. _____

_____ has demonstrated competency in caring for the patient being treated with a

strontium 90 applicator.

Evaluator _____   Date _____

Figure 19-4 • Critical skill evaluation checklist for radiation oncology nurse.

Figure 19-5 • Critical skill evaluation checklist for radiation oncology nurse.

GOAL: To demonstrate competency in caring for the patient receiving IV contrast material.

Evaluator
Initials

1. Explains procedure to patient/family. _____
2. Assesses patient's renal function as evidenced by serum creatinine of <1.5. (This value should be documented on chart.) _____
3. Verifies that patient is not allergic to contrast material or shellfish. _____
4. Takes and records patient's preprocedure vital signs. _____
5. Obtains written consent. _____
6. Places respiratory box, emergency drug box, and oxygen in procedure room. _____
7. Pages IV therapy nurse to insert patient's IV access device. _____
8. Prepares appropriate type and amount of IV contrast material (as prescribed by physician). _____
9. Administers IV contrast material. _____
10. Monitors patient for signs of allergic reaction. _____
11. Flushes IV device with 3.5 cc of NSS after administration of IV contrast material. _____
12. Calls Emergency Response Team in event of adverse patient reaction. _____
13. Takes and records patient's postprocedure vital signs. _____
14. Removes IV access device prior to patient's discharge from department. _____

_____ has demonstrated competency in caring for the patient receiving

IV contrast material.

Evaluator _____   Date _____

Table 19-1 • Cost-Savings Benefit of Time Management

Staff	Fiscal Year	OT Hrs	Fiscal Year	OT Hrs	Reduction in Hrs	Cost Savings
Secretaries	94	1331	95	360.25	970.75	9707.75
Nurses	94	394.75	95	52	342.75	6855
Totals		1725.75		412.25	1313.5	16,562.75

These factors prompted the nurse manager to explore alternative wage and salary strategies with the hospital's Human Resource Department. After consultation and subsequent discussion with both the nursing and secretarial staffs, the nurse manager exercised the option of changing the wage and salary category of the employees.

The nurses were reclassified as exempt employees who managed their own work and vacation time. As exempt employees, the nurses were still required to work their assigned hours; however, they did not have to sign in and sign out their time. In addition they had the option of working according to the patient care need of the day. For example, they might work 10 hours one day and 6 hours on another. Time management became their responsibility.

Because compensation laws differ for professional and support staff, the secretarial staff could not be classified as exempt employees. Instead, this group was recategorized as 40-hour work week nonexempt employees. Under these conditions, the secretarial staff had the option of flexing their work hours over the 40-hour work week. If a secretary needed to leave early one day, she could come in early or stay late on another day during the week. When a secretary requested a vacation day, it was her responsibility to provide the nurse manager with a coverage plan.

In addition to empowering the staff to manage their own time, the nurse manager also looked outside of the department for opportunities to "shift" processes. Were there other departments in the hospital performing similar processes on a reg-ular basis? Through networking and discussions with colleagues in other departments, the nurse manager outsourced the following processes: patient registration, insurance verification and treatment authorization, and transcription.

What measures of success are there for these empowerment and outsourcing activities? Measures include reports of greater employee satisfaction, greater customer (physician) satisfaction with transcription, and reduction in overtime hours. Table 19–1 illustrates the cost savings benefit of time management.

Parting Thoughts

Based on one department of radiation oncology's experience, the concepts of reengineering, cross-functional work teams, restructuring, rightsizing, empowerment, coaching, continuous process improvement, and zapping are more than just buzzwords. The few examples in this chapter have demonstrated that organizational change can be realized and the challenges of customer satisfaction and cost efficiency met by putting on different "thinking hats"—that is through creativity, staff participation, and patience.

References

Allen RE. (1994). *Winnie-the-Pooh on management.* New York: Penguin Books.

Blanchard K, Carlos J, Randolph A. (1996). *Empowerment takes more than a minute.* San Francisco: Berret-Koehler.

Byham W, Cox J. (1994). *Hero Z.* New York: Harmony Books.

Rural Care Issues in Radiation Oncology

JAYNE S. WARING

Oncology nursing focuses on the intertwined care of individuals, families, and groups within the community. The community may vary in size from a small rural settlement to a sprawling metropolis. Whereas the diversity of resources and opportunities attract people to urban areas, different resources and opportunities appeal to rural dwellers. The purpose of this chapter is to familiarize the reader with rural radiation oncology nursing issues, identify challenges that face patients and their families living in small-town USA, and describe the professional benefits of providing care in a rural setting. This chapter will address the challenges and distinct privileges of practicing as the single radiation oncology nurse in a private practice with a service population of 75,000.

Attitudes of Rural Consumers Toward Cancer

The rural community's attitude toward exercising health care options tend, for the most part, to be directed toward seeking care at large institutions or urban facilities for presumably the best health care. In addition, the rural hospital emergency room often experiences overcrowding due to its prevalent and inappropriate use as a primary-care facility. Consequently, long delays in care often result in a community's disgruntled view of that hospital. To further complicate matters, many rural dwellers continue to dread and fear cancer and radiation therapy. Despite the tremendous advances in the safety and delivery of radiation therapy over the years, there is still great fear and mystery attached to radiation as a viable treatment modality for cancer.

One of the many challenges for oncology care in rural settings is limited access to specialized health care (Curtiss, 1993). For example, there may be only a general surgeon available in the community when the need calls for a thoracic surgeon. Patients are referred to a tertiary-care facility for specialized care. However, diligent tracking and follow-up are necessary so that the patient can be returned to the community and home to receive further treatment and care. It is most appropriate for the oncologist, rather than a primary-care physician, to initiate a surgical referral so that the tertiary-care facility can refer the patient back home for cancer care. The oncology nurse must be cognizant of the differences between urban and rural care practice to advocate for patients and ease the communication process. Rural-care nurses are increasingly challenged not only to treat the cancer but also to assist rural health care consumers to understand that they do not have to seek cancer care far away from home and family.

Building the Foundation of Radiation Oncology in a Rural Setting

Setting up and starting a radiation therapy center in a rural setting can be a formidable task. Much research, planning, and marketing must go into making the center accessible and user friendly to patients and their families, and to the health care community in general. In addition, radiation therapy and other cancer treatments are often misunderstood and misrepresented by medical professionals themselves. Thus, education and re-assurance to both the medical and lay community about the disease and treatment options are vitally needed. Patient referrals from primary-practice physicians and surgeons require education, rein-forcement, and building of trust over time.

The traditional role of the registered nurse (RN) in a conventional medical office setting is to assist the physician/employer. However, this role is rapidly changing in a freestanding radiation therapy facility in a rural setting. In practice, there is generally one nurse and one radiation oncolo-gist. In order for a well-orchestrated practice to function, there must exist a collaborative relation-ship that is complementary and trusting. In a rural radiation oncology setting, the collegial relation-ship of the oncologist and radiation oncology nurse are both collaborative and independent (Hilderley, 1991).

Before the radiation oncology department be-gins accepting patients for care, it must make con-tinuous and routine appearances and contact with the acute care facility, multiple doctors' offices, and referral agencies. These same frequent con-tacts should continue for the purpose of reinforc-ing the role of cancer treatment and management of side effects. The primary-care physicians are an integral part of the management team, particularly in this era of managed care. Thus, visibility is a key ingredient to becoming familiar and staying con-nected with these physicians. Frequent visits to the local hospital to offer formal inservice pro-grams or informal exchange of cancer concerns, treatment modalities, or radiation safety concerns are also part of marketing the specialty, and prob-ably the most important when it comes to pro-moting good oncology patient care. Frequent con-tact also assures that one is viewed as a viable and valuable resource in oncology.

Individuals living at the periphery of the rural community present another challenge. Whereas the local folks may know about the oncology treat-ment facility, people living in the outlying perime-ter may not have any knowledge that a cancer treatment facility even exists. Thus, it takes a lot of creative marketing, persistence, and diligence to educate these rural dwellers about the services of the radiation oncology treatment facility.

Brachytherapy in a Rural Setting

Another challenge of working in a rural radiation oncology practice is in setting up a brachytherapy program. Close collaboration with hospital ad-ministration and the nuclear medicine department is vital to organizing in-house brachytherapy pro-cedures. The rural radiation oncology nurse must be cognizant of many rules, regulations, and pro-cedures in setting up collaborative services be-tween the acute-care facility and the radiation on-cology center. If the radiation oncology nurse is not an employee of the hospital, the nurse must obtain clinical privileges to coordinate and con-duct the necessary nursing care pertaining to brachytherapy procedures.

Providing information on brachytherapy re-quires diligent staff education, reinforcement, and patience on the part of the radiation oncology nurse. The various radioactive isotopes and im-plant procedures can be a source of confusion and fear among staff who are not familiar with radiation principles and practices (Sedhom & Yanni, 1985). Although the volume of brachytherapy procedures is smaller and less frequent than in an urban set-ting, the rural radiation oncology nurse must be present to teach, reinforce, and reassure the pa-tient, family, and staff each time a brachytherapy procedure is done.

It is also important to develop a relationship with the laboratory, pathology, radiology, materi-als management, billing, and admissions depart-ments at the hospital. In addition, the department of nursing, surgery, and medical records will be frequently called upon as the radiation oncology practice develops.

One of the benefits of practicing in a small community is knowing that one may also care for one's coworkers and their relatives and friends. Word-of-mouth marketing and visibility is of paramount importance for building trust, espe-cially in a small town. For example, in my setting, when I am not actually consulting on a patient in the hospital, I may go there to pick up x rays, ob-tain medical records, or simply to eat lunch. In walking to each destination, I will generally see an individual from any number of hospital depart-ments and will start conversations with them. At times, this exchange feels like "politicking," which in a way is true, as one is campaigning for excellence in oncology care.

Transportation Issues

In setting up a rural-based radiation oncology cen-ter, one must also consider developing a plan for transporting inpatients to and from the acute-care and extended-care facilities in the community.

For example, in my setting we coordinated an effort with the only local hospital to develop a contract plan with a transport company for the purpose of providing nonemergency stretcher and wheelchair transportation to and from the hospital for patients' daily radiation treatments. The transport company was made aware of the need for schedule adherence, intermittent machine maintenance, and occasional need for urgent transport.

Community Education and Support

There is a universal and ongoing need to provide education in the earlier detection and screening of cancer. The classic manner in which to attract attention to this issue is to offer free or low-cost screening in the communities of need. Once a cancer diagnosis is made, however, comes the challenge of providing appropriate treatment, especially for patients with limited financial resources. Forums, health fairs, and support groups are excellent strategies to educate, distribute key messages, and network with key members of the lay community. The oncology nurse serves as one of few resources the community has access to for cancer support groups and for screening and early detection programs. This results in the rural oncology nurse being the front-line educator and trainer to carry out these assignments.

It is often within the support group setting that tales of suffering and exaggerated misconceptions of cancer treatment are fostered, and it is within those same group settings that education and damage control can take place. Individualized education about the disease and treatment are available for each patient and friends or family members who accompany their loved ones for radiation treatment. However, fear of cancer treatment may prevent others from ever seeking health care. Thus, public gatherings may be our only link to some individuals. Unfortunately, we will never reach all people with cancer. Consequently, it is of utmost importance that we use the successfully treated and cured patients to deliver the accurate and true message through support groups and other forums.

It is also important for rural oncology nurses to know and respect their own limitations. Times do occur when they cannot be available for every community function or event. The main point is to learn to build trust and then to delegate to other appropriate resources so that the community's needs are met without compromising oneself.

Patient/Family Care Issues in the Rural Radiation Oncology Setting

The oncology nurse is responsible for the patient and family education related to cancer (ONS, 1995a). To carry out this standard, the oncology nurse must have knowledge about the patient, the treatment modalities, and the ever-changing resources in the local community. Patients come to the cancer experience with different agendas, educational background, life events, and emotional configurations. Building trust and offering individualized cancer instruction to everyone who seeks care can certainly be obtained, but it takes great commitment, teamwork, skill, and patience.

Financial Concerns

Many patients may arrive at their initial radiation treatment appointment with great anguish about their financial status, especially after they have had surgery and the necessary workup. It is necessary to initiate or continue to pursue ways to provide financial assistance or to set up and reassure a manageable financial payment plan before patients can even clear their mind to accept information and instruction about their disease and treatment options. At times, this financial concern involves primarily transportation issues (e.g., gas mileage, unreliable vehicle). Pointing out the patient's own resource systems (family, neighbors, church) is occasionally all that is needed. Linking them with the appropriate transportation source in a community that does not have a public transportation system is challenging but resolvable.

Managed health care is an issue in both large and small clinic settings. Preferred provider organizations (PPO), health maintenance organizations (HMO), and other health care coverage may be the primary or secondary payment source for the new oncology patient. For proper payment, and sometimes any payment at all, the rural radiation oncology nurse must be aware of their payor sources because they do not have the luxury of an on-site billing department within the rural radiation oncology center. Often, this means directly assisting the patient to seek and apply for aid so that the department can eventually be reimbursed for care.

Simulation

A unique issue in some rural radiation oncology centers is that the simulator for treatment planning is located off site. This fact can actually be a mixed blessing. As mentioned earlier, rural consumers may feel that urban areas hold the key to better health care. Informing patients that they have to make a fifty-mile journey to obtain their cancer treatment planning is a validation for some and a nemesis for others. Being able to instruct the new oncology patient as well as emphasize the need for this "mysterious process" so soon into the relationship, in addition to sending the patient out of town for simulation, takes the skill and collaboration of a good physician-nurse team.

Managing Side Effects of Treatment

A detailed informed consent procedure is an opportunity to instruct the patient about aspects of the particular disease process, the radiation treatment plan, and the rationale for many of the routine procedures that will take place during the treatment course. A patient booklet addressing treatment and management of side effects along with individualized therapy instructions helps patients to understand the individualized care plan (Strohl, 1988). Multiple questions are always addressed by the radiation oncologist and oncology nurse during consultation. Queries should always be encouraged and the department's phone number should be freely given to each patient and family member. When patients become part of the team, each team member, including the radiation oncologist and oncology nurse, must keep each other abreast of needs and changes. Weekly team meetings of the patient, nurse, and radiation oncologist help to assure continuity of care. The weekly visit provides an opportunity to discuss the patient's status, treatment tolerance, and side effect management. It also provides an opportunity to discuss emotional and personal issues. In my setting, if patients do not have any specific issues to discuss, we may initiate discussions about their grandchildren, the weather, or other day-to-day activities. Similar to every other aspect of life, these weekly (or more often when necessary) evaluations are unique to the individuals involved, regardless of treatment evaluation.

One of the routine procedures during the patient's treatment regime is laboratory testing to monitor the complete blood count (CBC). Until recently, it was thought necessary to monitor the CBC weekly. Current research, however, reveals that routine weekly monitoring of the CBC may not be necessary or cost effective in selected cases (Yang et al., 1995). Coordinating the relevant monitoring schedule, as well as using the patient's appropriate laboratory site, also falls into the category of nursing responsibilities in a rural treat

ment setting that does not house a laboratory of its own. In my setting, we have developed a tool to monitor frequency and compliance of lab work data that is readily available to multiple care providers.

One of the most important roles of the radiation therapy nurse is to be cognizant of each patient's anticipated side effects through the treatment plan and by attendance in chart rounds. Constant surveillance and verbalization to the patient and caregivers of their need to anticipate and prepare for these side effects is crucial to a successful treatment experience. When the treatment effects occur, counseling and coaching the patient and caregiver will assist them to cope effectively. Personalized, one-to-one care is the standard in the rural setting, thus allowing the patient to feel like an individual.

There are definite advantages to the patient and family in being treated in a small, rural treatment facility. Advantages include easy access and less confusion in locating a single building as opposed to a single department in a large hospital (Groenwald et al., 1992). Another intangible advantage is the fact that close relationships can develop with a small, unchanging staff. The patient and family are more aware of whom to call for information when there is a singular radiation therapy nurse. Even if the patients cannot remember the nurse's name, they will still be connected to the proper resource by asking for the nurse.

Concomitant and adjuvant chemotherapy are given in conjunction with radiation. Thus, coordination of care is vital. For example, in my practice, the rural radiation treatment center shares office space with a separate medical oncology practice. A very close collegial relationship developed between the nurses of these practices. Timing of laboratory appointments, nadir expectation, and coordination of treatments and office visits are among the data shared between the nurses. Because there are only two oncology nurses, we share a tremendous mutual respect that is a unique blessing of small-town oncology nursing.

Challenges Facing a Freestanding Rural Care Setting

In the rural clinic setting, the nurse may be designated to perform nonnursing functions. Among these are the interviewing of and monitoring of other personnel, which could include individuals applying for the front office to the cleaning service, as well as monitoring biohazardous waste and changing lightbulbs. In the larger health care setting, there are ancillary departments to initiate and monitor these services. In the small rural setting, responsibility for these functions must be addressed, and it is often most appropriate that the nurse be the arbitrator.

A rural radiation oncology center is limited in size and in the number of employees. The radiation therapists, who observe the patients on a daily basis, are alert to the need for nursing interventions. A treatment setting is extremely fortunate when blessed with the combination of appropriate personalities, high levels of technical skills, and befitting professionalism among all team members.

There are times in the rural setting that a patient may arrive for evaluation without having a tissue diagnosis. This can occur with a referral from a primary-care physician who needs assistance with the proper workup. At times, people may even walk in off the street with a "lump" or a "feeling" they have cancer. The oncology nurse is often the first to consult with the patient and must be knowledgeable of the cancer process as well as sensitive to patient concerns.

By virtue of the fact that it is an outpatient setting, the radiation oncology center has limited operating hours. Chronically and critically ill patients may need to use supplemental care services. An emergency answering service number should be made available to patients to reach the radiation oncologist on call after hours. They need to be educated and encouraged to contact their primary-care physician in other urgent situations.

Home health agencies offer acute and chronic care, and hospices offer chronic supportive care. Each could have a role in the care of the outpatient radiation therapy patient. Developing a knowledge of admission criteria and collegial relationships with the nursing staff of these service agencies is beneficial to both the professionals and the patients. The management of acute and long-term effects of radiation therapy can be taught to these professionals, thus extending and reinforcing care of the patient during and after the treatment course (Yannaco, 1993). Developing close ties with the hospice nursing staff also provides a valuable resource for pain management dilemmas for the nurse as well as a source for referral of patients and families.

Resources for the Rural Radiation Oncology Nurse

The sole nurse in a rural radiation oncology center must stay abreast of current care measures and issues. The rural oncology nurse is faced with limited opportunities for specialty education, few local colleagues, and unique care issues (Curtiss, 1993). The Oncology Nursing Society (ONS) is an invaluable source of information, resources, and direction for any aspect of oncology nursing or patient care. Membership in this organization brings current journal articles and issues to one's doorstep each month as well as a myriad of opportunities to further educate oneself in oncology nursing. Membership with a local chapter will also connect nurses with the finest oncology nurses in one's area. For example, my rural radiation oncology center is located fifty miles away from the local ONS chapter. I decided early on to travel those fifty miles so that I could enjoy collaboration with other oncology nurses on a regular basis. Shortly thereafter, other medical oncology nurses joined the monthly journey, so that the two-hour commute for chapter meetings is often felt to be too short. Much supportive interaction about patient care and professional issues takes place during those excursions.

The American Cancer Society (ACS) is also a tremendous asset for nurses and patients. Many patient resources are available through ACS, which will assist in educating patients and enhancing the quality of life for them and their families. The National Cancer Institute is another resource for both nurse and patient. The myriad of educational materials is appropriate to teach and reinforce information.

Another educational resource for nurse and the medical staff in my community was the development of a tumor board. The tumor board structure was modeled after similar boards in tertiary setting and uses the multidisciplinary oncology team to present and discuss specific cancer cases. The oncology nurse's role in this monthly tumor board is supportive and collaborative. In my experience, both hospital and community nurses also attend the tumor board meetings, which provides them with an opportunity to hear discussions about cancer diagnosis, treatment plan, prognosis, and specific patient issues.

Additional Affirmation

A validating, encouraging oncologist/colleague is ever important in the effectiveness, growth, and survival of the radiation oncology nurse in the rural setting. An oncologist who regards nursing as an enhancement to the patient care team, who is sensitive to the input of nursing even when it may differ from his or her viewpoint, and who encourages professional growth is a great catalyst for the survival and longevity of the oncology nurse, who might feel totally isolated otherwise.

Much impetus for the effectiveness of the nursing role lies in outside sources, as mentioned above. However, it is the sole responsibility of each nurse to seek the resources and to adapt them to each specific circumstance. Keeping an open mind to every challenge, using all available resources, and staying committed to optimum patient outcomes will allow the radiation oncology nurse, whether in the rural or urban setting, to thrive with honor.

References

Curtiss CP. (1993). Trends and issues for cancer care in rural communities. *Nursing Clinics of North America, 28*(1), 241–251.

Groenwald SL, Frogge MH, Goodman M. (eds.). (1992). Delivery systems for cancer care. In *Cancer Nursing: Principles and Practice* (2nd ed.), 1075–1147. Boston: Jones and Bartlett.

Hilderley, LJ. (1991). Nurse-physician collaborative practice: The clinical nurse specialist in a radiation oncology private practice. *Oncology Nursing Forum, 18*(3), 585–591.

Oncology Nursing Society. (1995a). *Standards of oncology education: Patient/family and public.* Pittsburgh: Author.

Oncology Nursing Society. (1995b). *Standards of oncology nursing education: Generalist and advanced practice levels.* Pittsburgh: Author.

Sedhom LN, Yanni MI. (1985). Radiation therapy and nurses' fears of radiation exposure. *Cancer Nursing, 8*(2), 129–134.

Strohl RA. (1988). The nursing role in radiation oncology: Symptom management of acute and chronic reactions. *Oncology Nursing Forum, 15*(4), 429–434.

Yang FE, Vaida F, Igancio L, et al. (1995). Analysis of weekly complete blood counts in patients receiving standard fractionated partial body radiation. *International Journal of Radiation Oncology, Biology, Physics, 33*(3), 607–617.

Yannaco TM. (1993). Radiation therapy: Implications for home care. *Caring, 12*(2), 38–62.

The Advanced Practice Nurse in Radiation Oncology

BARBARA E. BODANSKY

The twenty-first century is rapidly approaching. In the last decade of the twentieth century, dramatic changes in health care have begun to occur. The 1990s began with the Health Security Act proposal, and evolved into managed care, critical pathways, and "nurse extenders." This revolution is not yet concluded, and no one can know exactly what form the health care environment of the year 2000 and beyond will assume. However, through an understanding of current societal, economic, and political issues, we are better able to predict the future.

This is an especially critical time for the advanced practice nurse (APN). Will the role survive health care reform? What form will the future role take? What will we call ourselves—APN, clinical nurse specialist (CNS), nurse practitioner (NP), or some combination of the three?

An attempt to answer these questions and predict our future in health care reform can be made only after careful consideration of a variety of issues. It is important for the APN to understand how the role evolved, what circumstances gave rise to the role, the components of the role, and how legislation has affected the advanced practice nurse's ability to practice. It is through an understanding of where we have been that we can begin to predict where we are going.

This chapter will describe the history of advanced practice nursing, history of health care reform, future predictions for the APN in oncology—specifically in radiation therapy (RT), and finally issues relevant to the survival of advanced practice nurses. Although this is an uncertain time in health care, it is a time of opportunity. Advanced practice nurses must be prepared to seize the opportunities incurred by change.

The Clinical Nurse Specialist: Evolution of the Role

In the early 1900s educational preparation of the nurse was primarily by diploma and was received through hospital training. The expression "specialist" described the nurse who had developed expertise in a particular area such as private duty nursing (Hamric & Spross, 1989). The term *nurse clinician* was first used by Francis Reiter in the 1940s. Reiter described the nurse clinician as an individual who collaborated with the physician to deliver care, had achieved clinical competence, and had developed expertise in a variety of areas in the delivery of health care (Sparacino et al., 1990).

Peplau developed the first graduate program for the CNS at Rutgers University in 1954. This program for APNs educated CNSs in the subspecialty of psychiatry. The nurse had begun to move away from the purely functional role of past generations toward the role of clinical expert (Sparacino et al., 1990).

A number of events in the 1960s created an environment that popularized the role of the CNS. First, graduate nursing education programs began to expand. Programs for the CNS were developed in oncology and other subspecialty areas. Second, because of the nursing shortage of the 1960s, the federal government expanded its Professional Nurse Traineeship Program to include educational preparation for the CNS (Weiss, 1995). Finally, the CNS role was operationalized at two university hospitals in Washington and Michigan. These programs offered CNSs a unique format in which to perform their role with flexible work hours, less restricted practice areas, and the opportunity to act as change agents within the hospital system (Galassi & Wheeler, 1994). Although these changes have become commonplace in today's hospital environment, they were revolutionary at the time and were critical to the development of the CNS role. These changes allowed the nurse with the skills of the expert practitioner to remain at the bedside, unlike their predecessors, who advanced into hospital administration or teaching positions.

In the 1970s, a definition of the master's degree program for the oncology CNS was developed by the American Cancer Society (ACS). The American Nurse's Association (ANA) defined specialization in nursing in the 1980s (Hamric & Spross, 1989). Whereas the CNS role was traditionally performed in the inpatient hospital setting with a specific population of patients, the CNS is no longer tied to the inpatient practice setting. Currently the CNS role is fulfilled in outpatient settings, freestanding clinics, and home care agencies.

Role Components of the Clinical Nurse Specialist

The CNS role was characterized by four major subroles: expert clinician, consultant, educator, and researcher.

Expert Clinician

The subrole of expert clinician is the most central of the subroles and the one from which other aspects of the CNS role evolve. The expert clinician combines theory with practical experience. Through this knowledge the CNS is able to establish credibility with other members of the health care team, patients and families, administrators, and the community. The role of expert clinician is so vital to the role of the CNS that it must always remain a substantial percentage of the clinical nurse specialist's activities. By maintaining clinical expertise, the CNS enhances other subroles of the position (Sparacino et al., 1990). Clinical expertise enables the CNS to fulfill other aspects of the role such as standard development, research utilization and development, competencies, education, and certification (Hamric & Spross, 1989).

Consultant

In the role of consultant, the CNS provides information to other members of the health care team, administrators, and patients to assist them in resolving problems and making decisions. Sparacino et al. (1990) describe three types of consulta-

tive activities that the CNS engages in while performing the role. The expert consultant is viewed as possessing enough skills, experience, and education to be able to provide the consultee with alternative solutions or approaches to different clinical problems. The resource consultant provides a variety of alternatives from which the consultee may select to solve a particular problem. The process consultant brings change to a situation and, in so doing, allows the consultee to make decisions. Through education and practical experience, the CNS provides information to others to make changes and achieve goals.

Educator

The subrole of educator is critical to the role of the CNS. The clinical nurse specialist educates patients and family members with regard to health promotion, self-care activities, treatment modalities, medications, and a myriad of other subjects that arise from the CNS role as expert practitioner. With other nurses the CNS acts as preceptor for new employees or graduate students and provides inservices on new treatment modalities. In the community the CNS provides continuing education programs and support groups and represents nursing to the public (Hamric & Spross, 1989). In the academic environment the CNS holds appointments as clinical or associate faculty and provides classroom education to university students. Education, whether formal or informal, is a constant component of the clinical nurse specialist role.

Researcher

The role of researcher is often cited by the CNS as the most difficult subrole to fulfill due to lack of time, lack of administrative support, and minimal research education at the master's level. As part of the research component of the role, the CNS transmits information regarding research that affects current methods of practice. The CNS may conduct research, participate in research, or disseminate research findings (Sparacino et al., 1990). When conducting research, the CNS may be involved in nursing research or may collaborate with physicians or other members of the health care team. It is the responsibility of the CNS to be informed about current research that relates to their practice area and to share this information with other members of the health care team.

A review of the components of the CNS emphasizes its complexity and the integral relationship between the different aspects of the role.

The Nurse Practitioner: Evolution of the Role

The role of the nurse practitioner (NP) and the impetus that gave birth to this role developed in the 1960s, when changes in both American society and health care occurred simultaneously. The decade gave rise to soaring health care costs and diminishing numbers of primary-care physicians. The lack of sufficient health care in rural areas coincided with a trend among physicians to specialize (Weiss, 1995). At the same time the United States government instituted Medicaid and Medicare. The institution of these programs guaranteed subsidized health care to a significant number of American citizens (Safriet, 1992). As soldiers returned from the Vietnam War, physician assistant programs began to develop. It had become clear during the war that nonphysicians could provide medical care similar to the care that medics provided during the war (Inglis & Kjervik, 1993).

Two important additional developments occurred during the mid 1960s that established the NP role. The University of Colorado established the first NP program in pediatrics. At the University of Kansas Medical Center, nurses were put in charge of a clinic that provided health care to chronically ill women. An evaluation of the NPs' practice found that they provided more effective care for this population. Improved care resulted from better health education, superior health promotion and screening, and patient education that had not been previously provided (Weiss, 1995). Inglis and Kjervik (1993) indicate that without decreasing physician strength, increased demands for health care among rural and poor populations, and government's and businesses' desire to decrease health care costs, the role of the NP would not have survived.

Role Components of the Nurse Practitioner

The role of the NP has historically combined activities associated with the professions of both nursing and medicine. Traditionally, NPs provided counseling about prevention and early detection of illness, conducted physical exams, assessed and diagnosed patients, ordered laboratory and other diagnostic tests, and developed and implemented plans of care for individuals. Now NPs prescribe medications, monitor patients, educate and counsel, and consult and collaborate with physicians and other health care providers (Safriet, 1992).

At first glance it appears that NPs follow an orthodox medical model, but this is not the usual case. NPs have consistently operated under a nursing model of care where they provide counseling and preventive health care information.

The role of the NP was traditionally practiced in rural, often poor areas of the country where there was a dearth of primary-care physicians. Currently the NP practices in inpatient units, clinics, extended care facilities, ambulatory care, private offices, and in nursing centers of excellence.

Nurse Practice Act/ Legislative Issues

To understand the historical development of the APN and to predict where advanced practice nursing is heading in the year 2000 and beyond, it is important to gain an understanding of the Nurse Practice Act. Issues related to prescriptive privileges and reimbursement are governed by the Nurse Practice Act and are significant to the advanced practice role.

In the early 1900s nurses first received certification, which allowed anyone to practice nursing. However, the title of registered nurse was restricted to qualified practitioners (Safriet, 1992). Licensure for professionals arose out of the states' responsibility to protect the public and to guarantee that the licensee was able and qualified to practice (Inglis & Kjervik, 1993).

Physicians were the first health care professionals to become licensed in the early 1800s. The development of the physicians' scope of practice was to have a major impact on the scope of practice of nurses. Physicians defined their scope of practice to include curing, diagnosing, treating, and prescribing. This scope of practice made it illegal for any other health care profession to carry out these tasks. In the 1930s, when nursing was developing its scope of practice, it was restricted to defining itself outside of the domain of the physicians. Thus, nursing defined its scope of practice as encompassing the supervision of patients, the observation of symptoms and reactions, and the recording of facts. All other areas of the nurse's scope of practice fell under the supervision and direction of the physician (Inglis & Kjervik, 1993; Safriet, 1992).

In the 1950s the American Nurses Association redefined some nursing activities to exclude physician supervision. However, nurses continued to be restricted from prescribing, diagnosing, implementing, and administering medications or treatments unless prescribed by a physician (Safriet, 1992; Inglis & Kjervik, 1993).

Hospitals discovered that with the evolution of the profession of nursing, the definitions governing nurses' practices were too restrictive. Statements were developed that expanded the scope of practice of nurses to include initiating of cardiopulmonary resuscitation (CPR), starting intravenous lines, and performing defibrillation. In 1971, Idaho was the first state to recognize diagnosis and treatment statutorily as part of the APN scope of practice, although the nursing and medical boards continued to oversee nursing diagnosis and treatment (Inglis & Kjervik, 1993; Safriet, 1992).

In the 1970s the legislative bodies of the states expanded the functions of the registered nurse to allow for inclusion of the APN. These changes stipulated that the states' nursing boards would determine regulations that would govern the APN, expanded some behaviors that could be practiced by APNs, allowed physicians to delegate to nurses, and broadened the scope of practice legislatively (Weiss, 1995).

In the 1990s there are four major legislative categories under which advanced practice nurses may practice. All but five states provide APNs with title protection. Twenty states have designated the Board of Nursing as the sole authority in scope of practice. Seventeen states require that the scope of practice have a requirement for supervision or collaboration with a physician. In five states the APN's scope of practice is governed by both the Board of Nursing and the Board of Medicine. Thirty-four states recognize the CNS within the APN category, although in some states this is limited to the psychiatric/mental health CNS (Pearson, 1995).

The second major area of legislative importance for the advanced practice nurse is prescriptive privileges. A number of issues are involved in the states' decisions to grant these privileges and impose restrictions on the APN. Regulators determine who will be authorized to prescribe, what devices and drugs may be prescribed, how far the authority extends, whether the prescriptive authority will be limited to certain geographical regions, who will regulate the authority, what qualifications the APN must meet to gain prescriptive rights, and whether the authorization requires a separate form of certification (Safriet, 1992). As of 1995 there are five categories of prescriptive authority. In ten states APNs may prescribe all sub-

stances, including controlled substances, without the involvement of a physician in the prescription-writing process. Twenty-two states permit the APN to prescribe all drugs, including controlled substances, with some degree of physician involvement or delegation in prescription writing. Fifteen states permit the APN to prescribe with physician involvement or delegation, but exclude controlled substances. In twelve states advanced practice nurses have dispensing privileges. Three states have no statutory prescribing authority for the APN. As of this writing ten states are planning to introduce legislation for independent APN prescriptive authority or expanded prescriptive authority (Pearson, 1995).

It is important to understand current issues related to third-party reimbursement for the NP in order to better predict future trends for the role of the APN in practice. Questions that must be addressed include what services the NP will be reimbursed for, at what level the services will be reimbursed, and whether the reimbursement will be made directly to the provider or the NP must bill through the physician. Third-party reimbursement from private insurance is primarily dependent on state statutes (Safriet, 1992).

Medicaid reimbursement was originally limited to reimbursement for pediatric and family NPs. In 1995 reimbursement by Medicaid varies from state to state. This variation is directed toward the rate of reimbursement and what APN titles are reimbursed (Safriet, 1992).

Medicare reimbursement requires the NP to work in collaboration with the physician and within the NP's scope of practice. The provided services must fall into one of four categories: incidental to physician services, under contract to a health maintenance organization (HMO), in a skilled nursing facility, or in a rural area. Further restrictions are placed on amount of reimbursement relative to physician reimbursement, and direct reimbursement is provided only to NPs in rural areas (Haber, 1995; Safriet, 1992).

In 1995 all states with the exception of Ohio reimburse APNs directly for Medicaid services. Thirty-seven states specify that NPs are reimbursed at 80–100 percent of the amount paid to a physician billing for the same service. Thirty-five states either allow third-party reimbursement within the statute or have an "any willing provider statute," by which reimbursement may be limited to narrowly defined situations (Pearson, 1995).

Numerous studies were conducted during the 1980s to evaluate the care provided by the APN in comparison to the primary-care physician (Safriet,

1992). These studies concluded that the quality of care provided by the APN was equivalent to or better than that of the physician. Quality of care was measured by evaluating physical assessment, prescription of medications, short- and long-term patient compliance, resolution of acute problems, improvement in functional and psychosocial status, and reduction of pain. In analysis of patient satisfaction with the care provided, patients were as satisfied or more satisfied with the care provided by the APN than with physicians. Another study evaluated the use of diagnostic testing and found that the APN was less likely to use costly diagnostic procedures, thus reducing the cost of care. Finally, a limited number of studies examined issues related to malpractice and found that the incidence and successful conclusion of malpractice cases occurred less often with the advanced practice nurse (Inglis & Kjervik, 1993; Pearson, 1995; Safriet, 1992).

In the mid 1990s, the dramatic growth of hospital systems and the increasing number of acute care beds was halted. Hospitals began to close inpatient beds and lay off health care workers, including nurses. Provision of care has moved from the traditional inpatient setting into ambulatory and home care (Edwards & Horn, 1995). Hospitals of the future are predicted to provide care only in the form of intensive and emergency care. In oncology, many chemotherapeutic regimens that were previously administered inpatient are now administered in the outpatient setting, and this trend is rapidly growing (Xistris & Houlihan, 1994). In radiation oncology, procedures such as high-dose brachytherapy and stereotactic radiosurgery are administered almost entirely in an ambulatory setting. Early discharge and the movement of care delivery into the ambulatory setting has become the norm.

In the mid 1990s, retrospective payment systems became capped, prospective reimbursement arrangements (Edwards & Horn, 1995). The traditional fee-for-service method of payment proved too costly. This form of reimbursement rewarded the most costly behaviors through financial compensation but provided no reward for the delivery of economical care (Enthoven, 1994). In the new health care environment, insurance companies will shift from the philosophy of limiting access and reducing risk to focusing on diagnosis or community-based health care outcomes (Paris & Hines, 1995).

Health care appears to be more controlled by marketplace regulation, trending toward managed care and capitation of health care costs. In response to these trends, major cancer centers are formulating oncology critical pathways. With these pathways, the centers will develop networks of smaller, community hospitals that will employ these pathways to treat cancer patients (Harvey, 1994; Baird, 1995; Donley, 1995).

Questions that we are currently faced with are to determine where health care reform is going and how this will effect the delivery of cancer care—specifically the provision of radiation therapy. APNs must have a clear understanding of these trends and attempt to position themselves to meet the health care demands of the future.

Current Advanced Practice Roles in Radiation Oncology

In radiation oncology, whether part of a hospital or freestanding clinic, all radiation oncology nurses are involved in patient care and patient education. In addition, the APN's practice may include any or all of the following: administration, research, education, and consultation.

The oncology clinical nurse specialists (OCNSs) act as consultants to the staff, other health care team members, and the community. They provide inservices and precept new staff members and graduate students. OCNSs also develop and implement standards of care, policies, and procedures for individuals receiving radiation therapy. Continuous quality improvement (CQI) programs and nursing research activities are also responsibilities of the OCNS (Iwamoto & Gough, 1993).

Hilderley (1991) describes the role components for the OCNS in a freestanding radiation oncology practice as including evaluation and teaching of inpatients prior to formal consultation, telephone management, health history and assessment, side effect management, nutritional counseling, and adjustment of pain medications. Professional nursing activities include attendance at conferences, involvement in committee work, and financial support for continuing education activities.

The manager/clinical nurse specialist is another advanced role currently practiced in radiation oncology. This position combines the expert practitioner skills of the OCNS with those of nurse manager. The successful fulfillment of all the role requirements of this position can be difficult to meet. The OCNS/manager often carries a specific caseload of patients in addition to having responsibilities in staffing, discipline, CQI, policies, procedures, research, and other management obligations. This dual position has been successfully operationalized in radiation oncology; however, the risk in this position is an overabundance of diverse responsibilities and a lack of time to meet all the challenges of the role (Dudjak, 1992).

The nurse practitioner in radiation oncology performs physical and psychosocial assessments of patients and manages treatment of side effects. The NP provides comprehensive management, including nutrition and pain management, prescribes medications, and follows patients post-treatment (Iwamoto & Gough, 1993).

The future of the APN in radiation oncology is at a critical junction in preparing for the future. It behooves APNs to inform themselves about trends in health care as well as trends and proposed changes for the role of the APN. The following section will identify future trends in health care and what role the APN in radiation oncology can play in these changes.

Trends in Oncology Ambulatory Nursing

Decreasing hospital occupancy rates and the expansion of services into the ambulatory and home care settings have created a renewed focus on the provision of preventive and primary care services (Donley, 1995). Health promotion, health education, and self-help activities will hold primary positions in the provision of future health care. The primary goal of outpatient care is to provide the patient with the necessary tools to perform self-care. Education provided to the patient to meet this goal includes information about treatment options, specific treatments and diagnostic testing, symptom management, nutrition, pharmacology, available social services, technical skills, and how to access assistance when the patient is at home or during nonclinic hours (Lamkin, 1994). These activities encompass not only the prevention of illness but also the management of symptoms of disease and side effects related to treatment. The APN is perfectly suited to meeting the patient needs of the future (Miaskowski, 1993).

Critical Paths/ Case Management

Case management was first initiated at the New England Medical Center in 1985. The goal of this program was to identify a case manager, usually a registered nurse, who would monitor a group of patients throughout the illness continuum to ensure timely passage through the system. The goal of the case manager was to maintain outcomes within the prescribed framework (Hampton, 1993).

In 1995 critical pathway development in oncology is an aspect of managed care that is receiving increased attention. The concept of critical pathways includes the development of practice parameters (Stair, 1995). The pathway defines the care of the individual from entry into the health care system through diagnostic evaluation, treatment modalities, inpatient and outpatient care, and follow-up monitoring or supportive care.

The critical pathway framework identifies the processes required, necessary resources, expected costs, and desired outcomes within a designated time line. The decisions required to develop the critical pathway are made by a multidisciplinary group composed of physicians and nurses from multiple specialty areas, administration, and other health care team members. The multidisciplinary group reaches a consensus, based on practice and research, on what the daily or episodic experiences of the patient with a particular diagnosis must include. This information is then transferred into critical paths, flowcharts, and written descriptions. These interventions and activities are documented in conjunction with the development of a timeline. The purpose of these activities is to enable the group to define its care for a particular diagnostic group, determine a timeline for its management, determine the cost and resources needed to provide care, and outline the expected outcomes (Hampton, 1993).

Involvement in the development of critical pathways is an important activity for the APN in radiation oncology. The APN brings the necessary theoretical and practical expertise necessary to elucidate, to the multidisciplinary group, the nursing care required to efficiently move a patient through the radiation portion of the pathway.

In the Department of Radiation Oncology at Memorial Sloan-Kettering Cancer Center, the APNs are involved in the development of critical pathways. Their activities involve identifying the nursing care (education, symptom management, psychosocial activities) required for a patient with a particular diagnosis receiving radiation therapy. Decisions are based on the nursing standards of care developed by the nursing staff.

Positioning the APN role for the future requires not only participation in the development of critical pathways but also involvement in the next step of case management. Once critical pathways have been defined and agreed upon by the health care team, they direct the management of patient care. The APN in radiation oncology is in an excellent position to act as case manager for critical pathways. The role of case manager for patients receiving RT is an important position for the advanced practice nurse with the potential for future growth (Hamric, 1992).

Nurse-Managed Clinics/ Collaborative Practice

It is predicted that the APN will be managing nurse-run clinics where symptom management, health assessment, teaching, evaluation, maintenance, screening, and prevention will take place in medical, surgical, and radiation oncology practices (Lamkin, 1994). In a nurse-managed clinic, the APN is authorized by the physician(s) to perform some of the medical aspects of care. The APN orders lab work, assesses patients' response to treatment, administers treatments, monitors patients, and coordinates care. The APN's activities are usually guided by protocols of care that have been collaboratively developed with the physician(s) (Lamkin, 1993). These activities are currently performed by APNs in radiation oncology departments (J. Kelvin, personal communication, June 1992). Typically, patients receiving RT are assessed weekly during their treatment by the physician and the nurse. A likely future role for the APN will be that of collaborative practice with the radiation oncologist.

A recent trend in health care has been the movement of the NP from the primary-care setting into the acute-care setting. A number of forces have led to the creation of this phenomenon. Medical education has downsized with fewer residency programs, and therefore fewer residents to care for acutely ill inpatients. Limitations have been placed on the number of hours housestaff members may work. This has led to a gap in the provision of care and the movement of the nurse practitioner into tertiary care (El-Sherif, 1995; Galassi & Wheeler, 1994).

Advantages of this trend are the provision of care by an experienced NP as opposed to care by rotating, inexperienced housestaff. Although NPs receive higher salaries, they are able to provide improved quality and consistency of care. Potential disadvantages include on-the-job training that the NP must receive that may not be acceptable to the individual state board of nursing. Economically, nurses are paid more than residents; however, the question is whether they are paid commensurate to their level of responsibility. Finally, one must question whether these nurses are at greater risk for burn-out than their counterparts in primary care (Galassi & Wheeler, 1994).

To fulfill this position, the NP would assume many of the responsibilities that are currently those of the resident. This would include physical assessments, ordering and review of diagnostic tests and laboratory studies, management of patients during treatment and follow-up, medication management, hospital admissions, and inpatient rounds. Additionally, the APN would be responsible for providing some nursing care.

The benefits of this position for the APN would include greater autonomy in the care of patients, less time spent in procuring prescriptions for patients and requesting orders from physicians, and greater continuity of care for both patients and nurses. Potential negative aspects of the role to be considered include role ambiguity, the potential of creating a hierarchy of nurses, on-call schedules, additional education in radiographic interpretation, and difficulty in time management in relation to medical and nursing care. In the future, it is reasonable to contemplate the development of collaborative practice in radiation oncology. This role would be appropriately filled by the APN.

Documentation/Outcomes/ Continuous Quality Improvement

A major deficit in the advanced practice literature is research on outcomes. The changing health care environment demands now more than ever the need for APNs to validate their positions in relation to cost containment and patient outcomes (Powel & Mayer, 1992). APNs of the future can accomplish validation of their roles through pure research examining patient outcomes, or continuing quality improvement projects (Ponte et al., 1993).

Case management and critical pathways are the ideal venue by which the APN can demonstrate the cost effectiveness of the role and improvement in patient outcomes. As APNs in radiation oncology position themselves as case managers, they will be able to evaluate reasons why some patients do not achieve desired outcomes. They will be able to analyze variances, develop interventions, document system problems, and determine methods to improve patient care. In conjunction with these activities, APNs must critically examine their actions to determine what nursing interventions promote adherence to critical paths. When APNs can examine their actions within the context of case management and demonstrate improved outcomes, they will achieve concrete validation of their role. In this era of cost containment, this activity will become a vital research area for the APN.

Boyle (1995) identifies areas of documentation in evaluating and validating the APN role that require attention for the future. Documentation should include written description of APN activities, including interventions, how role responsibilities are executed, and what outcomes are achieved in the areas of practice, education, consultation, and research. These areas are significant because through documentation the APN clarifies the role of the APN and decreases role ambiguity. Thorough documentation validates provided care using the outcome parameters of quality, quantity, and cost. These activities substantiate the role of the APN and ensure its future survival.

Continued quality improvement (CQI) activities is another approach that APNs can use to critically examine their practice or system-related issues. CQI offers a number of advantages over research. The completion process for a CQI project is more rapid than that of a research study, resulting in faster outcome information. By definition, CQI projects are multidisciplinary; this encourages APNs to share their activities with a diverse group of health team members and promotes awareness of APN positions within the department or hospital.

At Memorial Sloan-Kettering Cancer Center, APNs in radiation oncology have conducted a number of CQI studies; these included evaluation of nutritional management of the head and neck patient, analysis of the process of inpatient consultation, and documentation of pain assessment and interventions for the patient receiving radiation therapy. In research, the APNs have been involved in a number of studies as principal or coprincipal investigators. The studies examine the comparison of skin moisturizers in the management of skin reactions, the evaluation of a mouth moisturizer in the relief of subjective symptoms of xerostomia, changes in sexual function related to three-dimensional conformal radiation therapy for prostate cancer, and quality-of-life issues for the lymphoma patient (J. Kelvin, personal communication, 1995). Conducting CQI projects or research studies highlights the role of the APN and results in improved care of the patient receiving radiation therapy.

Consultation and Education

The subroles of consultant and educator have consistently been part of the advanced practice role in radiation oncology. The future role of the APN must continue to emphasize these subroles. In the role of consultant and educator, the opportunity exists to go into the community and expand the public's understanding of the APN role and its contribution to health care. Among the medical and nursing communities there are frequently misconceptions about the delivery of radiation therapy and its associated side effects. Through the consultative and educative activities of the APN, opportunities exist to disseminate information to others about the modality, and its effects. As the focus of care moves into the home care environment, the APNs should avail themselves to provide consultation and education to visiting nurses and primary-care physicians. Improving public awareness is an important future role for the APN.

Issues for the APN of the Future

A review of recent nursing literature reveals an abundance of articles examining trends in advanced practice education and role evolvement. Williams and Valdivieso (1994) describe five models of advanced practice nursing that reflect current trends in these roles. The first model, the additive model, describes the current trend in graduate education that finds educationally prepared CNSs returning to school for postmaster's certification as NPs. The dual pathways model describes the assumption that educational preparation for either the CNS or the NP prepares the individual for the advanced practice role. This model is based on laws in some states that recognize both the CNS and NP as APNs. The third model is one of overlapping roles. This model acknowledges the unique positions of the CNS and NP yet recognizes educational trends that provide shared curriculum in preparation for advanced practice. The subsumed within the other model represents the trend in CNS graduate preparation to incorporate practitioner skills. In the blended role model, there is recognition of the development of graduate programs that will prepare the individual to assume either the CNS or the NP role. The blended role model describes the future of advanced practice nursing through the merging of the two roles in education and practice.

In preparing for the advanced practice roles of the future, and positioning the oncology APN for a place in the health care environment of the year 2000 and beyond, a number of issues must be addressed. The Oncology Nursing Society (ONS) has addressed the problems of titling, documentation and outcomes, education, prescriptive authority, reimbursement issues, second licensure, and certification in their Proceedings in the State-of-the-Knowledge Conference on Advanced Practice in Oncology Nursing (Carroll-Johnson, 1995).

Conclusion

As we prepare ourselves for the role of the APN of the future we must be cognizant of a number of relevant issues. Before we can predict our future path, we must understand how the APN evolved and how historical events influence our professional lives today. With this knowledge we can better predict future positions for the APN and the tools needed to meet the challenges of the future.

References

Baird SB. (1995). The impact of changing health care delivery on oncology practice. *Oncology Nursing: Patient Treatment and Support, 2*(3), 1–13.

Boyle DM. (1995). Documentation and outcomes of advanced nursing practice. *Oncology Nursing Forum, 22*(Suppl. 8), 11–17.

Carroll-Johnson RM (Ed.). (1995). Proceedings of the state-of-the-knowledge conference on advanced practice in oncology nursing. *Oncology Nursing Forum, 22*(8).

Donley R. (1995). Advanced practice nursing after health care reform. *Nursing Economics, 13*(2), 84–88.

Dudjak LA. (1992). Administration. In KH Dow, LJ Hilderley (Eds.). *Nursing care in radiation oncology*, 378–382. Philadelphia: W.B. Saunders.

Edwards DS, Horn PA. (1995). War on many fronts: Troubling trends in health care delivery. *Journal of Nursing Administration, 25*(5), 5–7.

El-Sherif C. (1995). Nurse practitioners: Where do they belong within the organizational structure of the acute care setting? *Nurse Practitioner, 20*(1), 62–65.

Enthoven AC. (1994). Health care reform and the future of managed care. *San Francisco Medicine, June–July*, 21–22.

Galassi A, Wheeler V. (1994). Advanced practice nursing: History and future trends. *Oncology Nursing: Patient Treatment and Support, 1*(5), 1–10.

Haber J. (1995). Legislative priorities for 1995: Medicare and Medicaid reimbursement. *Clinical Nurse Specialist, 9*(3), 143.

Hamric AB. (1992). Creating our future: Challenges and opportunities for the clinical nurse specialist. *Oncology Nursing Forum, 19*(Suppl. 1), 11–15.

Hamric AB, Spross JA. (1989). *The clinical nurse specialist in theory and practice* (2nd ed.). Philadelphia: W.B. Saunders.

Hampton DC. (1993). Implementing a managed care framework through care maps. *Journal of Nursing Administration, 23*(5), 21–27.

Harvey C. (1994). New systems: The restructuring of cancer care delivery and economics. *Oncology Nursing Forum, 21*(1), 72–76.

Hastings KE. (1995). Health care reform: We need it, but do we have the national will to shape our future? *Nurse Practitioner, 20*(1), 52–57.

Hilderley LJ. (1991). Nurse-physician collaborative practice: The clinical nurse specialist in a radiation oncology private practice. *Oncology Nursing Forum, 18*(3), 585–591.

Iglehart JK. (1994). Health policy report: physicians and the growth of managed care. *The New England Journal of Medicine, 331*(17), 1167–1171.

Inglis ADB & Kjervik DK. (1993). Empowerment of advanced practice nurses: Regulation reform needed to increase access to care. *The Journal of Law, Medicine, & Ethics, 21*(2), 193–205.

Iwamoto R & Gough S. (1993). Radiotherapy: Ambulatory care models. In PC Buchsel & CH Yarbro (Eds.), *Oncology nursing in the ambulatory setting issues and models of care* (pp. 133–164). Boston: Jones and Bartlett Publishers.

Jordan P. (1994). Heathcare reform: Current and proposed approaches. *Oncology Nursing Forum, 21*(7), 1215–1220.

Lamkin L. (1993). The new oncology ambulatory clinic. In PC Buchsel & CH Yarbro (Eds.) *Oncology nursing in the ambulatory setting issues and models of care* (pp. 107–131). Boston: Jones and Bartlett Publishers.

Lamkin L. (1994). Outpatient oncology settings: A variety of services. *Seminars in Oncology Nursing, 10*(4), 229–236.

McDermott KC. (1994). Healthcare reform: past and future. *Oncology Nursing Forum, 21*(5), 827-832.

Miaskowski C. (1993). Future trends in ambulatory care nursing. In PC Buchsel & CH Yarbro (Eds.), *Oncology nursing in the ambulatory setting issues and models of care* (pp. 341–351). Boston: Jones and Bartlett Publishers.

Paris NM & Hines J. (1995). Payer and provider relationships: The key to reshaping health care delivery. *Nursing Administration Quarterly, 19*(3), 13–17.

Pearson LJ. (1995). Annual update of how each state stands on legislative issues affecting advanced nursing practice. *Nurse Practitioner, 20*(1), 13–18.

Ponte PR, Higgins JM, James JR, Fay M, Madded MJ. (1993). Development needs of advance practice nurses in a managed care environment. *Journal of Nursing Administration, 23*(11), 13–19.

Powel LL & Mayer DK. (1992). The future of advanced clinical practice in oncology nursing. *Oncology Nursing Forum, 19* (Suppl. 1), 28–31.

Safriet B. (1992). Health care dollars and regulatory sense: The role of advanced practice nursing. *Yale Journal on Regulation, 9*(2).

Sparacino PS, Cooper DM, Minarick PA. (1990). *The clinical nurse specialist: Implementation and impact.* Norwalk, CT: Appleton & Lange.

Stair J. (1995). Oncology critical pathways. *Oncology Issues, July/August*, 20–21.

Weiss JP. (1995). Nursing practice: A legal and historical perspective. *Journal of Nursing Law, 2*(1), 17–35.

Williams CA, Valdivieso GC. (1994). Advanced practice models: Comparison of clinical nurse specialist and nurse practitioner activities. *Clinical Nurse Specialist, 8*(6), 311–317.

Xistris DM, Houlihan NG. (1994). Impact of reimbursement and health care reform on ambulatory oncology setting. *Seminars in Oncology Nursing, 10*(4), 281–287.

22

Administrative Issues in Today's Managed Care Environments

ELYSE SPORKIN

Administration in radiation therapy is changing and adapting to new methods brought about by the evolution of managed care. Traditional methods of delivering and charging for services are being replaced by new programs including HMOs and PPOs, capitation and case rates, and utilization review and gatekeepers, all of which are aimed at decreasing health care costs. Nurse administrators in radiation therapy are challenged to integrate established roles with innovative functions to ensure quality patient outcomes while controlling costs. Participation in managed care requires enhancing patient access to service, demonstrating patient outcomes, and documenting accountability and cost effectiveness to remain viable. Although the swift changes are creating uncertainty in radiation therapy administration, opportunities for advanced nursing practice abound in the areas of research and documentation of patient outcomes, development of clinical pathways, and collaborative practice.

To plan for the changes in health care, the nurse should have an understanding of the evolution of the system. In 1993, health care reform was a controversial topic, seen as a possible cure-all or as an evil of government intervention. President Clinton envisioned that the program, the Health Security Act of 1993, would control health care costs while attempting to ensure universal access to care. Health care costs in the United States are the highest in the world, yet millions of Americans lack insurance, and, consequently, many are unable to seek health care services. Proposed health care reform involved a complex system combining government regulation and competition (McDermott, 1994).

Although the Health Security Act of 1993 was not enacted, its influence has been evident. It is important to note, however, that changes in health care preceded the President's move for health care reform and have continued in its absence. Market conditions, whereby health care costs continue to grow, led to the development of managed care (Peters, 1995). Managed care has been defined as "an integration of health care financing with the provision of care" (Packard, 1993, p.8). Viewed simply, managed care is a system whereby payors and providers collaborate to deliver health care while controlling costs. Traditional health insurance, the indemnity plan, provides reimbursement for professional and technical services provided to individuals covered by the plan (Kelly et al., 1994).

Managed care's influence on health care in the United States is substantial and increasing. It has become the most prevalent method of controlling costs. Many regions of the United States, such as the West, have reached high levels of managed care coverage, whereas other regions, such as the South, have largely been unaffected. This disparity is expected to change. Current estimates show that approximately 50 percent of the United States population is enrolled in an HMO or PPO (Peters, 1995). Within the next 10 years, 90 percent of the population will be covered by managed care plans (Kerfoot, 1994).

Managed care provides incentives and disincentives to health care providers. It promotes the formation of networks that may save resources and prevent duplication of services. Managed care also discourages independent practice and use of many or excess resources. The insurance company does not participate in the decision making and accompanying financial risk, leaving these activities to the consumer and the provider. The assumption is that this arrangement will lead to changes in the way clinical decisions are made and resources are used. More data on how clinical decision making, patient outcomes, and costs are needed to measure the effectiveness of managed care (Packard, 1993).

One product of managed care is the dramatic shift from financing a fee-for-service model to discounted case rates and capitation contracts. In fee-for-service reimbursement, the physician or institution provides a service, bills an insurance company (third-party payor), and receives payment. Discounted case rates are negotiated between providers and payors for groups before services are initiated. Capitation contracts are agreements in which the provider is paid a fixed amount, usually per member per month, for all covered services (Kelly et al., 1994). A physician would, therefore, provide medical services to covered individuals with no additional charges. Physicians receive the fixed payment whether services are provided or not. From the payor's standpoint, these new systems make good financial sense and will likely increase in use (Peters, 1995). For radiation therapy, like all services, a capitated system forces renewed attention to cost. A fee-for-service model recognizes various procedures as reimbursable and revenue generating. Under capitation, services are delivered as part of a flat rate. The emphasis is on decreasing cost, often by limiting use of additional resources such as referrals to other specialists and use of more complex treatments when simpler approaches are sufficient, rather than increasing numbers of billable procedures.

Capitation could affect clinical and technical decisions in radiation therapy practice in many ways. For instance, ten fractions of radiation treatment for bone metastases might be replaced by two high-dose fractions (Peters, 1995) or by strontium injections, depending on cost effectiveness. In other cases, there could be a decrease in the number of custom blocks created in an effort to conserve resources and time. Alternative treatments such as stereotactic radiosurgery versus conventional external beam radiation therapy would also be weighed for their cost effectiveness.

Opinions over the effects of managed care on oncology and radiation oncology practices vary. Although some believe that the system will give priority to quality over cost containment, others worry that financial considerations will far outweigh clinical decisions. Radiation oncologists who participated in a 1994 survey about managed care expressed frustration with the new system (Taylor, 1994). Sixty-nine percent of the respondents feared that quality of care would decrease under managed care, whereas only 14 percent predicted an improvement in the quality. Delays in simulation were cited as examples of problems caused by extra paperwork and required documentation before approval for treatment is obtained. Radiation oncologists were also concerned about a slowing in the development of new technology due to the effects of managed care. Further, 45 percent of the respondents said they couldn't afford new technology under the new system. Despite the negatives, there is some support for the concept of patient advocacy and accountability under the managed care system.

Concerns about quality under managed care have led to the creation of new treatment guidelines. For example, a group of cancer centers formed the National Comprehensive Cancer Network and is developing cancer treatment guidelines for seven major cancer sites (McIntosh, 1995b). The American College of Radiology is also developing guidelines for the use of imaging and radiation therapy in four cancer sites: lung, breast, prostate, and bone metastasis. These proactive efforts were taken to ensure that the best treatment options are made available and become standardized (McIntosh, 1995a).

Clinical pathways are also being developed to standardize approaches to care (Sovie, 1995). They are aimed at providing patients with a treatment course that will result in the best possible outcome while using fewer resources and less time. For example, use of clinical pathways will aid in reducing the number of tests and procedures ordered, unless the need is specifically indicated. Such guidelines should also help to decrease or eliminate redundancy in documentation. Managed care companies are increasingly looking at standardization as an approach to modify costs and promote quality outcomes (McIntosh, 1995b; Rohrer et al., 1993; Sovie, 1995). Standardization is also aimed at preventing unexpected outcomes by decreasing variations in treatment patterns (Abbott, 1993).

Inherent in the development of critical pathways is multidisciplinary collaboration. Because no one group can successfully meet all the patient's needs, it is crucial that the appropriate team members have the opportunity to identify potential problems and plan for intervention. Teamwork takes priority in a patient-focused environment. Members of the various disciplines will collaborate throughout the treatment course from the initial consult through treatment and follow-up.

Documentation of quality patient care outcomes is a priority for managed care because it has become the predominant health care reimbursement scheme. Much has been written about patient care outcomes, but it is still early in the development of data collection, analysis, and evaluation. Outcomes research has been defined as "linking the type of care received by a variety of patients with a particular condition to positive and negative outcomes in order to identify what works best for which patients" (Guadagnoli & McNeil, 1994, p.14). Outcomes research offers the possibility of providing useful information to payers, providers, and consumers about types of care, costs of care, and alternatives to care. Because of a lack of standardization in health care, there has been increasing interest in examining outcomes. Studies are currently under way to determine whether analysis and use of outcomes data lead to decreased costs and improved quality of care (Guadagnoli & McNeil, 1994).

Radiation therapy must also demonstrate successful outcomes and control costs. Discounted case rates and capitation are realities in many insurance plans. Peters, in his 1994 American Society for Therapeutic Radiation Oncology Presidential Address, addressed the many issues facing radiation therapy in managed care evolution (Peters, 1995). He expressed concern that this specialty, which is procedure oriented, is not prepared for the capitation payment system. Peters stressed the need to obtain and use outcomes research to ensure that appropriate services are delivered to those who can benefit, while reducing excess services. He stressed that the use of technology must be driven by proven effectiveness instead of dictating treatment decisions. Peters stressed the need for practice patterns to be steered by data when alternatives or cost can be reduced. He emphasized the importance of outcomes research in terms of treatment efficacy when considered with quality of life issues such as function, morbidity, and survival. Finally, Peters described priority setting in radiation therapy to maximize use of limited resources (Peters, 1995).

Administrative Challenges

Administrators in radiation therapy have the opportunity to maximize patient care, but they face many challenges. Nurse administrators will be expected to have expertise in the collection and analysis of outcomes data and to be able to analyze the effectiveness and productivity of services (Packard, 1993). Familiarity with quality of life research will be another expectation as payors, providers, and consumers incorporate quality of life into their clinical decision making.

Excellent leadership in radiation therapy will need to support and guide services that are appropriate and efficient while decreasing or eliminating inefficient, nonproductive services. These efforts are necessary to achieve quality outcomes in an efficient environment. The manager must participate in plans such as development of clinical guidelines or critical pathways. The goals of such plans are to decrease variations in care and minimize problems that can lead to treatment delays, breaks in treatment, or costly medical interventions. Excellent collaboration is called for as nursing helps to identify the support services or members of the multidisciplinary team that can help accomplish the goals. Using clinical guidelines, nursing must be able to demonstrate its responsibility and accountability in patient care.

Nursing must take a strong role in assuring a fully coordinated treatment course while eliminating lapses and duplications in service. Good communication with the patient and family is essential throughout treatment to assure their understanding of the process and to gain their cooperation. Patient and family teaching is integral to the entire process beginning at the time of consultation and continuing through discharge and follow-up. Nurses must also direct efforts in patient and family teaching to anticipatory guidance. For example, the subject of symptom management must be redirected to prevention or reduction of symptoms.

Ability to reorganize services to adapt quickly and responsively to change is inherent in the managed care environment. Managed care contracts bring in groups of "covered lives," and radiation therapy must be positioned to provide care that is patient focused. Streamlined access to radiation therapy services should be every manager's goal. Processes and procedures necessary for making appointments, registration, coordination of other services, and communication flow should be seamless and transparent to the patient. Radiation therapy managers will need to ensure timely appointments, minimal waiting times, and prompt initiation of treatment when prescribed. Under managed care, these efforts will maximize successful outcomes and patient and payer satisfaction (Kerfoot, 1994).

Patient satisfaction surveys can be designed to elicit information about perceived or real delays and extended waiting times. Analysis of departmental information such as computerized data can also provide opportunities for improvement. The data may reveal questions regarding delays in scheduling or seeing new consults, delays in initiating treatment, or patients lost to follow-up. Information management systems such as IMPAC and VARIS have the ability to track many facets of the radiation therapy program and facilitate analysis of quality indicators.

Strategies for Success

When problems are identified, the staff must look for ways to solve them. Continuous process improvement (CPI) is one approach used to identify problems, develop potential solutions, and evaluate results. CPI is a process and outcome method for dealing with needed change. It has been described as both a philosophy and a methodology. It is driven by patient needs and guided by data sources. It requires input, planning, implementation, and evaluation by all members of the care team (University of Texas Medical Branch, 1994).

Documentation of quality patient outcomes is a high priority in managed care and will be necessary to remain competitive. Nursing must demonstrate effectiveness of radiation therapy by means of survival, morbidity (disease and treatment-related), and quality of life data (Peters, 1995). Providers who cannot document quality outcomes and patient satisfaction will have difficulty competing for contracts and may eventually cease to exist (Sovie, 1995).

Success under managed care demands renewed attention to the competency of all physicians, nurses, and allied health professionals in radiation therapy. The fact that professional nursing roles in radiation therapy are established is a definite advantage. Dudjak (1992) described the established roles of case manager, nurse manager, clinical nurse specialist, and clinical director. Enhancement of those roles and results-oriented evaluation will be important to demonstrate that they are cost effective and appropriate. Job descriptions and performance appraisals must reflect this attention to competency. The philosophy of patient-focused care should be reflected in job descriptions and performance goals and appraisals. For example, patient care should be age appropriate, with developmental abilities and limitations of patients taken into consideration. Job descriptions

and performance goals should be written to include care specific to patients across the life span.

Adequate staffing is another significant issue in radiation therapy. Administrative decisions regarding appropriate skill mix must be made based on analysis of workload, acuity, specific needs of patients, and quality, while balancing budgetary constraints. When advocating for professional nursing personnel, it is necessary to provide for adequate ancillary personnel to allow nurses to care for patients and their families. Although radiation therapy centers vary in their staffing patterns and needs depending on factors such as private practice versus academic settings, guidelines are available for staffing in radiation therapy, which can be used as a basis for planning. For example, the Report of the Inter-Society Council for Radiation Oncology (1991) or "blue book" provides "minimum personnel requirements" for radiation therapy. Other avenues for information include informal surveys and benchmarking. Benchmarking is a formal process of looking at industry standards and so-called best performers and using this comparative data as a goal in various areas of management (Sovie, 1995).

Nursing Roles in Managed Care

Although some nurses may fear that current economics will lead to a diminishing role for nursing in radiation therapy, it seems clear that nursing will become more important in the delivery of care that is appropriate and cost effective. To achieve quality outcomes, it is imperative that patients and families be included in all aspects of planning, including examining options and alternatives and understanding expected outcomes. Nurses' expertise in patient teaching and recognition and management of side effects, as well as their ability to intervene promptly, is integral to the attainment of high-quality patient outcomes.

The radiation therapy nurse will have increasing responsibility for documentation of patient outcomes. Use of documentation records such as the "Radiation Therapy Patient Care Record" (Oncology Nursing Society, 1994) enables the nurse to document assessment, patient teaching, and medications on one record. In addition, documentation of the plan of care, interventions, and evaluation of outcomes can be made. The record has been developed for seven treatment sites: brain, head and neck, breast, chest, abdomen, pelvis, and bone.

Nurses are increasingly the leaders in developing methods to contain and decrease costs in radiation therapy. By coordinating schedules and tests for patients, following up on lab and x rays, and decreasing use of little-used or inappropriate supplies, cost savings can be realized. Efficiencies in the way nurses manage caseloads or assignments in the clinic can be realized by a change of assignment. Telephone triage for patients may be used to decrease patient time spent traveling and waiting to see physicians, may identify problems earlier, and can prevent misuse of emergency departments.

Dudjak's (1992) description of the case manager includes the ability to identify problems early and intervene promptly. Missed treatments may result from a range of problems as diverse as lack of transportation, pain, or nausea and vomiting. The nurse's ability to intervene effectively and reestablish the patient's treatment schedule is integral to the patient's compliance with and successful completion of treatment. Ongoing patient teaching related to general and specific care issues affect the patient's ability to stay well, progress uneventfully through treatment, and remain symptom-free after treatment.

Case managers are in an excellent position to facilitate quality patient care. The case manager is expert in the use of existing resources while minimizing use of expensive or unnecessary resources. Referrals to agencies such as the American Cancer Society may be made for equipment loans, assistance in obtaining supplies, and emotional support through specific groups. Ongoing teaching and assessment can identify skin care, nutrition, fatigue, and pain issues early enough to intervene, possibly eliminating the need for more complex solutions later in the course of treatment.

Nurse managers' direction and leadership skills will be challenged under managed care as they deal with increased attention to patient outcomes balanced with budget constraints. Whereas all staff members will have responsibilities for cost containment, the nurse manager helps to keep plans and programs patient centered.

The clinical director's nursing background, combined with management skills, are strong assets in the changing managed care arena. Attention to cost, quality, and access will likely increase as the goal of cost-effective and appropriate care delivery is attained. By focusing on patients and the staff who care for them (Dudjak, 1992), the clinical director is able to view the program in its entirety. The ability to interact with other department heads and the radiation therapy medical director and staff is essential to facilitate collaboration.

Managed care also brings exciting opportunities for advanced practice nursing. The clinical nurse specialist (CNS) may need to develop new skills and expertise in this cost-conscious environment, but the benefits to patient and institution can be significant. The CNS must integrate the use of outcomes research as an essential part of practice. Such research can also be invaluable in documenting the role of the CNS in improving patient outcomes (McCaffrey-Boyle, 1994) in radiation therapy. Cost-effective methods for identifying patients at high risk will be extremely useful in promoting timely, appropriate care. For example, the nutritional status of head and neck patients should be evaluated before the start of treatment. Patients at high risk for weight loss would be started on supplements or have a feeding tube inserted to prevent problems serious enough to necessitate hospitalization and delay completion of the treatment course. Additionally, the CNS assists in assuring quality outcomes through the appropriate use of existing resources.

Higgins et al. (1994, p.166) believe that the "CNS has the expertise to meet the demands of aggregate patient populations for which hospitals choose to compete." The CNS must be able to prove cost effectiveness and competence. The CNS has a leadership role in the development of clinical guidelines or pathways and must be able to demonstrate how this effort influences outcomes. The CNS can provide expertise in documentation and evaluation methodology. The radiation therapy CNS also must be able to demonstrate expertise in caring for uniquely complicated cases.

The nurse practitioner also plays an important role in managed care in radiation therapy. Strong physical and psychosocial assessment skills will enable the nurse practitioner to identify possible high-risk issues before treatment begins. Interventions before and during the course of therapy may decrease problems and facilitate completion of therapy. Nurse practitioners' practice may be guided by clinical protocols that enable them to intervene promptly and efficiently. Their skills in patient and family teaching will be utilized fully under managed care, where the treatment course is streamlined and cost effective. Finally, past experience in collaborative practice will enhance the nurse practitioner's efficacy in the managed care environment.

Future Considerations

The advanced practice nurse should look to the future under managed care for new career directions. Opportunities for nursing research should be explored as a means to further efforts toward quality outcomes and to document effectiveness in the role. The fact that managed care contracts bring patients in aggregates leads to new interest in system management. Advance practice nurses should seek ways to further their role in system management to bring about change in patient care. Nurse-run clinics are being developed as cost-effective methods of managing patient care on a timely basis. There is also a trend toward the combination of medical oncology and radiation therapy clinics to facilitate patient care and decrease cost by eliminating duplication of services. The advanced practice nurse can perform very well in such an environment and promote the multidisciplinary approach to care. Finally, the advanced practice nurse should become a leader in information management in patient care (Ponte et al., 1993).

Successful administration of a radiation therapy department in the era of managed care will depend heavily on the ability to deliver care in a cost-effective manner. This will be accomplished by high productivity, efficiency, prevention of duplication of services, and decrease in unnecessary or nonproductive procedures. From a patient care standpoint, cost-effective care translates to keeping patients as healthy as possible, minimizing untoward treatment effects, and dealing promptly with symptoms to decrease the demand for additional services. There will be renewed efforts to teach patients, families, and the public about cancer prevention and early detection. These efforts will be especially important for cancers with familial tendencies. For radiation therapy, this also means treating patients efficiently and on a timely basis. The challenges for nursing and managers are many, but the opportunities to improve outcomes while managing costs are exciting and have long-range implications for health care.

References

Abbott J. (1993) Making the commitment to managed care. *Nursing Management, 24,* 36–37.

Dudjak L. (1992). Administration. In K Hassey Dow, L Hilderley (eds.). *Nursing care in radiation oncology,* 378–382. Philadelphia: W.B. Saunders.

Guadagnoli E, McNeil B. (1994) Outcomes research: Hope for the future or the latest rage? *Inquiry, 31,* 14–24.

Higgins J, Ponte P, James J, Fay M, Madden M. (1994) Restructuring the CNS role for a managed care environment. *Clinical Nurse Specialist, 8,* 163–166.

Inter-Society Council for Radiation Oncology. (1991). *Radiation oncology in integrated cancer management.* Philadelphia: Inter-Society Council for Radiation Oncology.

Kelly M, Bacon G, Mitchell J. (1994). Glossary of managed care terms. *Journal of Ambulatory Care Management, 17,* 70–76.

Kerfoot K. (1994). Health care futurists: the vision of the future and the nurse manager. *Nursing Economics, 12,* 235–236.

McCaffrey-Boyle D. (1994). Where is the missing piece of the jigsaw puzzle? *Clinical Nurse Specialist, 8,* 117–121.

McDermott K. (1994). Healthcare reform: Past and present. *Oncology Nursing Forum, 21,* 827–832.

McIntosh H. (1995a). Managed care brings major changes to cancer care. *Journal of the National Cancer Institute, 87,* 784–786.

McIntosh H. (1995b) Use of treatment guidelines surges as urge to manage care increases. *Journal of the National Cancer Institute, 87,* 1044–1047.

Oncology Nursing Society. (1994). *Radiation Therapy Patient Care Record: A tool for documenting patient care.* Pittsburgh: Radiation Therapy Special Interest Group Documentation Project Core Committee.

Packard N. (1993). The price of choice: Managed care in America. *Nursing Administration Quarterly, 17,* 8–15.

Peters L. (1995). Through a glass darkly: Predicting the future of radiation oncology. *International Journal of Radiation Oncology, Biology, Physics, 31,* 219–225.

Ponte PR, Higgins JM, James JR, Fay M, Madden MJ. (1993). Development needs of advance practice nurses in a managed care environment. *Journal of Nursing Administration,* 23(11), 13-19.

Rohrer K, Poppe M, Noel L. (1993). Staff preparation for managed care. *Nursing Administration Quarterly, 17,* 74–78.

Sovie M. (1995). Tailoring hospitals for managed care and integrated health systems. *Nursing Economics, 13,* 72–83.

Taylor K. (1994). Survey: Oncologists frustrated with managed care hurdles. *Hospitals and Health Networks, 68,* 78.

University of Texas Medical Branch, Galveston (1994). Staff training in CPI techniques. (Correspondence to staff from Micky Moore, Galveston, TX: 1994.)

Radiation Oncology Nursing Documentation

ALLISON BLACKMAR

Nursing documentation is an essential component of clinical nursing practice. It is the fundamental method by which nurses communicate patient status and record responses to nursing interventions. An entire team of health care providers including nurses, physicians, nutritionists, physical therapists, social workers, and counselors relies on accurate and thorough nursing documentation. In addition, the medical record is important to administration because it enables the institution to evaluate the care given and to meet standards of care required for continued accreditation. In today's health care market, this means that the medical record is necessary for reimbursement and thus is directly linked to the viability of the institution.

Nursing documentation provides written evidence of clinical nursing practice. Researchers estimate that 15 to 20 percent of work time is spent documenting patient care and that documentation is the most common cause of nursing overtime (Moody & Synder, 1995). Nursing documentation in radiation therapy has and continues to challenge nurses. High patient-to-nurse ratios, managing numerous nursing and nonnursing duties, and cost containment issues greatly affect documentation systems in radiation therapy. Numerous tools are available to assist nurses in accurately and thoroughly recording the care they give to patients receiving radiation therapy. This chapter will discuss these documentation tools, educate the reader on the principles of nursing documentation, and describe the related administrative and clinical issues. Documentation of nursing care has long been considered a cumbersome and time-consuming task. However, given the availability of current and upcoming resources,

nurses practicing in radiation oncology may find it no longer an arduous responsibility.

Documentation and Nursing Practice

Throughout nursing school curriculum's students learn the nursing process and the importance of documenting nursing care. Yet when confronted with the realities of clinical practice, nurses often prioritize patient care over record keeping. A complete and concise medical record, however, is an invaluable asset to the patient, health care providers, administration, and insurance companies.

Principles of Nursing Documentation

Nursing documentation is an important portion of the medical record. The medical record serves many purposes, the most significant of which is communication. It is a method of recording and communicating pertinent information about the patient and reflects everything seen, heard, smelled, and felt, as well as actions taken (Feutz-Harter, 1989). Another significant purpose for documenting nursing care relates to an institution's financial reimbursement. Given today's health care situation, accurate and complete record keeping is of utmost importance to administrators as they strive to acquire reimbursement from the government and insurance companies. Currently, administrators are limited in the ways in which they can capture charges for nursing care in radiation therapy. This will most likely change, however, as the surge toward capitated care continues. Administrators will need to know exactly what is required to deliver care for a particular diagnosis. Although these organizational changes challenge radiation oncology nurses to do more with less, they also provide an opportunity to define for administration exactly what is needed to provide quality care to patients receiving radiation therapy. Thorough documentation of clinical nursing practice can serve as a mechanism for supporting the nurse in this endeavor.

Information recorded in the medical record demonstrates not only patient status but also nursing interventions and a patient's response to the care. Data recorded in the medical record provides members of the health care team a method of tracking a patient's progress toward expected outcomes. It contributes to the continuity of care and enables an institution to monitor and evaluate services delivered to meet standards of care required for accreditation (Butler, 1991). In addition, recorded data serves as a mechanism for clinical research. Standardized methods of documenting nursing care can provide a database of information for clinical research and quality improvement studies.

Lastly, the medical record is a legal document that can be used in a variety of legal proceedings and provide important information regarding the standard of care given (Butler, 1991; Feutz-Harter, 1989). Nurses have long since heard the adage "if it wasn't charted, it wasn't done." The literature, however, supports a shift in the legal ramifications of nursing documentation. According to Butler (1991), numerous cases demonstrate that the courts are aware of the demands placed on nurses by the nursing shortage and organizational restructuring. If the focus of a lawsuit is inadequate nursing documentation, the court will often look for evidence to support the inference that care was actually given (Butler, 1991). Documents used to demonstrate that care was provided include flow sheets, medication records, procedures, protocols, and nursing care plans. Thus, nursing documentation of care can be performed in a number of methods and is supported by accreditation agencies, insurance companies, and the legal system. A complete medical record is a vital document for the entire health care team. Fortunately, nurses can be creative and diverse in their methods of documenting care and patients' responses to care.

Documentation in Oncology Nursing

A review of the literature over the last five years demonstrates that documentation of clinical nursing practice is a universal concern of oncology nurses (Behrend, 1994; Cushman, 1991; Dudjak, 1988; Hirshfield-Bartek et al., 1990; Lynch & Yanes, 1991; Moore & Knobf, 1991; Pevny, 1993; Pfeifer, 1992; Pickett, 1992). Many documentation tools are available to assist nurses in a variety of clinical settings. Most prevalent in the literature are tools to assist nurses working in medical oncology, specifically flow sheets for documenting chemotherapy administration and education (Cushman, 1991; Lynch & Yanes, 1991; Moore & Knobf, 1991; Pfeifer, 1992; Pickett, 1992). Documentation tools to expedite intake of basic health history and psychosocial information are also available (Skinn & Stacey, 1994). It is evident from the literature that oncology nurses from a diverse array of clinical settings struggle with documentation issues and continue to create tools for recording information in thorough yet time-sparing ways.

A variety of documentation formats are used in the ambulatory oncology setting. A wide range of tools have been developed to assist nurses in documenting oncology nursing practice. There is no one right way to document nursing care. Instead, using more than one method to record clinical information may result in improved data collection and record keeping. It is important that documentation formats are concise, timely, effective, and capable of being adapted to a variety of clinical settings (Behrend, 1994). Methods of documentation include written narrative notes and flow sheets. Narrative notes provide subjective information and are useful in reporting the necessary detailed commentary required for unusual occurrences in daily clinical practice (Moore & Knobf, 1991). Flow sheets enable oncology nurses to record data with greater efficiency, to track specific clinical data by patient population, and to provide objective information (Moore & Knobf, 1991). Others report that flow sheets facilitate continuity of care and patient education and help to identify critical indicators affecting quality of care (Behrend, 1994; Edelstein, 1990; Lynch & Yanes, 1991; Pevny, 1993). Still other styles of documentation include dictated progress notes and charting by exception (Behrend, 1994). Charting by exception refers to the practice by which standard nursing care is recorded in the nursing care plans and any unusual or unexpected occurrence that is not delineated in the care plan is recorded.

Documentation in Radiation Oncology

Radiation oncology is a unique and diverse specialty. The roles and responsibilities of radiation oncology nurses vary based on the type of clinical setting (Bruner, 1993; Bucholtz, 1987; Hilderley, 1980; Strohl, 1991). Nurses may work within an academically affiliated university, a community hospital, a rural setting, or freestanding clinics. High patient-to-nurse ratios, limited staffing patterns, multiple roles and responsibilities, and organizational restructuring greatly influence the accuracy and consistency of nursing documentation in radiation oncology. As a result, a variety of documentation formats are currently used, including hand-written narrative notes, SOAP notes, flow sheets, dictated progress notes, and computerized spreadsheets (Blackmar, personal communication, 1992).

Although it is not documented in the clinical literature, standardized methods of documenting care is a common concern verbalized by radiation oncology nurses attending professional meetings. Before 1994, two tools were published, each addressing the need to improve the efficiency and timeliness of nursing documentation in radiation oncology. One was a comprehensive flow sheet enabling nurses to document assessments, patient education, and evaluation (Dudjak, 1988). The other was an innovative patient self-assessment tool and standardized flow sheet incorporating frequently used nursing diagnoses and potential nursing interventions in radiation oncology (Hirshfield-Bartek et al., 1990). The authors reported a decrease in documentation time, an increase in the quality of information documented, and more effective use of nursing time for patient support and education (Hirshfield-Bartek et al., 1990).

Recognizing the wide disparity of documentation methods and the need for standardization, in 1990 the Radiation Therapy Special Interest Group (SIG) organized a group of radiation oncology nurses to address this issue. The goal was to create a tool that was comprehensive, time sparing, and useful in a variety of clinical settings. After much research and collaboration, the first standardized radiation therapy nursing documentation tool was published in 1994. The ONS *Radiation Therapy Patient Care Record: A Tool for Documenting Nursing Care* is a set of eight comprehensive, anatomically site-specific forms designed for use in their entirety or as a guide for creation of institution-specific tools. The tool enables the nurse to document radiation-induced side effects according to standardized site-specific assessment parameters (Figures 23-1 and 23-2) and site-specific education (Figure 23-3). In addition, a comprehensive medication form is available

to facilitate thorough documentation of medications prescribed during therapy (Figure 23-4). Nurses using the tool in a pilot study evaluating the prepublished tool reported that it is comprehensive yet concise and time sparing. Others identify that the standardized assessment parameters have greatly reduced the subjectivity of nursing assessments.

Another resource available to nurses seeking examples of institution-specific documentation tools is the *Documentation Manual for Radiation Oncology Nursing* (Bruner & Slivjak, 1994). The manual contains a variety of tools designed to assist radiation oncology nurses in documenting the clinical aspects of nursing care, including consultation, assessment, consent to treatment, patient education, and follow-up forms.

Documentation and Quality Assurance in Radiation Oncology

The Joint Commission on Accreditation of Health Care Organizations (JCAHO) was established in 1953 and has been the motivating force in regulating the standard of care delivered by health care organizations. Recently, a shift took place within the quality review process. Instead of determining whether an organization provides quality care (quality assurance), JCAHO is now more concerned with whether an organization is consistently making efforts to improve the care it provides (quality improvement) (Thomas, 1994). JCAHO provides national standards of care to guide and instruct organizations in developing quality improvement (QI) programs. In nursing practice, professional organizations such as the Oncology Nursing Society have established standards of care to serve as the basic unit of measurement and evaluation of clinical nursing practice (Oncology Nursing Society, 1987). In addition, health care facilities often develop institution-specific standards of care for managers to use in monitoring and evaluating nursing practice and clinical outcomes. Regulatory agencies demand that the quality and appropriateness of patient care be monitored and evaluated (Edelstein, 1990). The available standards of care guide nurses in developing systems and tools to meet these regulatory requirements.

Continuity of care and consistency of nursing assessment, interventions, and evaluation can easily be recognized through well-designed and organized documentation tools (Pevny, 1993). The challenge for radiation oncology nurses is identi-

Dx _____

Site _____

Name   MR #/RT #

Assessments (Date/rad or Gy)										
Comfort Alteration Fatigue										
Pain rating										
Pain treatment										
Pain relief										
Mucous Membrane Alteration Esophagitis/Pharyngitis										
Laryngitis										
Mucositis										
Taste changes										
Xerostomia										
Nutrition Alteration Anorexia										
Nausea										
Vomiting										
Weight										
Sensory Alteration Hearing Changes										
Skin Alteration Skin reaction										
Injury, Potential CBC DATE **Bleeding/Infection** WBC										
Hemoglobin/ Hematocrit										
Platelets										
Other										
INITIALS										

Pre-existing Conditions/Medical Information
Date: Ht =   BP =   P =   R =   Concurrent Chemotherapy: Yes   No

_____ (___) _____ (___) _____ (___)
Signature   Initials   Signature   Initials   Signature   Initials

Figure 23-1 • Radiation Therapy Patient Care Record: Head and Neck. Used with permission from the Oncology Nursing Society. Original appears in Radiation Therapy Special Interest Group Documentation Project Core Committee. (1994). *Radiation Therapy Patient Care Record: A Tool for Documenting Nursing Care.* Pittsburgh: ONS.

fying the pertinent outcomes to monitor and the development of tools to capture and report this information. This challenge is coupled with the need to provide documentation that not only reflects JCAHO, professional, and institution-specific standards of care, but do so in a way that results in minimal time expenditure and paper work. Bruner (1990) cites an example of an institution-specific, three-phase plan in which a quality assurance program for radiation oncology nursing was developed based on national guidelines for nursing practice.

CNS Alteration

DYSPHASIA
0—None, normal speech
1—Slowed or slightly slurred speech
2—Long pauses in speech
3—Unable to select right words when speaking
4—Unable to speak

BOWEL INCONTINENCE
0—None
1—One to two episodes of bowel incontinence in 24 hours
2—Three to five episodes of bowel incontinence in 24 hours
3—Complete loss of bowel control

HEMIPARESIS
0—None
1—Weakness with no impairment in function
2—Weakness with impairment of function
3—Complete loss of function

LEVEL OF CONSCIOUSNESS
0—Alert; responds briskly, appropriately with minimal stimulus
1—Sleeping; responds appropriately with minimal stimulus
2—Sleeping; requires moderate amount of stimuli to elicit response
3—Sleeping; makes no verbal response to forceful, painful stimuli
4—No response when maximally stimulated

ORIENTATION
0—Oriented in three spheres of person, place, time
1—Oriented in two spheres of person, place, time
2—Oriented in one sphere of person, place, time
3—Disoriented in all three spheres of person, place, time

SEIZURE ACTIVITY
0—None
Use a check mark to indicate seizure activity and describe in plan/interventions/outcomes.

SLEEP DISTURBANCE
0—Able to sleep through the night without awakening
1—Awakens less than 2 times per night and stays awake for more than 60 minutes
2—Awakens more than 2 times per night and stays awake for more than 60 minutes
3—Unable to sleep throughout night

URINARY INCONTINENCE
0—None
1—Stress incontinence
2—One to two episodes of urinary incontinence in 24 hours
3—Three to five episodes of urinary incontinence in 24 hours
4—Complete loss of bladder control

VISUAL DISTURBANCE
0—None
1—Visual changes reported; able to perform daily activities
2—Visual changes reported; unable to perform daily activities
3—Blindness in one or both eyes

Sensory Alteration

HEARING CHANGES
0—None
1—Reduced hearing; able to perform daily activities
2—Reduced hearing; unable to perform daily activities
3—Complete hearing loss

Mucous Membrane Alteration

ESOPHAGITIS/PHARYNGITIS
0—None
1—Tolerates regular diet
2—Tolerates soft diet
3—Tolerates liquids only
4—Chokes and/or coughs when swallows liquids

LARYNGITIS
0—None
1—Intermittent hoarseness
2—Persistent hoarseness
3—Whispered speech

MUCOSITIS
0—None
1—Generalized erythema
2—Isolated small ulcerations and/or white patches
3—Confluent ulcerations and white patches
4—Hemorrhage or necrosis

TASTE CHANGES
0—None
1—Loss of one of the taste sensations (sweet, sour, salty, bitter)
2—Loss of any two of the taste sensations
3—Loss of any three of the taste sensations
4—Complete loss of taste

VAGINAL DISCHARGE
0—None
1—Contained in panty shield
2—Contained in sanitary napkin
3—Not contained in sanitary napkin

XEROSTOMIA
0—None
1—Mild mouth dryness; slightly thickened saliva
2—Moderate mouth dryness; thick, sticky saliva
3—Complete dryness of the mouth

Figure 23-2 • Assessment parameters: CNS, sensory, and mucous membrane. Used with permission from the Oncology Nursing Society. Original appears in Radiation Therapy Special Interest Group Documentation Project Core Committee. (1994). *Radiation Therapy Patient Care Record: A Tool for Documenting Nursing Care.* Pittsburgh: ONS

Name: _____   MR #/RT #: _____

	Date/ Initials	METH	EVAL	PLAN	Date/ Initials	METH	EVAL	PLAN	Educational Materials
GENERAL Simulation									
Initial treatment									
Self care information									
Nutrition									
Social service									
Discharge instructions									
SITE-SPECIFIC Side effects									
Dental hygiene									
Esophagitis management									
Fatigue management									
Hearing loss management									
Laryngitis management									
Mucositis management									
Pain management									
Skin/scalp care									
Taste management									
Xerostomia management									
Weight loss management									
OTHER/PREVENTION BSE/TSE									
Smoking cessation									

Method Codes:
A. Person: Person Session
B. Family Conference
C. Booklet (specify)
D. Demonstration
E. Audio/Visual

Evaluation Codes:
UE: Unable to evaluate (explain)
V: Verbalizes concept accurately
D: Demonstrates skill accurately
R: Needs review
NR: Not receptive to learning at this time (explain)

Plan Codes:
RC: Reinforce Concept
RD: Return Demonstration
LOM: Learning objective met
RF: Referral to other health care givers (specify)
O: Other (specify)

Date	Comments

_____ (   )   _____ (   )   _____ (   )
Signature   Initials   Signature   Initials   Signature   Initials

Figure 23-3 • Teaching and instructions: Head and Neck. Used with permission from the Oncology Nursing Society. Original appears in Radiation Therapy Special Interest Group Documentation Project Core Committee. (1994). *Radiation Therapy Patient Care Record: A Tool for Documenting Nursing Care.* Pittsburgh: ONS.

Name _____   MR #/RT # _____   Date _____

Allergies _____

Chemotherapy

Prior to XRT (P) Concurrent (C)	Drugs	Last Course	Future Course(s)
P C			
P C			
P C			
P C			

Medications Prior to Starting Treatment

Medication	Dose	Route	Freq	DC'D	INIT	DR	Refilled #/Date/INT

Medications Prescribed During Treatment

Date	Medication	Dose	Route	Freq	#/Oz	DC'D	INIT	DR	Refilled #/Date/INT

Samples Given During Treatment

Date	Medication	Dose	Route	Freq	#/Oz	Lot #	INIT	DR	Refilled #/Date/INT

_____   (   )   _____   (   )   _____   (   )
    Signature   Initials   Signature   Initials   Signature   Initials

Figure 23-4 • Patient medication record. Used with permission from the Oncology Nursing Society. Original appears in Radiation Therapy Special Interest Group Documentation Project Core Committee. (1994). *Radiation Therapy Patient Care Record: A Tool for Documenting Nursing Care.* Pittsburgh: ONS.

Information Systems in Radiation Oncology

Computers are being used more and more in the health care market. Organizations, hospitals, and ambulatory clinics are acquiring new and larger information systems. Within nursing practice, computers are being used widely throughout clinical settings. Nurses are now able to chart at the bedside, order laboratory studies, implement physician's orders, order supplies, fax reports, and even send electronic mail via computer terminals. Benefits related to automation for health care organizations include improved patient care, refined quality documentation, and reduction of time required for documentation (Couillard-Getreuer, 1994). Computers assist nurses in providing patient care through automated care planning, discharge planning, monitoring, and patient education (Hendrickson et al., 1991). A comprehensive automated system should be able to provide on-line care plans and discharge plans as well as incorporate national and institutional standards of care.

Computers offer particular benefits to nurses working in oncology, given its multidisciplinary nature. Computers enable nurses to plan, direct, and evaluate care. Computers are now being used in creative ways in radiation oncology. Companies specializing in radiation therapy computer software have developed programs that link computers to linear accelerators to verify and record treatment data and capture treatment-related charges. Some radiation therapy centers are presently in the process of moving from a paper chart to a completely electronic chart. When using an electronic charting system, physicians no longer record treatment prescriptions on paper but instead enter it into a computer. With the record and verify system, treatment deviations are practically eliminated, thus greatly improving the quality of therapy. In addition, treatment and follow-up appointment schedules are on line, which results in improved scheduling of patients and reduced delays in appointments. Departments are more organized and efficient as a result of department-wide radiation oncology information systems.

Presently, some office-based computer software programs have scheduling and documentation capabilities. The documentation tools used in these products are either general oncology flow sheets or specific to medical oncology and the delivery of chemotherapy. In the near future, the ONS *Radiation Therapy Patient Care Record* will be available on line to improve nursing documentation of assessments, side effect management, and patient education. In addition, the information collected in a database will assist nurses in deriving specialized reports that measure expected clinical outcomes. This will greatly enhance the ability to conduct nursing research studies. Ultimately, medical oncology and radiation oncology departments will be integrated and share automated patient care information.

Future Trends in Radiation Oncology Nursing Documentation

Many opportunities lie ahead in radiation oncology nursing documentation. With the publication of the ONS *Radiation Therapy Patient Care Record* nurses will have a standardized, comprehensive tool to facilitate efficient and objective data collection specific to radiation oncology. The tool will need to be reviewed and refined in the future to better meet the ever-changing needs of radiation oncology nurses. During this revision and in the creation of other tools, nurses must begin thinking toward information systems, because the key to the future of quality documentation is in automation. Nurses will need to create tools that collect measurable, objective data that can be evaluated and sorted in numerous ways. Information systems will need to be integrated and communicated to other systems so data can be shared and compiled. The potential and need for nursing research in the field of radiation oncology is vast. With the creation of large databases, multisite and multi-institutional studies can be performed, providing valuable information to clinicians in the management of radiation-induced side effects. As nurses begin using computers to develop reports that capture data, new and innovative ideas will emerge regarding documentation. As computer technology increases, more opportunities for nursing documentation and clinical research in radiation oncology will emerge.

References

Behrend SW. (1994). Documentation in the ambulatory setting. *Seminars in Oncology Nursing, 10*(4), 264–280.

Blackmar A. (1992). Chair of the Oncology Nursing Society's Radiation Therapy Special Interest Group Documentation Project.

Bruner DW. (1990). Model quality assurance program for radiation oncology nursing. *Cancer Nursing, 13*(6), 335–338.

Bruner DW. (1993). Radiation oncology nurses: Staffing patterns and role development. *Oncology Nursing Forum, 20*(4), 651–655.

Bruner DW & Slivjak A. (1994). *Documentation manual for radiation oncology nursing.* Philadelphia: Fox Chase Cancer Center.

Bucholtz J. (1987). Radiation therapy. In C Ziegfeld (ed.). *Core curriculum for oncology nursing,* 207–224. Philadelphia: Saunders.

Butler PL. (1991). The nursing shortage: The legal impact on documentation. *Journal of Continuing Education in Nursing, 22*(5), 189–191.

Couillard-Getreuer D. (1994). Informatics and information in nursing. *Cancer Nursing Practice Update, 2*(1), 1–11.

Cushman KE. (1991). A tool for documenting chemotherapy administration quickly and completely. *Oncology Nursing Forum, 18*(3), 599–600.

Dudjak LA. (1988). Radiation therapy nursing care record: A tool for documentation. *Oncology Nursing Forum, 15*(6), 763–777.

Edelstein J. (1990). A study of nursing documentation. *Nursing Management, 21*(11), 40–46.

Feutz-Harter S. (1989). Documentation principles and pitfalls. *Journal of Nursing Administration, 19*(12), 7–9.

Hendrickson G, Kelly JB, & Citrin L. (1991). Computers in oncology nursing: Present use and future potential. *Oncology Nursing Forum, 18*(4), 715–723.

Hilderley L. (1991). The role of the nurse in radiation oncology. *Seminars in Oncology, 7*(1), 39–47.

Hirshfield-Bartek J, Dow KH, & Creaton E. (1990). Decreasing documentation time using a patient self-assessment tool. *Oncology Nursing Forum, 17*(2), 251–255.

Lynch M, Yanes L. (1991). Flow sheet documentation of chemotherapy administration and patient teaching. *Oncology Nursing Forum, 18*(4), 777–783.

Moody L, Synder PE. (1995). Hospital provider satisfaction with a new documentation system. *Nursing Economics, 13*(1), 1–31.

Moore JM, Knobf MT. (1991). A nursing flow sheet for documentation of ambulatory oncology. *Oncology Nursing Forum, 18*(5), 933–939.

Oncology Nursing Society. (1994). *Radiation therapy patient care record: A tool for documenting nursing care.* Pittsburgh: Author.

Pevny V. (1993). Outcome of a quality assurance review: Development of a documentation tool for chemotherapy administration. *Oncology Nursing Forum, 20*(3), 535–541.

Pfeifer P. (1992). Documentation of care in an oncology outpatient setting. *Oncology Nursing Forum, 19*(5), 809–818.

Pickett RR. (1992). Outpatient oncology chemotherapy documentation tool. *Oncology Nursing Forum, 19*(3), 515–517.

Skinn B, Stacey D. (1994). Establishing an integrated framework for documentation: Use of a self-reporting health history and outpatient oncology record. *Oncology Nursing Forum, 21*(9), 1557–1566.

Strohl R. (1991). The nursing role in radiation oncology: Symptom management and chronic reactions. *Oncology Nursing Forum, 15*(4), 429–434.

Thomas D. (1994). Quality assessment and improvement via the ten-step model. *Oncology Issues, 9*(2), 21–23.

Care Maps in Radiation Oncology

PATRICIA BIECK, MICHELE HALLER, KAREN KUGEL, LINDA PRICE,
AND VICKIE K. FIELER

Over the last 15 years, health care institutions have been challenged by the rapid changes occurring in our health care system. In response to cost containment, technological advances, increasing acuity, and higher consumer expectations, hospitals have restructured their patient care delivery systems. Various care delivery models have been developed based on individual institution needs. Although different terms have been used to describe these models—such as case management or collaborative care—all share a multidisciplinary, outcome-oriented approach to quality patient care while making more efficient use of clinical resources. Inpatient, acute-care units have been the setting for the development of these models. It is only over the last few years that outpatient settings have begun to explore incorporating and adopting this model to meet their patients' needs. For this chapter, we will focus on the Collaborative Care model at Strong Memorial Hospital and how it was modified for use at the University of Rochester Cancer Center in Rochester, New York, primarily an outpatient setting.

The purpose of this chapter is to (1) provide information and share our experiences regarding the development and implementation of care maps as part of a collaborative care approach to patient care and (2) describe the relationship to quality improvement and nursing research in radiation oncology. By the end of this chapter, the reader will be able to identify the key components of a care map or critical pathway, develop a care map for a radiation therapy patient group, and discuss ways of integrating quality improvements using care maps.

Rapid changes in health care have forced hospitals and other institutions to critically explore alternative models of patient care delivery. These new care delivery models emphasize more efficient and effective use of clinical resources and redirect the focus of care to improving patient outcomes and satisfaction.

Case management or collaborative care is based on an interdisciplinary collaboration among health care team members that provide care to a specific patient population. The case manager or care coordinator is an experienced nurse or an advanced practice nurse with clinical expertise for a specific group of patients. Patients are usually grouped by diagnosis. This nurse is responsible for the overall coordination of care for a group of patients. Ongoing collaboration with physicians and other health care team members and advanced planning ensure the timely integration of patient care. The case manager or coordinator is not necessarily responsible for the direct care for patients but rather assists others to provide patient care consistent with the standards set in a critical pathway or care map.

Many terms have been used to describe these innovative models of care delivery. *Case management, managed care,* and *collaborative care,* the most common terms used in the literature, are often used interchangeably. Although these terms have slightly different definitions, all focus on improved patient outcomes using a multidisciplinary approach. Models focusing on patient outcomes and managed care were introduced in 1985 at the New England Medical Center (Giuliano & Poirier, 1991). At Strong Memorial Hospital, the terms *collaborative care* and *care coordinator* were chosen and will be used throughout this chapter.

Critical pathways or care maps replace the traditional nursing care plan and nursing history and are a permanent part of the medical record. A care map is used to identify specific patient care needs and to plan interventions accordingly. The chronological organization of the interventions and patient education allow any member of the health care team to look at the care map and identify the course of care. All education and interventions are documented on the care map.

Development of a Collaborative Care Model

In January 1991, Strong Memorial Hospital in Rochester, New York, was funded by the New York State Department of Health to develop, implement, and evaluate a case management approach to care delivery in an acute care inpatient setting. Patient, nurse, and physician surveys were conducted to identify the areas that could most benefit from a collaborative care model. Criteria included patient length of stay greater than state and national norms, professional nurse turnover rate greater than 20 percent, opportunities for improvement in communication among health care team members, and problem areas identified by patient satisfaction surveys.

Two major focus areas were identified: patient/caregiver and system goals. The patient/caregiver goals included obtaining improved patient outcomes, timely discharge from the hospital, and increased patient satisfaction. The system goals were to increase collaboration among members of the health care team, increase staff satisfaction, and implement continuous quality improvement. Three components of a collaborative care model include (1) developing care maps, (2) defining the role of the care coordinator, and (3) development of variance analysis. A variance analysis is a method to determine whether patients are achieving outcomes that health care professionals have set as standards. For example, a group of patients undergoing surgery might have an outcome goal of discharge from the hospital after three days. In order to achieve that goal, specific interventions will need to occur at specific times. For example, the patients may need to ambulate in the first 12 hours after surgery. These interventions are written on the care map. A method to measure how long each patient stays in the hospital needs to be developed or put into place. Data are collected either for a specific period of time or until a target number of patients has been reached. During data collection, if a patient exceeds the time frames for an intervention or for an outcome, the care coordinator investigates why the problem occurred and documents it on the variance analysis form. Using the surgical example, perhaps three patients did not ambulate within the first 12 hours. One

did not ambulate because he had a surgical complication, and two did not ambulate because the unit was short staffed. At the end of the data collection period, the care coordinator summarizes the findings. What percentage of patients were able to be discharged in three days? For the patients who did not meet the outcome, what contributed to the failure? Was it the three patients who did not ambulate in the recommended time? If a common problem is identified, is there a common cause to the problem (e.g., short staffing)? Are there ways to modify the care map, increase resources, or modify the standards of care so that the desired outcomes can be achieved? To complete the variance analysis process, changes are implemented into patient care and outcomes are measured again.

Evaluation of this model focused on achieving positive patient outcomes determined for a specific population of patients, decreasing length of stay, and cost containment. The demonstration project was completed in December 1993. At that time, there were 25 care coordinators working in seven different clinical areas, and 65 care maps in use. A decision was made to implement the model throughout the hospital, including the ambulatory care areas.

Historically at the University of Rochester Cancer Center, primary nursing was the care delivery system. Although it was considered to be an effective method of nursing care delivery, it is not always efficient. Early in 1993, a decision was made to conduct a trial of a collaborative care project in the Cancer Center. A work group was formed consisting of an advanced practice nurse, a nurse leader, and staff nurses from each area.

The purpose of this group was to identify the goals of collaborative care in the Cancer Center, implement a trial project, and evaluate the achievement of the goals. The goals were to develop a care delivery system that promotes positive patient outcomes through the development of specific standards of care, enhance patient and care provider satisfaction through increased interdisciplinary collaboration, and achieve more efficient use of resources (University of Rochester Cancer Center, 1993). One method to meet the goals was the development of diagnosis-specific care maps. Care maps provide a streamlined documentation process that consists of patient care outcomes developed by the clinical care providers of this group of patients. Care coordinators were identified, and they organized the effort to write the first care maps in their own areas (medical oncology, radiation oncology, and gynecologic oncology). The care coordinators were experienced staff nurses with the following responsibilities:

- communicating with other health team members regarding patient progress and assuming responsibility of the overall plan of care
- serving as an educator and resource person to clinical staff and providing information regarding the use of the care map and the variance analysis tool
- monitoring patients' progress through the use of a variance analysis and incorporating variance resolution into the quality improvement program.

Care maps were developed for patients receiving radiation therapy to the breast and to the pelvis in late 1994 and early 1995. Revisions were recently made to the existing care maps, reflecting the new and changing needs of the radiation oncology department, and new care maps are being added.

We have recently completed an evaluation of the effectiveness of the care maps in radiation oncology. Based on the results, we have listed the positive and negative outcomes (Table 24-1).

Development of Care Maps

One of the first decisions to make when implementing collaborative care is what patient population to use (Ferguson, 1993). The two tenets of managed care are high volume and high risk (Jones & Mullikin, 1994). In reviewing our population of patients, it was easy to identify the high-volume groups: breast and prostate cancer patients. Identifying our high-risk patients required

Table 24-1 • Positive and Negative Outcomes of Collaborative Care

Positive Outcomes	Negative Outcomes
Streamlined documentation	Primarily used by nursing rather than all team members
Standardized plan of care	
Identification of early trends and patterns in patient outcomes	Resident rotations necessitate frequent changes on care maps
Facilitation of cross-coverage for nursing	Difficulty in getting physicians to participate
Ease in orienting new staff nurses	Major time commitment to develop a new care map
Improved continuity of care	Printed on extra-large paper that does not easily fit into patient records
Positive patient outcomes	

additional discussions. High risk has been defined as a patient group that requires a wide variety of health care practitioners, resources, and services (Petryshen & Petryshen, 1992) or a patient group with high cost such that the cost of providing care exceeds the amount of reimbursement (Jones & Mullikin, 1994). In radiation oncology, we determined our high-risk patients to be patients with head and neck cancer and patients with lung cancer. Because of the complexity of care required by high-risk patients, we decided to start with our high-volume groups.

The first care maps were begun by gathering a multidisciplinary group. The care coordinator prepared an outline in advance in order to have a starting point for the group. Team members included a radiation oncology resident, a staff nurse, an advanced practice nurse, a social worker, and a radiation therapist. A rough care map was created in about an hour. Everyone's ideas were incorporated. The care coordinator then revised the care map and circulated it to the team members until everyone was in agreement. This took about 10 weeks, which was longer than anticipated. The care map was implemented and, over the course of two years, has undergone several revisions.

Currently, a template is available to start a care map, and existing care maps serve as a framework. Rather than having a work group meet at the same time, one or two individuals, usually nurses, draft a care map and circulate it to other team members for input and approval. With the existing care maps and the template, the time it takes to develop a new map has been shortened from 10 weeks to about 6 weeks. We have also used the strategy of giving the reviewers a specific deadline to make changes on the care map, about 1 week. If they have not responded by the deadline, we assume that they are in agreement with the draft.

An example of how our care maps have changed over time can be seen in the change from a care map for prostate cancer to a care map for patients receiving radiation to the pelvis. The staff nurses identified that all patients receiving radiation to the pelvis had similar side effects and a similar course of treatment. Rather than create many care maps with small differences among them, it was more efficient to have a few care maps and be able to individualize them. In contrast, we decided not to combine the care maps for patients receiving radiation therapy for breast cancer and those receiving radiation therapy to the chest. Although the two are considered similar in anatomical area, the radiation treatment techniques vary as do the expected side effects, potential complications, and the psychosocial issues each group may be struggling with. It is not an expectation that every group of patients will have a specific care map. For patients with unusual diagnoses such as a malignant melanoma, it is not cost effective to take the time to develop a preprinted care map. However, one way to address care for these patients is to use a blank care map or to develop a generic care map.

Typically, to develop a care map, a problem list is developed (Petryshen & Petryshen, 1992). One major difference that we have incorporated into our care maps is rather than starting with a patient problem list, we start with the eleven Standards of Oncology Nursing Practice (1987). These constitute the categories on the care maps. We chose this method because even if one of the outcome standards does not address a common complication of radiation therapy for a specific group of patients, it still needs to be assessed, and there needs to be a way to individualize and document on care maps, particularly for patients with other chronic diseases. For example, on the care map for patient receiving radiation to the pelvis, the cardiovascular standard is included. In addition, the use of the ONS Standards have provided a way for the care maps to become our standards of nursing care. They document when and how often to do nursing assessments and interventions and what the content of our interventions are. The care maps ensure that we provide consistency and continuity of care.

In order to decrease the size of the care maps, we have also developed formal protocols for discharge instructions at the end of treatment and for the content of the patient teaching modules. These activities are listed on the care map at the appropriate time intervals, but the nurses refer to standardized protocols kept on file for the actual content.

Clinical Use of Care Maps in Radiation Oncology

During the development of the care maps, a strong effort was made to facilitate documentation. Our goal was that all routine documentation would be done directly on the care maps and progress notes would be used only for unusual problems or in instances where more space was needed. As a result, our care maps are large, but we have been able to streamline documentation tremendously. A recent idea was to incorporate the nursing history and assessment onto the care map. This eliminates the separate nursing history form and keeps the assessment information easily available.

Incorporating our patient education program into the collaborative care model was easily accomplished. We had been participating in nursing research studies using an informational intervention to assist patients in coping with the experience of receiving radiation therapy (Johnson et al., 1987; Johnson et al., 1989). As part of one study, we had broken up our patient teaching into four modules that were given at different points in time during treatment. The purpose of breaking up the information into segments is to provide patients with the information they need, right before they need it, rather than providing it all at the start of radiation treatment. It was very simple to identify on the care maps when each of the appropriate teaching sessions was to be given (Table 24–2).

The care maps were also designed to be easily individualized. Space was included to write short notes such as what skin care products were being used or whether the patient was on a specific type of diet. Special needs can also be incorporated. For example, some breast cancer patients receive radiation treatment after a mastectomy and require range of motion assessments and exercises. Additional tests, medications, blood work, consulta-

Table 24-2 • Patient Education Sessions

Teaching Session	When	Content
Presimulation	Presimulation	General information about RT department, personnel, and resources for the patient. Sensory information about the simulation and first treatment. Overview of treatment course.
Side effects and self-care management	First week of treatment	Site-specific side effects and self-care information
Treatment completion	Last week of treatment	Resolution of side effects, common emotional reactions to finishing treatment, return to normal activities, discharge instructions
Follow-up	One-month follow-up visit	Assessment of side effects and problems, prevention and early detection activities, survivorship issues, community resources

tions, and transportation arrangements can all be written on the care map.

Care maps are meant to be working tools. In our experience, they are most helpful if they are allowed to evolve over time. The care coordinators and the collaborative care team have the authority to modify and change the care maps as their clinical practice changes. Copies of the care maps are kept on a computer disk so that changes can easily be incorporated into the printed forms.

Care Maps and Quality Improvement

The variance analysis tool is an integral component of collaborative care and has also gone through several revisions. When we developed the first care maps, we began with the care that patients were currently receiving. In other words, we did not change our care to be more efficient or to improve patient outcomes. We started by documenting what our current care was and by determining what patient outcomes we wanted to collect data on. Over time, we have been modifying our patient care using incremental changes and monitoring for changes in patient outcomes.

One of the first ideas we had for improving the efficiency of our care was to measure the number of times patients had unplanned visits or phone calls. In radiation oncology, this was difficult to measure. Because our patients come in daily, they will stop the nurses or physicians in the hall, or ask a secretary to page them whenever they need additional information or care. Patients are scheduled to meet with the physicians and nurses every week. The patient teaching sessions with the nurses are also scheduled appointments. We wanted to track how much additional time patients needed from us. These unplanned interactions interrupted scheduled activities and consumed a significant amount of nursing and secretarial time.

We began by asking the nurses to track unplanned interactions with patients on a specific variance form. Purely social interactions with patients were not included. The breast cancer care map was the first map we had implemented. We chose an arbitrary goal of ten patients for data collection and tracked data on the unplanned interactions. Our results indicated that this group of patients requested frequent additional interactions with staff. The primary reason for patients' requests were for psychosocial support. The nurses also acknowledged that they underdocumented the patient encounters—they would forget to document the encounter if the variance form was not immediately available. Therefore we assumed that the number of unplanned interactions was underestimated.

After reviewing the data, a team meeting was held to discuss ideas to reduce the number of unplanned interactions. A plan was made to have the social worker contact each breast cancer patient early in treatment, offer her services, and inform patients about the available support groups.

Data were again collected. Unfortunately, only a minimal reduction was seen. We are now looking to identify other methods of reducing unplanned visits, one of which is to include more planned patient visits with nursing staff.

Another focus of variance analysis is to improve patient outcomes. We have begun discussions about variance analysis for a new care map for patients receiving radiation to the chest. We have discussed reducing dyspnea as a patient outcome. We have some prior research data that indicates that dyspnea is a significant side effect of disease for this group of patients (King et al., 1985). We proposed whether teaching patients breathing techniques identified in the pulmonary rehabilitation literature, such as the tripod breathing position, would improve patients' perceptions of dyspnea.

Over the past year, we have also changed the way we collect variance data. Currently, instead of using a separate form, the outcomes identified for monitoring are put in boldface type on the care maps. While this practice change makes it easier for the staff to document variances, it requires a little more work for the care coordinator to track the data. Although the words *variance analysis* can cause groans among staff, it can also be quite creative and exciting to look at how such an analysis can influence patient outcomes.

Future Directions

We anticipate being able to use care maps in creative ways in the future and look forward to when they can be incorporated into a clinical information system. From a nursing management perspective, care maps might be an innovative way to develop an outpatient acuity system by monitoring the number and type of care maps in use. Many types of quality improvement activities are possible. Care maps may also be useful as data collection tools for nursing research, particularly in

Text Continued on page 420

UNIVERSITY OF ROCHESTER/STRONG MEMORIAL HOSPITAL
SMH 630
PATIENT CARE MAP

PATIENT NAME: _____ UNIT# _____
COMORBIDITIES: _____

FOR: __Breast Cancer Patients Receiving Radiation Therapy__
MD: _____ **PRIMARY NURSE:** _____
CARE COORDINATOR: _____
ALLERGIES: _____
REFERRALS: SSW _____ CHN _____ OTHER _____

IV INSERTIONS
DATE: _____ SITE: _____ TYPE: _____ BY: _____
DATE: _____ SITE: _____ TYPE: _____ BY: _____
DATE: _____ SITE: _____ TYPE: _____ BY: _____
AGE: _____ DIAGNOSIS: _____

PATIENT NEEDS	DATE Consult/Assessment	DATE Pre-Simulation	DATE 1st Week
VENTILATION	Respirations regular WNL Y N		
CIRCULATORY/NEUROLOGICAL	No evidence of lymphedema on affected side Y N B/P Cardiovascular status WNL specify Neuro status WNL specify		Lymphedema: None 1+ +2 +3

MOBILITY/SELF CARE/ MENTAL STATUS
 	
Transportation Needs:
None
Specify:
	Pt demonstrates adequate ROM of affected side Y N
	ROM instructions reviewed Y N
	Self care ability:
	    Independent Requires Asst.
	Fatigue: None Mild Moderate Severe
	Mental Status: A O X 3
		Demonstrates adequate ROM of affected side and ROM exercises Y N Plan:
		Fatigue: None Mild
		Moderate Severe
			Self care abilities: Independent
			    Requires assistance
			Fatigue: None Mild
			Moderate Severe

ELIMINATION: Bowel Renal/Bladder	Bowel movement: Baseline urination:		

COMFORT/SLEEP	Pain: None Severity
	Location:
	Management:
	Sleeping difficulty: None Plan:
		Sleeping difficulty
		    None Plan:
			Sleeping difficulty
			    None Plan:

NUTRITION	Weight: Appetite Stable → Diet: Wt change: _____ #'s Lost/gained time: _____		Comfortable at current weight Y N Plan:
PROTECTIVE MECHANISMS	Well healed lumpectomy scar	Incision well healed w/o	

SEXUAL REPRODUCTIVE	Sexually active Y N Specify Concerns about body image N Plan Hot flashes N Plan	s/s of infection Y No Δ Plan:	Discuss possible concerns r/t changes in body image

COPING	Financial concerns
	Referred to financial consultant
	Retired Employed Disability
	Support Systems:
	Psychiatric/Emotional Hx N Specify:
		Verbalizes concerns & questions
		  No Yes Plan:
		
		Anxiety level: Mild Moderate
		Severe Plan:
		Society work need/offered
		  Y N
			Verbalizes concerns & questions No Yes
			Plan:
			
			Anxiety level: Mild Moderate Severe
			Plan:
			Society work need/offered
			  Y N

INFORMATIONAL NEEDS	Informed re: SW, URCC library,
	  community resources
	Bill of Rights received
	Pt/family mutually agree to plan of care
		Presimulation teaching
		completed/written materials
		given Y N
		
		Verbalizes understanding
		  Y Plan:
			Side effect intervention completed/written
			material given #2
			  Y Plan
			
			Verbalizes understanding Y Plan
			Pt/family agree with plan of care

TESTS: Bloodwork		CBC/diff, platelet count WNL Y N NA Verbalizes understanding of planning CT Yes N/A	CBC/diff, platelet count weekly if receiving chemo/post BMT otherwise prn Y N
MEDICATIONS/TREATMENTS	Current chemo: N Specify Previous chemo: N Specify Previous Surgery: N Specify Current Meds:	Tamoxifen Y Not Planned	
PREVENTION/DETECTION	Primary MD: Alcohol use: None Occasional Specify Drug use: None Specify Annual physicals N Y BSE Y No Routine Pap Y N Mammogram Y N		Discuss possible benefit of low fat/high fiber diet
RN Signature/Initials			

UNIVERSITY OF ROCHESTER/STRONG MEMORIAL HOSPITAL
SMH 630
PATIENT CARE MAP

PATIENT NAME: _____ UNIT# _____
COMORBIDITIES: _____

FOR: _Breast Cancer Patients Receiving Radiation Therapy_
MD: _____ PRIMARY NURSE: _____
CARE COORDINATOR: _____
ALLERGIES: _____
REFERRALS: SSW _____ CHN _____ OTHER _____
AGE _____

IV INSERTIONS

DATE:	SITE:	TYPE:	BY:
DATE:	SITE:	TYPE:	BY:
DATE:	SITE:	TYPE:	BY:
DATE:	SITE:	TYPE:	BY:
DATE:	SITE:	TYPE:	BY:
DATE:	SITE:	TYPE:	BY:
DATE:	SITE:	TYPE:	BY:
DATE:	SITE:	TYPE:	BY:
DATE:	SITE:	TYPE:	BY:

PATIENT NEEDS	DATE _____ 2nd Week	DATE _____ 3rd Week	DATE _____ 4th Week
VENTILATION			
CIRCULATORY/NEUROLOGICAL	Lymphedema: None 1+ 2+ 3+ Plan:		
MOBILITY/SELF CARE/ MENTAL STATUS	Fatigue None Mild Moderate Severe	Fatigue None Mild Moderate Severe	Fatigue None Mild Moderate Severe
ELIMINATION: Bowel Renal/Bladder			
COMFORT/SLEEP	Sleeping difficulty None Plan: Breast discomfort related to treatment None Plan:	Sleeping difficulty None Plan: Breast discomfort related to treatment None Plan:	Sleeping difficulty None Plan: Breast discomfort related to treatment None Plan:
NUTRITION			
PROTECTIVE MECHANISMS	Skin Reaction None Mild Moderate Severe Moist Plan:	Skin Reaction None Mild Moderate Severe Moist Plan:	Skin Reaction None Mild Moderate Severe Moist Plan:

	Visit 1	Visit 2	Visit 3
SEXUAL REPRODUCTIVE		Hot flashes None Plan:	
COPING	Verbalizes concerns/questions Yes Plan: Anxiety Level None Mild Moderate Severe Plan:	Verbalizes concerns/questions Yes Plan: Anxiety Level None Mild Moderate Severe Plan:	Verbalizes concerns/questions Yes Plan: Anxiety Level None Mild Moderate Severe Plan:
INFORMATIONAL NEEDS	Reinforce side effect teaching	Restates self-care measures Yes Plan:	Instructed on changes in plan of care Restates self-care measures Yes Plan:
TESTS: Bloodwork	Reinforce rational for treatment planning CT		
MEDICATIONS/TREATMENTS			
PREVENTION/DETECTION			
RN Signature/Initials			

UNIVERSITY OF ROCHESTER/STRONG MEMORIAL HOSPITAL
SMH 630
PATIENT CARE MAP

PATIENT NAME: _____ UNIT# _____
COMORBIDITIES: _____

FOR: _Breast Cancer Patients Receiving Radiation Therapy_
MD: _____ PRIMARY NURSE: _____
CARE COORDINATOR: _____
ALLERGIES: _____
REFERRALS: SSW _____ CHN _____ OTHER _____

IV INSERTIONS

DATE:	SITE:	TYPE:	BY:
DATE:	SITE:	TYPE:	BY:
DATE:	SITE:	TYPE:	BY:
DATE:	SITE:	TYPE:	BY:
DATE:	SITE:	TYPE:	BY:
DATE:	SITE:	TYPE:	BY:
DATE:	SITE:	TYPE:	BY:
DATE:	SITE:	TYPE:	BY:
DATE:	SITE:	TYPE:	BY:
DATE:	SITE:	TYPE:	BY:

PATIENT NEEDS	DATE	DATE	DATE
	5th Week	6th Week	Treatment Completion
VENTILATION			
CIRCULATORY/NEUROLOGICAL			Lymphadema: None 1+ 2+ 3+ Plan:
MOBILITY/SELF CARE/ MENTAL STATUS	Fatigue None Mild Moderate Severe	Fatigue None Mild Moderate Severe	Fatigue None Mild Moderate Severe
ELIMINATION: Bowel Renal/Bladder			
COMFORT/SLEEP	Sleeping difficulty None Plan: Breast discomfort related to treatment None Plan:	Sleeping difficulty None Plan: Breast discomfort related to treatment None Plan:	Sleeping difficulty None Plan: Breast discomfort related to treatment None Plan:
NUTRITION		Comfortable at current wt. Yes Plan:	
PROTECTIVE MECHANISMS	Skin Reaction None Mild Moderate Severe	Skin Reaction None Mild Moderate Severe	Skin Reaction None Mild Moderate Severe Moist Plan:

SEXUAL REPRODUCTIVE	Moist Plan:	Moist Plan:	
		Hot flashes None Plan:	
COPING	**Pt adjusting to diagnosis &** **treatment Yes Plan:** S.O. adjusting to diagnosis & treatment Yes Plan:	**Pt adjusting to diagnosis & treatment** **Yes Plan:** S.O. adjusting to diagnosis & treatment Yes Plan:	**Pt able to verbalize feelings and ask questions** **Discuss emotional impact of treatment ending**

INFORMATIONAL NEEDS	Restates self-care measures	Restates self-care measures	Intervention # 3 completed
			 Pt. verbalizes
			   Plan for follow-up
			   Symptoms to report

TESTS: Bloodwork			
MEDICATIONS/TREATMENTS			Follow-up in medical oncology Y N Date of appointment _____
PREVENTION/DETECTION			
RN Signature/Initials			

411

UNIVERSITY OF ROCHESTER/STRONG MEMORIAL HOSPITAL
SMH 630
PATIENT CARE MAP

PATIENT NAME: _____ UNIT# _____
COMORBIDITIES: _____

FOR: ___ Breast Cancer Patients Receiving Radiation Therapy ___
MD: _____ PRIMARY NURSE: _____
CARE COORDINATOR: _____
ALLERGIES: _____
REFERRALS: SSW _____ CHN _____ OTHER _____

IV INSERTIONS
DATE: _____ SITE: _____ TYPE: _____ BY: _____
DATE: _____ SITE: _____ TYPE: _____ BY: _____
DATE: _____ SITE: _____ TYPE: _____ BY: _____
DATE: _____ SITE: _____ TYPE: _____ BY: _____
DATE: _____ SITE: _____ TYPE: _____ BY: _____
DATE: _____ SITE: _____ TYPE: _____ BY: _____
DATE: _____ SITE: _____ TYPE: _____ BY: _____
DATE: _____ SITE: _____ TYPE: _____ BY: _____
DATE: _____ SITE: _____ TYPE: _____ BY: _____

PATIENT NEEDS	DATE 1st F/U Visit	DATE	DATE
VENTILATION			
CIRCULATORY/NEUROLOGICAL	Lymphedema Y N		
MOBILITY/SELF CARE/ MENTAL STATUS	Fatigue None Mild Moderate Severe		
ELIMINATION: Bowel Renal/Bladder			
COMFORT/SLEEP	Sleeping difficulty None Plan: Breast discomfort related to treatment None Plan:		
NUTRITION	Comfortable at current wt Y Plan:		

412

PROTECTIVE MECHANISMS	Skin Reaction Resolved Plan:					
SEXUAL REPRODUCTIVE	Discuss concerns related to sexuality after treatment completion Returning to role functions					
COPING	Reinforce availability of support groups Discuss survivorship issues Return to normal activities Y N					

INFORMATIONAL NEEDS	Follow-up intervention completed
	Pt. verbalizes
	  plan for follow-up
	  community resources					

TESTS: Bloodwork						
MEDICATIONS/TREATMENTS						
PREVENTION/DETECTION	BSE demonstrated correctly Y N Reinforce importance of BSE/ mammograms schedule Reinforce possible benefits of low fat/high fiber diet.					
RN Signature/Initials						

University of Rochester Cancer Center / Strong Memorial Hospital

SMH 630

Patient Care Map

				IV therapy		
Patient Name:	Age:	Unit #				
Comorbidities:						

Patient Name: _____ Age: ____ Unit # _____   Date: _____ Site: _____ Type: _____ Site ✓ Patency: _____ By: _____
                                                      Date: _____ Site: _____ Type: _____ Site ✓ Patency: _____ By: _____
                                                      Date: _____ Site: _____ Type: _____ Site ✓ Patency: _____ By: _____
                                                      Date: _____ Site: _____ Type: _____ Site ✓ Patency: _____ By: _____

For: Patients receiving Radiation Therapy to the Pelvis:

MD: _____ Primary Nurse: _____ Age: ____

Care Coordinator: _____ Diagnosis: _____

Allergies: _____

Referrals: SW: ____ CHN ____ Other: ____

	Pre Simulation Assessment Date:	Week #1 Date:	Week #2 Date:
Ventilation	R ____ SOB ☐ N ☐Specify Cough ☐ N ☐Specify Oxygen ☐ N ☐Specify Smoking Hx: ☐ N ☐Specify		
Circulatory/ Neurological	BP ____ P ____ Cardiovascular Status WNL Specify Neuro Status WNL Specify		
Mobility/ Self Care/ Mental Status	Self care ability: Independent Requires Assistance Fatigue: None Mild Moderate Severe Transportation Needs: None Specify Mental Status: A&O x3	Fatigue: ☐ None ☐Mild ☐Moderate ☐Severe Verbalizes methods to manage fatigue. Neuro Status WNL Y N No △	Fatigue: ☐ None ☐Mild ☐Moderate ☐Severe Verbalizes methods to manage fatigue. Neuro Status WNL Y N No △
Elimination: Bowel Bladder	Baseline bowel movements: Baseline urination:	Bowel fx WNL ☐ Y ☐N ☐No △ Bladder fx WNL ☐ Y ☐N ☐No △	Bowel fx WNL ☐ Y ☐N ☐No △ Bladder fx WNL ☐ Y ☐N ☐No △
Comfort/ Sleep	Pain: None Severity: ____ Location: ____ Management: Simulation: ☐Tolerated ☐Specify: Sleeping difficulty: None Plan:	Pain: ☐ Absent ☐ Stable ☐ ↑ ☐ ↓ Management Plan: ☐N/A ☐Continue ☐△ Sleeping pattern WNL ☐Y ☐N ☐No △	Pain: ☐ Absent ☐ Stable ☐ ↑ ☐ ↓ Management Plan: ☐N/A ☐Continue ☐△ RT tx administered w/o discomfort. Sleeping pattern WNL ☐ Y ☐N ☐No △
Nutrition	Wt ____ Appetite ☐Stable ☐ ↓ Diet: Wt change: ____ #'s lost gained time: ____ Nausea / Vomiting ☐ None Stable ☐Specify:	Wt ☐ Stable ____↓ lb. ____↑lb. Appetite ☐Stable ☐ ↓ Nausea / Vomiting ☐None ☐Stable ☐Specify:	Wt ☐ Stable ____↓ lb. ____↑lb. Appetite ☐Stable ☐ ↓ Nausea / Vomiting ☐None ☐ Stable ☐Specify: Low fiber required Y N

Category	Assessment/Interventions	Outcomes	Outcomes
Protective Mechanisms	Afebrile □Y □Specify Skin Intact: □ Y □Specify	Skin Intact □ Y □N □Specify Erythema: □None □ Mild □ Moderate □Severe Skin Care:	Skin Intact □ Y □N □Specify Erythema: □None□ Mild□ Moderate □Severe Skin Care:
Sexual/ Reproductive	Sexuality/ Reproductive concerns □ N □Specify Potential Alopecia □ N □Specify Concerns about body image □N □Specify	Pt. verbalizes understanding of RT impact on sexual function. "Sexuality and You" booklet given.	
Coping	Financial Concerns: None Referred to financial counselor Retired Employed Disability Support System :_____ Psychiatric/Emotional Hx □ N □Specify	Patient able to verbalize feelings and ask questions Exhibiting adequate adjustment to tx and dx. Social Work Referral □ Y □N/A	Patient able to verbalize feelings and ask questions Exhibiting adequate adjustment to tx and dx.
Informational Needs	Pre sim teaching completed Informed re: SW,URCC library, community resources Bill of Rights received. Pt/family mutually agree to plan of care	Side effect teaching completed & written information given. Pt verbalizes understanding.	Restates appropriate side effect management.
Tests: Bloodwork	CBC w/plt & diff □ Y □N □N/A SMA 6 & 12 & Aly □ Y □N □N/A		
Medications/ Treatments RT Field	Concurrent Chemo: □ None □Specify Previous Chemo □ None □Specify Previous Surgery □ None □Specify Hormone Tx: None Specify Current Meds:	Pt verbalizes understanding of rationale for RT Tx with full bladder. Y N NA	
Prevention/ Early Detection	Recent exposure to communicable disease: None Primary MD:_____ Alcohol Use: None Occasional Specify: Drug Use: None Specify: Annual Physicals □ N □Y BSE/ TSE □Y □N Routine Pap □ Y □N □N/A Mammogram□ Y □N □N/A		
RN Signature			

SMH 630
Patient Care Map

Date:	Site:	Type:	By:

Patient Name: _____ Unit # _____

Date:	Site:	Type:	By:

Comorbidities: _____

Date:	Site:	Type:	By:

For: Patients receiving Radiation Therapy to the Pelvis:

Date:	Site:	Type:	By:

MD: _____ Primary Nurse: _____ Age: _____

Care Coordinator: _____ Diagnosis: _____

Allergies: _____

Referrals: SW: _____ CHN _____ Other: _____

	Week #3 Date:	Week #4 Date:	Week #5 Date:
Ventilation			
Circulatory/ Neurological			
Mobility/Self Care/ Mental Status	Fatigue: ☐ None ☐Mild ☐Moderate ☐Severe Verbalizes methods to manage fatigue. Neuro status WNL Y N No Δ	Fatigue: ☐ None ☐Mild ☐Moderate ☐Severe Verbalizes methods to manage fatigue. Neuro status WNL Y N No Δ	Fatigue: ☐ None ☐Mild ☐Moderate ☐Severe Verbalizes methods to manage fatigue. Neuro status WNL Y N No Δ
Elimination: Bowel	Bowel fx WNL ☐ Y ☐N ☐No Δ	Bowel fx WNL ☐ Y ☐N ☐No Δ	Bowel fx WNL ☐ Y ☐N ☐No Δ
Bladder	Bladder fx WNL ☐ Y ☐N ☐No Δ Pt verbalizes methods to manage Δ's in bowel and bladder habits Y N	Bladder fx WNL ☐ Y ☐N ☐No Δ	Bladder fx WNL ☐ Y ☐N ☐No Δ
Comfort/ Sleep	Pain: ☐ Absent ☐ Stable ☐ ↑ ☐ ↓ Management Plan: ☐N/A ☐Continue ☐Δ RT tx administered w/o discomfort. Sleeping pattern WNL ☐ Y ☐N ☐No Δ	Pain: ☐ Absent ☐ Stable ☐ ↑ ☐ ↓ Management Plan: ☐N/A ☐Continue ☐Δ RT tx administered w/o discomfort. Sleeping pattern WNL ☐ Y ☐N ☐No Δ	Pain: ☐ Absent ☐ Stable ☐ ↑ ☐ ↓ Management Plan: ☐N/A ☐Continue ☐Δ RT tx administered w/o discomfort. Sleeping pattern WNL ☐ Y ☐N ☐No Δ

Nutrition	Wt □ Stable ↓ lb. □ ↑lb. Appetite □Stable Nausea / Vomiting □None □ Stable □Specify: Low fiber diet required Y N	Wt □ Stable ↓ lb. □ ↑lb. Appetite □Stable Nausea / Vomiting □None □ Stable □Specify: Low fiber diet required Y N	Wt □ Stable ↓ lb. □ ↑lb. Appetite □Stable Nausea / Vomiting □None □ Stable □Specify: Low fiber diet required Y N		
Protective Mechanisms	Skin Intact □ Y □No Δ □ Specify Erythema: □None □ Mild □ Moderate □Severe Skin Care:	Skin Intact □ Y □No Δ □ Specify Erythema: □None□ Mild□ Moderate □Severe Skin Care:	Skin Intact □ Y □No Δ □Specify Erythema: □None □ Mild □ Moderate □Severe Skin Care:		
Sexual/ Reproductive					
Coping	Patient able to verbalize feelings and ask questions Exhibiting adequate adjustment to tx and dx.	Patient able to verbalize feelings and ask questions Exhibiting adequate adjustment to tx and dx.	Patient continuing to adjust to dx and prognosis.		
Informational Needs	Restates appropriate side effect management.	Restates appropriate side effect management.	Restates appropriate side effect management.		
Tests: Bloodwork					
Medications/ Treatments					
Prevention/ Early Detection					
RN Signature					

University of Rochester Cancer Center / Strong Memorial Hospital
SMH 630
Patient Care Map
Patient Name: _____ Unit # _____
Comorbidities: _____
For: **Patients receiving Radiation Therapy to the Pelvis:**
MD: _____ Primary Nurse: _____
Care Coordinator: _____ Diagnosis: _____
Allergies: _____
Referrals: SW: _____ CHN _____ Other: _____

IV therapy

Date: _____	Site: _____	Type: _____	Patency: _____	By: _____
Date: _____	Site: _____	Type: _____	Patency: _____	By: _____
Date: _____	Site: _____	Type: _____	Patency: _____	By: _____
Date: _____	Site: _____	Type: _____	Patency: _____	By: _____
	Site ✓			
	Site ✓			
	Site ✓			
	Site ✓			

Age: _____

	Week #6 Date:	Treatment Completion Week #7 Date:	First Follow up
Ventilation			
Circulatory/ Neurological			
Mobility/ Self Care/ Mental Status	Fatigue: ☐ None ☐Mild ☐Moderate ☐Severe Verbalizes methods to manage fatigue.	Fatigue: ☐ None ☐Mild ☐Moderate ☐Severe Verbalizes methods to manage fatigue. Neuro Status WNL Y N No △	Fatigue: ☐ None ☐Mild ☐Moderate ☐Severe Verbalizes methods to manage fatigue. Neuro Status WNL Y N No △
Elimination: Bowel	Bowel fx WNL ☐Y ☐N ☐No △	Bowel fx WNL ☐Y ☐N ☐No △	Bowel fx WNL ☐Y ☐N ☐No △
Bladder	Bladder fx WNL ☐Y ☐N ☐No △	Bladder fx WNL ☐Y ☐N ☐No △	Bladder fx WNL ☐Y ☐N ☐No △
Comfort/ Sleep	**Pain: ☐ Absent** ☐ Stable ☐↑ ☐↓ Management Plan: ☐N/A ☐Continue ☐△ RT tx administered w/o discomfort. Sleeping pattern WNL ☐ Y ☐N ☐No △	RT tx administered w/o discomfort. Evaluate Overall Pain Management: ☐Not required ☐Unchanged through treatment ☐Initiated during treatment **☐Revised during treatment** Managed by: ☐RT ☐PCP ☐PTC ☐MO Sleeping pattern WNL ☐ Y ☐N ☐No △	Pain: ☐ None ☐ Stable ☐↑ ☐↓ Management Plan: ☐N/A ☐Continue ☐△ Sleeping pattern WNL ☐ Y ☐N ☐No △
Nutrition	Wt ☐ Stable ↓ lb. _____ ↑lb. Appetite ☐Stable ☐↓ Nausea / Vomiting ☐None ☐ No △ ☐Specify: Low fiber diet required Y N	Wt ☐ Stable ↓ lb. _____ ↑lb. Appetite ☐Stable ☐↓ Nausea / Vomiting ☐None ☐ No △ ☐Specify: Low fiber diet required Y N	Wt ☐ Stable ↓ lb. _____ ↑lb. Appetite ☐Stable ☐↓ Nausea / Vomiting ☐None ☐ No △ ☐Specify: Tolerating regular diet Y N

418

	Column 1	Column 2	Column 3
Protective Mechanisms	Skin Intact ☐ Y ☐ No Δ ☐ Specify Erythema: ☐None ☐ Mild ☐ Moderate ☐Severe Skin Care:	Skin Intact ☐ Y ☐No Δ ☐ Specify Erythema: ☐None ☐ Mild ☐ Moderate ☐Severe Skin Care:	Skin Intact ☐ Y ☐ No Δ ☐Specify Erythema: ☐None ☐ Mild ☐ Moderate ☐Severe Skin Care:
Sexual/ Reproductive		Discuss concerns r/t sexuality post - RT Pt comfortable with current sexual function	Verbalizes undeerstanding of long term effects of RT on sexual function Vaginal dilator teaching done Y N NA
Coping	Patient able to verbalize feelings and ask questions Exhibiting adequate adjustment to tx and dx.	Patient able to verbalize feelings and ask questions Exhibiting adequate adjustment to tx and dx.	Patient able to verbalize feelngs and ask questions. Exhibiting adequate adequate adjustment to dx and prognosis.
Informational Needs	Restates appropriate side effect management.	Treatment completion teaching done (i.e. resolution of side effect, reaction to end of tx, return to normal diet and activities) Pt verbalizes understanding Y N	Follow up intervention completed. Y N See RT follow up protocol.
Tests: Bloodwork			PSA Y N NA CBC w/plt & diff Y N NA
Medications/ Treatments			
Prevention/Early Detection			Verbalizes understanding of rationale for f/u visits, screening Y N
RN Signature			

the area of symptom management. Linked with inpatient care maps, they can serve to direct patient care across the continuum of patient care and can be the core of developing work redesign projects that combine inpatient and outpatient care into one unit. Although predicting what will happen in the future related to health care systems is very risky, collaborative care and care maps are here to stay.

References

Ferguson LE. (1993). Steps to developing a critical pathway. *Nursing Administration Quarterly, 17,* 58–62.

Giuliano KK, Poirier CE. (1991). Nursing case management: Critical pathways to desirable outcomes. *Nursing Management, 22,* 52–55.

Johnson JE, Lauver D, Nail LM. (1989). Process of coping with radiation therapy. *Journal of Consulting and Clinical Psychology, 57,* 358–364.

Johnson JE, Nail LM, Lauver D, King KB, Keys H. (1987). Reducing the negative impact of radiation therapy on functional status. *Cancer, 61,* 46–51.

Jones RA, Mullikin CW. (1994). Collaborative care: Pathways to quality outcomes. *Journal for Healthcare Quality, 16,* 10–13.

Oncology Nursing Society (1987). Standards of oncology nursing practice. Pittsburgh: Author.

Petryshen PR, Petryshen PM. (1992). The case management model: An innovative approach to the delivery of patient care. *Journal of Advanced Nursing, 17,* 1188–1194.

Strong Memorial Hospital. (1994). Collaborative care manual. Rochester, NY: Strong Memorial Hospital.

University of Rochester Cancer Center. (1993). Collaborative care manual. Rochester, NY: University of Rochester Cancer Center.

Nursing Research
in Radiation Oncology

KAREN HASSEY DOW

Overview of Oncology Nursing Research

Nursing research is defined as the scientific investigation of questions related to the diagnosis and treatment of human responses to actual or potential health problems (Burns & Grove, 1993; Hinshaw, 1988; Merritt, 1986). This scientific inquiry includes an examination of the fundamental biomedical and behavioral processes relevant to nursing and to the various aspects of the nursing process involved in caring for patients. Nursing research focuses on problems of patients as they respond to their disease and to treatment. The specialty of oncology provides an excellent background for the conduct of nursing research. Although nursing research is in its infancy when compared to biomedical research, there continues to be a steady improvement of clinically relevant studies conducted within the specialty of oncology nursing. This development has led to the need to develop depth in research and to target high priority areas of research. Since 1978, top research priorities for cancer nursing research priorities have been published (Grant & Stromborg, 1981; McGuire et al., 1985). A comparative listing of research priorities from 1981 to 1995 are listed in Table 25-1.

Role of the Radiation Oncology Nurse in Research

The specialty of radiation oncology nursing has developed significantly over the past 20 years (Hilderley, 1980). In 1989 the Radiation Special Interest Group (SIG) became one of the first eleven SIGs approved by the Oncology Nursing Society (ONS). Starting with 137 initial members, the Radiation SIG now has 423 members, (C. De-Marco, Oncology Nursing Society, personal communication, 1996). Radiation oncology nurses were organized to provide support, foster professional development and education, and develop guidelines for care of patients receiving radiation therapy. In addition, there have been several SIG-associated research activities including skin care protocol management. In addition, a research work group is working to develop a research plan using ideas from a Radiation SIG patient education survey (Radiation SIG, 1996).

Many early oncology nursing studies conducted within radiation or with radiation patients were largely descriptive studies. Sources for identification of relevant studies include the Cumulative Index to Nursing and Allied Health Literature (CINAHL) and research abstracts from relevant oncology meetings. The following section contains a synopsis of published studies related to radiation oncology. These studies are clustered around the topics of information, education, symptom management, and late effects and survivorship issues. Identified areas of self-care management, intervention, and research utilization are also covered.

Studies Conducted in Radiation Therapy

Information

Dodd and Ahmed (1987) determined preferred type of information (cognitive versus behavioral) among patients starting a course of radiation therapy. Using a longitudinal research design, 60

Table 25-1 • Comparison of Oncology Nursing Society's Top Ten Research Priorities—1988–1995

1988	1991	1995
Prevention and early detection	Quality of life	Pain
Symptom management	Symptom management	Cancer prevention
Pain control and management	Outcome measures for intervention	Quality of life
Patient/health education	Pain control and management	Risk reduction/cancer screening
Coping and stress management	Cancer survivorship	Ethical issues
Home care	Prevention and early detection	Neutropenia/immunosuppression
Economic influences	Research utilization	Patient education
Cancer rehabilitation	Cost containment	Stress, coping, adaptation
AIDS	Economic influences	Cancer detection
Compliance with treatment	Family issues	Cost containment

Data from SW Funkhouser & MM Grant. (1989). ONS survey of research priorities. *Oncology Nursing Forum 16*(3), 413–416. K Mooney, B Ferrell, L Nail, S Benedict, & M Haberman. (1991). Oncology Nursing Society research priorities survey. *Oncology Nursing Forum 18*(8): 1381–1390. K Stetz, M Haberman, J Holcombe, & L Jones. (1995). 1994 Oncology Nursing Society research priorities. *Oncology Nursing Forum 22*(5):785–789.

subjects were interviewed at the start and end of radiation. The investigators used the Health Opinion Survey and the Health Care Preference Survey to determine subjects' preference for type of information. Findings revealed that the majority of subjects (n = 38) preferred cognitive information. In addition, control, anxiety, and demographic variables were significantly associated with the preference for type of information. The investigators concluded that there was need for additional research to evaluate how to better measure the complexities in information preferences.

With the increased use of breast-conserving surgery and radiation therapy for breast cancer, Harrison-Woermke and Graydon (1993) assessed perceived informational needs of breast cancer patients receiving radiation therapy after breast-conserving surgery. Two groups of 20 subjects (women receiving radiation therapy during the first week and women who had completed their radiation course) were interviewed using an investigator-developed Information Needs Questionnaire (INQ). The INQ assessed women's informational needs about diagnosis, investigative tests, treatment, physical and psychological functioning, family, and financial resources. Although subjects in both groups reported informational needs across the seven domains, they scored highest in the need for information on treatment and physical effects. Results suggest that during the illness experience, women seek specific information about their treatment and care and provide a research basis for developing targeted information.

In another study of information, preferences or choice concerning treatment were evaluated (Ward et al., 1989). The investigators interviewed 22 women who had a choice of receiving either modified radical mastectomy (MRM) or breast-conserving surgery (BC) for stage I or II breast cancer. Half of the women preferred modified radical mastectomy and the other half selected breast-conserving surgery. Findings relevant to the role of the radiation nurse focus on the perceptions of the patients in both groups regarding radiation therapy, and the nature and kind of information the patient used in decision making. Concern about radiation therapy was the first reason expressed by subjects in the MRM group (p = 0.003) compared with desire to maintain body integrity identified by subjects in the BC group (p = 0.04). Additional factors identified by patients selecting BC included equal survival rates for the two types of surgery, concern about losing a breast, and feasibility of breast reconstruction. An additional trend in the BC group revealed concern for the partner's feelings about breast removal. Patients in both groups wanted to be involved in the decision-making process, and there was a trend for patients who chose MRM to want the decision to be fully their own and for women who chose BC to want to share the decision with someone else. Findings revealed that the physician and nurse, in that order, were the most frequently identified sources of information used in the decision-making process. In addition, people sources were considered more important than other sources, such as reading materials, television and radio, and visual materials.

A comparison of responses of younger and older patients undergoing radiation therapy was the focus of another study by Campbell-Forsyth (1990). The purpose of this study was to compare differences in perceived knowledge and perceived learning needs about radiation treatment both between and within younger and older age groups. Forty subjects between the ages of 25 and 39 were compared with 40 subjects between the ages of 60 and 83. No significant differences were found in relation to overall perceived knowledge and in overall perceived learning needs about radiation therapy between older and younger patients. Results of this study pose interesting concerns and deserve further examination. Because age-related concerns are often noted in the clinical setting, it would be helpful to conduct additional studies using larger numbers of subjects across a multitude of radiation settings.

Education

A series of studies have been conducted evaluating different educational approaches to side effect management in radiation therapy patients. One of the first publications of this group reported on the ability of patients to learn facts about radiation therapy via a slide-tape program (Israel & Mood, 1982). The three slide-tape presentations developed focused on a pretreatment orientation, common side effects, and usual emotional reactions. The therapy time period for which these three slide-tape series was developed corresponded to the first week of therapy, the third week of therapy, and just before the end of therapy. The tapes were used in teaching 36 radiation therapy patients of varying ages, ethnicity, and prognoses. Results were measured via patients' answers to standardized knowledge questions posed by the data collectors. In general, results indicated that the audiovisual tapes were effective in teaching radiation therapy patients information about treatment and self-care. In addition, anecdotal information revealed that the patients were interested in the learning sessions and learned a lot about treatment and self-care. Additional studies were conducted by Mood et al. (1986) to test the impact of this approach versus other educational interventions on increasing patients' self-care behaviors.

Hagopian (1991) also investigated the effects of a weekly radiation therapy newsletter on patients' knowledge, self-care behaviors, and side effect outcomes. She used a posttest-only control group design and found that subjects who read the newsletter scored significantly higher on the knowledge test. However, there were no significant differences in helpfulness or number of self-care behaviors or severity of side effects. She concluded that patient education via newsletter can be beneficial in reducing anxiety.

Patients undergoing pelvic radiation were tested by another group of investigators to determine the impact of educational approaches on patients' compliance with the treatment plan and with recommended health maintenance behaviors (Padilla & Grant, 1987). A self-directed audiovisual slide-tape learning program was compared with a nurse-directed nurse-patient discussion of the same material. Content included general information on radiation therapy as well as self-care activities related to lifestyle, nutrition and hydration, skin, stress and tension, sexual concerns, and pain. The 190 subjects were randomized into 62 self-directed participants, 63 nurse-directed participants, and 65 controls. Initial analysis of variance revealed a main effect for the type of education program ($p = 0.001$), with the self-directed group missing the least number of appointments and the control group missing the most. Accurate records of side effects and related health maintenance behaviors occurred more significantly in the nurse-directed group ($p = 0.02$). Compliance with general health maintenance prescriptions was significantly higher for the self-directed group than for the nurse-directed or control groups ($p = 0.03$). From these initial findings it appears that both self-directed and nurse-directed patient education approaches show beginning effectiveness in helping patients comply with treatment regimens and recommended health maintenance behaviors during radiation therapy.

More recently, Llewellyn-Thomas et al. (1995) assessed the effects of two teaching approaches about a clinical trial in relationship to patient satisfaction, information understanding, and decisions about entering a clinical trial. One hundred patients receiving radiation therapy were randomized to receive information about a hypothetical trial into one of two groups: audiotape or interactive computer instruction. Their information understanding was evaluated one day later. Subjects' method satisfaction and decisions as to whether they would enter a trial were assessed. Results showed that there was no difference between the groups in terms of understanding or satisfaction. Subjects in the computer instruction group were found to have a more positive attitude toward entering a trial than the audiotaped instruction group. Results indicated that teaching using interactive video may not adversely affect accrual into clinical trials.

Poroch (1995) tested the effectiveness of preparatory patient education in reducing anxiety and improving satisfaction among adult Australian patients during radiation treatment. Using a quasi-experimental design, the investigator compared two groups of 25 patients who were starting the first course of radiation treatment. Based on Johnson's framework on preparatory information, the experimental group received two structured teaching interventions that incorporated sensory and procedural information. The control group received standard teaching information. The Spielberger State-Trait Anxiety Inventory (STAI) and the Pienschke Patient Satisfaction Questionnaire (PPSQ) were used. Results showed that the experimental group was significantly less anxious and more satisfied during radiation treatment when compared to their control group counterparts. In addition, the effects of the preparatory patient education was consistent throughout a seven-week treatment period.

Patient Experiences During Radiation

Historically, patients have voiced many concerns about receiving radiation therapy, and several studies were conducted to describe the radiation therapy experience from the patient's perspective. As early as 1984, Kubricht used a descriptive survey design to identify therapeutic self-care demands expressed by outpatients receiving radiation therapy (Kubricht, 1984). Using an open-ended interview, 30 participants were asked to express changes that had occurred in their lives since the beginning of radiation therapy. Orem's self-care model was used as the study framework. Results revealed the following specific concerns in descending order: tiredness or fatigue, awareness of mortality, belief in a supreme being, the need to rest, depression, loss of appetite, loss of weight, cough, being careful not to wash off the red lines (markings), skin redness and dryness, diarrhea, inability to do things he or she used to do, pushing oneself to be with friends, and shortness of breath. It is interesting to note that this initial descriptive survey outlined an array of concerns ranging from physical (tiredness, fatigue, loss of appetite) to psychological (interference with social activities) to spiritual (awareness of mortality, belief in a supreme being) that are enduring concerns of patients receiving radiation therapy today.

In a study by King et al. (1985), 106 patients undergoing radiation therapy were interviewed weekly during treatment and monthly for 3 months after treatment. The purpose of the study was to describe symptoms experienced by radiation therapy patients during and following treatment. Subjects rated the following symptoms

weekly on a five-point Likert scale: sleep difficulties, fatigue, skin changes, anorexia, nausea, vomiting, indigestion, diarrhea, constipation, sore throat, cough, difficulty swallowing, and changes in saliva. The primary symptom experienced by all of the patients was fatigue, and this symptom persisted in a large number of subjects until 3 months after treatment ended. These results supported the frequent occurrence of fatigue initially reported by Haylock and Hart (1979). In addition, fatigue research continues as a major research priority within oncology nursing.

In a prospective, longitudinal study, Larson et al. (1993) examined differences between older (<65 years) and younger patients with lung cancer receiving radiation therapy. Results indicated that there was no statistically significant differences between the two groups based on caloric intake, adequacy of energy intake, total radiation dose, concurrent illnesses, and social support. In addition, there were no outcome differences in weight, body mass index, and multidimensional functional status. Results also suggested that subjects with lower social support perceived themselves to have better functional status. There was no relationship found between social support and functional status in the younger patients. Findings suggest that chronological age alone may not be a sufficient factor in making decisions about treatment or as a predictor for side effects.

Nutrition

Nutrition problems are among the most frequent and difficult challenges of nurses working with radiation therapy patients. Several studies have reflected this area of concern. In an exploratory study of 24 patients receiving radiation therapy to the chest and abdomen, Welch (1980) examined radiation-related nausea and vomiting. Seventy-nine percent of subjects reported some degree of nausea and vomiting. Antiemetics were used by some of the patients but were not consistently used to prevent these symptoms and were more likely to be used as needed or on a once-daily basis. Examination of potential predictive factors revealed that patients who had recurrent disease, who received their therapy earlier in the day, and who had a larger cumulative dose of radiation over a longer number of treatment days were most likely to experience nausea and vomiting. Patients identified specific nursing approaches that would best help them with nausea and vomiting management, and high ratings occurred for receiving instructions about what to eat and what not to eat and for having the nurse explain why these symptoms occur. In the intervening years since this study was first published, the increased use of serotonin antagonists as standard antiemetic treatment have helped to decrease nausea and vomiting among patients receiving chemotherapy. Less attention has focused on the use of serotonin antagonists in radiation-induced emesis.

In a longitudinal study of patterns of anorexia occurring in head and neck cancer patients undergoing radiation therapy, appetite scores were rated by patients on a 100-mm analog scale (Grant et al., 1991). At the beginning of radiation therapy, scores were already depressed from normal (mean score of 50 on the 100-point scale) but deteriorated during therapy, reaching a low mean score of 40 by the end of treatment. By the 3-month follow-up visit, scores had begun to return to normal but were still below the scores at the beginning of therapy. By the 18-month follow-up visit, appetite scores were above (mean score of 65) pretreatment scores but had not yet returned to appetite scores before disease. These findings illustrate the persistent pattern of anorexia in head and neck cancer patients and point to the need for nutritional counseling and coaching to prevent and manage undesired weight loss.

For this same group of patients, oral problems are common and may lead to profound nutrition problems. Dudjak (1987) compared two protocols for oral care for patients undergoing head and neck radiation therapy. Fifteen patients were randomly assigned to one of two specific mouth care protocols: half-strength hydrogen peroxide or a solution of baking soda and water. Stomatitis ratings included the physical condition of the mouth and the perception of mouth comfort by the patient. Findings revealed no differences between groups on physical condition but significantly lower scores on perception of mouth comfort by the hydrogen peroxide group. Study findings need replication in larger populations of patients.

Skin Care Management

Radiation skin reactions present continuing challenges for nurses and patients. Numerous skin preparations and dressings have been used to care for various levels of skin reactions, from dry desquamation to open draining wounds. One of the earliest published studies on skin care management was a prospective randomized trial on the use of moisture vapor permeable (MVP) dressings for patients with moderately severe skin reactions ranging from dry scaling desquamation

and brisk erythema to severe reactions consisting of vesicle formation, moist desquamation, full-thickness skin loss, and pronounced erythema (Shell et al., 1986). Twenty-one patients were followed—five with moderately severe reactions and sixteen with severe reactions. Patients were randomized to either the MVP dressing or a hydrous lanolin gauze group. Five patients were eliminated from the study because of significant wound complications. Wounds were rated for wound severity and grade, color and character of exudate, and leukocyte counts. Data were analyzed for healing rate indicated by the number of days to the complete return of skin integrity. The MVP group healed on an average of 19 days versus the gauze group with an average of 24 days. This difference, however, was not statistically significant. Results may be related to the small sample size, and trends in shorter healing time for the MVP group point to the need for larger-scale replication studies.

In a noncomparative descriptive study of 20 patients using hydrocolloid occlusive dressings, Margolin et al. (1990) investigated whether moist occlusive healing would be beneficial. Factors evaluated included healing time, safety, wound temperature, bacterial growth, and comfort. Data were collected by a variety of means: photographs, bacterial cultures, temperature probes, and patient evaluation. Results showed that the mean healing time was 12 days with a mean wound temperature relative to body core temperature of $-0.8°C$ on day 1 and $-1.2°C$ on the healed site. Fifteen patients reported that comfort was either excellent or good. The results of this study showed that the use of a hydrocolloid occlusive dressing can be an effective aid in healing moist skin reactions to radiation therapy, and study results warrant further exploration of the problem of skin care management.

Fatigue

Fatigue as a research area of interest was first identified by Haylock and Hart (1979) in a seminal study of patients receiving radiation therapy. Since that time, several multisite investigations have been conducted evaluating fatigue among cancer patients.

Graydon (1994) assessed the quality of life of 53 women having breast-conserving surgery and radiation therapy for breast cancer. She interviewed the women a mean of 7 weeks after radiation therapy based on the following parameters: function (Sickness Impact Profile), emotional distress (Profile of Mood States), and symptoms

(Symptom Distress Scale). Results showed that the women did not report significant emotional distress or symptoms. However, they experienced significant fatigue. Subjects with the greatest fatigue had the most reported symptoms and the poorest level of functioning.

In a follow-up study, Graydon et al. (1995) sought to determine which strategies were most effective in relieving fatigue among women receiving either chemotherapy or radiation therapy. Ninety-nine subjects were interviewed at two time points to evaluate their level of fatigue and the effectiveness of strategies they used to relieve fatigue. Women receiving radiation therapy were interviewed at the start and end of their radiation therapy. Subjects completed the Pearson Byars Fatigue Feeling Checklist and the Fatigue Relief Scale. At the second time point, subjects reported significantly more fatigue than at the first time point (p < 0.0001). Results showed that subjects used similar fatigue-reducing strategies at both time points: sleep and exercise. However, the study investigators noted a wide range of variability as to the effectiveness of the strategies. Results are preliminary and suggest two potential strategies that clinical nurses can use to reduce fatigue during treatment.

Mock et al. (1996) evaluated the effects of a walking exercise program for women with breast cancer who were receiving radiation therapy after breast-conserving surgery. Using an experimental design, they tested the hypothesis that women who participated in a walking exercise program would have higher levels of physical functioning, lower levels of symptom intensity, and higher quality of life than women who did not participate in the exercise program. The experimental intervention was a progressive, regular (4 to 5 times per week) self-paced program consisting of a brisk, incremental 10- to 45-minute walk, plus cool-down. A convenience sample of 50 women aged 35 to 65 (mean age: 49 years) was stratified according to type of medical treatment and randomly assigned to the experimental program (EX) or usual care (UC). A telephone intervention was used to monitor subjects' responses to exercise and to encourage adherence. Data were collected before treatment, midway through treatment, and at the end of radiation therapy. Instruments included the 12-Minute Walk Test, Symptom Assessment Scales, Piper Fatigue Scale, and Ferrans and Powers Quality of Life Index. In addition the Dow Adaptation Profile was given to subjects at the completion of treatment. Results indicated improved physical performance, decreased symptom

intensity, and higher quality of life in the exercise group. Study results demonstrated that breast cancer patients receiving radiation therapy may safely acquire physical and psychosocial benefit from a modest exercise program.

Coping and Comfort

Patients undergoing radiation therapy may experience anxiety and tension related to both the disease and the therapy. A responsibility of nursing care during therapy is to increase the patient's comfort and to ease tension and anxiety. Several studies have focused on patients' emotional responses during radiation therapy.

In a study of 84 patients undergoing radiation therapy for prostate cancer, Johnson et al. (1989) tested the effects of an information intervention on outcomes of coping with radiation therapy. The randomly assigned intervention included descriptions of the experience in concrete, objective terms. Results were analyzed to test two theories: the self-regulation theory and the emotional-drive theory. Findings supported self-regulation theory, illustrated by significantly lower scores on disruption in recreation and pastime activities in the experimental group. This finding is consistent with previous research of these investigators and supports the use of information interventions in increasing patients' ability to cope with stressful experiences.

In a study of 55 patients undergoing external beam radiation therapy for cure or control of cancer, patients' responses were described and compared in relation to the influence of uncertainty, hope, preference for control, and symptom severity on psychosocial adjustment while undergoing radiation therapy (Christman, 1990). Findings revealed that greater uncertainty and less hope were associated with most adjustment problems for patients. In addition, as symptom severity increased, adjustment difficulty at treatment completion was more likely. Concepts of uncertainty and preference for control did not provide any evidence of positive effects for this group of patients. Results underscore the need for further studies on the effect of symptoms and their relationship to patients' social adjustment to radiation therapy.

A third study on psychosocial responses involved a description of the burden of self-care, stress, and mood in a group of 72 adults with a variety of cancers receiving radiation therapy by Oberst et al. (1991). Self-care burden was predicted to be a function of illness factors, personal factors, and available resources. Self-care burden was also predicted to be a strong predictor of stress appraisal, and mood dysfunction was predicted to be a result of a stressful appraisal. Results did not meet the predictions but resulted in a revised model to predict psychosocial responses. Symptom distress was sufficient to produce significant disruption in daily activities for patients and led to considerable self-burden. This burden was perceived by patients as very stressful, both in itself and related to the therapy. Findings suggest that clinicians need to evaluate patients carefully and assist them to find better methods of symptom management, especially for fatigue and related problems.

In a recent meta-analysis of the effect of psychoeducational care on adults with cancer, Devine and Westlake (1995) evaluated how educational and psychosocial care affects seven outcomes of anxiety, depression, mood, nausea, vomiting, pain, and knowledge. The investigators calculated a standardized mean difference between treatment and control group for 98 studies that were published between 1976 and 1993, which included data on 5,326 subjects. Results indicated a statistically significant beneficial effect of psychoeducational care in relation to all seven outcome criteria. The investigators were not able to differentiate among the effectiveness of the different psychoeducational programs (e.g., individual and group counseling, cognitive behavior therapy, psychoeducational support, adult-oriented teaching/learning, biofeedback, biobehavioral interventions, muscle relaxation, and music therapy). They recommended that additional research is needed to evaluate the relative effectiveness of different types of psychoeducational care. The study investigators concluded that a strong research base is evident in the beneficial effects of psychoeducational care.

Late Effects and Survivorship Issues

The last group of nursing studies reviewed here focuses on the late effects of radiation therapy and survivorship issues after treatment. Two aspects of late effects were explored: cosmetic effect of radiation therapy for breast cancer and the cognitive functioning effect of prophylactic leukemia therapy. In a study of breast cancer patients, 32 patients were asked to rate the cosmetic outcomes following breast-preserving radiation therapy for cancer (Patterson et al., 1985). The average patient participated 19 months after completion of therapy. The patient-rated questionnaire consisted of ratings on the appearance of the treated breast, the degree of difference between breasts, and overall satisfaction with the cosmetic effect. Appearance of the treated breast was rated good to excellent by 94 percent of the subjects, with 88 percent noting a difference of slight to moderate degree between the treated and untreated breasts. Satisfaction was rated high (extremely to very satisfied) by 78 percent of the subjects and moderate by another 19 percent. Reasons for dissatisfaction included chronic breast pain in three patients, breast edema in one patient, and arm edema in one patient. Results point to a high degree of satisfaction with breast-preserving radiation therapy as a primary treatment for cancer.

Another late effect is related to the impact of therapy on cognitive functioning. In a study of effects of prophylactic leukemia therapy on cognitive functioning, 31 long-term survivors of childhood cancer were evaluated via school history and standardized measures of general intellectual ability, academic achievement, and vasomotor skills (Moore et al., 1986). Central nervous system (CNS) prophylaxis was composed of administration of intrathecal methotrexate and cranial or spinocranial radiation. Three groups of children participated. The first group was composed of 10 children who had received CNS prophylaxis during a vulnerable period of brain development; the second group was of 9 children who had received CNS prophylaxis after the age of brain growth spurt; the third group was of 12 children treated systematically for solid tumors and who did not receive any CNS treatment. The third group acted as a control group for the effects of systemic therapy and the presence of a life-threatening disease. Results supported the hypotheses posed and demonstrated lower levels of general intelligence, academic achievement, school performance, and deficits in visuomotor integration for those patients receiving CNS prophylactic treatment. In addition, deficits were more pronounced in the group treated during the vulnerable period of brain development. These results point to the need for follow-up testing in patients receiving CNS radiation therapy and a structured counseling program to help patients and their families adapt to the CNS deficits. Education of the teachers of these children is needed as well to provide an educational environment that supports the cancer-surviving child.

Dow (1994) conducted a qualitative study of 16 women having children after early-stage breast cancer who became pregnant after breast-conserving surgery and radiation therapy. The purposes of the study were to identify reasons why young women decide to become pregnant after breast cancer, to describe their personal concerns about pregnancy subsequent to breast cancer, to describe helpful behaviors in decision-making, and to explore the meaning of having children after breast cancer. Participants consented to a semistructured interview, and qualitative data were content analyzed. Results indicated that pregnancy subsequent to breast cancer provided a reason to look to the future. The reasons for subsequent pregnancy related to the participants' developmental age. Young women expressed concerns about the potential for disease recurrence, breast self-examination and mammography during pregnancy, and being able to live long enough to see their children grow up. Perceived helpful behaviors included the development of a realistic perspective on life, living with uncertainty, having love and support from one's spouse, and being able to delineate the differences between personal and medical decision making.

Interventions During Treatment

Self-Care Behaviors During Radiation Therapy

Although the majority of studies were descriptive in nature, several studies looked at ways to manage treatment-related effects—by either patient- or nurse-instituted management. Dodd (1984) conducted a series of studies of self-care among cancer patients, one of which focused on patients receiving radiation therapy. A convenience sample of 30 patients was followed to determine what self-care behaviors were demonstrated during a course of radiation therapy. Results revealed that most patients reported an average of 3.3 side effects (mean = 1.6, s.d. = 0.80) and initiated very few self-care management activities of those side effects. Patients also reported that they were the most common source of information used to provide self-care, followed by the physician and then the nurse. Results point to a continued need for nurses to become more visible and active in teaching patients self-care monitoring and interventions.

Hanucharurnkul (1989) followed a group of 112 patients receiving radiation therapy for cervical or head and neck cancers to determine factors predictive of self-care. The sample was drawn from three hospitals in Bangkok, Thailand. Results of the multiple regression analysis revealed that socioeconomic status and social support (by family and health care providers) were significant predictors of self-care. Other less important but interesting predictors included stage and site of cancer. Findings indicate the value of nurse involvement in the adaptation of the patient to radiation therapy.

Evaluation of Nursing Care Studies

Weintraub and Hagopian (1990) examined the effect of nursing consultation sessions on anxiety, side effects experienced, and helpfulness of self-care strategies used by patients receiving radiation therapy. The researchers used an experimental design to randomly assign 56 subjects into one of three groups: control, health education, and nursing consultation. Instruments used were the Side Effects Profile (SEP) and Spielberger's State-Trait Anxiety Inventory (STAI). A power analysis was not reported. Study findings demonstrated no significant differences among the groups. However, mean state-anxiety scores were consistently lower for the nursing consultation group. Findings indicate that nurses can have a positive influence on patients' anxiety.

Rose et al. (1996) used a nurse-managed telephone interview to identify patients' symptoms after completing a course of radiation therapy. One hundred eleven subjects who were treated with radiation therapy for a multitude of primary cancers (prostate, head and neck, lung, and breast) were drawn from a community hospital setting. Data were collected at two time points: an end-of-treatment symptom evaluation within 5 days of completing therapy and a telephone interview 14 to 21 days post-therapy. Interview questions were individually derived based on the subjects' end-of-treatment evaluation. Results indicated that 945 of patients experienced symptoms at the end of treatment. Nurses contacted 95 percent of patients by telephone and assessed symptoms in 79 percent of subjects. Eighteen percent of subjects reported new symptom development in the intervening time period. Nursing independently managed the patient symptoms. Findings indicate that telephone follow-up interviews are a good mechanism to evaluate short-term side effects and provides another vehicle for nurses to intervene with patients. Findings also demonstrate that a nurse-managed telephone follow-up program can be a useful component of continuous process improvement to provide ongoing assessment of patients' symptoms after therapy.

Methodologic Studies with Radiation Patients

Although the majority of studies focused on patient care and symptom management, a few methodologic studies were also reported using patients receiving radiation therapy. For example, Johnson et al. (1983) tested the Sickness Impact Profile, a standard tool for measuring functional status. The study of radiation therapy patients tested two different formats of the tool: the original format with statements stated in the first person ("I have attempted suicide") and one in an adapted, less personal format ("Have you attempted suicide?"). The purpose of the study was to compare the two formats, noting whether there were differences in patients' responses and whether patients were more prone to favor one approach rather than the other. Results indicated a high correlation within patients for the two formats (r = 0.943); that is, patients responded in a similar fashion to both approaches. In addition, either interview format was acceptable to the patients. The authors' recommend using the Sickness Impact Profile as a measure of functional status and underscored the need for a careful, complete explanation before the testing is started.

Quality of life (QOL) instruments have been used with patients receiving radiation therapy. QOL responses of patients receiving radiation therapy were compared with outpatients receiving chemotherapy, inpatients receiving chemotherapy, and a control group of healthy volunteers (Padilla et al., 1983). The Quality of Life Index consists of 14 linear analog items contained within three QOL subscales of psychological well-being, physical well-being, and symptom control. Scores ranged from 0 to 100, with the higher scores indicating a higher QOL. Results demonstrated that the chemotherapy inpatient group had the poorest quality of life scores, with a mean score of 55. The nonpatient population had the highest scores, with a mean score of 91. Radiation patients were grouped with chemotherapy outpatients and fell between the two extremes, with a mean score of 71.

Research Utilization

Although there is beginning evidence of nursing studies conducted by nurses in the area of radiation therapy, there is need for improved means of research utilization. Research utilization was iden-

tified as a top research priority in the 1991 ONS Survey, but there are no reported studies of effective research utilization within radiation oncology. Historically, there are many barriers to using research in the clinical setting. These barriers include lack of knowledge about research, lack of time to investigate research findings for a clinical problem, and lack of rewards for applying research in the clinical setting (Walczak et al., 1994). Although the research process is often considered complicated, when it is viewed as a framework similar to the problem solving or nursing process, there are fewer areas of confusion. A comparison of these processes is given in Table 25-2.

Initiating Nursing Research Activities

Characteristics of the role and the treatment modality make radiation nursing a unique specialty. The treatment setting is primarily an ambulatory setting, with daily treatments providing opportunities to get to know individual patients. The treatment plan is carried out over a circumscribed time period, generally 4 to 6 weeks, long enough to provide an opportunity for nurses to assist patients to prevent and manage treatment-related problems. In addition, the treatment period is short enough to provide an opportunity to test different interventions without the need for long-term follow-up studies or cross-sectional de-

Table 25-2 • Comparison of Problem-Solving Process, Nursing Process, and Research Process

Problem-Solving Process	Nursing Process	Research Process
Data collection	Assessment Data collection Data interpretation	Knowledge of the world of nursing Clinical experience Literature review
Problem definition	Nursing diagnosis	Problem and purpose identification
Plan Goal setting Identify solution	Plan Goal setting Planned interventions	Methodology Design Sample Methods of measurement
Implementation	Implementation	Data collection and analysis
Evaluate and revise process	Evaluation and modification	Outcomes and dissemination of findings

From Burns N & Grove S. (1993). *The practice of nursing research* (2nd ed.). Philadelphia: WB Saunders. Reproduced with permission.

signs. The treatment modality builds on a multidisciplinary approach (physicians, nurses, therapists, physicists, dosimetrists, social workers, and nutritionists), which results in a multidisciplinary team that works together daily. This team approach can foster a supportive and positive attitude that is important for the conduct of clinical studies by any of the team members.

Summary and Future Directions

Nursing research related to radiation therapy continues to develop in the areas of symptom management, patient education, and research utilization. Several studies describe the experience of radiation therapy as perceived by patients. These studies include descriptions of side effects, satisfaction with the radiation personnel, impact on quality of life, and functional status changes. These studies provide an excellent background from which to test various nursing interventions aimed at improving the patients' responses to the radiation therapy experience.

A beginning research foundation for radiation nursing is evolving. Continuing to add replication and extension studies to the areas of exploration discussed here will assist greatly in moving this foundation forward. Nurses in the radiation therapy setting are well positioned to initiate and participate in nursing research studies.

References

Burns N, Grove S. (1993). The practice of nursing research (2nd ed.). Philadelphia: Saunders.

Campbell-Forsyth C. (1990). Patients' perceived knowledge and learning needs concerning radiation therapy. *Cancer Nursing, 13*(2), 81–89.

Christman NJ. (1990).Uncertainty and adjustment during radiotherapy. *Nursing Research, 39*(1), 17–20.

Devine EC, Westlake SK. (1995). The effects of psychoeducational care provided to adults with cancer: Meta-analysis of 116 studies. *Oncology Nursing Forum, 22*(9), 1369–1381.

Dodd MJ. (1984). Patterns of self-care in cancer patients receiving radiation therapy. *Oncology Nursing Forum, 11*(3), 23–27.

Dodd MJ, Ahmed N. (1987). Preference for type of information in cancer patients receiving radiation therapy. *Cancer Nursing, 10*(5), 244–251.

Dow KH. (1994). Having children after breast cancer. *Cancer Practice, 2*(6), 407–413.

Dudjak LA. (1987). Mouth care for mucositis due to radiation therapy. *Cancer Nursing, 13*(3), 131–140.

Funkhouser SW, Grant MM. (1989). ONS survey of research priorities. *Oncology Nursing Forum, 16*(3), 413–416.

Grant M, Padilla G, Rhiner M. (1991). Patterns of anorexia in cancer patients: Maintaining nutritional status in patients with cancer. Pub. No. 91-25. M-332. 03-PE Atlanta: American Cancer Society.

Grant M, Stromborg M. (1981). Promoting research collaboration: ONS research committee survey. *Oncology Nursing Forum, 8*(2), 48–53.

Graydon J. (1994). Women with breast cancer: Their quality of life following a course of radiation therapy. *Journal of Advanced Nursing 19*(4), 617–622.

Graydon J, Bubela N, Irvine D, Vincent L. (1995). Fatigue-reducing strategies used by patients receiving treatment for cancer. *Cancer Nursing 18*(1), 23–28.

Hagopian G. (1991). The effects of a weekly radiation therapy newsletter on patients. *Oncology Nursing Forum, 18*(7), 1199–1203.

Hanucharurnkul S. (1989). Predictors of self-care in cancer patients receiving radiotherapy. *Cancer Nursing, 12*(1), 21–27.

Harrison-Woermke D, Graydon J. (1993). Perceived informational needs of breast cancer patients receiving radiation therapy after excisional biopsy and axillary node dissection. *Cancer Nursing 16*(6), 444–455.

Haylock PJ, Hart LK. (1979). Fatigue in patients receiving localized radiation. *Cancer Nursing, 2,* 461–467.

Hilderley LJ. (1980). The role of the nurse in radiation oncology. *Seminars in Oncology, 7*(1), 39–47.

Hinshaw AS. (1988). The new national center for nursing research: Patient care research programs. *Applied Nursing Research, 1,* 2–4.

Israel MJ, Mood DW. (1982). Three media presentations for patients receiving radiation therapy. *Cancer Nursing, 5*(1), 57–63.

Johnson JE, King KB, Murray RA. (1983). Measuring the impact of sickness on usual functions of radiation therapy patients. *Oncology Nursing Forum, 10*(4), 36–39.

Johnson JE, Lauver DR, Nail LM. (1989). Process of coping with radiation therapy. *Journal of Consulting and Clinical Psychology, 57*(3), 358–364.

King KB, Nail LM, Kraemer K, Strohl RA, Johnson JE. (1985). Patients' descriptions of the experience of receiving radiation therapy. *Oncology Nursing Forum, 12*(4), 55–61.

Kubricht DW. (1984). Therapeutic self-care demands expressed by outpatients receiving external radiation therapy. *Cancer Nursing, 7*(1), 43–52.

Larson O, Lindsay A, Dodd M, Brecht M, Packer A. (1993). Influence of age on problems experienced by patients with lung cancer undergoing radiation therapy. *Oncology Nursing Forum, 20*(3), 473–480.

Llewelyn-Thomas H, Thiel E, Sem F, Woermke D. (1995). Presenting clinical trial information: A comparison of methods. *Patient Education and Counseling, 25*(2), 97–107.

Margolin S, Breneman J, Denman D, LaChapelle P, Weckbach L. (1990). Management of radiation-induced moist skin desquamation using hydrocolloid dressing. *Cancer Nursing, 13*(2), 71–80.

McGuire D, Stromborg M, Varricchio C. (1985). 1984 ONS Research Committee survey of membership's research interests and involvements. *Oncology Nursing Forum, 12*(2), 99–103.

Merritt DH. (1986). The National Center for Nursing Research. *Image, 18*(3), 84–85.

Mock V, Dow KH, Meares C. (1996). Exercise effects on fatigue, physical functioning, and emotional distress during radiotherapy treatment for breast cancer. In *Proceedings 8th International Research Congress,* Sigma Theta Tau International.

Mood DW, Horowitz LB, Chadwell DK, Cook CA. (1986). Increasing patients' understanding of radiation therapy. Meeting abstract. *International Journal of Radiation Oncology, Biology, Physics, 12*(supp.), 168.

Mooney K, Ferrell B, Nail L, Benedict S, Haberman M. (1991). Oncology Nursing Society research priorities survey. *Oncology Nursing Forum, 18*(8), 1381–1390.

Moore IJ, Kramer J, Ablin A. (1986). Late effects of central nervous system prophylactic leukemia therapy on cognitive functions. *Oncology Nursing Forum, 13*(4), 45–51.

Oberst MT, Hughes SH, Chang AS, McCubbin MA. (1991). Self-care burden, stress appraisal, and mood among persons receiving radiotherapy. *Cancer Nursing, 14*(2), 71–78.

Padilla GV, Grant M. (1987). Compliance strategies for cancer therapy. Final report submitted to the National Cancer Institute, R18 CA 31164.

Padilla GV, Present C, Grant MM, Metter G, Lipsett J, Heide F. (1983). Quality of life index for patients with cancer. *Research in Nursing and Health, 6*, 117–126.

Patterson MP, Lipsett JA, Michel M, Archambeau JO. (1981). Cancer patients and informed consent: A study of relationships between comprehension of information, perceived ambiguity, and stress during radiotherapy. Meeting abstract. *International Journal of Radiation Oncology, Biology, Physics, 7*(supp.), 108.

Patterson MP, Pezner RD, Hill LR, Vora NL, Desai KR, Lipsett JA. (1985). Patient self-evaluation of cosmetic outcome of breast-preserving cancer treatment. *International Journal of Radiation Oncology, Biology, Physics,* 11, 1849–1852.

Poroch D. (1995). The effect of preparatory patient education on the anxiety and satisfaction of cancer patients receiving radiation therapy. *Cancer Nursing 18*(3), 206–214.

Radiation SIG. (1996). Research work group in Radiation SIG newsletter, 7(2), 1.

Rose MA, Shrader-Bogen C, Korlath G, Priem J, Larson L. (1996). Identifying patient symptoms after radiotherapy using a nurse-managed telephone interview. *Oncology Nursing Forum* 23(1), 99–102.

Shell JA, Stanutz F, Grimm J. (1986). Comparison of moisture vapor permeable (MVP) dressings to conventional dressings for management of radiation skin reactions. *Oncology Nursing Forum, 13*(1), 11–16.

Steinfeld A, Hanlon A, Pajak T, Hanks G. (1995). Gender as a determinant of palliative radiotherapy: A pattern of care study analysis. *Journal of Women's Health.*

Stetz K, Haberman M, Holcombe J, Jones L. (1995). 1994 Oncology Nursing Society research priorities. *Oncology Nursing Forum* 22(5), 785–789.

Walczak J, McGuire D, Haisfield M, Beezley A. (1994). A survey of research-related activities and perceived barriers to research utilization among professional oncology nurses. *Oncology Nursing Forum,* 21, 710–714.

Ward S, Heidrich S, Wolberg W. (1989). Factors women take into account when deciding upon type of surgery for breast cancer. *Cancer Nursing, 12*(6), 344–351.

Weintraub F, Hagopian G. (1990). The effect of nursing consultation on anxiety, side effects, and self-care of patients receiving radiation therapy. *Oncology Nursing Forum,* 17(3), Suppl, 31–36.

Welch DA. (1980). Assessment of nausea and vomiting in cancer patients undergoing external beam radiotherapy. *Cancer Nursing, 3*, 365–371.

Index

Note: Page numbers in *italics* refer to illustrations; page numbers followed by t refer to tables.

ISBN 0-7216-2347-6